FUNCTIONAL HISTOLOGY

D0865304

FUNCTIONAL HISTOLOGY

THIRD EDITION

Myrin Borysenko, Ph.D.

Associate Professor,
Department of Anatomy and Cellular Biology,
Tufts University School of Medicine, Boston

Theodore Beringer, Ph.D.

Associate Professor,
Division of Structural and Systems Biology,
School of Basic Life Sciences, University of Missouri—
Kansas City, Kansas City

LITTLE, BROWN AND COMPANY   Boston/Toronto/London

Copyright © 1989 by Myrin Borysenko and
Theodore Beringer
Third Edition
Previous editions copyright © 1984, 1979 by
Little, Brown and Company (Inc.)

All rights reserved. No part of this book may be
reproduced in any form or by any electronic or
mechanical means, including information storage
and retrieval systems, without permission in writing
from the publisher, except by a reviewer who may
quote brief passages in a review.

Library of Congress Catalog Card No. 89-80094

ISBN 0-316-10301-2

Printed in the United States of America

MV-NY

Contents

Preface

This book was originally developed from a syllabus that has been distributed with favorable response to students of medicine and dentistry at Tufts University. Its value stems from a concise presentation of material that integrates histology with corresponding biologic functions. We have tried to establish a conceptual understanding of the histologic organization of cells, tissues, and organ systems through the use of representative diagrams. This book provides a manageable reading load in today's stacked curriculum, allowing the student to concentrate on lectures rather than on the production of copious notes that often must be interpreted later.

During the years following the first and second editions we received many comments, suggestions, and criticisms from both students and colleagues that have contributed significantly to the third edition. We believe that we have succeeded in producing a *practical* textbook, one that is both concise and comprehensive, functionally oriented, and well illustrated. The incorporation of new photomicrographs and additional diagrams is intended to complement the text and emphasize the link between structure and function. *Functional Histology* provides the student with a core of relevant information that can serve as a foundation for many other biomedical courses.

The reader who is familiar with past editions of *Functional Histology* will immediately recognize that, in addition to the revisions in the text, a question bank with annotated answers appears at the end of each chapter. The decision to include questions sparked a lively dialogue between the authors. The controversy centered around some students' tendency of using question banks to learn the subject rather than to assess whether the material has been learned. The student of histology is cautioned to use the self-examination questions for the latter purpose. In addition, it should be assumed that an unsuccessfully answered question is an indication that other related concepts may also be incompletely understood. Since the annotated answers may falsely reinforce the student's sense of security that learning from studying questions and answers is effective, the student is encouraged to return to the chapter and reread appropriate material to expand understanding in weak areas. To aid this process, occasional references are made to page numbers within the text for more information than can possibly be included in the annotations.

We are indebted to many people for their continued interest and dedication to the educational process. Bryan Toole, Ph.D., Chairperson of the Tufts Department of Anatomy and Cellular Biology, has been constantly supportive of our efforts and has done much to expedite the book's production through the use of departmental facilities. We gratefully acknowledge the original contributions of Joan Borysenko, Ph.D., and Alvar Gustafson, Ph.D., who were among the authors of the first edition but have now moved on to other worthwhile endeavors. Finally, we thank all those, too numerous to name, who have kindly provided us with diagrams and micrographs of their original work and who have given us help and encouragement in the evolution of this book.

M. B.
T. B.

FUNCTIONAL HISTOLOGY

1 A Brief Introduction to Histologic Organization and Techniques of Microscopy

---

Objectives

You will learn the following in this chapter:

General organization of biologic tissues

Preparation of biologic tissues for examination with the light microscope and electron microscope

Methods of tissue staining to enhance visibility of cellular and extracellular structures when viewed with the microscope

Principles of optics used in microscopy

Factors that affect microscopic resolution of cellular detail

---

OVERVIEW OF THE RELATIONSHIP AMONG CELLS, TISSUES, AND ORGANS

The Cell

Cytology is the study of the cell, which is the basic unit of living matter. Unicellular organisms like amebae or paramecia are capable of carrying out all metabolic processes and reproduction alone. Even in this simple context, however, cells begin to cooperate to enhance their chances of survival, as shown by the phenomenon of conjugation between paramecia. Simple cells may aggregate into colonies, such as volvox, to which the beginnings of multicellular organisms may be traced. As cells begin to cooperate and to share labor among themselves, different cells become suited to carrying out particular functions. This functional diversity is reflected by the diversity of cell structure (morphology). Even in a two cell layered organism, such as a hydroid, some cells are differentiated into digestive cells, while others function as a combined muscle and covering cell. Certain of these two basic cell types differentiate further to become either reproductive cells or a special kind of defense cell. In this way, each cell type in the organism develops its own special functional priority. When structurally and functionally similar cells form groups within the organism, those groups of cells are known as distinct tissues. The different types of tissues become arranged into various organs. While these specialized cells have lost a multifunctional capacity in favor of fewer emphasized properties, their organization into tissues and organs allow the organism to perform biologic functions with greater economy.

The Tissues

In more complex species, three cell (germ) layers develop in the embryo; these are endoderm (inner), mesoderm (middle), and ectoderm (outer) cell layers. These basic layers give rise to four functional groupings of similar cells, called **tissues.** Study of the four tissue types and their particular specializations is called **histology.** The tissue types and their basic germ layer derivations are as follows:

1. Epithelium: arises from all three primary cell layers
   Endoderm: epithelium lining the digestive tract and its glands, epithelium of respiratory tract and its glands, epithelium of bladder and certain parts of the urinary and reproductive systems
   Mesoderm: epithelium (endothelium) lining the blood vessels, mesothelium lining serous membranes (pleural cavity, pericardium, peritoneum), epithelium of a large portion of the urogenital system
   Ectoderm: epithelium covering the body surface (skin), epithelium of the anus and oral cavity glands opening into the mouth, taste buds, enamel of teeth, and epithelium lining parts of the eye, ear, and nose
2. Connective tissue: primarily mesodermal, except some of the neuroglia
3. Muscle: mesodermal, except for the smooth muscle of sweat glands and pupillary muscles of the eye
4. Nerve: ectodermal

Each tissue can be further subdivided, resulting in variations on a basic theme. For instance, there are three types of muscle tissue that vary in the organization of the major contractile protein filaments, actin and myosin. The muscle proteins are best organized in the fast-contracting skeletal muscle fibers, whereas the slow, rhythmic contraction of smooth muscle is subserved by a more diffuse arrangement of component filaments. The intrinsic rhythmicity of cardiac muscle, however, relies both on the relationship between nerve and muscle cells, and also on the particular arrangement of protein filaments within the cells. In all cases, the important message to grasp is that **structure follows function.** Through the ages, organisms have evolved that are best able to adapt to the environment; this is also true on the cellular level. The various parts present within a cell reflect the function that these parts have evolved to perform. Therefore, simple examination of cell's component parts will reveal its particular function. When a functional approach is used in the study of histology, cell physiology will naturally unfold because the two together form a unified whole, and the need to memorize will be largely replaced by simple deductive logic.

The Organs

The four tissue types are further organized into **organs** and **organ systems.** For example, the digestive system is a series of hollow tubular organs with regional functional specializations of the component tissue types to form esophagus, stomach, and intestines. In addition, the large epithelially derived glands, liver and pancreas, as well as the gallbladder, contribute secretions to the digestive tract. The entire organ system functions in the intake, breakdown (digestion), and absorption of food. The human body is composed of several organ systems, which can be explored from the gross to the cellular level. Control and integration of the various systems are functions of both the nervous and endocrine systems. A basic knowledge of histology, therefore, provides both **morphologic** (structural) and **physiologic** (functional) understanding of the delicate homeostatic mechanisms involved in the interaction of an organism with the environment.

TECHNIQUES OF MICROSCOPY
The Light Microscope

The basic light microscope is constructed of three lenses arranged in sequence: the condenser lens, the objective lens, and the ocular

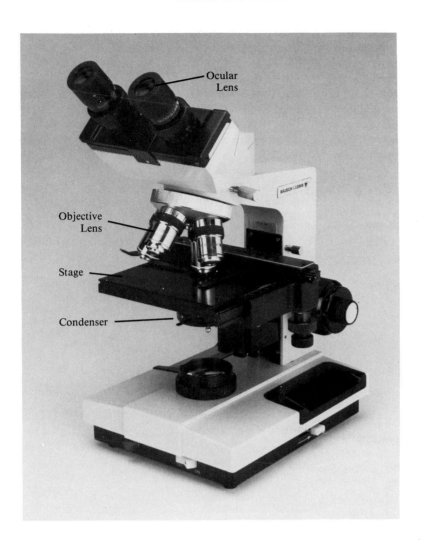

Fig. 1-1. The Galen III light microscope by Bausch & Lomb. The illuminating light source comes from the base of the microscope and rises in succession through the condenser, objective lens, and finally the optic lens. The microscope slide is mounted on the stage but not shown here. (Courtesy of Bausch & Lomb.)

lens. The condenser focuses the beam from a light source into a cone of light that shines upon the tissue section, which lays flat on a transparent glass slide. The correct positioning of the condenser imparts appropriate contrast to the visual image. The objective lens is deployed on the opposite side of the tissue section and collects light that has been transmitted through the section from the condenser lens. The objective lens magnifies the image of light and directs it to the ocular lens, which magnifies to a lesser extent and directs the image to the viewer's eye (in some cases, a photographic plate in a camera) (Fig. 1-1).

A variety of microscopes makes it possible to see not only cells but also their intracellular organelles that conduct various cellular activities. These different types of organelles often change their size in response to changing demands upon their functional roles in the cell at any given time. Consequently, references to their size are made frequently throughout this book according to a system of metric measurements listed in the scale below.

1 inch = 2.54 centimeters (cm)
1 cm   = 10 millimeters (mm)
1 mm   = 10^3 micrometers (μm; formerly micron, μ)
1 μm = 10^3 nanometers (nm; formerly millimicron, mμ)
1 nm   = 10 angstroms (Å, no longer used in the international system of units)
1 Å   = 10^{-7} mm

As a reference point appreciate that most human cells vary in size between 5 and 100 μm, although certain muscle and nerve cells have considerably larger dimensions. Furthermore, intracellular structures and organelles are even smaller. By comparison most bacteria have dimensions between 0.3 and 10 μm; and most viruses have dimensions between 1 and 50 nm. Since the smallest structure the unaided human eye can see is about 40 μm in diameter, the importance of magnification provided by the microscope is evident.

However, another characteristic of the microscope is more important than magnification, that is, **resolution.** Resolution is the smallest distance that can be seen between two visibly separate objects. For the light microscope the best effective resolution obtainable is about 0.25 μm. The equation defining resolution is:

$$R = \frac{0.61 \times \lambda}{NA}$$

The resolution (R) is directly proportional to the **wavelength of light** (λ) and indirectly proportional to the **numerical aperture** (NA). The most visible wavelength for white light is 0.55 μm, the yellow-green shade often used to make fire engines and ambulances more visible. The NA depends on the particular objective lens being used but it is defined as the sinc of the angle of light entering between the middle and the edge of the objective lens. Each objective lens has its NA engraved on it, usually to the right of its indicated magnification. When these values for wavelength and NA are inserted into the equation for resolution, it becomes apparent that larger NAs produce better resolution. As the resolution improves, more details are visible in the image of the tissue specimen.

TISSUE PREPARATION

Biological tissues are prepared in a variety of ways on glass slides which pathologists and students study in schools of medicine and dentistry. They are prepared according to the following basic protocol.

Fixation

Initially the tissue must be fixed before or after removal from the body to arrest intracellular enzymatic degradation that would normally cause putrefaction of the tissue and destruction of cellular detail. Certain chemical fixatives, such as picric acid, preserve tissues but also denature proteins. These types of fixatives introduce alterations in intermolecular organization that can sometimes be visible with the light microscope but are tolerated for limited purposes of microscopy where resolution is not extremely important. One drawback to this type of fixation is that advanced histochemical procedures cannot be used to study cellular processes because denatured proteins lose their normal molecular functions.

More frequently these types of fixatives have been replaced by formalin, a concentrated formaldehyde solution, which causes less artifactual change in the tissue because it does not generally denature proteins or alter tissue and cellular structure as severely. This fixative is commonly used in hospitals for routine preservation of pathologic specimens. Researchers are more likely to use fixatives such as paraformaldehyde and glutaraldehyde. These fixatives cross-link proteins through their amine groups. They will also denature proteins but not to the same extent as formalin or picric acid. In many cases they retain the antigenicity of the tissue so that immunocytochemical studies can be conducted to localize some cellular protein that an antibody has been formed against. In order to preserve full enzymatic activity of a tissue it must be rapidly frozen in liquid nitrogen or liquid helium.

Dehydration, Clearing, Embedding, and Sectioning

Since tissue must be thin enough to transmit light to be examined with conventional light microscopes, it must be sectioned in thin slices from 1 to 20 μm in thickness, the exception being when a layer or two of cells grown on a coverslip in a culture dish is to be examined; the latter is already thin enough to transmit light. Sectioning requires that the tissue have support or it will be compressed during the cutting action of the knife. Therefore tissues are embedded in a support such as wax (paraffin) or epoxy. Epoxy is much harder and is used where sections of 1 μm are to be cut or where the much thinner sections required for electron microscopy are cut. First, however, the tissue must be dehydrated since water in the tissue would prevent the paraffin or epoxy from entering the tissue.

Dehydration is usually accomplished by immersing the tissue in a series of increasingly concentrated solvents such as ethyl alcohol. If the tissue is to be embedded in paraffin, the alcohol is followed by benzene (a clearing agent) since the benzene is miscible with paraffin whereas alcohol is not. If the tissue is to be embedded in epoxy the alcohol is followed by propylene oxide, which is miscible with epoxy. It should be recognized that these solvents extract most of the lipids from the tissue causing artifactually produced gaps where lipids had resided in the living

state. This artifact is most prominent in fat cells, which lose their stored fat droplets during this dehydration step and will be seen in the microscope to have large, round vacant spaces where the lipid droplet was extracted. This is only one of many artifacts introduced into the tissue as a result of processing for microscopic viewing. Another artifact of dehydration is a certain amount of shrinkage, which is frequently observed in tissue sections as spaces where water has been removed and tissue components have pulled apart from each other. Once the tissue is embedded, it is sectioned with a microtome. The sections are then mounted on a glass slide. While on the glass slide the sections will be stained prior to viewing with the microscope.

Staining

Since the refractive index of different cell types and their intracellular organelles are very similar, they must be stained with dyes to help distinguish them and to make them more visible to the microscopist. Dyes absorb light in part of the visible spectrum and allow the complementary color to pass through the tissue. For instance, a blue dye absorbs yellow light and confers a blue color to any tissue element which the dye attaches to. Most dyes attach to cells by electrostatic attraction, which involves bonding between a dye and cell component of opposite charge. For this reason an acid dye and a basic dye of different colors are usually used in combination to color substances in the cell with different isoelectric points, which will have different affinities for the two dyes based upon charge and, consequently, different colors after staining. Recall that a protein that is found in a cell or tissue has a net neutral charge at its isoelectric point (pI). Above its pI a protein will be negatively charged; below its pI it will be positively charged. Consequently, a cationic dye (positive charge) will attach to negatively charged cellular substances; an anionic dye (negative charge) will attach to positively charged substances.

The portion of a dye that absorbs light and imparts the color to a dye is the **chromophore.** The chromophore is part of a larger ionizable chemical structure which over a broad range of pH is either a basic dye (such as methylene blue) or an acid dye (such as eosin). A basic dye is composed of a cationic chromophore and a colorless acid radical; an acid dye is composed of an anionic chromophore and a colorless basic radical. Since methylene blue is blue and eosin is a reddish-orange, tissue components having different charges will stain different colors when these two dyes are used. In this case negatively charged tissue components staining blue would be referred to as **basophilic** because they stain with the basic dye methylene blue (a cationic dye); positively charged tissue components staining reddish-orange would be referred to as **acidophilic** because they stain with the acidic eosin (an anionic dye). Under conditions of pH where most staining is performed, examples of acidophilia are collagen, mitochondria, and the hemoglobin of erythrocytes. Examples of basophilia include nuclear chromatin and ribosomes. In the latter, binding occurs with the acidic phosphate groups of the DNA and RNA respectively. The extracellular matrix of cartilage also stains with basic dyes due to the high concentration of negatively charged sulfate groups present on sulfated proteoglycans.

Because hematoxylin is a commonly used dye but is somewhat different in character than the dyes described above, it will be described briefly. It must be oxidized to hematin before use and has no staining properties until it is complexed with a heavy metal such as iron. The iron is referred to as a **mordant.** The iron confers a positive charge to hematin which then allows it to act as a cationic dye. The iron chelates or binds to negatively charged tissue components. By convention, tissue components stained with iron-mordanted hematin are then referred to as basophilic. Hematin is a dark-bluish color and is usually used in conjunction with eosin as a counterstain.

Certain dyes such as toluidine blue are called **metachromatic** because they stain with a different color when they are grouped closely together from when they are dispersed. Toluidine blue is a basic dye which binds to negatively charged tissue components, staining them blue when these tissue components are dispersed. When bound to polyanions like heparin or nucleoprotein which have closely spaced negative charges, toluidine blue aggregates into a polymer which absorbs light at a lower wavelength emitting a reddish or purplish light instead of blue. Consequently the tissue containing closely spaced anionic charges will stain reddish instead of blue. This phenomenon is called **metachromasia.**

Other stains are described as they are encountered in applications throughout the text.

OTHER TYPES OF LIGHT MICROSCOPY

Fluorescence Microscopy

Fluorescence microscopy has become an extremely valuable research and clinical tool because it allows molecules that have been tagged with fluorescent markers to be located within the cell. One particularly useful application of this technique employs fluorescent-tagged antibodies which can be synthesized against any given protein that one wishes to study. Since the antibody will attach to the protein, the small fluorescent tag on the antibody allows a researcher to determine the exact location of that protein within the cell. This technique, when used in conjunction with a highly sensitive television camera fitted to the microscope, can effectively increase the resolution of the light microscope somewhat more.

Unlike conventional light microscopy, fluorescence microscopy uses ultraviolet (UV) light. An exciter filter or dichroic beam splitter is used to project a particular wavelength of UV light onto the tissue section. A particular exciter filter is selected to produce a wavelength of UV light which will excite a known fluorescent tag located somewhere in the tissue section. The fluorescent tag responds to this exciting wavelength by emitting a longer wavelength of visible light (fluorescence) which passes through the objective and ocular lenses to be seen by the viewer. Since UV light damages the retina and can cause blindness, a barrier filter which eliminates any UV light but allows fluorescence light to pass through is placed in the final light path before reaching the ocular lens. Two excellent examples of fluorescence micrographs are found in Chapter 2 (see Figs. 2-27, 2-30).

Phase Contrast Microscopy

Although most conventional tissue sections are stained with different colored dyes to render cells and their organelles more visible and distinguishable from one another, a special pair of condenser and objective lens makes staining unnecessary. This type of optical system is referred to as phase contrast microscopy. It amplifies differences in refractive index between cellular organelles adding variable contrast to different organelles and increasing light intensity passing through areas with less refractive index. This technique is especially suitable for examining living cells in culture where staining may disturb cellular activity or even obscure it. An especially effective form of phase contrast microscopy is differential interference contrast (Nomarski optics) Examples of it are shown in Chapters 2 and 11 (see Figs. 2-38, 11-3).

Electron Microscopy

TRANSMISSION ELECTRON MICROSCOPY

Unlike light microscopy, electron microscopy employs an electron beam to "illuminate" the tissue. There is a substantial improvement of resolution since the wavelength of an electron beam accelerated by 100 kV is about 0.04 Å. When working with biologic tissue the attainable resolution is about 1 nm although theoretically it is even smaller. Instead of using glass lenses as in the light microscope, the electron microscope shapes the electron beam with electromagnets to provide magnification (Fig. 1-2). Staining is accomplished by using heavy metals such as uranyl and

osmium ions which obstruct the passage of electrons through the tissue section. Deflected electrons are eliminated by a metal aperture. Areas not specifically stained with the heavy metal allow the electron beam to pass through the section. Since the various parts of the cell in the tissue section have different affinities for the metal ions, cellular components exhibit different contrasts which generate a two-dimensional image of varying electron density. Since an electron beam is invisible to the eye, the beam, after passing through the tissue section, impacts on a fluorescent screen which is excited by the electrons. In this way a fluorescent image is generated to make the tissue image visible to the microscope operator. A permanent record of the image is made by exposing special photographic plates to the electron beam image to produce a negative from which black and white prints can be made.

Since the electron beam on conventional electron microscopes does not have high penetrating capabilities, tissue sections must be much thinner than for light microscopy. Consequently sections are cut as thin as 60 to 100 nm on a special ultramicrotome. The thinness of the section generates nearly a two-dimensional image. Although this characteristic has its limitations, the resolution of fine details is valuable. For examples of electron micrographs, see Figures 2-14 and 2-15 in Chapter 2. In high-voltage electron microscopy the electrons are accelerated at 1000 kV. This not only improves resolution, since the wavelength of the accelerated electron beam is smaller, but also improves penetrating power so that thicker sections comparable to those used with the light microscope can be viewed. The result is a more extensive morphologic picture providing more three-dimensional information than can be acquired from thinner sections.

SCANNING ELECTRON MICROSCOPY

Scanning electron microscopy differs from transmission electron microscopy in that only the surface architecture of cells is visualized. A gold rep-

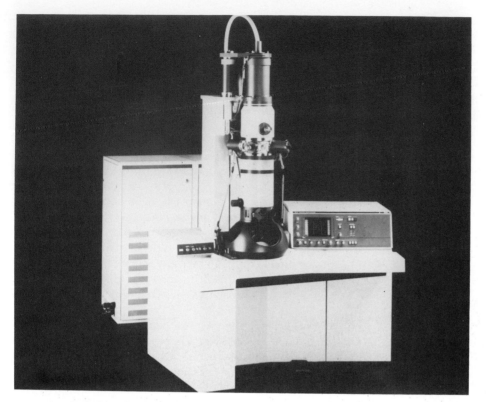

Fig. 1-2. The Philips CM10 transmission electron microscope. The specimen is mounted in the column. The electron beam is accelerated down the column from above. Magnification of the image is accomplished by electromagnetic lenses which shape the electron beam. (Courtesy of Philips Electronic Instruments, Inc.)

lica is made of the cellular surface by evaporating gold in a vacuum on the tissue. When the replica is viewed in the scanning electron microscope the electron beam provokes secondary emission of electrons which are detected by a cathode ray tube producing a three-dimensional–appearing image of the cellular surface. The resolution of the scanning electron microscope is about 5 nm, somewhat inferior to the transmission electron

microscope but advantageous for generating a surface landscape of the cell. For a comparison of scanning and transmission electronmicrographs, see Figure 5-11 in Chapter 5.

FREEZE-FRACTURE TECHNIQUE

In recent years the freeze-fracture (freeze-cleave) technique has come into wide use. A tissue specimen is frozen in liquid nitrogen–cooled isopentane and then fractured with a blade; the resulting fracture face is replicated under a high vacuum with platinum (at a 45-degree angle) and carbon. The platinum shadowing creates an effect similar to a snowfall propelled by a stiff wind. The platinum, like snow, accumulates on the near side of elevations and is absent on the far side. Conversely, the near side of a depression would be empty, while platinum would pile up on the far side. After the tissue has been dissolved away, the platinum replica can be viewed in the transmission electron microscope. When viewed in the transmission electron microscope, areas where platinum has accumulated will impede the flow of electrons and appear dark; areas devoid of platinum appear as white shadows. The carbon does not yield further electron density, but acts to stabilize the platinum-shadowed replica of the fractured surface after the tissue has been dissolved away. The advantage of this technique is that fracture occurs along the plane of least resistance, and in cells, one such area is between the hydrophobic acyl tails of membrane phospholipids. Thus the cell membrane is split down its middle exposing large macromolecular structures within the membrane (see Chap. 2, Figs. 2-2, 2-3).

NATIONAL BOARD TYPE QUESTIONS

Select the single best response for each of the following.

1. A cationic dye
   A. has a net negative charge.
   B. has an anionic chromophore.
   C. binds to positively charged tissue components.
   D. binds to negatively charged tissue components.
2. The resolution obtained with the electron microscope is superior to that obtained with the light microscope primarily because
   A. sections for electron microscopy are generally thinner.
   B. superior dyes are used in electron microscopy.
   C. the wavelength of the electron beam is shorter than the wavelength of visible light.
   D. the wavelength of the electron beam is longer than the wavelength of visible light.
3. Fixatives such as glutaraldehyde and paraformaldehyde
   A. act by cross-linking proteins through their amino groups.
   B. severely denature all cell proteins.
   C. completely fail to prevent intracellular enzymatic degradation.
   D. also impart a stain to the tissue specimen.
4. Occasionally, closely associated tissue components are stained a different color than the color of the dye attached to them. This phenomenon is
   A. mordanting.
   B. metachromasia.
   C. acidophilia.
   D. staining with acid dyes.
5. Which of the following is used to generate contrast in sections viewed with the electron microscope?
   A. Hematoxylin
   B. Eosin
   C. Methylene blue
   D. Uranyl and osmium ions

ANNOTATED ANSWERS

1. D. At the pH prevailing during staining a positively charged dye will have an electrostatic attraction to negatively charged tissue components.
2. C. Resolution is improved by shorter wavelengths. Read the discussion of resolution on page 4.
3. A. Covalent bonds formed, especially with intracellular enzymes, prevent enzymatic degradation of the cell after fixation.
4. B. Metachromatic dyes when closely packed absorb light at lower wavelengths than in the dispersed state.
5. D. Uranyl and osmium ions are large enough that their positively charged nuclei deflect electrons in the tissue where uranyl and osmium are deposited.

BIBLIOGRAPHY

Barka, T., and P. J. Anderson. *Histochemistry—Theory, Practice and Bibliography.* New York: Hoeber, 1963.

Bergeron, J. A., and M. Singer. Metachromasia: An experimental and theoretical reevaluation. *J. Biophys. Biochem. Cytol.* 4:443, 1958.

Caro, L. G., and G. E. Palade. Protein synthesis, storage, and discharge in the pancreatic exocrine cell. A radiographic study. *J. Cell Biol.* 20:473, 1964.

Conn, H. J. *Biological Stains* (9th ed.) Baltimore: Williams & Wilkins, 1977.

Deane, H. Intracellular Lipids: Their Detection and Significance. In S. L. Palay (ed), *Frontiers in Cytology.* New Haven: Yale University Press, 1958.

Essner, E. Hemoproteins. In M. A. Hayat (ed.), *Electron Microscopy of Enzymes.* Princeton, N.J.: Princeton U, 1974.

Everhart, T. E. and T. L. Hayes. The scanning electron microscope. *Sci. Am.* 226:55, 1972.

Glauert, A. M. Fixation, dehydration and embedding of biological specimens. In A. M. Glauert (ed.), *Practical Methods in Electron Microscopy.* Vol. 3, part 1. Amsterdam: North Holland, 1975.

Kasten, F. H. The chemistry of Schiff's reagent. *Int. Rev. Cytol.* 10:1, 1960.

Koehler, J. K. The technique and application of freeze-etching in ultrastructure research. *Adv. Biol. Med. Phys.* 12:1, 1968.

Pearse, A. G. E. *Histochemistry—Theoretical and Applied* (3rd ed.), Boston: Little, Brown, 1968 and 1972, Vols. 1 and 2.

Sabatini, D. D., K. Bensch, and R. J. Barrnett. Cytochemistry and electron microscopy. The preservation of cellular ultrastructure and enzymatic activity by aldehyde fixation. *J. Cell Biol.* 17:19, 1963.

Salpeter, M. M., L. Bachmann, and E. E. Salpeter. Resolution in electron microscope radioautography. *J. Cell Biol.* 41:1, 1969.

Singer, M. Factors which control the staining of tissue sections with acid and basic dyes. *Int. Rev. Cytol.* 1:211, 1952.

Sterberger, L. A. *Immunocytochemistry* (2nd ed.) New York: Wiley, 1979.

I Cells and Tissues

2 Cytology

Objectives

You will learn the following in this chapter:

Morphologic features of all cellular organelles when seen through various types of micro-

scopes including conventional light microscopy and electron microscopy

Cellular functions conducted by cellular organelles and their functional interrelationships

The cell can be viewed as a microcosm of the body, with organelles that are analogous to the bodily organ systems. The central coordinator of the cell and the archive of genetic information is the **nucleus.** The cell is capable of receiving and reacting to a wide range of stimuli that trigger nuclear control mechanisms. Different genes become activated or repressed, and the genetic message is relayed to the cytoplasm, where it is converted into an appropriate response. The delicate balance within the cell and the organelles responsible for maintenance of this balance are the subject of this chapter.

The cell is a mass of **protoplasm** surrounded by a cell membrane called the **plasmalemma** (or **plasma membrane**). The cell's protoplasm is divided into two compartments: (1) **cytoplasm,** that which lies between the cell membrane and the nuclear membrane, and (2) **nucleoplasm** (karyoplasm), that which fills the nucleus (Fig. 2-1). These "plasms" are colloidal in that they may occur in the form of sols or gels and are combinations of various organic molecules, salts, and water. Protoplasm is the medium in which the specific cellular machinery, the *organelles*, is suspended and constitutes the primordial "elec-

trolyte sea" or intracellular environment. The organelles that are suspended in this protoplasm conduct specific cellular activities.

CYTOPLASMIC ORGANELLES
The Concept of Membrane

The most ubiquitous structure in the cell is membrane. All cells are separated from the external environment by the plasmalemma, which acts as a selective barrier, recognizing and admitting some molecules while excluding others. In addition, the diversity of functions performed by each cell require compartmentalization within the cytoplasm to spatially segregate different classes of cellular activities. This compartmentalization is achieved through a system of intracellular membranous organelles. Membranes can enclose specific regions of cytoplasm and actively modify the environment they enclose through a variety of transport systems suited to the particular need of the organelle in question. The plasmalemma and the membranous organelles are complex structures composed of a **lipid bilayer** that is integrated with a variety of struc-

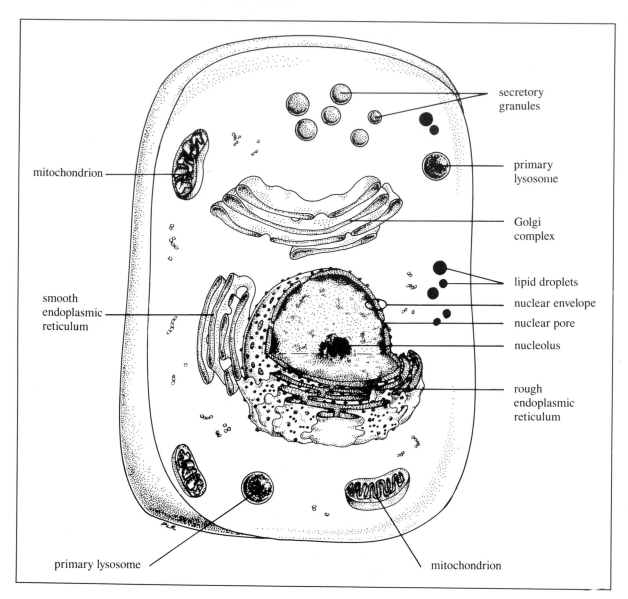

secretory
granules

primary
lysosome

mitochondrion

Golgi
complex

lipid droplets

nuclear envelope

smooth
endoplasmic
reticulum

nuclear pore

nucleolus

rough
endoplasmic
reticulum

primary lysosome

mitochondrion

Fig. 2-1. A cell. The major organelles and some inclusions are shown.

tural and functional proteins. The general composition of the plasmalemma is similar to that of internal membranes, but it differs in the types of lipid and protein present and in the additional presence of carbohydrate groups that project from the cell surface; these carbohydrate groups serve as receptors important in the recognition of

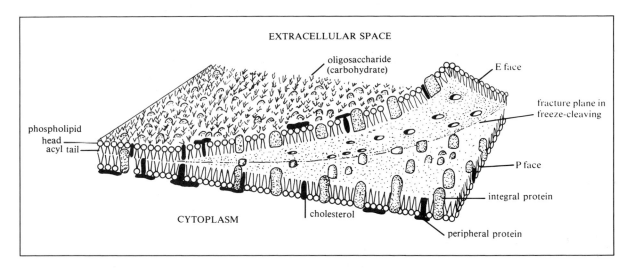

EXTRACELLULAR SPACE

oligosaccharide (carbohydrate)

E face

fracture plane in freeze-cleaving

phospholipid head

acyl tail

P face

integral protein

CYTOPLASM

cholesterol

peripheral protein

Fig. 2-2. The cell membrane or plasmalemma. In freeze-cleaving, the membrane is fractured along the lipid bilayer between the nonpolar acyl tails. The half of the membrane facing the cytoplasm is referred to as the P or protoplasmic face and retains most of the integral membrane proteins which give it a particle-rich appearance. The other half of the membrane facing the extracellular space is called the E face and is usually particle poor.

molecular signals, such as hormones, impinging on the cell from its external environment.

Specific membrane proteins, which either are integral parts of the membrane or merely associated with its surface through relatively weak molecular bonds, are responsible for most of the physiologic activities conducted by that membrane. Hence, the membranes of different organelles that perform different functions within the cell are biochemically distinct with regard to at least some types of membrane proteins. Furthermore, regions of a membrane may exhibit molecular domains preferentially occupied by aggregates of one type of membrane protein that may be sparse or absent elsewhere in the same membrane. This has the effect of focusing membrane activities in specific sites and is only one example of the complex level of organization displayed by the cell (Figs. 2-2, 2-3).

Another level of functional and structural organization is found within the cell's **cytoskeleton.** The cytoskeleton is composed of a variety of protein filaments that confer structural support and help direct the functions of the organelles to specific cellular localities.

This section describes the various organelles beginning with the plasmalemma. The cytoskeleton, sometimes referred to as a nonmembranous organelle, is described in a following section.

Membranous Organelles

CELL MEMBRANE (PLASMALEMMA)

The cell membrane (Fig. 2-4) is not visible with the light microscope but can be visualized with the electron microscope as a set of electron-dense lines, separated by a clear or lucent space. This "unit membrane" has been compared to railroad tracks; the width of this three-layered structure is usually 7 to 8 nm. The field of membrane science has advanced rapidly in the past 10 years with the advent of several specialized physical techniques to explore the arrangement of lipids and protein within the membrane. These physical methods, coupled with direct observation of the membrane interior through freeze-fracture electron microscopy, have yielded new concepts of membrane structure that are still evolving.

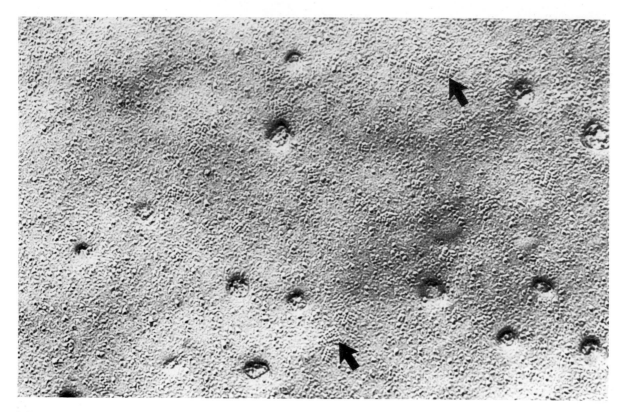

Fig. 2-3. Freeze-fractured replica of muscle cell plasmalemma. The outer or E-face leaflet of the plasmalemma has been fractured away to reveal intramembranous particles embedded in the protoplasmic
leaflet of the plasmalemma. These particles are believed to represent macromolecules within the membrane. Some of the particles are aggregated into clusters (*arrows*), but most have a less organized
distribution.

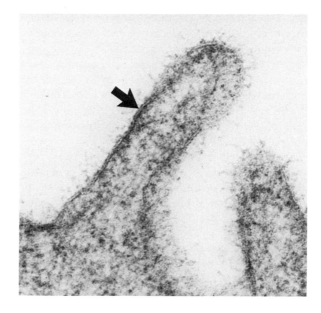

Fig. 2-4. Electron micrograph of the plasmalemma
from a kidney cell. The plasmalemma is resolved into
two electron dense lines separated by an electron lucent space (*arrow*). Also apparent as a result of
tannic acid staining are fine filamentous projections
from the outer surface of the membrane. These are
probably carbohydrate constituents anchored to
membrane molecules.

It should be stressed that many models exist for possible arrangements of membrane molecules and that currently there is no one model that is satisfactory on all fronts. At a very basic level, however, the cell membrane can be described as follows:

1. **A bimolecular leaflet of phospholipids** is the backbone of the membrane (see Fig. 2-2). Hydrophilic phosphate head groups are attached to long hydrophobic hydrocarbon tails (fatty acids). The hydrophilic (polar) heads are directed outward to abut on the aqueous cell cytoplasm or external milieu. The nonpolar hydrocarbon tails point inward, creating a hydrophobic environment sequestered in the membrane interior. These fatty acid tails can exist either as a rigid crystalline lattice or as a fluid phase in which the hydrocarbon tails are more freely mobile. This property, which can affect the location of membrane proteins that are inserted into the bilayer, forms the basis of some of the newer membrane models.

2. **Protein molecules,** which account for 60 to 70 percent of the membrane mass, are associated with the lipid bilayer in two ways:
   a. **Peripheral proteins** are external to the bilayer. They are associated with the polar lipid head groups by a variety of weak bonds, which can be broken by changing the pH or ionic strength.
   b. **Integral proteins,** on the other hand, can be liberated from the membrane only by the use of drastic measures such as detergents, which break up the lipids into micelles. Even this harsh treatment may not fully separate proteins from lipids. Integral proteins are actually inserted directly into the bilayer and extend either partly or completely through the lipid layer. These proteins are **amphipathic,** containing both hydrophilic and hydrophobic regions that allow them to penetrate the bilayer. Freeze-fracture electron micrographs reveal the inner region of the membrane because the fracture occurs along the pathway of least resistance—between the nonpolar lipid tails (see Figs. 2-2, 2-3). Such micrographs reveal numerous particles within the membrane that have diameters of 7 nm; these particles have been identified as membrane proteins. Membrane proteins have a variety of functions, many of which are enzymatic. They participate in a wide range of activities, from maintaining different ion concentrations on opposite sides of the membrane to transducing messages impinging on the cell surface into molecules that can trigger a specific nuclear or cytoplasmic response.

3. **Cholesterol** is a lipid that is present in nearly the same molar concentration as phospholipids in most cell membranes. Intracellular membranes, however, generally contain far less cholesterol. The cholesterol molecule readily associates with the fatty acid tails of membrane phospholipids and changes their molecular motions. In other words, cholesterol can determine whether the fatty acids are in crystalline or "loose" packing, and it is critical in determining how fluid the membrane is. The more cholesterol, the more fluid the membrane becomes.

4. **Carbohydrates** are linked to either proteins or lipids, primarily on the **outer** surface of the membrane abutting the external environment. These sugars serve as specific receptor sites for a host of incoming stimuli and also bear a net negative charge that is carried mainly by the amino sugar, sialic acid. The binding of particular molecules, such as hormones, to their specific receptor sites brings about local changes within adjacent membrane proteins (enzymes), which release messenger molecules such as the cyclic nucleotides (cyclic AMP and cyclic GMP) into the cytoplasm. These molecules can then trigger intracellular responses appropriate to the given stimulus.

The membrane is now viewed as potentially "fluid" in nature; that is, the lipids and also the proteins are capable of some degree of lateral motion. Certain proteins and species of lipid may occupy different sites, or **domains,** in the membrane, which can provide a functional mosaic displaying various receptor sites and enzymes (see Fig. 2-3). This dynamic concept of two-dimensional fluidity is known as the **fluid-mosaic** model of membrane structure. Although the membrane can behave as a fluid mosaic, the control mechanisms governing the disposition of the membrane proteins and the mechanics of membrane flow from the cell membrane to cytoplasmic membranous organelles are just beginning to yield to investigation.

Structural Specializations of the Plasmalemma

In electron micrographs the plasmalemma appears as two electron-dense lines separated by an electron-lucent line. That picture is slightly embellished after staining with tannic acid, which is believed to emphasize certain carbohydrate moieties that project away from the extracellular surface of the plasmalemma (see Fig. 2-4).

Another morphologic specialization of the plasmalemma is the **gap junction (nexus).** Gap junctions are specialized areas of plasmalemma involving contiguous surfaces of adjacent cells. The gap junctions permit the flow of ions and substances of very small molecular weight between adjacent cells. For this reason they are sometimes referred to as **communicating junctions.** Since ions can pass from one cell to another through gap junctions, an electric current can be distributed throughout layers of communicating cells. By this mechanism a layer of smooth muscle cells can respond when only a small percentage of the cells are in direct contact with nerves. In this instance a nerve impulse may directly provoke contraction of a single smooth muscle cell, but the depolarization spreads through contiguous noninnervated smooth muscle cells owing to the flow of potassium through the low-resistance pathway provided by gap junctions between the cells. This ionic flow is probably influenced by calcium or hydrogen ions, which seem to alter

permeability of the gap junctions. In this way cells can alter the resistance of their gap junctions from a low state to a high state so that intercellular communication can be regulated. Gap junctions permit selective flow of other substances, such as cyclic AMP and various regulatory molecules as well. Gap junctions are especially common between epithelial cells, liver cells, nerve cells, and smooth and cardiac muscle cells.

Gap junctions cannot be resolved with the light microscope. However, in electron micrographs, a thin section through a gap junction reveals that the plasmalemmas of adjacent cells approach to within 2 nm of each other (Fig. 2-5A, B). This narrow intercellular space between plasmalemmas is spanned by numerous bridging structures. In freeze-fractured gap junctions, these bridging structures (**connexons**) appear as intramembranous particles (Fig. 2-6A, B). In conventional transmission electron micrographs using negative staining, an electron-dense, water-soluble material can be introduced to infiltrate the gap junction wherever water is allowed. This approach delineates the connexons within the gap junction. Gap junctions prepared in this way reveal a central hydrophilic channel or annulus which occupies the central axis of each connexon. The connexon appears to be constructed of six subunits arranged around the annulus. This hydrophilic annulus, when open, would provide an unimpeded channel for the flow of appropriately small ions or molecules between cells (Figs. 2-7, 2-8).

Another structural specialization of the plasmalemma is the **zona occludens (tight junction).** The zona occludens consists of a thread-like constituent of the plasmalemma that courses around the entire circumference of a cell interlocking with threadlike elements within the plasmalemma of contiguous cells. The word **zonula** is derived from the belt that forms around the entire cell circumference. The result is the fusion of adjacent plasmalemma between participating cells. A sheet of cells bonded together in this way is relatively impermeable because it limits the passage of fluid between cells.

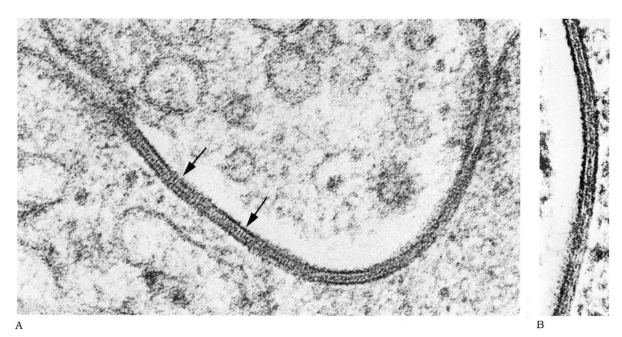

A   B

Fig. 2-5. Gap junctions between ovarian granulosa cells of the rat. A. Tangentially sectioned gap junction revealing regular series of parallel lines (*arrows*) 4 to 5 nm apart produced by connexons, which are believed to be low-resistance channels between interiors of adjacent cells ($\times$210,000 before reduction). B. Transversely sectioned gap junction. The central lucent zone, which lies between the outer lamellae of the two adjoining plasmalemmas, is the "gap." The term *gap junction,* however, is a misnomer because the space is occupied by the connexons and is therefore not a true gap ($\times$232,000 before reduction). (From F. B. Merk, J. T. Albright, and C. R. Botticelli, The fine structure of granulosa cell nexuses in rat ovarian follicles. *Anat. Rec.* 175:107, 1973.)

An occluding junction composed of a single threadlike element or strand is not completely impermeable but becomes more impermeable when several strands are involved in the fusion of plasmalemmas. The zonula occludens is a specialization of epithelial cells, sheets of cells that line the various hollow organs and cavities of the body. The zonula occludens provides an epithelial permeability seal that separates the lumen of a cavity or organ from the extracellular space between and beneath epithelial cells lining that cavity (Figs. 2-9, 2-10).

In electron micrographs, a sectioned zonula occludens appears as a fusion of the outer leaflets of plasmalemma of contiguous cells (see Fig. 2-9). In freeze-fractured preparations, the strands of the occludens appear to be composed of fused interlocking intramembranous particles contributed by adjacent cells. It has been compared to a zipper. In the most impermeable occluding junctions, these strands or filaments anastomose to form an elaborate network (see Fig. 2-10).

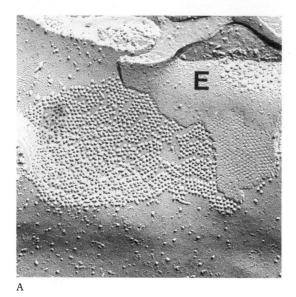

A

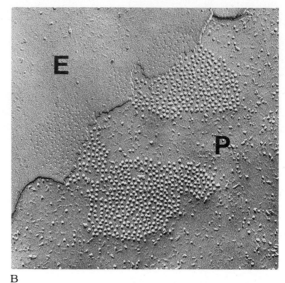

B

Fig. 2-6. Freeze-fracture replica of gap junctions. A. The particles of the gap junction are revealed where the E face (*E*) of one cell's plasmalemma has been cleaved away to reveal the P face of the adjacent cell's plasmalemma (*P*). The particles represent the connexons that link the plasmalemma of adjacent cells. B. The gap junction in this micrograph has been exposed to increased calcium concentrations, which causes the gap junction particles to aggregate into small groups of hexagonally packed arrays. This spatial relationship parallels that observed when gap junctions have been electrically uncoupled. This phenomenon may be similar to the mechanism employed by the cell to regulate the resistance of its gap junctions. (From C. Peracchia and L. Peracchia, Gap junction dynamics: Reversible effects of divalent cations. *J. Cell Biol.* 87:708, 1980. Reproduced by copyright permission of The Rockefeller University Press.)

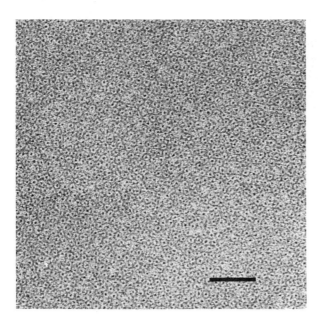

Fig. 2-7. Electron micrograph of gap junctions isolated from mouse liver and negatively stained with uranyl acetate. The stain delineates the connexons and occupies their central hydrophilic channels, which appear as dense dots. *Bar* = 50 nm. (From D. Goodenough, Gap junction dynamics and intercellular communication. *Pharmacol. Rev.* 30:383, 1979. © 1979 American Society for Pharmacological and Experimental Therapeutics.)

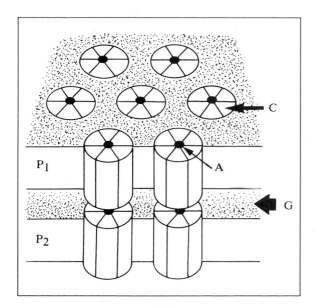

Fig. 2-8. Gap junction linking the plasmalemmas (P_1 and P_2) of adjacent cells. Each connexon (C) consists of six subunits arranged around a central hydrophilic channel or annulus (A). The connexons are drawn slightly separated in the 2-nm gap between plasmalemmas to show their three-dimensional relationship in the gap (G).

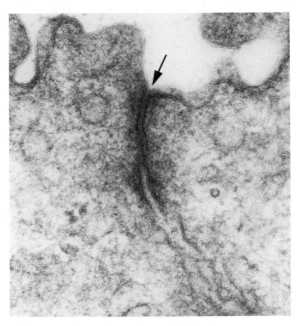

Fig. 2-9. Electron micrograph of a zonula occludens junction connecting the lateral plasmalemmas of adjacent epithelial cells lining a renal collecting duct. The arrow points to the occluding junction but is positioned within the lumen of the duct. The fused plasmalemmas seal the lumen of the duct off from the intercellular space between the lateral surfaces of the cells.

MITOCHONDRIA

Mitochondria are the major energy providers of the cell, utilizing an orderly sequence of membrane-bound enzymes to generate adenosine triphosphate (ATP) by the process of **oxidative phosphorylation.** In addition to providing energy, these organelles also actively sequester calcium ions, which are stored within their matrix as granules of $(CaPO_4)_2$ and are released in response to the cell's changing needs. When living cells are observed with a phase contrast microscope, mitochondria appear as threads that are

about 0.2 μm in diameter and up to several micrometers in length. They can be observed to move around within the cytoplasm in quite an autonomous manner and also to divide by binary fission. The **matrix** of the mitochondria contains closed loops of deoxyribonucleic acid (DNA) similar to those of bacteria, as well as particles resembling ribosomes. These molecules allow mitochondria to function as partially independent organelles, since they can self-replicate and synthesize some of the proteins they require to function.

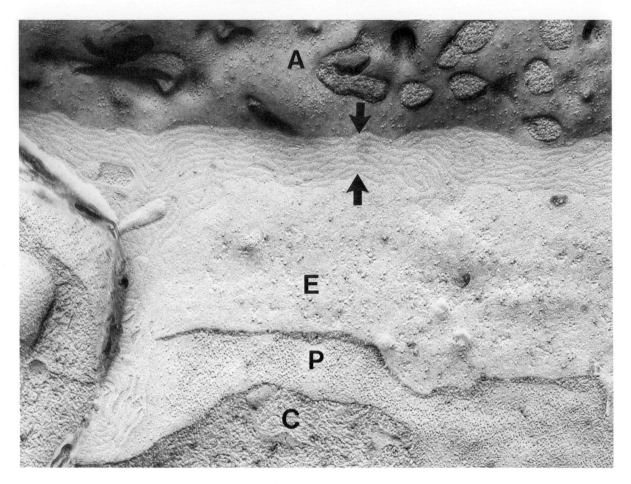

Fig. 2-10. Replica of freeze-fractured epithelial cells from renal collecting duct. An elaborate zonula occludens (*arrows*) is revealed in the extracellular leaflet (*E*) of the lateral plasmalemma of one cell. A small portion of the protoplasmic leaflet (*P*) of the lateral plasmalemma of the adjacent cell and its cytoplasm (*C*) is also visible. *A* = apical surface of adjacent cell.

When viewed with the electron microscope (Fig. 2-11), mitochondria show a highly plicated (folded) membranous structure, which mirrors their function as generators of ATP. These organelles are composed of two membranes, a smooth outer limiting membrane and an inner membrane convoluted into a series of folds or **cristae.** The numerous cristae dramatically increase the surface area available for the disposition of the respiratory chain enzymes involved in the generation of ATP. The surface of the cristae facing the interior of the mitochondrion is further studded with a series of particles similar in shape to lollipops, the **elementary particles.** The

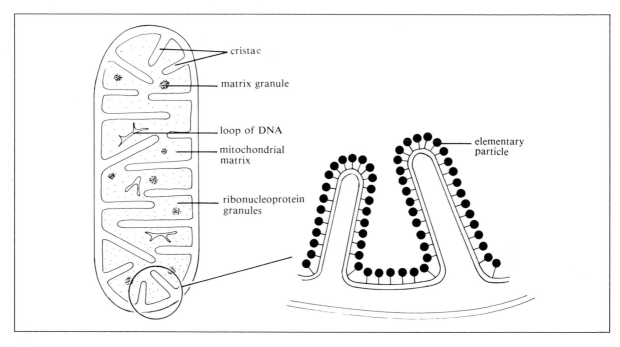

Fig. 2-11. A mitochondrion.

round 10-nm head of the elementary particle is attached by a slender stalk to the inner membrane. The region of the mitochondrion enclosed by the folded inner membrane houses the matrix.

⌐Mitochondria receive **pyruvate,** which has been generated from the metabolism of glucose, and they generate ATP by the process of oxidative phosphorylation.⌐The final generation of ATP occurs in a series of steps that are localized to certain compartments of the mitochondrion (see Fig. 2-11), as follows:

1. Krebs cycle enzymes are located in the mitochondrial matrix. Pyruvate is converted to carbon dioxide and reduced coenzyme (NADH).
2. Respiratory chain enzymes (dehydrogenase, flavoproteins, cytochromes) occupy the inner mitochondrial membranes (cristae). For each pair of hydrogen ions entering the chain as

reduced coenzyme, three ATP molecules will ultimately be generated.
3. The elementary particles house the actual enzymes of oxidative phosphorylation and adenosine triphosphatase (ATPase). Energy released from the respiratory chain oxidation-reduction reactions is stored as a high-energy phosphate bond in ATP. The energy required for the actual phosphorylation of ADP to ATP is now thought to result from a **chemiosmotic gradient** created by the respiratory chain enzymes, which pump their H^+ ions unidirectionally across the inner and outer membranes to the cytoplasm (Mitchell's chemiosmotic theory). The resultant gradient appears to drive the synthesis of ATP, which occurs in the elementary particles.

LYSOSOMES

Lysosomes are a morphologically heterogeneous class of organelle participating in cellular functions that involve enzymatic digestion of intracellular or extracellular material. Lysosomes are responsible for the resorption of tissue that is no longer needed by the organism, such as regression of the mammary glands following weaning or the resorption of the tadpole tail during metamorphosis. Generally, lysosomal enzymes degrade a variety of substances that would otherwise accumulate to the detriment of the cell. Congenital absence of particular lysosomal enzymes results in an accumulation of their substrates within the cell, producing a wide variety of storage diseases. One well-known example of this type of deficiency is Tay-Sachs disease, in which a particular type of lipid (ganglioside) cannot be degraded and becomes concentrated within nerve cells, leading to a fatal malfunctioning of the nervous system. Gaucher's disease is another lysosomal disorder. It is characterized by a deficiency of glucocerebrosidase and an abnormal accumulation of glucocerebrosides.

While inconspicuous with the light microscope, lysosomes appear in electron micrographs as membrane-bound vacuoles about 0.25 to 0.50 μm in diameter. Since their contents are morphologically variable or amorphous, histochemical techniques for acid phosphatase are usually necessary for positive identification of lysosomes since they contain hydrolytic enzymes with acid pH optima. A lysosome may contain one or more of 50 known acid hydrolases. The lysosomal membrane confines these enzymes within the lysosome, thereby protecting the other cytoplasmic structures that would be degraded by the action of these enzymes. The lysosome can direct its degradative action either against its own cellular material and organelles (**autophagy**) or against extracellular materials (**heterophagy**). Autophagy is a normal cellular activity by which lysosomes dismantle damaged or worn-out organelles. During autophagy of a mitochondrion, for instance, the mitochondrion is engulfed by the lysosome and digested entirely within the lysosome. During heterophagy, material obtained from the cell's external environment is digested. Extracellular fluids and extracellular particulates are internalized by becoming captured within an invagination of the plasmalemma, which detaches from the cell surface to become a mem-

brane-bound vesicle (endosome, endocytic vesicle) suspended within the cytoplasm. This vesicle is a **pinocytotic vesicle** if it contains fluid predominantly or a **phagocytic vesicle** (**phagosome**) if it contains particulate material predominantly. In both instances these vesicles fuse with a lysosome, and their contents are exposed to the hydrolytic action of lysosomal enzymes (Fig. 2-12).

Several morphologic structures have been identified at each of the stages of lysosomal activity. Lysosomes that have recently been formed from the Golgi apparatus but that contain no ingested or digested material are referred to as **primary lysosomes.** After fusing with material of any kind, the lysosome is called a **secondary lysosome.** A secondary lysosome displays various morphologic appearances depending on whether it has fused with another organelle, with a phagosome, or with pinocytotic vesicles. At the early stages of autophagy or heterophagy, the

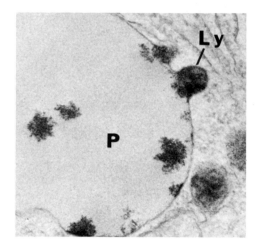

Fig. 2-12 Phagolysosome (P) or secondary lysosome formed by the fusion of a lysosome (Ly) with a phagosome. The lysosome is densely stained by a cytochemical process for trimetaphosphatase. (From A. F. Payer, C. L. Battle, and R. L. Peake, Ultrastructural and cytochemical effects of trypan blue on TSH stimulation of thyroid follicular cells. *Cell Tissue Res.* 218:547, 1981.)

material within the lysosome can frequently be identified. A bacteria or red blood cell may be visible within a **phagosome;** a mitochondrion may be visible within an **autophagic vacuole;** and in some instances pinocytotic vesicles may be visible within **multivesicular bodies,** although there are probably other explanations for the formation of multivesicular bodies (Fig. 2-13). All of these structures are different morphologic manifestations of secondary lysosomes. Late in the digestive phase, the material within the lysosome becomes unrecognizable, degraded debris. These structures are referred to as **residual bodies.** Residual bodies contain indigestible residues that the lysosome cannot further degrade (see Fig. 2-18). The cell disposes of the material within residual bodies by **exocytosis.** The residual body migrates to the plasmalemma, fuses to it, and ruptures, releasing its contents extracellularly. In certain cell types (e.g., nerve cells and cardiac muscle cells), residual bodies accumulate with age because they cannot be disposed of by exocytosis. The accumulated residual bodies contain a residue called **lipofuscin,** a golden brown pigment.

PEROXISOMES

Peroxisomes are organelles which engage in various oxidative degradation reactions that produce hydrogen peroxide. Since hydrogen peroxide is very toxic to the cell, peroxisomes also contain catalase, a heme enzyme which metabolizes peroxides to water and oxygen. In fact 40 percent of the enzyme content of the peroxisome is catalase. It is also effective in metabolizing the peroxide produced by mitochondria during their enzymatic activity associated with the electron transport chain and other oxidative reactions. This protection provided by peroxisomes is necessary for survival of the cell, especially any cell engaged in high-volume aerobic activity. Peroxisomes also account for considerable beta-oxidation of fatty acids and are exceeded in this activity only by mitochondria.

Peroxisomes are approximately 0.5 μm in diameter and similar in appearance to lysosomes. They are limited by a single membrane which encloses a uniform granular matrix. The granular matrix is separated from the membrane by a narrow translucent space. In some animals a crystalline lattice, believed to represent urate oxidase, is present in the matrix (Fig. 2-14). Neither this enzyme nor the crystalline inclusion are in human peroxisomes. Consequently the substrate for this enzyme, uric acid, is released into the urine without further modification in humans.

Peroxisomes are formed by budding from the smooth endoplasmic reticulum. Catalase, after being synthesized in the cytoplasm by free ribosomes, is transported into the peroxisome. Cytochemical reactions for catalase are frequently used to identify peroxisomes with certainty for electron microscopy.

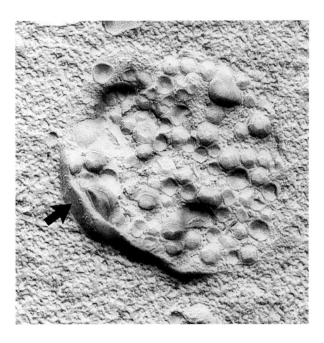

Fig. 2-13. Freeze-cleave replica of a multivesicular body that has been fractured open to expose numerous vesicles occupying its interior. The multivesicular body is believed to be a form of secondary lysosome containing vesicles that may have originated from the cell's plasmalemma. The fractured limiting membrane of the lysosome is indicated by the arrow.

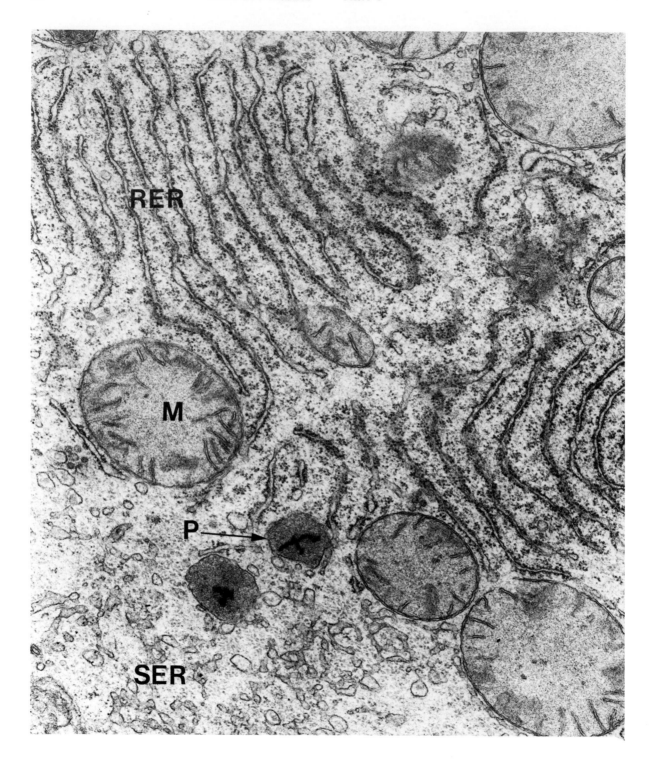

SMOOTH ENDOPLASMIC RETICULUM

The **smooth (agranular) endoplasmic reticulum** (SER) is a delicate branching network of **tubules** that ramify through the cytoplasm (see Fig. 2-14). The extent of its development depends both on cell type and on functional need. The slender processes can only be seen in the electron microscope. The function of SER varies in different cell types, examples of which are listed below:

1. Cells producing steroid hormones have abundant SER, in which cholesterol is stored as a precursor for steroidogenesis.
2. Liver cells (hepatocytes) are situated in the portal circulation and have many responsibilities, one of which is the detoxification of lipid-soluble chemicals arriving from the gastrointestinal tract. The enzymes that hydroxylate these substances and thus inactivate them are located in the SER and are inducible. Therefore, if a given dose of a drug such as phenobarbital is taken on day 1, the hepatocyte SER will begin to hypertrophy (increase in size), and more hydroxylating enzymes will be present on each subsequent day of drug intake. After several days, SER may be the predominant cellular organelle, and the phenobarbital will be rapidly inactivated. Therefore, as time goes on, progressively more drug is required to achieve the same therapeutic effect. This phenomenon is known as **induced drug tolerance.**
3. Striated muscle cells have a highly developed system of SER known as **sarcoplasmic (sarco = muscle) reticulum.** This organelle has a very specialized function in the uptake and release of intracellular CA^{++} ions, which control muscle contraction and relaxation (see Muscle, Chap. 7).

Fig. 2-14. Electron micrograph of Chinese hamster cell showing mitochondria (*M*), rough endoplasmic reticulum (*RER*), smooth endoplasmic reticulum (*SER*), and peroxisomes (*P*). (Courtesy of W. Duane Belt).

RIBOSOMES AND ROUGH ENDOPLASMIC RETICULUM IN POLYPEPTIDE SYNTHESIS

All cells synthesize proteins either for their internal use or for export (secretion). In both instances, amino acids are assembled into proteins by ribosomes, which translate the genetic message from messenger RNA (mRNA). Cells that synthesize protein in greater quantity contain proportionately higher amounts of ribosomes in their cytoplasm. Ribosomes have a high affinity for basic dyes because they consist of 35 percent RNA. Their negatively charged phosphate groups attract positively charged dyes. Consequently, areas of the cell with a large number of ribosomes appear as small clumps of basophilic material with the light microscope. With the superior resolution of the electron microscope, ribosomes are visualized either as free in the cytoplasm or as attached to membranes (Figs. 2-14, 2-15, 2-16). The unattached ribosomes assemble proteins for the cell's internal use, including structural proteins forming the cell's cytoskeleton, various enzymes, and proteins required for the repair and manufacture of organelles. The ribosomes attached to membranes assemble proteins destined for secretion, such as the digestive enzymes of the pancreatic exocrine cells, which are secreted into the small intestine. The membrane, together with its associated ribosomes, constitutes the **rough endoplasmic reticulum** (RER). With electron microscopy, the membrane of the RER (sometimes called granular endoplasmic reticulum) is shown to be a complex intracellular network of long, branching tubules and flattened saccules or cisternae. The tubules and cisternae interconnect and form an elaborate channel throughout much of the cytoplasm. The ribosomes appear as granules 15 nm in diameter adhering to the outer surface of the membrane facing the cytoplasm (Fig. 2-17; see also Figs. 2-15, 2-16). The RER is most abundant in cells that synthesize large quantities of protein for secretion.

The ribosome consists of two subunits with different sedimentation coefficients (S): a 60S

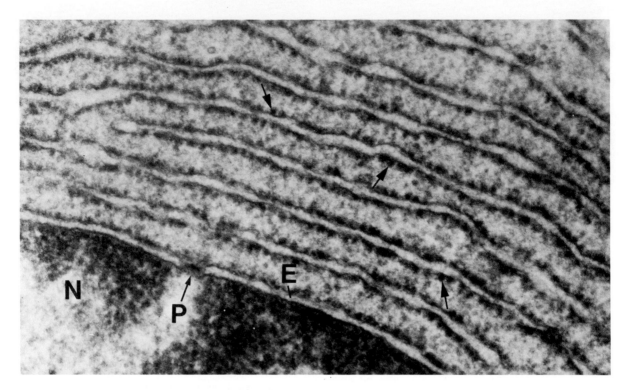

Fig. 2-15. Transmission electron micrograph of rough endoplasmic reticulum (RER) near the nucleus (*N*). The RER is sectioned to show longitudinal profiles of cisterna, whose limiting membrane is studded with ribosomes (*arrows*). The nuclear envelope (*E*) is conspicuous also. Its outer membrane is studded with ribosomes; its inner membrane has clumps of heterochromatin associated with it. *P* = nuclear pore. (Courtesy of W. Duane Belt.)

and 40S subunit. In the specific instance of the RER, ribosomes are attached to the reticulum membrane by their larger subunit. The small ribosomal subunit is associated with a strand of mRNA whose size is just barely within the resolving power of the best electron microscopes. In most electron micrographs, mRNA is not visible. ⌈Several ribosomes attached to a strand of mRNA constitute a polysome.⌋ The mRNA provides the genetic information to the ribosomes regarding the amino acid sequence of the particular protein to be translated. The peptidyltransferase center is located on the large ribosomal subunit. Peptidyltransferase catalyzes the formation of peptide bonds to elongate the nascent polypeptide. As the polypeptide is assembled by the ribosomes, it remains attached to the large subunit and to mRNA through cognate transfer RNA (tRNA) (see Fig. 2-17). When assembly of lysosomal enzymes, secretory proteins, and plasmalemmal proteins are completed, each will have a hydrophobic amino terminal signal peptide. This signal peptide will interact with a signal recognition particle of the ribosome that initiates vectorial transport of the newly synthesized proteins through a channel in the large ribosomal

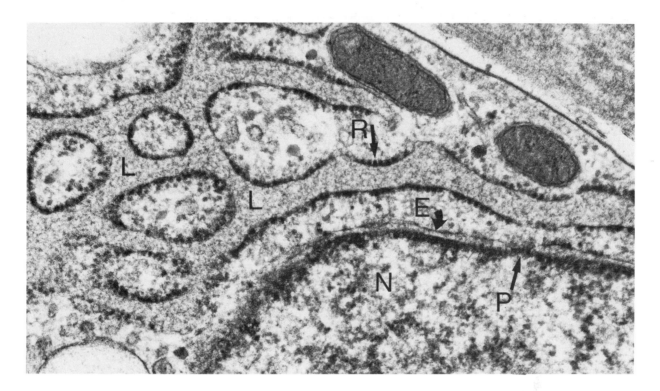

Fig. 2-16. Human cultured fibroblast showing an area of rough endoplasmic reticulum near the nucleus (*N*). The lumen (*L*) of the rough endoplasmic reticulum is dilated with flocculent material representing nascent polypeptides. Ribosomes (*R*) are visible on the outer surface of the reticulum. In addition, the outer membrane of the nuclear envelope (*E*) is visible near a nuclear pore (*P*).

subunit into the lumen of the RER. While still within the lumen of the RER, all these mixed proteins will undergo posttranslational glycosylation, resulting in the addition of an oligosaccharide. After further modification the glycopeptides are transported to the Golgi apparatus. They are apparently transported by vesicles that bud from a transitional element of the RER, which lacks ribosomes on one surface and migrate to the Golgi. However, an additional route may follow

direct tubular connections between the transitional RER and the Golgi.

GOLGI APPARATUS (COMPLEX)

The Golgi apparatus receives proteins from the cisternae of the RER for required posttranslational modification before distributing them to multiple destinations within the cell. For example, after emerging from the Golgi apparatus, acid hydrolase enzymes will be shuttled to lysosomes by coated vesicles; secretory proteins will be sorted into secretory vesicles; and plasmalemmal proteins will be deployed along the cell surface membrane.

The Golgi apparatus usually occupies a location between the RER and the plasmalemma. It is

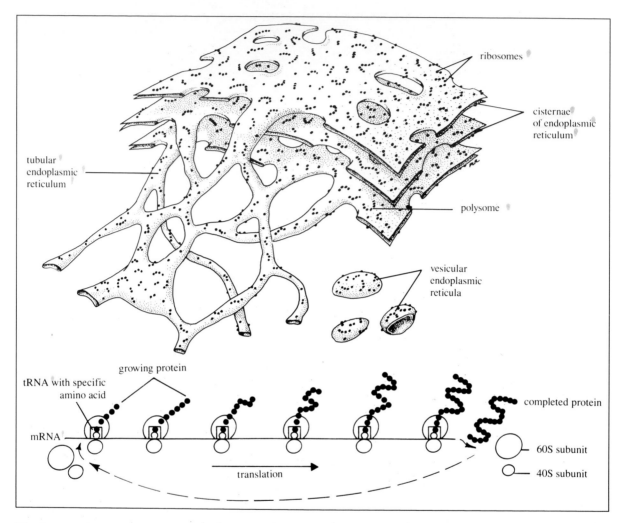

Fig. 2-17. The interconnected cisternae and tubules of RER. A polysome of six ribosomes is also depicted, each ribosome translating a complete copy of a protein from a strand of messenger RNA (*mRNA*). The ribosome attaches to the mRNA at one end, acting as a scaffolding on which the appropriate transfer RNA molecules (*tRNA*) can be oriented to read the base sequence on the mRNA, attaching the appropriate amino acids. The ribosome moves down the mRNA strand while more amino acids are added sequentially. At the end of the strand, both ribosome and completed protein are released. The ribosome splits into its component subunits, which are used to form new ribosomes. (From W. M. Copenhaver, R. P. Bunge, and M. B. Bunge [eds.], *Bailey's Textbook of Histology* [16th ed.]. Baltimore: Williams & Wilkins, 1971. Reproduced with permission.)

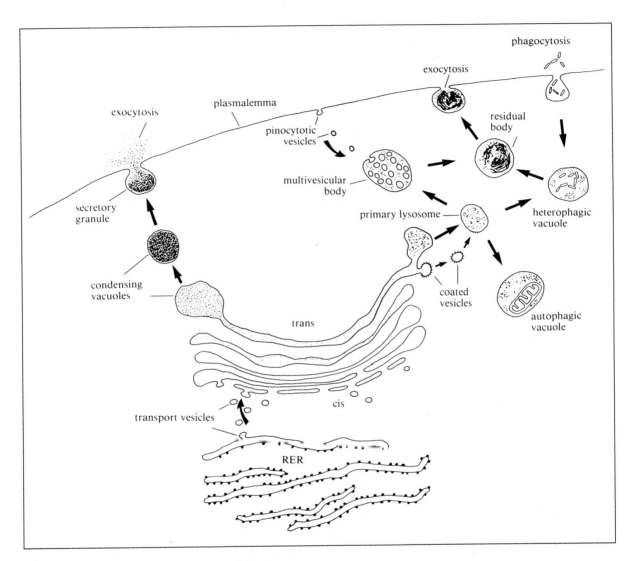

Fig. 2-18. Various cellular activities involving the Golgi apparatus. The secretory pathway is depicted on the left; the lysosomal pathway is depicted on the right.

composed of smooth-surfaced membrane organized into a stack of parallel, flattened cisternae or saccules. The cisternae are all slightly curved, producing a convex side (cis side) that faces the RER, and a concave side (trans side) (see Figs. 2-18, 2-19, 2-23). In the light microscope the Golgi apparatus does not stain well with conventional stains; in fact, this absence of staining usually identifies the location of the Golgi apparatus within the cell as a relatively translucent space, sometimes referred to as a negative image (see Fig. 6-8). Since the Golgi reduces metal salts to dense metallic deposits, it can be effectively stained with osmium, silver, or lead. Because it is actively engaged in carbohydrate attachment

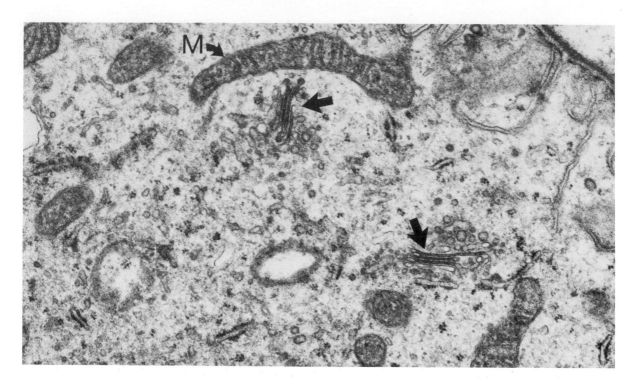

Fig. 2-19. The two Golgi complexes in this photo (*arrows*) are not as magnified as in figures 2-20, 2-21, and 2-22 and give an appreciation for their relative size compared with neighboring mitochondria (*M*) in the same cell.

to proteins arriving from the RER, the periodic acid-Schiff reaction will stain the Golgi apparatus red if sufficient carbohydrate is present. The size of the Golgi body fluctuates with its current activity and therefore can be conspicuous or inconspicuous. Also, the full extent of its elaborate three-dimensional geometry is difficult to appreciate with the conventional thin sections used for electron microscopy.

The Golgi apparatus processes secretory products in one or more of the following ways: (1) glycosylation and sulfation of glycoproteins and glycolipids; (2) proteolytic processing of presec-

retory proteins; and (3) concentration and packaging of secretory products into membrane-bound secretory vesicles.

Since newly synthesized polypeptides destined for secretion must be processed by the Golgi apparatus, they must be shuttled from the RER to the Golgi apparatus (Figs. 2-18, 2-20). This function is performed by **transitional vesicles,** which pinch off from small portions of the RER devoid of ribosomes. These membranous vesicles containing the nascent polypeptide migrate to the Golgi apparatus and fuse with the dilated rims of some of its saccules, frequently the outermost saccule on the cis side. In electron micrographs, several transitional vesicles are usually found in transit between the nearby RER and the cis face (forming face) of the Golgi. Once within the Golgi, the polypeptides may be modified by sulfation, glycosylation, or hydrolysis into biologically active molecules. The enzymes performing these modifications in the nascent polypeptide are

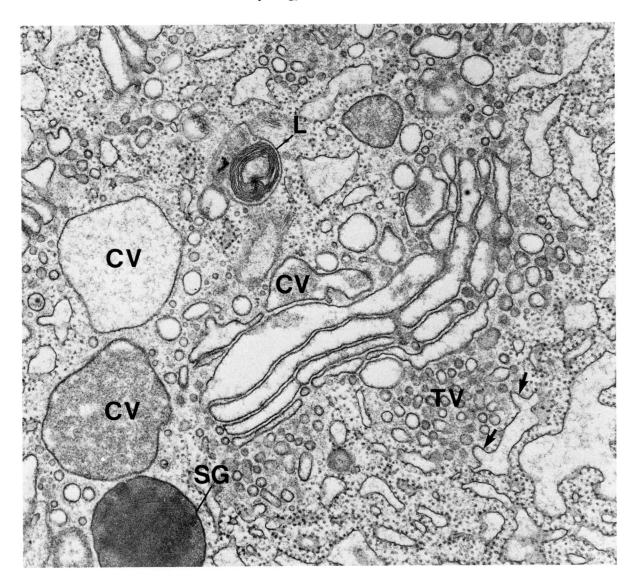

Fig. 2-20. Golgi area in an exocrine pancreatic cell of the guinea pig. This Golgi apparatus consists of four cisternae with condensing vacuoles (*CV*) on its trans side and transport vesicles (*TV*) on its cis side. The transport vesicles are presumed to originate from transitional elements (*arrows*) of the RER and fuse with the cis side of the Golgi. The condensing vacuoles are presumed to emerge from the trans side and contain secretory proteins that gradually become concentrated into secretory granules (*SG*) or zymogen granules. *L* = secondary lysosome or autophagic vacuole containing a myelin figure. (From M. G. Farquhar and G. E. Palade, The Golgi apparatus [complex]—[1954–1981]—from artifact to center stage. *J. Cell Biol.* 91:77s,1981. Reproduced by copyright permission of The Rockefeller University Press.)

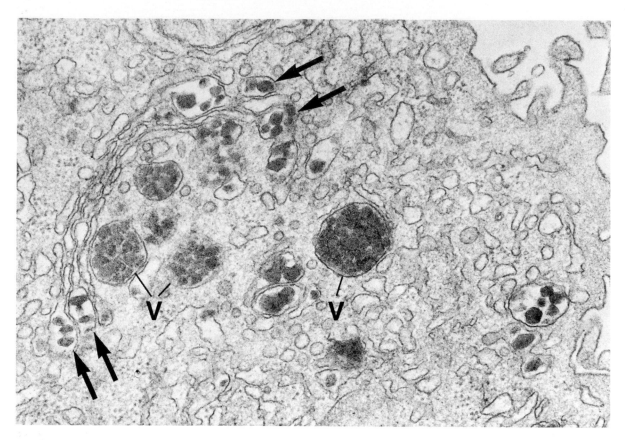

Fig. 2-21. Golgi apparatus from liver cell (hepatocyte). Clusters of dense lipoprotein particles occupy the dilated rims of the Golgi cisternae (*arrows*) and numerous secretory vesicles (*V*) located on the trans side of the complex. (From M. G. Farquhar and G. E. Palade, The Golgi apparatus [complex]—[1954–1981] —from artifact to center stage. *J. Cell Biol.* 91:77s, 1981. Reproduced by copyright permission of The Rockefeller University Press.)

housed in the Golgi membranes. The nascent polypeptide apparently travels sequentially through the cisternae until it emerges within a membrane-bound **condensing vacuole** from the dilated rims of the trans cisternae (maturing face). The proteins will be concentrated within this vacuole by elimination of water until a final,

smaller **secretory vesicle** is formed (Figs. 2-18, 2-20, 2-21). The secretory vesicle will eventually fuse to the plasmalemma and rupture, releasing its contents to the exterior of the cell (a process termed **exocytosis**).

The Golgi apparatus also processes other cell products, including lysosomal enzymes. Since virtually all lysosomal enzymes are glycoproteins, they are glycosylated in the Golgi apparatus. In order to protect secretory proteins from the lytic action of lysosomal enzymes, the Golgi apparatus must be capable of processing them in a segregated fashion. A specialized portion of the Golgi apparatus has been implicated in the processing of lysosomal enzymes. It is called GERL, an acronym for *G*olgi, *e*ndoplasmic *r*eticulum, *ly*sosomal system. The lysosome emerges from the trans side of the Golgi by pinching off from one of the dilated rims of the cisternae (Fig. 2-22; see also Fig. 2-23 for general organization of the Golgi apparatus). There is also evidence that newly synthesized lysosomal enzymes can be transported from the Golgi apparatus to the primary lysosome by **coated vesicles** (vesicles with a conspicuous external, hexagonal scaffolding that may also be involved in ferrying substances between the Golgi and plasmalemma).

Newly synthesized polypeptides to be secreted are distinguished from lysosomal enzymes destined for incorporation into lysosomes by molecular signals that are tagged onto these nascent polypeptides in the RER and serve to sort them on their way through the Golgi apparatus. These molecular signals are modified sugar residues that direct molecular traffic along a secretory pathway through the Golgi or a lysosomal path-

way through the GERL. In the neutrophil, one of the white blood cells, segregation of lysosomal enzymes from nonlysosomal proteins within the Golgi apparatus is accomplished by synthesizing them at different times. In this particular instance, the two different protein products emerge from opposite sides of the Golgi apparatus (see Fig. 2-22).

Fig. 2-22. A developing neutrophil, one of the white blood cells, showing the formation of lysosomes (*arrows*) along the trans side of the Golgi complex. (From D. F. Bainton and M. G. Farquhar, Origin of granules in polymorphonuclear leukocytes: Two types derived from opposite faces of the Golgi complex in developing granulocytes. *J. Cell Biol.* 28:277, 1966. Reproduced by copyright permission of The Rockefeller University Press.)

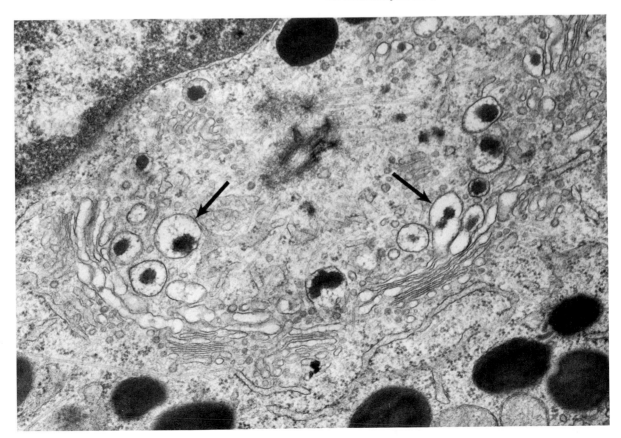

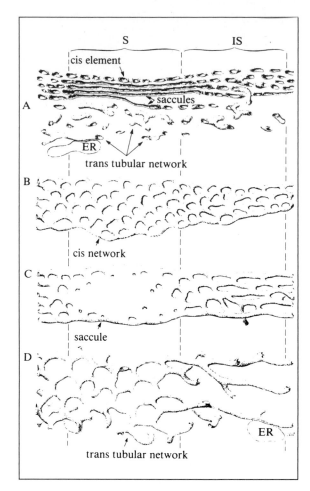

Fig. 2-23. The morphology of various components of the Golgi apparatus. A = the appearance of the Golgi apparatus sectioned perpendicular to its stack of saccules. B, C, and D represent three-dimensional face views of each component of the Golgi complex. *ER* = endoplasmic reticulum; *IS* = intersaccular region; *S* = saccular region. (From A. Rambourg, Y. Clermont, and L. Hermo, Three-dimensional architecture of the Golgi apparatus in Sertoli cells of the rat. *Am. J. Anat.* 154:455, 1979.)

Since all transmembrane proteins of the plasmalemma have oligosaccharide chains, it is assumed that the Golgi complex is involved in biogenesis of many membrane components because the Golgi apparatus is the main site of terminal glycosylation in the cell. Autoradiographic evidence has shown that certain plasmalemmal molecules, such as the acetylcholine receptor in the muscle cell plasmalemma, are present in the Golgi complex before their insertion into the plasmalemma. Consequently, the Golgi apparatus not only sorts secretory proteins from lysosomal proteins by directing the former to secretory vesicles and the latter to lysosomes, but also directs certain transmembrane proteins to their destination in the endoplasmic reticulum or plasmalemma.

Distinct functional properties have been localized to three compartments within the Golgi apparatus. These compartments are the cis lamellae, the trans lamellae, and the medial lamellae, which are sandwiched between the cis and trans lamellae. It appears that glycoproteins (i.e., secretory proteins, lysosomal proteins, and plasmalemmal proteins) traverse the Golgi, completely or partially, by riding in transport vesicles that bud off from one lamella and fuse with the next. This vesicular transport mechanism carries glycoprotein from the cisternae of the cis lamellae through the medial and trans cisternae sequentially. The enzymes on the inner surface of each lamella modify the glycoprotein in different ways.

Glycoproteins such as the acid hydrolase enzymes, destined to be carried by coated vesicles to lysosomes, are phosphorylated within the cisternae of the cis lamellae. Mannose-6-phosphate residues are the recognition signal identifying lysosomal enzymes. The cis lamellae also contain the mannose-6-phosphate receptor, which is responsible for binding to these enzymes via their mannose-6-phosphate residues for specific distribution to lysosomes via coated vesicles. Coated vesicles carrying lysosomal enzymes will bud off from the cis lamellae and shuttle these enzymes to lysosomes.

Within the cisternae of medial lamellae *N-*

acetylglucosamine residues are added to the carbohydrate chain of the glycoprotein by a variety of transferases. Subsequently these carbohydrate chains are elongated within the cisternae of the trans lamellae by glycosyltransferases that first attach galactose residues followed by a terminal sialic acid residue. This terminal sialic acid residue will be directed to the plasmalemma where it will be inserted into the plasmalemma as an integral membrane glycoprotein. These post-translational modifications of the carbohydrate chains of glycoproteins are crucial identification signals, not only for their correct distribution to intracellular destinations but also for their recognition by other cells in the body. For example, glycoproteins with mannose-6-phosphate residues are recognized as lysosomal hydrolases and will be retrieved by certain cell types and shuttled to their lysosomes. This process is prominent among phagocytic cells like macrophages. Another example are glycoproteins with terminal sialic acid residues, which circulate within the bloodstream conducting their various functions. If the terminal sialic acid residue is removed exposing the penultimate galactose, that glycoprotein will be removed from the circulation by hepatocytes.

Endocytosis

All cells must internalize substances from their environment that are required for the cell's survival. Several different methods of internalization are used. Lipid-soluble substances such as oxygen enter the cell by simply diffusing across the plasmalemma. Various ions are partitioned across the plasmalemma through specific channels driven either by differences in ion concentrations across the plasmalemma or by ion pumps such as sodium-ATPase which pumps sodium outside of the cell. Additionally, *endocytosis* is a fundamental mechanism utilizing various morphologic entities visible with the electron microscope. Endocytosis includes **phagocytosis, pinocytosis,** and **receptor-mediated endocytosis.** Phagocytosis is the entrapment of particles, pinocytosis is the incorporation of bulk

fluid, and receptor-mediated endocytosis is the incorporation of specific molecules in high concentration relative to other inadvertently incorporated solutes. All three processes involve specializations of the plasmalemma.

During phagocytosis, an evagination of the plasmalemma surrounds the particle equally on all sides until it completely engulfs it. The particle becomes completely enclosed in an intracellular vesicle as that portion of the plasmalemma pinches off from the rest of the uninvolved plasmalemma to become fully internalized. The particle and its investing membrane derived from the plasmalemma is referred to as a phagosome.

During pinocytosis (sometimes referred to as macropinocytosis), a small volume of extracellular fluid is trapped by a ruffle of the plasmalemma in a wavelike fashion. The fluid becomes internalized in a vesicle as that portion of the plasmalemma pinches off from the rest of the uninvolved plasmalemma. The fluid plus its surrounding membrane derived from the plasmalemma is referred to as a pinosome.

Both of the above methods of incorporation are believed to be relatively unspecific processes. However, receptor-mediated endocytosis is a specific mechanism that incorporates high concentrations of a particular substance to the relative exclusion of other substances. This mechanism incorporates several hormones such as insulin, various serum components such as transferrin, low-density lipoproteins, mannose-terminated and galactose-terminated glycoproteins, and undesirable entities such as viruses, which also use the mechanism to enter cells. The selectivity of receptor-mediated endocytosis depends on the prior insertion of specific receptor molecules into the plasmalemma. Although the receptor molecule is anchored in the plasmalemma, the receptor portion projects onto the extracellular surface of the plasmalemma where it can bind to a particular ligand such as insulin. Originally the membrane receptor is distributed diffusely throughout the plane of the plasmalemma, but as the receptors become occupied by ligand they are sequestered into highly concentrated areas of the plasmalemma. These areas of the plasmalemma become slightly indented forming coated pits.

Coated pits are identified in the electron microscope by the scaffolding attached to the cytoplasmic surface of the plasmalemma where the pit is forming (Fig. 2-24A). As the pit invaginates further, the receptor-occupied surface of the plasmalemma becomes the internal surface of the coated vesicle which apparently retains its connection to the plasmalemma by a narrow neck of membrane (Figs. 2-24A and 2-25). Within freeze-fractured cells viewed with the electron mi-

croscope, this scaffolding around the pit and vesicle appears as a lattice of hexagons and occasional five-sided and seven-sided polygons (Fig. 2-24B). The coat that invests the vesicle and pit consists of a protein called **clathrin.** Its function has not been clarified but it appears to be involved in formation of the coated pit and coated vesicle.

Shortly after formation of the coated vesicle, the receptor and attached ligand appears in a smooth-surfaced vesicle of larger diameter called the **receptosome** or **endosome.** The interior of the endosome is rapidly acidified by ATP-dependent proton pumps which lower the pH of the endosome interior. In most instances the acidic pH causes uncoupling or dissociation of the ligand from its receptor. Although the endosome is acidic it does not contain any of the hydrolytic enzymes produced in the lysosome unless they are ligands being taken up from the exterior environment by receptor-mediated endocytosis also. The endosome may become larger by fusing with other endosomes. The endosome is shuttled along a track of microtubules to a pre-

Fig. 2-24. A. Various stages of endocytosis. The arrows indicate coated pits which are forming prior to the formation of coated vesicles. The coat or basket formed by clathrin is not conspicuous in this photo. B. However, when baskets or scaffolding surrounding coated vesicles are isolated and viewed with the electron microscope, the polygonal baskets are conspicuous, as shown here. (Figure 2-24B produced by Dr. John E. Heuser of Washington University School of Medicine, St. Louis, Missouri. From *J. Cell Biology* 84:560, 1980. Reproduced by copyright permission of The Rockefeller University Press.)

A

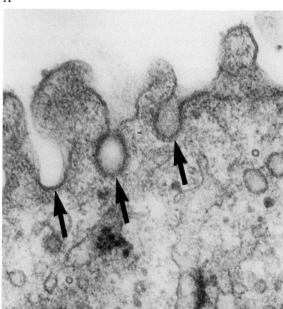

B

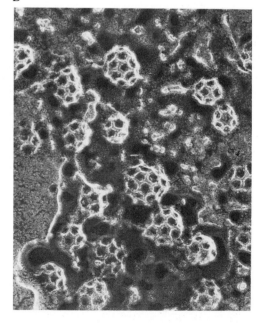

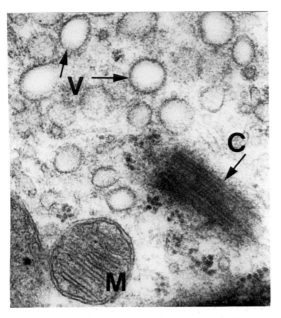

Fig. 2-25. Electron micrograph of coated vesicles (*V*), a mitochondrion (*M*), and a centriole (*C*) sectioned along its long axis.

lysosomal compartment believed to be either a specific portion of the endoplasmic reticulum or the trans-Golgi tubules.

The prelysosomal compartment apparently recognizes and distinguishes ligand from receptor and sorts them to different destinations. The ligand is first found within a coated pit on the Golgi which then becomes a coated vesicle shuttling the ligand to fuse with the lysosome where it is degraded. The receptor is sent back to the plasmalemma probably in the membrane of a smooth vesicle which pinches off from the Golgi and fuses with the plasmalemma, thereby escaping lysosomal degradation. This recycling of the receptor is economical but there are instances when the receptor is also shuttled to the lysosome and degraded. In addition, there are a few ligands which are recycled back to the plasmalemma without lysosomal degradation. An example is transferrin.

It should also be appreciated that extensive amounts of membrane are exchanging places within the active cell and, if membrane were not recycled, there would be considerable accumulation at certain sites. This is known as **membrane flow.** Consequently, the net flow of membrane is balanced between the amount of Golgi membrane lost in the formation of secretory vesicles that become incorporated into the plasmalemma during exocytosis and the amount of membrane received by the Golgi apparatus either directly as an endocytic vesicle returning from the plasmalemma or indirectly after the endocytic vesicle first fuses with the lysosome. The Golgi apparatus also receives membrane from the transitional vesicles that arrive from the RER.

Cytoskeleton

If it were not for an internal cytoplasmic support system called the **cytoskeleton,** cells would be unable to maintain control of their shape. The cytoskeleton consists of several classes of structural elements: **microtubules, thick filaments, intermediate filaments,** and **microfilaments.** Although none of these structures can be resolved by the light microscope unless they are present in thick aggregates or bundles, their influence on cell shape is often strikingly evident.

Microtubules are slim, hollow tubes involved in several aspects of cell motility, including (1) changes in cell shape and (2) the movement of organelles throughout the cytoplasm. Perhaps the most striking effect of microtubules that is visible with the light microscope is their control over precise movements of chromosomes during cell division (**mitosis**). Microtubules have also been implicated in the movement of secretory vesicles to the plasmalemma prior to exocytosis, since microtubule-binding drugs interfere with cell secretion. Accumulating evidence indicates that microtubules are involved in maintaining the precise location and distribution of membrane molecules within the plasmalemma, probably through some interaction with other elements of the cytoskeleton.

In electron micrographs, microtubules are about 25 nm in diameter with a wall 5 nm thick surrounding a lumen 15 nm in diameter (Fig. 2-26). They vary in length up to several microns and extend to all regions of the cytoplasm (Figs. 2-27, 2-28).

All microtubules are composed of tubulin, a glubular protein that is associated in pairs or dimers. The dimers are organized into a helix of protofilaments, 13 of which form the wall of the microtubule. Microtubules are very labile structures that can change length by polymerization and depolymerization. Their depolymerization is triggered by elevated concentrations of cytoplasmic calcium. This ability to change length is ultimately responsible for their role in movement of cytoplasmic organelles. However, they act in conjunction with other elements of the cytoskeleton in ways that remain to be clarified.

Fig. 2-26. Electron micrograph of cell process containing many microtubules (*arrows*).

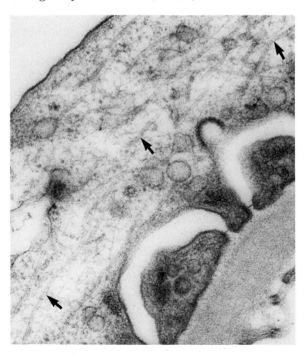

Microtubules are also the multiple constituents of other organelles, including the **centriole, basal body, cilia,** and **flagella.** The centriole is a short blind-ended cylindrical structure composed of nine sets of three microtubules each (Fig. 2-29). Centrioles are about 150 nm in diameter and 300 to 500 nm long (see Fig. 2-25). They occur in pairs (called **centrosomes** or **diplosomes**) with their long axes oriented at 90 degrees with respect to each other. When cross-sectioned, the profiles of nine sets of triplet microtubules are visible (see Fig. 2-29). Such a view reveals that each triplet of microtubules consists of one whole microtubule (the innermost of each set) and two that are incomplete to the extent that they share part of the wall of the adjacent tubule. The nine sets of triplets are aligned at 30 degrees to one another. The centrosome and poorly characterized material surrounding it represent a microtubule organizing center (MOC). In the interphase cell (one of the stages of a cell between cell divisions) the majority of cytoplasmic microtubules have grown out from this MOC. The Golgi apparatus is often located very near the centrosome. Since this tendency to be located as neighbors within the cell is lost after microtubules have been artificially disrupted by researchers, it is believed that microtubules govern the location of the Golgi apparatus within the cell. The participation of the centriole in cell division is described in a following section.

In addition to their role in cell division, centrioles proliferate to form structurally identical **basal bodies,** the nucleation sites for the microtubules located within the core of cilia. Cilia are fingerlike projections from the apical cell surface that beat in coordinated fashion to move a film of fluid along the surfaces of certain epithelial cells. The formation of cilia begins when basal bodies are replicated in large numbers from centrioles in the nondividing cell. These newly formed basal bodies migrate to the apical surface and become deployed at the origin or base of each presumptive cilium, where they initiate the polymerization of microtubules. The microtubules grow into the core of each cilium and form the

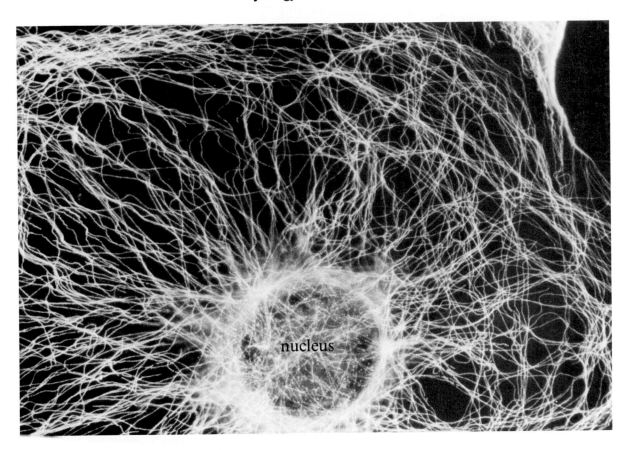

nucleus

Fig. 2-27. Fluorescence micrograph of mouse fibroblast reacted with a fluorescein-tagged antibody against tubulin to demonstrate the elaborate distribution of microtubules within the cell. Note how the microtubules converge upon the nucleus. (From M. Osborn and K. Weber, The display of microtubules in transformed cells. *Cell* 12:561, 1977. Copyright M.I.T.)

ciliary shaft or **axoneme.** The axoneme consists of nine pairs of microtubules or doublets organized around a central pair of single microtubules (see Fig. 3-11 in Chap. 3). The doublet microtubules grow out from the inner two microtubules of each triplet of the basal body. The third or outermost microtubule of each triplet does not contribute a microtubule to the axoneme nor do the central microtubules. The A subfiber of each doublet is attached by a radial spoke to the central pair of single microtubules; it also has two short arms, which project tangentially away from itself toward the adjacent doublet. These arms are composed of dynein. Dynein possesses ATPase activity. The hydrolysis of ATP by dynein produces a beating motion of the cilia. This is known as mechanochemical coupling. During hydrolysis of ATP the microtubules composing the cilia are displaced relative to one another. This displacement is generated by transient cross-bridges that form between the dynein arms of each A subfiber and the B subfiber microtubules. This produces a stiff bending motion in the cilia that moves a film of mucus along the

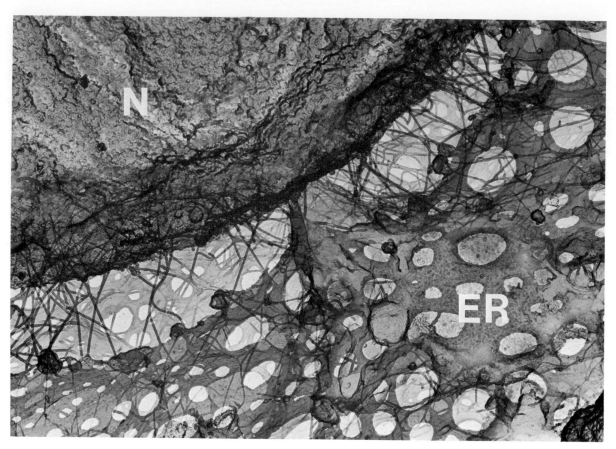

Fig. 2-28. Perinuclear region of the cytoplasm of a cell that has been rotary shadowed with carbon and platinum. The nucleus (*N*) fills most of upper field. Many cytoplasmic filaments appear to pierce the nuclear envelope and also encase much of the nucleus. Observe the continuity of the endoplasmic reticulum (*ER*) with the nuclear envelope. (Courtesy of Bruce Batten.)

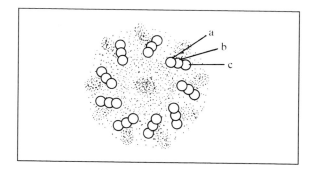

Fig. 2-29. Cross section of a centriole, showing nine sets of triplet microtubules. The innermost microtubule of each triplet is designated *subfiber a*. Subfibers *b* and *c* are incomplete and share walls along their innermost aspects.

surface of the cell in one direction. The recoil beat is a limp one that does not interfere with the unidirectional movement of mucus. For further structural-functional details on cilia and flagella, see Chapter 3.

A similar microtubule assembly called a flagellum exists in the tail of the spermatozoa, conferring the ability to swim. It will be described in the chapter dealing with the male reproductive system (Chap. 18).

The other elements of the cytoskeleton are filamentous. Thick filaments, 15 nm thick, consist of **myosin,** one of the principal proteins involved in muscle contraction. Microfilaments are 6 nm thick and consist of **actin,** the other principle protein involved in muscle contraction. However, both these protein filaments also exist in noncontractile cells, where they have been implicated in intracellular exertion of force for maintenance of cell shape and movement of membrane proteins within the plasmalemma. The exact mechanism is still poorly understood. The details of myosin-actin interaction will be more completely described in the discussion of muscle tissue, in which their actions are more completely known (Chap. 7). However, the general mechanism of myosin-actin interaction in muscle cells is referred to as the sliding filament mechanism. Cross-bridges of myosin filaments possess intrinsic ATPase activity and can bind to the actin filament. The energy derived from hydrolysis of ATP allows the myosin cross-bridges to move the actin filament relative to the myosin filament. This is another example of mechanochemical coupling similar to the interaction of dynein-tubulin in the microtubules of cilia. It is unclear to what extent this contractile mechanism of muscle cells operates in noncontractile cells. However, it is known that unlike muscle cells, where myosin is the more abundant contractile protein, nonmuscle cells contain relatively small amounts of myosin compared to actin.

Bundles of actin filaments are particularly abundant just beneath the plasmalemma of many nonmuscle cells, where they are responsible for maintaining or changing cell shape (Figs. 2-30, 2-31). For instance, actin filaments form a

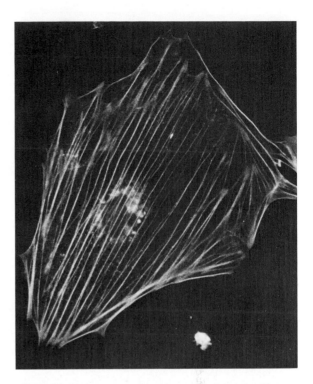

Fig. 2-30. Rat ovarian granulosa cell stained with fluorescent NBD-phallicidin, which binds specifically to filamentous actin. The actin filaments are the bright lines extending across the cell. There is also some diffuse fluorescence associated with the nucleus. It is obvious from the taut appearance of these filaments why they are referred to as *stress filaments*. (Courtesy of David Albertini.)

three-dimensional network within the pseudopod, a projection of cytoplasm involved in ameboid locomotion displayed by certain mammalian cells such as the white blood cell. They are also abundant in cytoplasmic areas involved in phagocytosis. Another change in cell shape involving actin filaments is cytokinesis, the final stage in cell division when a constriction develops in the cytoplasm called a cleavage furrow, which separates a dividing cell into two daughter cells (see Fig. 2-36).

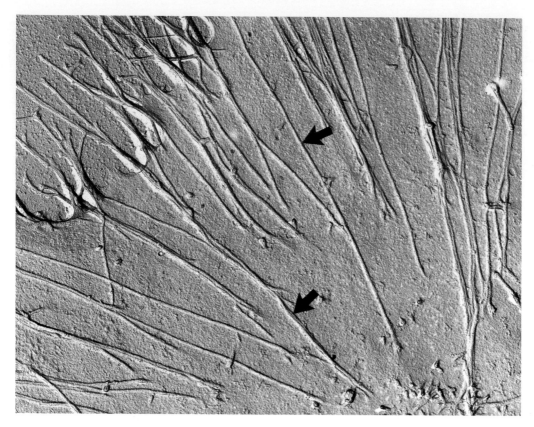

Fig. 2-31. Surface replica of fibroblast in culture dish. The stress fibers are the linear elements radiating throughout the cytoplasm (*arrows*). The stress fibers look like raised elements because the cell has shrunk down upon them as a result of dehydration associated with making a replica of the cell surface. (Courtesy of Joan Borysenko.)

Actin filaments also form the structural core of the microvilli. Microvilli are multiple, fingerlike projections of the plasmalemma that increase the surface area of the plasmalemma of certain epithelial cells for absorption. The actin filaments are anchored to the plasmalemma in the tips of the microvilli. From here actin filaments extend through the core of the microvilli into a transverse array of filaments located at the base of the microvilli and called the **terminal web.** Within the terminal web actin filaments become associated with myosin. These two contractile proteins are probably responsible for the movement of microvilli observed along the brush border in the small intestine. However, most of the terminal web is constructed of intermediate filaments which are anchored in the zonula adherens of the lateral plasmalemma. Microvilli are described in more detail in the chapter concerned with epithelium (Chap. 3).

Besides actin, another important microfilament is **spectrin,** which was first discovered in the red blood cell. However, structurally and functionally similar protein filaments have been discovered in many other cell types also. In the red blood cell, spectrin is responsible for linking actin to a membrane protein called **ankyrin** located in the red cell plasmalemma. Thus, spectrin is the basis for actin's influence on the topology of the red cell's surface membrane and on the distribution of membrane proteins within the cell's plasmalemma. Since spectrin also has affinity for microtubules, continuing research seeks to understand the complex interrelationships of these various filaments in the function of the cell's plasmalemma. It is not known at this point whether spectrin is associated with actin in all of actin's membrane-associated functions.

Intermediate filaments (8–10 nm thick) are a biochemically diverse class of filaments intermediate in size between myosin (thick filaments) and microfilaments. Unlike the contractile functions performed by actin and myosin, intermediate filaments appear to be purely structural elements. They are organized into five distinct classes: (1) **tonofilaments (keratan filaments)** found in epithelial cells; (2) **desmin filaments,** found primarily in muscle cells; (3) **vimentin filaments,** found in mesenchymal cells or mesenchymally derived cells, (4) **neurofilaments,** found in nerve cells; and (5) **glial filaments,** found in the glial cells, the supporting cells of nerve cells. Commonly, two of these filaments will be located in the same cell type. These filaments are discussed in more detail in appropriate chapters dealing with cells in which they are located. However, their common function is to provide three-dimensional support within the cell.

THE NUCLEUS

The nucleus is visibly the most prominent structure within the cell. It is usually an ovoid structure with an affinity for basic dyes because it contains DNA. The nucleus within every cell of an organism contains the same genetic information coded within its DNA. Only part of that information is expressed in any cell, determining that cell's structural and functional identity. The portion of genetic information expressed in any cell depends on a complex series of events, which allows only certain segments of the genetic code to be transcribed from DNA into messenger ribonu-

cleic acid (mRNA). Through the variable expression of the cell's genes, the nucleus initiates and coordinates cytoplasmic activities. It accomplishes this task not only by transcribing mRNA from its DNA, but also by producing ribosomal RNA (rRNA) and transfer RNA (tRNA), the two forms of RNA involved in the translation of mRNA into proteins within the cytoplasm.

With the resolution of electron microscopy, the nucleus is seen to consist of **chromatin** and a **nucleolus;** it is circumscribed by a double membrane called the nuclear envelope, which segregates it from the cytoplasm (Fig. 2-32, see also Fig. 2-15, 2-16).

Chromatin

Chromatin consists of strands of DNA and its associated proteins. These strands are about 20 nm in diameter and occupy the entire nucleus including the interstices of the nucleolus. Chromatin occurs in either a condensed or an extended state, depending on the prevailing rate of transcription occurring in the nucleus. Extended chromatin represents the form that DNA and its associated proteins assume when actively transcribing genetic information into mRNA. Condensed chromatin represents the form that DNA and its associated proteins assume when the rate of transcription is suppressed. The nucleus of any cell usually displays variable amounts of both extended and condensed forms of chromatin. The preponderance of one form over the other provides a rough index of the rate of transcription occurring in that nucleus. The histologic terms for these two appearances of chromatin in section are **euchromatin** (extended chromatin) and **heterochromatin** (condensed chromatin). Since euchromatin does not stain well, its location within the nucleus is apparent only as poorly stained regions between heterochromatin. Heterochromatin is stained conspicuously with basic dyes, which have high affinity for the many negatively charged phosphate groups along the DNA molecule. Heterochromatin usually involves only a segment of any particular **chromosome,** indicating that genetic

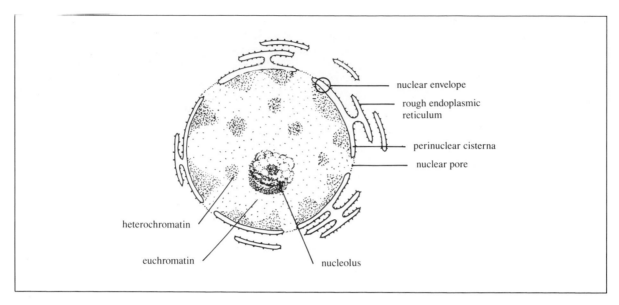

Fig. 2-32. The nucleus and the relationship of its nuclear envelope to the rough endoplasmic reticulum.

expression of the cistrons of DNA located there is suppressed. However, heterochromatin may also involve an entire maternal or paternal chromosome. For example, in the somatic cells of females, one of the two X chromosomes (sex chromatin) is inactivated during ontogenesis. This X chromosome is visible as a convex clump of heterochromatin (Barr body) usually situated against the nuclear envelope but occasionally visible as a small rounded appendage of the nucleolus as in nerve cells. Ninety percent of female somatic cells have Barr bodies; ten percent of male somatic cells contain them. In general, most heterochromatin is located at two sites, adhering either to the nuclear envelope or to the nucleolus (Fig. 2-33; see also Fig. 2-15, 2-16).

In dying cells, the nucleus consists predominantly of heterochromatin, which reflects that cell's diminished ability to express any portion of its genome. The nuclei of dead cells are usually shrunken and completely heterochromatic. Such nuclei are referred to as **pyknotic.**

In healthy cells, heterochromatin is densest during cell division, when the chromatin condenses into the individual **chromosomes** observable with the light microscope. In fact, these chromosomes can be isolated from dividing cells and identified according to their various sizes and lengths. This procedure is called **karyotyping** and provides a simple method for detecting some of the more obvious chromosomal abnormalities, such as deformed chromosomes or inappropriate numbers of chromosomes.

There are two copies of each chromosome in every somatic cell, since the maternal and paternal germ cells each contribute 23 chromosomes to the zygote from which all somatic cells are derived (Fig. 2-34). **Haploid** refers to the 23 chromosomes contributed by each germ cell. Consequently, every somatic cell contains twice that number or 23 pairs of homologous chromosomes. **Diploid** refers to the fact that there are 23 pairs of chromosomes present in each somatic cell. Sometimes a cell may have more than the normal diploid complement of chromosomes. When this excess number is a multiple of the

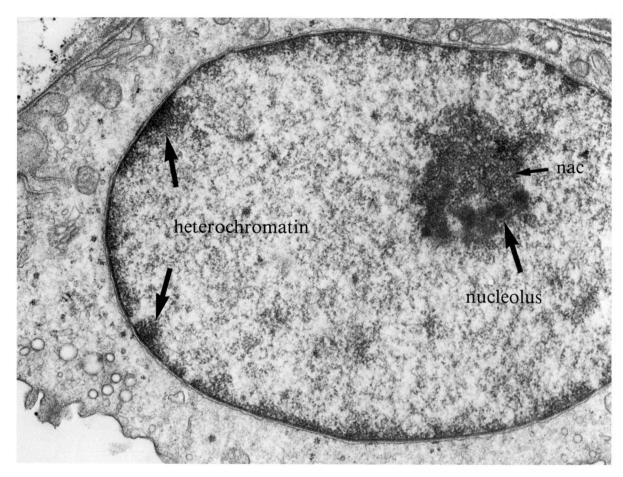

Fig. 2-33. A low power electron micrograph of the nucleus showing the densely stained heterochromatin condensed against the inner membrane of the nuclear envelope. A portion of the nucleolus is also present with its nucleolar associated chromatin (*nac*).

haploid number of chromosomes, it is referred to as polyploid. Occasionally, even normal cells are polyploid. Cells whose nuclei contain a number of chromosomes that are not an exact multiple of the haploid number of 23 are termed aneuploid. Malignant cells often contain aneuploid nuclei.

Certain congenital abnormalities have been correlated with a particular aberrant karyotype.

For example, Down's syndrome (mongolism) is the result of trisomy, in which three copies of chromosome number 21 are present in the cell instead of the usual diploid complement of two. The recent advent of amniocentesis, a procedure in which amniotic fluid is aspirated from the amnion through a needle, has allowed recovery of suspended embryonic cells that can be cultured so that karyotypes can be prepared and examined for diagnosis before birth.

Nucleolus

The nucleolus is a nonmembranous, intranuclear organelle responsible for the synthesis of ribosomal RNA (rRNA) and ultimately the bio-

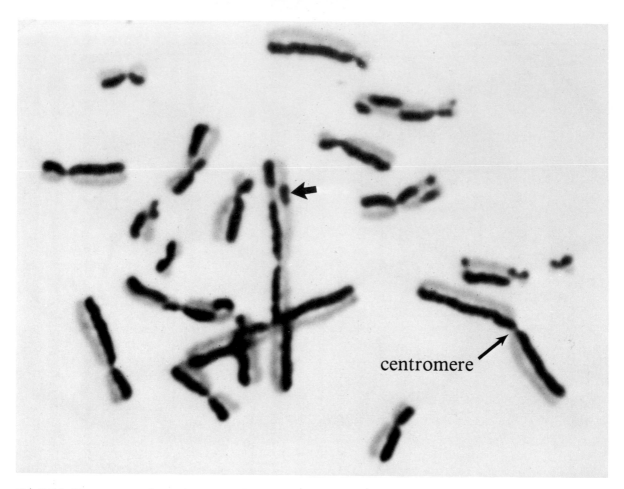

centromere

Fig. 2-34. Chromosomes from a hamster ovary cell stained by the fluorescent-plus Giemsa technique to display sister chromatids. The cell was arrested in metaphase after undergoing two rounds of DNA synthesis in the presence of the base analogue 5-bromodeoxyuridine (BrUrd). The chromatid that incorporated BrUrd into both its DNA strands is less condensed and stains weaker with Giemsa than its sister chromatid, which incorporated BrUrd into only one strand of DNA. The contrast in staining of paired sister chromatids is striking and makes areas of chromatid exchange easily identifiable (*arrow*). This exchange does not normally occur during mitosis. (From S. Wolff and P. Perry, Differential Giemsa staining of sister chromatids and the study of sister chromatid exchanges without autoradiography. *Chromosoma* 48:341, 1974.)

genesis of ribosomes. With the light microscope most cells have one or more nucleoli. They are ovoid in shape and stain with basic dyes because of their high content of RNA. A patch of heterochromatin is closely applied to the perimeter of the nucleolus as the nucleolar-associated chromatin (see Fig. 2-33). Generally, the size of the nucleolus reflects the level of rRNA synthesis occurring in that cell and, indirectly, the level of protein synthesis since proteins are subsequently translated from mRNA by ribosomes in the cytoplasm. Therefore some cells have conspicuous nucleoli, while the nucleoli in other cells are inconspicuous. Consequently, cells with large well-developed nucleoli often have abundant ribosomes (free or attached to RER) in their cytoplasm. In the light microscope cells with large nucleoli have cytoplasm loaded with areas of basophilia representing rRNA.

With the electron microscope nucleoli can be resolved into two distinct components: a fibrillar component called the **nucleolonema,** and a granular component called the **pars granulosa.** In the active interphase nucleus, the fibrillar component represents about 15 percent of the nucleolus by volume; the granular component represents about 75 percent of the nucleolus. The fibrillar component corresponds to transcribed ribosomal chromatin; the granular component represents preribosomes at different stages of maturation as well as some ribosomes.

The genes for rRNA are found in at least one or more loci on each chromosome called **nucleolus organizers.** During mitosis the nucleolus organizers (containing the rRNA genes active in the nucleolus of the previous interphase nucleus) are seen as secondary constrictions in the chromosomes. (The centromere is the primary constriction.) These nucleolar organizers form nucleoli during the telophase stage of mitosis. In other words, the nucleolus is transcribed from rRNA genes (rDNA repeating units) contributed by each chromosome. The fibrillar component is the first distinctive structure formed and it remains continuous with the nucleolus organizer. The granular components appear next. They are the preribosomes transcribed from genes in the nucleolus organizer. This transcription of rRNA genes is the initial step in ribosomal biogenesis. These preribosomes will undergo various modifications collectively referred to as **maturation.** Most of this maturation of preribosomes into the large and small ribosomal particles occurs in the nucleolus. Subsequently the ribosomes are transported to the cytoplasm.

The ratio of fibrillar to granular elements constituting the nucleolus informs the microscopist about the activity of the cell. If transcription of rRNA genes was suspended long enough for existing transcripts of rRNA to mature and enter the cytoplasm, the granular components of the nucleolus would disappear. The morphologic ap-

pearance and size of the nucleolus is an index of the cell's health and activity.

The nucleolonema consists of densely packed filaments. These filaments are composed of ribonucleoprotein and are considered to contain the 45S rRNA synthesized from nucleolar DNA cistrons. These strands may subsequently undergo a series of cleavages into smaller molecules that are coupled to protein, some of which may form the granular elements of the pars granulosa. An 18S fragment of the original 45S rRNA is coupled to protein and passes quickly to the cytoplasm for incorporation into the smaller ribosomal subunit.

The granularity of the pars granulosa is attributed to the presence of ribonucleoprotein particles containing the 32S rRNA. This 32S rRNA is cleaved to the 28S rRNA fragment, which becomes incorporated into the larger ribosomal subunit.

The interface between the fibrillar and granular components of the nucleolus is not always distinct. In addition, some extended intranucleolar chromatin is interspersed among the fibrillar elements.

The nucleoli disperse during cell division and reform in the reconstituting nuclei of the daughter cells. The nucleoli reform at areas of chromosomes called **nucleolus organizing centers.** The DNA contained within the chromatin of the nucleolar organizers of each chromosome that codes for rRNA is the only permanent component of the nucleolus. Near the end of mitosis, the nucleolonema is reconstructed around nucleolar organizing chromatin. Following this, the pars granulosa appears.

Nuclear Envelope

The nucleus is enclosed and separated from the cytoplasm by a nuclear envelope. The nuclear envelope has three structural components: the **inner** and **outer nuclear membranes,** the **nuclear pore complexes,** and the **nuclear lamina.** The envelope consists of two 7.5-nm membranes separated by a narrow space called the **perinuclear cistern** (see Figs. 2-15, 2-16, 2-32). The outer membrane is continuous with the RER and frequently has ribosomes attached to its cytoplasmic surface. The inner surface of the inner membrane has no associated ribosomes but is characteristically adorned by clumps of heterochromatin. The inner and outer membranes are interrupted at the nuclear pores where active and passive nucleocytoplasmic exchange occurs. The pore is an octagonal structure with an estimated effective 90-Å-diameter annulus. The pore complex consists of two rings of eight globular subunits, one ring on the nuclear side of the pore and the other ring on the cytoplasmic side. The center of the pore contains a central granule apparently attached by spokes to the outer ring of globular subunits. Ions and small molecules can pass through the pore passively, but mRNA, tRNA, ribosomal subunits, and large proteins are transported by active transport into the cytoplasm.

The nuclear lamina is a mesh of intermediate filaments consisting of lamin B which form an orthogonal network of intersecting filaments attached to the nucleoplasmic side of the inner nuclear membrane. The nuclear lamina assists in the reorganization of the nuclear envelope during telophase of mitosis, serves as an anchoring site for interphase chromosomes, and is also attached to the nuclear pores.

CYTOPLASMIC INCLUSIONS

Unlike organelles, inclusions are variably present within cells. They may occur only in specific cell types or only in association with a particular stage of functional activity. Examples of cytoplasmic inclusions are pigment, lipid, and glycogen.

Pigment

MELANIN

Melanocytes and certain other cells—such as those in the iris of the eye, others in the basal layers of the epidermis, and a specialized layer of cells in the eye (pigment epithelium)—contain membrane-bounded granules of black melanin pigment. The pigment is contained within membrane-limited granules called **melanosomes,** and the number of these melanosomes present in cells from various locations determines skin, hair, and eye color. Melanin also shields the body from overexposure to UV light.

LIPOFUSCIN

Lipofuscin pigment has already been described in conjunction with lysosomes. This golden-brown pigment is an end product of lysosomal activity that accumulates in cells as they age. It is, therefore, particularly evident in postmitotic cells (those that do not undergo mitosis in the adult), such as cardiac muscle and neutrons. Such lipofuscin is derived from lysosomes, it too is membrane-bounded.

HEMOSIDERIN

Hemoglobin from aged red blood cells that have been filtered out of the circulation and destroyed by phagocytosis is degraded to a golden-brown pigment called **hemosiderin,** which is rich in iron. It can be distinguished from lipofuscin in the light microscope. Hemosiderin is easily distinguished in the electron microscope by the presence of 9-nm dense particles that are formed by polymerization of nonferritin micellar iron with protein. This pigment normally occurs in phagocytes of the bone marrow, spleen, and liver in the free (unbounded) state.

Lipid

Oil droplets within the cytoplasm of cells serve as energy stores and sources of lipid for turnover of membrane. Unless specially preserved and stained, lipid droplets are dissolved away in the organic solvents used for tissue processing, and they appear as round holes under the light microscope. Fat cells, in which the cytoplasm is occupied chiefly by one enormous lipid droplet, appear entirely empty. In the electron microscope lipid droplets are often preserved by osmium and appear black and spherical. They are not membrane-bounded.

Glycogen

Glycogen is a polymer of glucose that is present in the cytoplasm of a wide range of cell types as a storage form of carbohydrate. Unless specifically preserved and stained, glycogen will dissolve out when a section is prepared for the light microscope, leaving ragged, irregular spaces. It can be demonstrated with a histochemical reaction known as the **periodic acid–Schiff (PAS) reaction,** which will stain it crimson. Glycogen appears in the electron microscope as free, dense, irregular particles 15 to 30 nm in diameter. Isolated particles are called **α particles,** and large aggregates of these particles in the form of rosettes are called **β particles.**

CELL DIVISION (MITOSIS)

Mitosis refers to the mechanism by which somatic cells divide and distribute nuclear and cytoplasmic material to their daughter cells. A variation of cell division involving the germ cells (oocytes and spermatocytes), referred to as **meiosis,** is described in the discussion of the male reproductive system (Chap. 18). Somatic cells include the fertilized ovum and all the cells that result from its subsequent divisions. Mitosis is required to supply adequate numbers of cells during embryonic development and future growth and to maintain cell populations by replacing injured or dead cells.

The longevity of different cell types varies widely. For example, some cells, like those lining the stomach and intestines, have a lifetime of only 3 to 5 days, and a high rate of mitosis is required to replace the cells that die. Most cells are capable of replenishing their number by mitosis and are referred to as **renewing cell populations.** At the other end of the scale are **postmitotic cells,** such as nerve cells and cardiac muscle cells. These cells are no longer capable of mitosis once their adult populations are established by mitosis of precursor cells. Adult nerve and cardiac muscle cells lost through attrition are never replaced through mitosis; their populations diminish with advancing age.

When a cell is not dividing, it exhibits relatively predictable activities that alternate with mitosis. These repetitive cellular activities alternating with mitosis occur during **interphase,** the stage between mitotic divisions. Three stages of cellular activity occur during interphase and together with mitosis constitute the cell cycle (Fig. 2-35):

M   Mitosis or cell division producing daughter cells.

G_1 First gap, the interval between mitosis and DNA synthesis when the daughter cells synthesize protein and other molecules and grow in size.

S   Period of DNA synthesis when one or both daughter cells duplicate the DNA in preparation for mitosis of the next cycle.

G_2 Second gap, the interval between DNA synthesis and the onset of mitosis. During this short stage a few proteins that participate in cell division of the next cell cycle will be synthesized.

Fig. 2-35. The cell cycle.

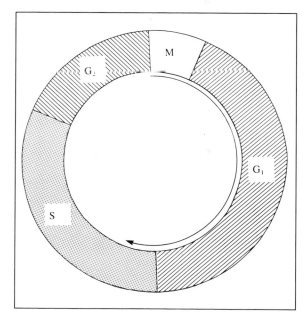

The length of time that different cell types spend in each phase of the cell cycle varies considerably. Cells that do not divide frequently spend most of their time in G_1 while rapidly dividing malignant cells exhibit a G_1 stage of short duration.

The normal somatic cell in G_1 contains 23 pairs of homologous chromosomes—namely, one chromosome of each pair contributed by the maternal germ cell (oocyte) and the other chromosome of each pair contributed by the paternal germ cell (spermatozoa). Twenty-two pairs are somatic chromosomes and one pair is the sex chromosome. During the S phase of the cell cycle, the number of chromosomes is replicated, resulting in 23 pairs but now consisting of two chromatids each. Longitudinal splitting of each chromosome occurs during the S and G_2 phases but is not visibly apparent until early stages of mitosis. The two chromatids remain attached to each other at the centromere but entirely detach and separate from each other during a later stage of mitosis. During the G_2 phase of the cell cycle, the centrioles replicate themselves, each serving as a template for assembly of another at right angles to itself, producing two pairs.

Four consecutive stages occur during mitosis that are easily recognizable with the light microscope: **prophase, metaphase, anaphase,** and **telophase** (Fig. 2-36).

Prophase

Prophase begins as the two pairs of centrioles separate from each other and migrate to opposite poles of the cell. The mechanism believed to be responsible for pushing these centrioles apart is the polymerization of microtubules between centrioles. A small area on one side of each centriole serves as a **microtubule organizing center** from which the lengthening microtubules are assembled. Since these microtubules are connected to the microtubule organizing centers of both centrioles, the increasing length of microtubules pushes the centrioles apart. These are usually called **continuous microtubules** or **interpolar microtubules.** Continuous microtubules plus chromosomal microtubules form the **mitotic spindle,** which can be observed in phase contrast microscopy. A less conspicuous array of microtubules, the **astral rays,** fans out from each centriole pair and connects the centriole to the plasmalemma at their respective cell poles. Gradually the nuclear membrane breaks down; the nucleus and nucleolus disappear as cytologically distinct structures since their chromatin begins to condense into threadlike structures corresponding to the 46 pairs of chromosomes (see Fig. 2-36).

Metaphase

During metaphase the condensation of these threadlike chromosomes continues until they become shorter and denser and occupy a central plane in the cell, transverse to the long axis of the mitotic spindle. These metaphase chromosomes can be isolated by experimental methods and scrutinized more closely. Each of the 46 chromosome pairs appear as two dense lengths, each a homologous chromosome (**chromatid**) attached to the other at one point called the **centromere** (see Fig. 2-34). With the electron microscope the centromere has two small disk-shaped areas known as **kinetochores.** Kinetochores are microtubule organizing centers from which **chromosomal microtubules** are assembled. The fully assembled chromosomal microtubules connect the kinetochores of each pair of chromatids to centrioles in opposite poles of the cell. Although the mechanism is not clear, the centromeres of all 46 pairs of chromatids line up within the equatorial plane of the cell. Pairs of chromatids remain attached at their centromeres but are separated throughout the rest of their length and oriented toward opposite poles of the cell. This distinctive configuration characterizes the cell in metaphase (Figs. 2-36, 2-37, 2-38).

Anaphase

Anaphase begins as the centromeres joining paired chromatids divide to produce 92 individual chromatids (chromosomes). Beginning im-

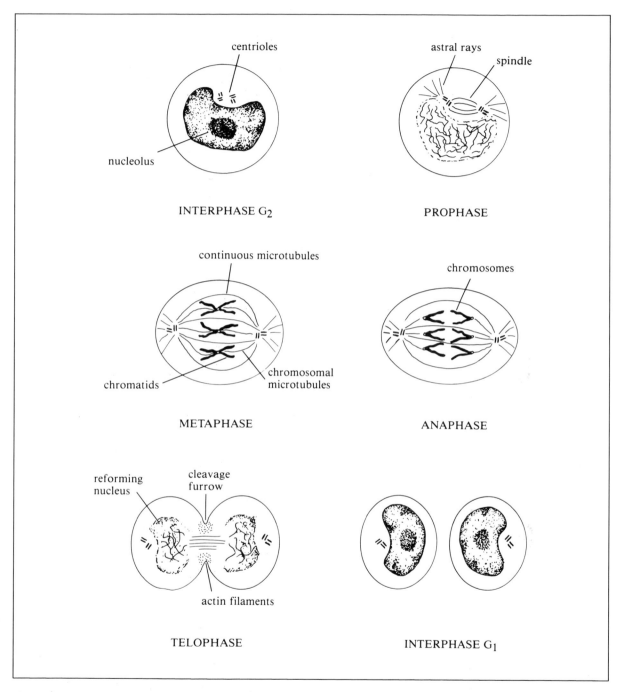

Fig. 2-36. Sequential stages in mitosis: interphase
G_2; prophase; metaphase; anaphase; telophase; and
interphase G_1.

Fig. 2-37. Two fish gastrula cells during the meta-phase stage of mitosis. The chromosomes are lined up within the equatorial plane of the cells (C). The astral rays are visible at both poles of the cell (AR). The chromosomal microtubules linking the chromosomes to the centrioles within the astral rays are visible as the mitotic spindle. (MS).

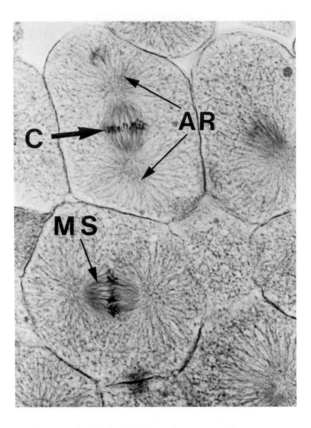

Fig. 2-38. Isolated mitotic spindle in metaphase from a dividing sea urchin embryo viewed with polarized light (right) and differential interference contrast (left) microscopy. A = astral ray; S = mitotic spindle consisting of interpolar and chromosomal micro-tubules; C = chromosomes. (From E. D. Salmon and R. R. Segall, Calcium-labile mitotic spindles isolated from sea urchin eggs [Lytechinus variegatus]. *J. Cell Biol.* 86:355, 1980. Reproduced by copyright permission of The Rockefeller University Press.)

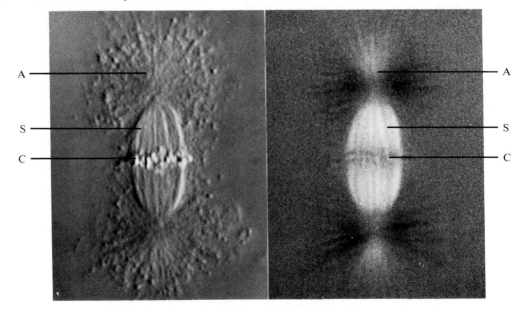

mediately but proceeding at a slow pace, 46 chromosomes move toward one pole of the cell and 46 move toward the other pole (see Figs. 2-36, 2-39). The precise mechanism for segregating chromosomes into opposite poles of the cell remains to be established. However, it appears that anaphase chromosome movement is affected by a net disassembly of the chromosomal microtubules and a net lengthening of the continuous microtubules. During anaphase, daughter chromosomes move to opposite poles of the cell along stationary microtubules (kinetochore microtubules) which shorten by depolymerization at the kinetochore. Since chromosomal microtubules are attached to chromosomes at their kinetochores, chromosomes are actively pulled toward the cell pole as the microtubules shorten. This disassembly would also provide tubulin for lengthening the continuous microtubules between centrioles, thereby separating the spindle poles and completing karyokinesis. The possible interaction of myosin and actin with these microtubules has not been ruled out.

Telophase

As the elongated cell enters telophase, nuclear membranes begin to reform around the segregated chromosomes in each pole. Almost immediately the chromosomes begin to uncoil, appearing less like discrete entities and more like the extended chromatin network of the interphase nucleus. The nucleolus reappears, forming from nucleolar organizing centers in each chromosome that were visible as secondary constrictions in the metaphase chromosomes. The separation and segregation of nuclear material into two separate nuclei is called **karyokinesis.**

At the same time that these nuclear events are occurring, cytoplasmic separation takes place (**cytokinesis**). Cytokinesis commences when a cytoplasmic constriction develops in the midportion of the cell, called a **cleavage furrow,** which will eventually separate the dividing cell into two daughter cells (Figs. 2-36, 2-40). In the initial stages of cytokinesis a contractile ring of parallel actin filaments encircles the equator of the cell. It

Fig. 2-39. A typical cell during anaphase. The daughter chromosomes have migrated to opposite poles of the cell.

Fig. 2-40. A typical cell during telophase. The cell membrane has begun constricting in the middle of the cell as cytokinesis begins.

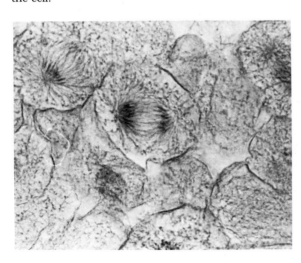

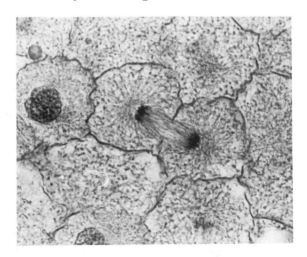

is believed that the cleavage furrow forms during an interaction of actin with myosin, but most details of this part of the mechanism remain to be clarified. Immediately prior to separation of daughter cells, microtubules of the spindle are still present within the narrow cytoplasmic bridge remaining between daughter cells (see Fig. 2-36).

NATIONAL BOARD TYPE QUESTIONS

For the following, select

    A. if only *1, 2, and 3* are correct.
    B. if only *1 and 3* are correct.
    C. if only *2 and 4* are correct.
    D. if only *4* is correct.
    E. if *all* are correct.

1. The nuclear envelope
   1. disassembles during cell division.
   2. has an outer membrane with ribosomes attached to it.
   3. has an outer membrane that is continuous with the rough endoplasmic reticulum.
   4. contains pores believed to be involved in nucleocytoplasmic exchange.

2. Gap junctions
   1. are specialized areas of plasmalemma of adjacent cells permitting the regulated flow of ions between involved cells.
   2. consist of threadlike components of the plasmalemma that involve the entire circumference of the cells.
   3. contain connexons, each consisting of six subunits arranged around a hydrophilic pore or annulus.
   4. establish a permeability seal that fuses the plasmalemma of adjacent epithelial cells, thereby preventing the flow of fluid from the lumen between epithelial cells.

3. Which of the following events accurately characterizes the somatic cell cycle?
   1. Replication of centrioles occurs during the G_2 phase.
   2. Rapidly dividing malignant cells spend only a short time in the G_1 phase.
   3. Postmitotic cells spend all their time in the G_1 phase.
   4. During the S phase, the nucleus of a normal cell changes from haploid to diploid.

4. The inner mitochondrial membrane
   1. contains enzymes of the electron transport system.
   2. consists of elementary particles with ATPase activity projecting into the matrix.
   3. is impermeable to most ions.
   4. contains most of the enzymes of the tricarboxylic acid cycle.

5. Receptor-mediated endocytosis is characterized by
   1. ligand-receptor complexes that become concentrated in coated pits.
   2. a coated vesicle scaffolding consisting of clathrin.
   3. dissociation of ligand-receptor complexes in acidified endosomes.
   4. a wavelike evagination of the plasmalemma which traps the receptor.

6. Which of the following statements concerning the nucleolus is (are) correct?
   1. Its granular component represents 15 percent of the nucleolar volume in a healthy cell.
   2. Nucleoli are formed from nucleolar organizers of each chromosome during telophase.
   3. During re-formation of the nucleolus, the fibrillar component is formed after the granular component is formed.
   4. The granular component represents preribosomes at different stages of maturation.

7. Peroxisomes
   1. are distinguished from other organelles by a positive histochemical reaction for catalase.
   2. are distinguished from lysosomes by a positive histochemical reaction for acid phosphatase.

3. contain a granular matrix enclosed by a translucent space and a single membrane.
4. are formed by budding from the Golgi apparatus.

8. Secretory proteins
   1. are synthesized by the rough endoplasmic reticulum.
   2. are carried by transport vesicles from the rough endoplasmic reticulum to the forming face of the Golgi apparatus.
   3. are terminally glycosylated with sialic acid in the trans lamella of the Golgi apparatus.
   4. emerge from the maturing face (trans) of the Golgi apparatus in a condensing vacuole.

9. Identify examples of condensed (coiled) DNA in the cell.
   1. Pyknotic nucleus
   2. Barr body
   3. Metaphase chromosomes
   4. Areas of the nucleus which do not stain with basic dyes

10. The terminal web
    1. consists of filaments that are anchored in desmosomes.
    2. has actin filaments from microvilli anchored in it.
    3. consists of microtubules.
    4. has filaments that are anchored in the zonula adherens.

11. Organelles consisting of nine triplets of microtubules include
    1. axonemes of cilia.
    2. basal bodies.
    3. axonemes of flagella.
    4. centrioles.

12. Which of the following statements concerning microtubules are correct?
    1. During anaphase they are attached to the kinetochore of each chromatid as chromatids migrate to opposite poles of the cell.
    2. During metaphase kinetochores of attached chromatids are connected by microtubules to centrioles in opposite poles of the cell.
    3. They are involved in the mechanism responsible for movement of organelles within the cell.
    4. They are composed of actin dimers.

ANNOTATED ANSWERS

1. E. For further discussion, refer to Nuclear Envelope on page 45 and Prophase on page 52.
2. B. If you are confusing gap junctions with zonula occludens, refer to Structural Specializations of the Plasmalemma on page 18.
3. A. During the S phase of a somatic cell, the cell changes from diploid to tetraploid before being restored to diploid during mitosis.
4. A. Remember that the enzymes of the Krebs cycle are located in the mitochondrial matrix.
5. A. Wavelike evaginations of the plasmalemma are characteristic of pinocytosis.
6. C. For further discussion, refer to Nucleolus on page 47.
7. B. If you are confusing peroxisomes with lysosomes, refer to Peroxisomes on page 25.
8. E.
9. A. Unstained nuclear areas represent sites of active uncondensed DNA.
10. C. The terminal web is associated with microvilli and zonula adherens by intersecting cytoskeletal elements.
11. C. Axonemes are composed of microtubule doublets.
12. A. Microtubules consist of tubulin dimers arranged into a helix.

BIBLIOGRAPHY

Back, F. The variable condition of euchromatin and heterochromatin. *Int. Rev. Cytol.* 45:25, 1976.
Bainton, D. F. The discovery of lysosomes. *J Cell Biol.* 91 (3, Pt. 2):66s, 1981.

Bainton, D. F., and M. G. Farquhar. Origin of granules in polymorphonuclear leukocytes: Two types derived from opposite faces of the Golgi complex in developing granulocytes. *J. Cell Biol.* 28:277, 1966.

Borysenko, J. Z., and J. P. Revel. Experimental manipulation of desmosome structure. *Am. J. Anat.* 137:403, 1973.

Bretscher, M. S., J. N. Thomson, and B. M. F. Pearse. Coated pits act as molecular filters. *Proc. Natl. Acad. Sci. U.S.A.* 77:4156, 1980.

Brown, M. S. Receptor-mediated endocytosis. *Proc. Natl. Acad. Sci. U.S.A.* 76:3330, 1979.

Caro, L. G., and G. E. Palade. Protein synthesis, storage and discharge in the pancreatic exocrine cell: A radiographic study. *J. Cell Biol.* 20:473, 1964.

Ernster, L., and G. Schatz. Mitochondria: A historical review. *J. Cell Biol.* 91 (3, Pt. 2):227s, 1981.

Farquhar, M. G., and G. E. Palade. The Golgi apparatus (complex)–(1954–1981)–from artifact to center stage. *J. Cell Biol.* 91 (3, Pt. 2):77s, 1981.

Friend, D. S., and M. G. Farquhar. Functions of coated vesicles during protein absorption in the rat vas deferens. *J. Cell Biol.* 35:357, 1967.

Ghosh, S. The nucleolar structure. *Int. Rev. Cytol.* 44:1, 1976.

Glaumann, H., J. L. E. Ericson, and L. Marzella. Mechanisms of intralysosomal degradation with special reference to autophagocytosis and heterophagocytosis of cell organelles. *Int. Rev. Cytol.* 73:149, 1981.

Hadjiolov, A. A. *The Nvcleolus and Ribosome Biogenesis.* New York: Springer-Verlag, 1985.

Haimo, L. T., and J. L. Rosenbaum. Cilia, flagella, and microtubules. *J. Cell Biol.* 91 (3, Pt. 2):125s, 1981.

Hand, A. R. Cytochemical differentiation of the Golgi apparatus from GERL. *J. Histochem. Cytochem.* 28:82, 1980.

Hay, E. Extracellular matrix. *J. Cell Biol.* 91 (3, Pt. 2):205s, 1981.

Herzog. The secretory process as studied by the localization of endogenous peroxidase. *J. Histochem. Cytochem.* 27:1360, 1979.

Heuser, J., and L. Evans. Three-dimensional visualization of coated vesicle formation in fibroblasts. *J. Cell Biol.* 84:560, 1980.

Heuser, J. E., and M. W. Kirschner. Filament organization revealed in platinum replicas of freeze-dried cytoskeletons. *J. Cell Biol.* 86:212, 1980.

Heuser, J. E., and T. S. Reese. Structural changes after transmitter release at the frog neuromuscular junction. *J. Cell Biol.* 88:564, 1981.

Hsieh, P., R. Segal, and L. B. Chen. Studies of fibronectin matrices in living cells with fluoresceinated gelatin. *J. Cell Biol.* 87:14, 1980.

Inoué, S. Cell division and the mitotic spindle. *J. Cell Biol.* 91 (3, Pt. 2):131s, 1981.

Kanaseki, T., and K. Kadota. The "vesicle in a basket." A morphological study of the coated vesicle isolated from nerve endings of the guinea pig brain, with special reference to the mechanism of membrane movements. *J. Cell Biol.* 42:202, 1969.

Lazarides, E. Intermediate filaments as mechanical integrators of cellular space. *Nature* 283:249, 1980.

Lehninger, A. L. *The Mitochondrion: Molecular Basis of Structure and Function.* Menlo Park. Calif.: Benjamin, 1964.

Luft, J. H. The structure and properties of the cell surface coat. *Int. Rev. Cytol.* 45:291, 1976.

McNutt, N. S., and R. S. Weinstein. Membrane ultrastructure at mammalian intercellular junctions. *Prog. Biophys. Mol. Biol.* 26:45, 1973.

Mazia, D. The cell cycle. *Sci. Am.* 230:54, 1974.

Morré, D. J., and L. Ovtracht. Dynamics of the Golgi apparatus: Membrane differentiation and membrane flow. *Int. Rev. Cytol.* 5 (Suppl.):61, 1977.

Novikoff, P. M., et al. Golgi apparatus, GERL, and lysosomes of neurons in rat dorsal root ganglia, studied by thick section and thin section cytochemistry. *J. Cell Biol.* 50:859, 1971.

Novikoff, P. M., and A. Yam. Sites of lipoprotein particles in normal rat hepatocytes. *J. Cell Biol.* 76:1, 1978.

Palade, G. Intracellular aspects of the process of protein synthesis. *Science* 189:347, 1975.

Peracchia, C. Structural correlates of gap junction permeation. *Int. Rev. Cytol.* 66:81, 1980.

Rambourg, A., Y. Clermont, and A. Marraud. Three-dimensional structure of the osmium-impregnated Golgi apparatus as seen in the high voltage electron microscope. *Am. J. Anat.* 140:27, 1974.

Siekevitz, P., and P. C. Zamecnik. Ribosomes and protein synthesis. *J. Cell Biol.* 91 (3, Pt. 2):53s, 1981.

Soifer, D. (ed.). The Biology of Cytoplasmic Microtubules. *Ann. N. Y. Acad. Sci.* 253, 1975.

Staehelin, L. A., and B. E. Hull. Junctions between living cells. *Sci. Am.* 238:140, 1978.

Unwin, P. N. T., and G. Zampighi. Structure of the junction between communicating cells. *Nature* 283:545, 1980.

Wade, J. B., and M. J. Karnovsky. The structure of the zonula occludens: A single fibril model based on freeze-fracture. *J. Cell Biol.* 60:168, 1974.

Warner, F. D., and D. R. Mitchel. Dynein: The mechanochemical coupling adenosine triphosphatase of microtubule-based sliding filament mechanisms. *Int. Rev. Cytol.* 66:1, 1980.

Whaley, W. G., and M. Dauwalder. The Golgi apparatus, the plasma membrane, and functional integration. *Int. Rev. Cytol.* 58:199, 1979.

Zampighi, G., J. M. Corless, and J. D. Robertson. On gap junction structure. *J. Cell Biol.* 86:190, 1980.

Zanetti, N. C., D. R. Mitchell, and F. D. Warner. Effects of divalent cations on dynein cross bridging and ciliary microtubule sliding. *J. Cell Biol.* 80:573, 1979.

3 Epithelium

Objectives

You will learn the following in this chapter:

How to identify the four basic tissue categories

Some general features of epithelia (e.g., origins, distribution, variations, functions)

Classification of surface epithelia in terms of their appearance, location, and function

The three major criteria for classification of glandular epithelia

Some varieties of glandular secretion and the modes by which they are secreted

Three apical surface specializations and a primary function for each

The four types of cell junctions and their locations and functions

How to identify and describe two specializations of the cytoskeleton that are prominent in some epithelia

---

Having been introduced in the preceding chapter to the cytoarchitecture that subserves cellular functions, one should recognize that no single cell can possess all of the structures or specializations that are required to carry out the diverse functions in higher organisms ranging from sustenance to reproduction. Certainly, individual cells possess the ability for deriving sustenance from their immediate environment (e.g., diffusion, active transport, endocytosis) and to a lesser extent for their own reproduction (mitosis). Yet when one considers such functions of the multicellular organism in toto, no single differentiated cell is capable of such a task—partly because of that particular cell's location in the organism with respect to various microenvironments, but also because it is just not economically feasible for the cell or the organism. Therefore, a **division of labor** exists in such organisms, whereby certain cells are specialized for specific roles and as a result usually exhibit a particular structure. An examination of large and complex organisms reveals that cells are organized into "fabrics" that effectuate this division of labor. The microscopic examination of the functional fabric of specialized cells is the core of **histology**—the study of tissues.

ORGANIZATION OF CELLS INTO TISSUES

A tissue is a functional collection of cells and associated intercellular material that is specialized to carry out a specific role. Although tissues were first recognized by gross anatomists as the various "fabrics" of the body that could be dissected and separated, it was the use of microscopic techniques that enabled histologists to realize that these fabrics were actually organizations of specialized cells or cell products.

CLASSIFICATION OF THE BASIC TISSUES

There are four basic tissue categories, outlined as follows. Although some authors consider blood as a fifth category, this cellular fluid is treated as a connective tissue in this summary.

I. Epithelial tissue
   A. Surface epithelia
   B. Glandular epithelia
   C. Special epithelia
II. Connective tissue
   A. Connective tissue proper
     1. Loose connective tissue
     2. Dense connective tissue (regular, irregular)
     3. Special connective tissues
   B. Hemopoietic tissue
   C. Blood and lymph
   D. Supportive tissue
     1. Cartilage
     2. Bone
III. Muscular tissue
   A. Smooth
   B. Skeletal
   C. Cardiac
IV. Nerve tissue

The remainder of this chapter and those immediately following describe the fundamental tissues. With an adequate understanding of the structure and function of tissues, one will later be able to understand more easily the organs and systems as they are encountered.

GENERAL FEATURES OF EPITHELIA

Epithelia are unilaminar or multilaminar sheets of cells in which the cells are closely apposed to one another with little intercellular material. As a class, the epithelial tissues are the most diverse in function, a property that no doubt contributes to their wide structural multiformity. Some features of epithelia are summarized in the following outline:

1. All surfaces in the body, excluding the joint cavities, are covered or lined by an epithelium; epithelia, therefore, serve as barrier membranes to seal and separate the organism from various external and internal environments. An epithelium (a) covers the entire exterior surface of the body (the epidermis and its appendages, the cornea); (b) lines all passages that connect directly or indirectly with the exterior (digestive, respiratory, and urogenital systems); (c) lines all closed coelomic cavities (pleural, pericardial, peritoneal, where the epithelium is termed **mesothelium**); (d) lines the cardiovascular channels (where the epithelium is termed **endothelium**); and (e) lines all derivatives of the surface epithelial layers that developmentally were formed by invagination into the underlying connective tissue (e.g., glands).

2. Epithelia rest on a **basement membrane** (see Epithelial Specializations) and an underlying connective tissue.

3. Epithelia are generally avascular; the blood vessels of the subjacent connective tissue do not enter the epithelial membrane. Nourishment of an epithelium occurs by diffusion from the underlying connective tissue vasculature.

4. The majority of glands develop as epithelial outgrowths into the subjacent connective tissue; connections (ducts) to the surface are retained in the **exocrine** glands and normally lost in **endocrine** glands.

5. All body surfaces are more or less "active," with a continuous flux of materials—either unidirectional or bidirectional—across the epithelium; virtually everything that enters or leaves the body passes through, is modified by, or is synthesized by an epithelium.

6. Epithelial tissues possess a remarkable capability for renewal and regeneration. For example, epithelia of the skin or digestive tract are constantly renewed. Monitoring the sloughed cells of such an epithelium forms the basis for a diagnostic aspect of cytomorphology called **exfoliative cytology;** one group

of widely used exfoliative techniques includes the Papanicolaou procedures (Pap smear) for cancer and precancer diagnosis.

7. Epithelial tissues also possess the ability to undergo morphologic and functional change from one type of epithelium to another (**metaplasia**) when local environmental conditions become chronically altered. In essence, epithelia are more plastic than most other tissue groups.

8. Epithelia are diverse in origin; they are derived from all three primary germ layers (ectoderm, mesoderm, and endoderm), a property that also contributes to their structural multiformity.

9. Finally, the diversity of epithelial function includes protection, lubrication, secretion, digestion, absorption, transport, excretion, sensory reception and transduction, and reproduction. Epithelial "glands" produce sweat, sebum, milk, mucus, hydrochloric acid, enzymes, hormones, bile salts, urine, and reproductive cells.

CLASSIFICATION OF EPITHELIA

Although all epithelia are surface epithelia in the sense that they cover or line some surface in the body, certain of them are structurally modified to perform highly specialized functions, such as secretion, sensory reception, and gamete production. Therefore, it is convenient to consider three types of epithelia: (1) **surface epithelia,** (2) **glandular epithelia,** and (3) **special epithelia.**

Surface Epithelia

Surface epithelia are distinguished and classified primarily on the basis of two major characteristics:

1. The number of cell layers in the epithelium (simple vs. stratified)
2. The height and shape of the surface layer of cells in the epithelium (squamous vs. cuboidal vs. columnar)

Additionally, in certain epithelia the free surface of the outermost cells may be structurally specialized for particular functions; in such cases these characteristics may also be used in classifying the epithelium.

Eight types of surface epithelia—four simple and four stratified—can be described.

SIMPLE EPITHELIA

In a simple epithelium there is one layer of cells resting on the basement membrane; according to the shape of these cells a **simple squamous, simple cuboidal,** or **simple columnar** epithelium can be differentiated. The fourth variety is termed **pseudostratified;** despite an apparently stratified appearance, all cells rest on the basement membrane. Simple epithelia are functionally the most diverse.

1. Simple Squamous Epithelium

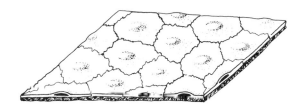

This epithelial variety is termed **squamous** (scalelike) because the flattened, platelike cells resemble scales in their surface aspect. Frequently, the nuclei are plumper than the cells are high, which causes the plasma membranes above and below to bulge slightly (Fig. 3-1A).

Sample locations: glandular ducts of small caliber; lining the pleural, pericardial, and peritoneal cavities (**mesothelium**); lining the cardiovascular and lymph channels (**endothelium**); respiratory bronchioles and alveoli of the lungs; Bowman's capsule (parietal layer) and loop of Henle (thin segment) in the kidneys; the inner aspect of the tympanic membrane.

Functionally, this epithelium is well suited for sites of fluid, metabolite, or gas exchange, where such exchange may occur across or between the cells.

2. Simple Cuboidal Epithelium

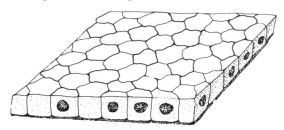

The cells of this epithelium are so named because they usually appear as high as they are wide in profile. However, a surface view reveals that they are actually more hexagonal in this aspect. The spherical nuclei are normally centrally positioned (Fig. 3-1B).

Sample locations: ducts of many glands; lining certain kidney tubules; rete testis; covering the free surface of the ovary.

Some authors consider the secretory cells in many glandular termini and the liver parenchymal cells as cuboidal, although these cells are probably best described as pyramidal and polyhedral, respectively.

Functionally, this epithelium may simply serve as lining cells in conducting passageways (e.g., glandular ducts) or it may be structurally adapted to play important roles in secretion or absorption (e.g., the proximal and distal convoluted tubules of the kidney).

3. Simple Columnar Epithelium

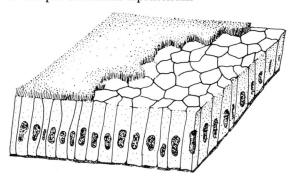

Although a surface view reveals that the cells in this epithelium have a polygonal outline similar to the cuboidal variety, their name is derived from the profile view, which exhibits cells that are taller than they are wide. These columnlike cells typically possess an ovoid, basally located nucleus (Fig. 3-1C).

Sample locations: ducts of many glands; much of the digestive tract (stomach, intestines, gallbladder); small bronchi of the lungs; portions of the female reproductive tract (oviducts and uterus).

Functionally, this epithelial type is primarily associated with secretion (e.g., intestinal goblet cells, oviduct and uterine secretory cells) and absorption (e.g., intestinal absorptive cells, gallbladder).

4. Pseudostratified Columnar Epithelium

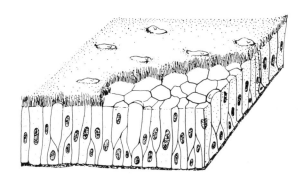

This epithelial variety appears stratified because (1) not all of the cells reach the free surface, (2) the nuclei are "stratified," being at two or more levels, and (3) the cells appear crowded due to varying cellular shapes. However, since all the cells touch the basement membrane, this type is considered to be a simple epithelium of differing cell heights (Fig. 3-1D).

Sample locations: large portion of the respiratory passages; eustachian tube and part of the middle ear; portions of the male accessory apparatus; portions of the male and female urethrae.

In the respiratory passages this epithelium is abundantly ciliated and contains numerous goblet cells, so that a **pseudostratified ciliated columnar epithelium with goblet cells** is named based on these structural modifications. Likewise, the epithelial cells in the ductus epididymidis and the ductus deferens of the male reproductive system have unusually long microvilli on their luminal surfaces, so that a **pseudostratified columnar epithelium with stereocilia** is also named. The term **stereocilia** is derived from early light microscopic observations, which suggested that these surface specializations were nonmotile cilia; the electron microscope has shown that they are actually microvilli (see Epithelial Specializations).

Functionally, this epithelium has lining, secretory, and absorptive roles. In addition, the ciliated variety is capable of moving material across its surface (see Epithelial Specializations).

STRATIFIED EPITHELIA

In a stratified epithelium there are two or more layers of cells; only the basal (lowermost) layer of cells rests on the basement membrane. According to the shape of the surface (outermost) layer of cells, a **stratified squamous, stratified cuboidal,** or **stratified columnar** epithelium can be distinguished. A fourth variety of stratified epithelia is termed **transitional.** As a group these epithelia are largely protective, covering areas that are subject to wear, tear, stress, or strain.

1. Stratified Squamous Epithelium
   This multilayered epithelium derives its name from the squamous appearance of the outermost layers of cells. Subjacent layers, from the most basal to the more superficial, contain cells that vary in shape from cuboidal or columnar to polyhedral; the closer they are to the surface, the more flattened the cells become. Two variations of stratified squamous epithelium occur:

a. Mucous type (nonkeratinized)

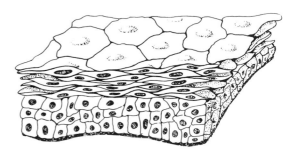

The surface cells in this epithelium are viable and contain nuclei, but they lack keratin (Fig. 3-1E).

Locations: on the surfaces of moist cavities or orifices that open onto the body surface, such as the mouth, pharynx, esophagus, vagina, and urethra.

b. Cutaneous type (keratinized)

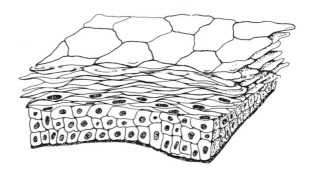

Surface layers of this epithelium, while still squamous, are dead and anucleate; at this stage the cells are veritable "bags" of the protein keratin.

Locations: covering the entire exposed surface of the body (except for the cornea); in man, certain areas of the oral cavity (the gingiva and portions of the hard palate) may become keratinized due, in part, to diet or techniques of oral hygiene; in many mammals whose diets contain highly abrasive components, the majority of the upper gastrointestinal tract may be keratinized.

Functionally, this variety is particularly well adapted to such physical insults as abrasion and desiccation.

2. Stratified Cuboidal Epithelium

This epithelium has a very limited distribution, but where it is found there are usually two layers of cuboidal cells.

Locations: may be found in the glandular ducts of larger caliber; some authors consider the granulosa cells of the ovarian follicle to be of this variety when two or more layers of cells exist.

3. Stratified Columnar Epithelium

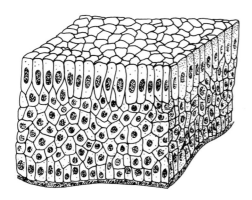

This type also has a limited distribution. Only the cells of the surface layer are columnar, with those in subjacent layers varying in shape from cuboidal to polyhedral.

Locations: small portions of the pharynx and larynx; glandular ducts of large caliber; portions of the male urethra.

Apart from functioning as a lining in major ducts, this epithelium occurs at interfaces or regions of epithelial transition, being interposed between two other varieties of epithelia.

4. Transitional Epithelium

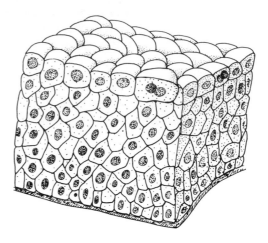

Originally this epithelium was termed transitional because it was considered to be an intermediate between stratified squamous and stratified columnar—essentially, a stratified cuboidal epithelium. Now, this epithelial type is recognized for its unique flexible qualities. The appearance of this epithelium varies tremendously depending on whether it is in its contracted or expanded state. Hence, the term **transitional** has taken on a new, but still appropriate meaning.

This multilayered epithelium is characterized by its surface layer of dome-shaped cells. Occasionally two nuclei per cell are observed. Subjacent layers contain cells that may be cuboidal, columnar, or polyhedral in shape (Fig. 3-1F).

Location: limited to lining some portions of the urinary tract, namely, the renal pelves, ureters, urinary bladder, and the initial part of the urethra.

Functionally, this epithelium is specifically adapted to stretching. Due to the functional state of the bladder in particular, at the time of removal and fixation, the transitional epithelium can show a variable appearance. In the nondistended (contracted) state, the epithelium may be four to six or more cell layers thick, with the surface layer exhibiting the typical dome cells. In the distended (stretched) condition, however, an epithelium of only two or three cell layers may be present. The surface layer in the distended condition is typically of the squamous or low cuboidal variety. In going from the contracted to the stretched state, the epithelial cells presumably slide past one another; electron microscopic observations show few cell-to-cell contacts in the form of desmosomes—a condition that apparently facilitates freer sliding movement. Fine structural studies also suggest that a membrane storage phenomenon occurs in surface cells when the epithelium is in the contracted state. This observation may explain how the surface layers deal with "extra" membrane when the bladder decreases in size on emptying. Finally, it is probable that the surface cell membranes are specialized in chemical structure and act as an exosmotic barrier to prevent diffusion of water into the lumen and resultant dilution of the hypertonic urine.

On reading the organ systems section of this book, it will become evident that epithelia are an integral component of most organs where they perform a variety of important physiologic functions. These functions are largely reflected in the epithelium's cellular organization and composition, its secretory products, and the surface specializations of the constituent cells. Examples of the most common types of epithelia are shown in Figure 3-1.

Glandular Epithelia

Single cells or groups of cells which are specialized for secretion are called **glands.** Secretion is the active process whereby certain cells take up precursor (building block) molecules from their surrounding environs and transform them biochemically into some product that is discharged from the cell. This discharge may be accomplished by release into the duct system (**ex-ocrine glands**) or ultimately into the bloodstream (**endocrine glands**). The exocrine glands are described here because they are all epithelial derivatives. The endocrine glands, not all of which are epithelial structures, are studied in future chapters, either as individual organs or in association with the organs or systems in which they are found.

EXOCRINE GLANDS

Exocrine glands can be classified on the basis of four factors:

1. The number of cells (unicellular vs. multicellular)
2. The duct system (simple vs. compound) and secretory portion (tubular vs. alveolar vs. tubuloalveolar)
3. The nature of the secretion (mucous vs. serous vs. seromucous)
4. The mode of secretion (merocrine vs. apocrine vs. holocrine)

Number of Cells

A **unicellular gland** (Fig. 3-2A; example: mucous goblet cell) is a single secretory cell interposed in an epithelium between cells of other functions.

Multicellular glands vary in complexity and may occur as (1) epithelial sheet glands (Fig. 3-2B; example: surface mucous cells of the stomach), (2) intraepithelial glands (Fig. 3-2C; example: urethral mucous glands), or (3) complex glands with ducts (Fig. 3-2D). The complex multicellular glands with ducts are by far the most numerous type and are distinguished by the appearance of both their duct systems and secretory portions.

Duct System and Secretory Portion

Based on the duct system alone, glands are considered **simple** (Fig. 3-3A), or **compound** (Fig. 3-3B) if the duct is unbranched or branched, respectively.

Based on the organization of the epithelium in

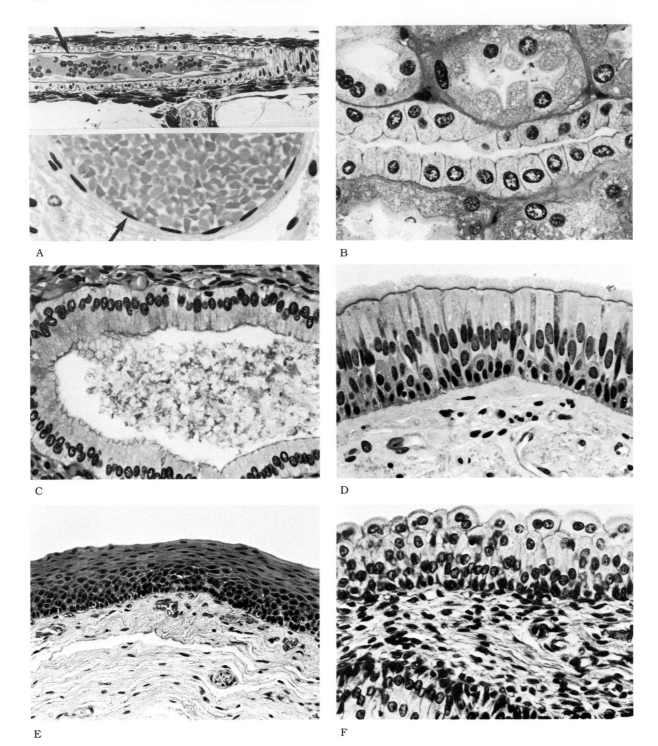

A

B

C

D

E

F

Fig. 3-1. Composite of the more common epithelial types. A. Simple squamous epithelium (endothelium) lining blood vessels. Thin plastic preparation (*above*) shows longitudinal section of a small artery. Endothelial cells line the lumen (*arrow*). To the right, the artery is cut obliquely through its wall. The middle layer is composed of smooth muscle, the outer wall of the connective tissue. A standard paraffin preparation (*below*) of a small vein in cross section. Only the nuclei of the endothelial cells are clearly discernible (*arrow*). B. Simple cuboidal epithelium of kidney tubules. The cells are outlined clearly in the longitudinally cut duct passing through the center of the field. C. Simple columnar epithelium of a pancreatic duct. The precipitate in the lumen is composed of digestive enzymes on their way to the duodenum.

D. Pseudostratified columnar epithelium of the trachea (respiratory epithelium). Note the cilia at the apical surface. The dense line subjacent to the cell surface represents the basal bodies from which the cilia arise. The small cells in the basal region are immature cells, which give rise to the tall ciliated cells, and goblet cells, which have no cilia (tall dark cells). E. Stratified squamous epithelium of the esophagus. The cells at the basal legion are cuboidal, while those in the more superficial layers are flat. This epithelium is nonkeratinized. The underlying connective tissue is dense and contains a few small vessels. F. Transitional epithelium of the urinary bladder in a contracted state. Most of the dome-shaped surface cells are binucleate. When the bladder is expanded, the cells stretch and appear flat.

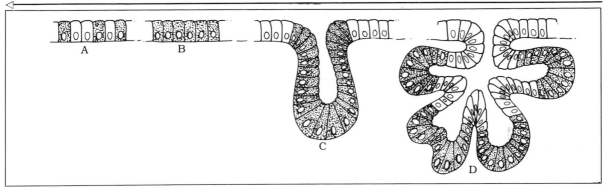

Fig. 3-2. Unicellular versus multicellular glands. Glandular cells are stippled; nonglandular surface cells and duct cells are clear. (A) unicellular glands; (B) epithelial sheet gland; (C) intraepithelial gland; (D) complex multicellular gland with ducts.

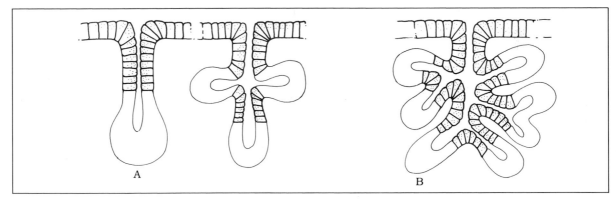

Fig. 3-3. Variations in complex multicellular glands based on the structure of the ducts. (A) simple glands; (B) compound gland.

the secretory portion alone (Fig. 3-4), glands are considered **tubular, alveolar** (acinar), or **tubuloalveolar** (tubuloacinar). The shape of the secretory unit in complex glands can be compared to the shape of certain pieces of laboratory glassware, namely, test tubes (tubular types) and flasks of the Florence and Erlenmeyer varieties (alveolar types).

Examples of simple and compound glands are given in the following outline:

I. Simple glands (Fig. 3-5)
  A. Simple tubular glands
    Example: crypts of Lieberkühn in the intestine (Fig. 3-5A)
  B. Simple coiled tubular glands
    Example: eccrine sweat glands (Fig. 3-5B)
  C. Simple branched tubular glands
    Examples: fundic glands of the stomach (Fig. 3-5C); Brunner's glands of the duodenum

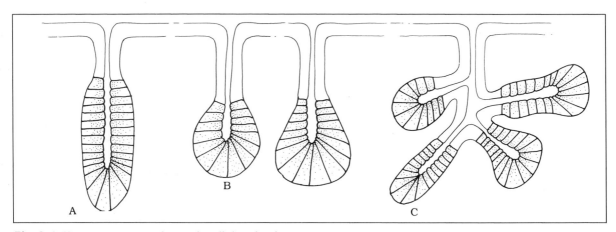

Fig. 3-4. Variations in complex multicellular glands based on the structure of the secretory portions. (A) tubular type; (B) alveolar types; (C) tubuloalveolar type.

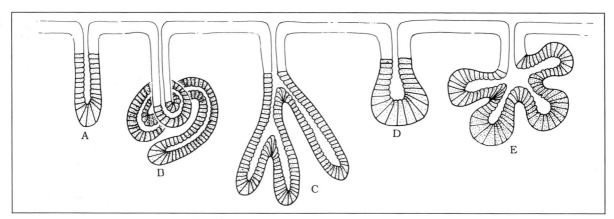

Fig. 3-5. Types of simple glands. (A) simple tubular; (B) simple coiled tubular; (C) simple branched tubular; (D) simple alveolar; (E) simple branched alveolar.

D. Simple alveolar (acinar) glands
Example: poison glands in certain amphibians (Fig. 3-5D); may not occur in mammals

E. Simple branched alveolar (acinar) glands
Example: sebaceous glands (Fig. 3-5E)

II. Compound glands (Fig. 3-6)

A. Compound tubular glands
Example: cardiac glands of the stomach (Fig. 3-6A)

B. Compound tubuloalveolar glands
Examples: salivary glands, pancreas (Fig. 3-6B)

Nature of the Secretion

Based on the nature of the secretion, glands are described as **mucous, serous,** or **mixed (seromucous).**

1. Mucous glands. As the name suggests, the mucous gland secretes the glycoprotein mucin (mucin + water = mucus). The light microscopic appearance of the plump secretory cell is distinctive (Fig. 3-7), with a light-staining cytoplasm due to the large quantity of mucigen and a well-flattened nucleus that is "forced" against the basal portion of the cell.

2. Serous glands. The serous (wheylike) secretion is a clear, watery fluid containing a proteinaceous component. Serous secretory cells (see Fig. 3-7) are easily distinguished from their mucous counterparts by perinuclear cytoplasmic basophilia (rough endoplasmic reticulum) and a nucleus that is basally placed but well rounded.

3. Mixed (seromucous) glands. This gland type (see Fig. 3-7) has both a serous and mucous component to its secretion, in that both types of secretory units occur as either mixed alveoli or mucous units with serous "caps" (**demilunes**). The submandibular salivary gland is a mixed seromucous gland (Fig. 3-8).

Functionally, the mucous secretion is both lubricating and protective; the serous secretion may be lubricating, may serve to cleanse epithelial surfaces, and often contains enzymes.

Mode of Secretion

Based on the mode of secretion, glands are described as **merocrine, apocrine,** and **holocrine.**

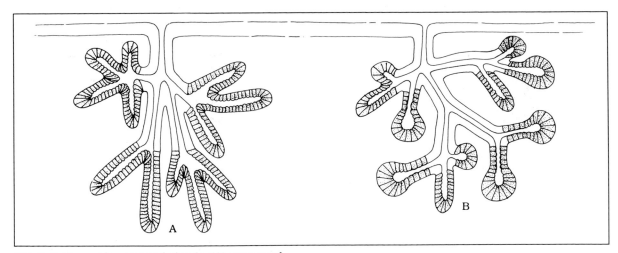

Fig. 3-6. Types of compound glands. (A) compound tubular; (B) compound tubuloalveolar.

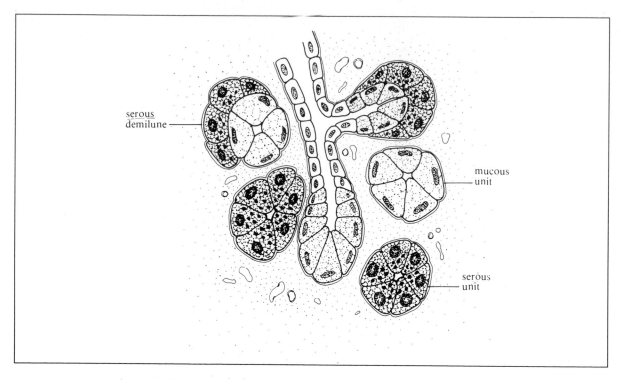

serous
demilune

mucous
unit

serous
unit

Fig. 3-7. Mucous, serous, and seromucous glandular units.

In merocrine secretion, the secretory product is "separated" by release through the cell membrane; the cell itself remains essentially intact. The mechanism involves fusion of the boundary membrane of the secretory granule with the plasma membrane and resultant discharge of granular contents into the lumen. This mode of secretion is typical of glands involved in protein or mucin release. Examples of merocrine secretion are the salivary glands and the pancreas.

Apocrine secretion is a "separating off" of the secretory product involving a loss of part of the apical cytoplasm. Essentially, the secretion product "lifts off" at the apical surface of the cell **together** with either a thin rim of the surrounding cytoplasm or a larger cap of luminal cytoplasm. Examples of apocrine secretion are the apocrine sweat glands, lipid secretion in the mammary glands, and the ceruminous glands.

Holocrine secretion involves the release of entire cells and contained secretory product into the glandular lamina. Accumulation of secretory product in these cells results in organelle disintegration and eventual cell destruction. The sebaceous glands are an example of this type of secretion. The testis and ovary may be considered as special types of holocrine glands in that whole **living** cells (spermatozoa and ova) are "secreted," a process that is sometimes referred to as **cytogenous secretion.**

MYOEPITHELIAL CELLS

Situated between the basal portions of the secretory cells and the basement membrane in certain glands (sweat, salivary, mammary, ceruminous, and lacrimal) are special cells that are contractile in function, known as **myoepithelial cells** (basal

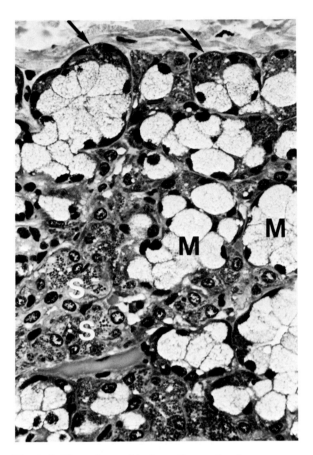

Fig. 3-8. The submandibular salivary gland contains serous (*S*) and mucous (*M*) acini as well as mixed units with serous caps (*arrows*). The mucin-producing cells are pale with dark basal nuclei. The nuclei of the serous cells are less dense. Serous granules are visible in their cytoplasm.

cells, basket cells). These **myoid** (musclelike) cells have been shown to contain myofibrils, but unlike the mesodermally derived muscular tissues, they are ectodermal in origin. This origin no doubt accounts for their location within the limits of the basement membrane. In specially stained whole mount preparations of glandular termini, these cells are shown to extend their delicate processes around the secretory units in

such a way as to resemble a loosely woven basket. Functionally, these contractile elements are thought to aid in the expression of secretory product into the glandular ducts.

Special Epithelia

In addition to the surface epithelia and those that are specialized wholly for secretion, a few others possess unique structure and special properties. The most notable of these "special" epithelia are concerned with sensory perception (olfactory, gustatory, visual, and auditory epithelia) and reproduction (germinal epithelium lining the seminiferous tubules of the testis). These types of epithelia are considered in detail when studied in appropriate later chapters.

EPITHELIAL SPECIALIZATIONS

It has already been stated that the epithelia, as a class of tissues, are the most diverse in function. Related to this property—and probably to the wide germ layer origin of epithelia as well—is the structural multiformity of the various epithelial membranes described in previous sections. Likewise, the individual cells that make up these membranes possess specializations of structure that allow or enhance epithelial functions, coherence, communication, and structural integrity.

The fundamental property that reflects these functions is the polarized organization of epithelial cells in terms of their organelle distribution and surface specializations. Organelles are usually arranged in a line perpendicular to the basement membrane. This imaginary line is referred to as the **cell axis.**

Cytologic specializations of epithelia (Fig. 3-9) may occur at the various interfacial areas of (1) the cell and the surface environment (apical cell surface), (2) the cell and adjacent members of the epithelium (lateral cell surfaces), and (3) the cell and the underlying connective tissue (basal cell surface). In addition, there may be specializations for intracellular support (cytoskeleton) that are often intimately associated with the interfacial structures.

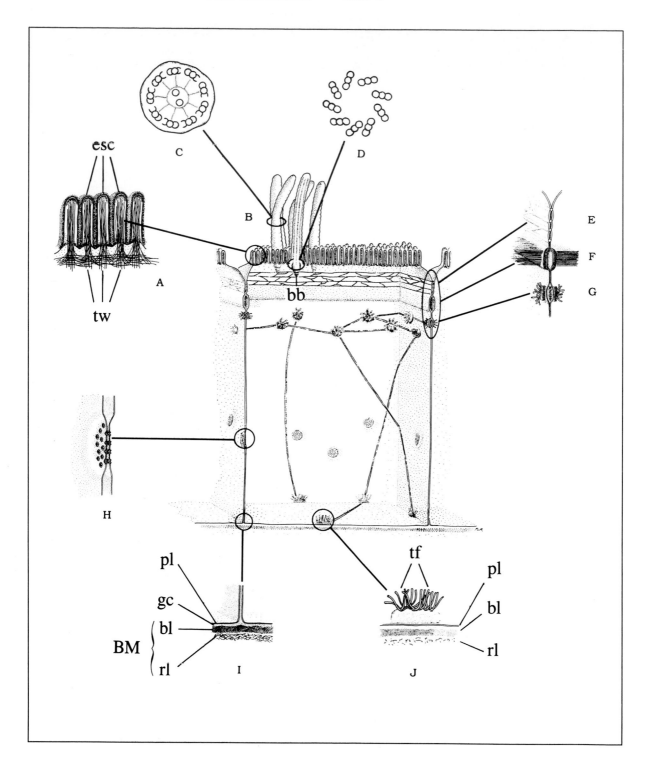

Fig. 3-9. An idealized epithelium, with the various specializations of the apical, lateral, and basal surfaces of the cells as well as those of the cytoskeleton. The epithelium is shown in three dimensions representing a face view of the cells. (A) Microvilli; (B) cilia; (C) cross section of cilium; (D) cross section of basal body; (E) zonula occludens; (F) zonula adherens; (G) macula adherens; (H) macula communicans; (I) basement membrane; (J) hemidesmosome. *bb* = basal body; *bl* = basal lamina; *BM* = basement membrane; *esc* = enteric surface coat; *gc* = glycocalyx; *pl* = cell membrane; *rl* = reticular lamina; *tf* = tonofilaments; *tw* = terminal web.

◁——————————————————————

Other specializations include the degree of development and arrangement of the various intracellular organelles and other structures that were described in Chapter 2. These specializations are examined in later chapters when epithelial function is described in relation to organ function as a whole.

Although many of the specializations to be discussed here are not unique to epithelia, overall they are probably the best developed in this class of tissues. Finally, it should be pointed out that an appreciation of the true structure of epithelial specializations has been possible only with the aid of the electron microscope.

Specializations of the Apical (Free) Surface

MICROVILLI

Before the development of the electron microscope, it had long been recognized that the apical surfaces of certain epithelial cells possessed a border of delicate striae or appendages. Based on their appearance in the light microscope, some of these surface specializations were named **striated border** (intestinal absorptive cells), **brush border** (proximal kidney tubules), and **stereocilia** (appendages on principal cells of the ductus epididymidis and ductus deferens) (see Fig. 3-12). However, stereocilia are much larger and more specialized than typical microvilli found

elsewhere. Electron microscopy has now shown that these surface specializations are all composed of similar structures called microvilli.

Microvilli are delicate fingerlike or hairlike projections from the surface of the cell (Fig. 3-10; see also Fig. 3-9A) formed by multiple evaginations of the plasma membrane and underlying cytoplasm. They contain a core of fine, 6-nm filaments running in their longitudinal axes and perpendicular to the cell surface. Most, if not all, of these filaments have been shown to be actin filaments. The **actin bundle** is attached to the plasma membrane at the apical tip of the villus in a dense structure (**dense tip**). Cross-bridges attach the actin bundle to the membrane. The basal portions of the filamentous cores are embedded in and interconnected with a meshwork of other filaments that excludes other organelles (the **terminal web;** see Specializations of the Cytoskeleton). This meshwork lies just beneath the cell surface and is arranged perpendicularly to the microvilli.

Recent studies have shown that microvilli of intestinal epithelial cells are capable of movement; their contraction is presumably mediated by actomyosin. In the terminal web, actin filaments and myosin-containing filaments run horizontal to the cell surface and perpendicular to the microvillar actin bundles (Fig. 3-10). Thus, the myosin of the terminal web in association with the microvillar actin bundles may constitute a U-shaped "sarcomere" capable of contraction and relaxation, similar to the sliding filament mechanism of actin-myosin interaction in muscle contraction proposed by Huxley (discussed in Chap. 7).

In epithelia, microvilli are found on the surfaces of many different types of cells, but are most abundant and well developed on those cells concerned with secretion and absorption. Functionally, these appendages greatly increase the apical surface area of cells, thereby enhancing the secretory or absorptive processes.

In the small intestine, the plasma membranes of microvilli are also associated with enzymes which carry out the final steps in the digestion of carbohydrates. Thus, the intestinal brush border

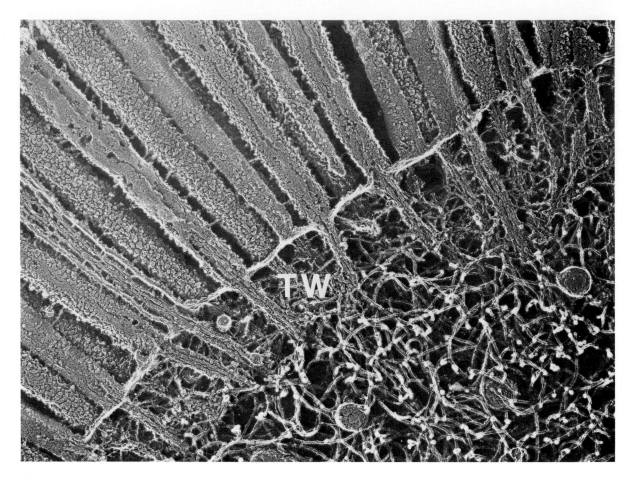

Fig. 3-10. A freeze-fracture shadow cast replica of the apical portion of a mouse epithelial cell as it appears under the electron microscope. Most of the cytoplasmic proteins are extracted from the cells that were sheared open before freezing. This reveals a filamentous cytoskeleton composed of a bed of intermediate filaments (*lower right*) upon which rest the bundles of microfilaments that form the cores within the microvilli (*upper left*). They form a meshwork just beneath the cell surface, called the terminal web (*TW*). (From N. Hirokowa and J. E. Heuser, Quick-freeze, deep-etch visualization of cytoskeleton beneath surface differentiations of intestinal epithelial cells. *J. Cell Biol.* 91:399, 1981. By permission of The Rockefeller University Press.)

promotes the digestive and absorptive efficiency of the epithelium. The enzymes protrude into the surface coat referred to as the **glycocalyx.**

CILIA

Cilia (and flagella) are motile, lashlike projections from the cell surface that are visible with the light microscope. Like microvilli, these cellular appendages are also plasmalemma-covered evaginations of the cell surface (see Fig. 3-1D, 3-9B). However, the electron microscope has shown that their internal structure (Fig. 3-11A, B; see also Fig. 3-9C) is composed of microtubules typically arranged as nine doublets surrounding a central pair (**axoneme:** 9 + 2 complex). The axoneme is common to all cilia and flagella found in

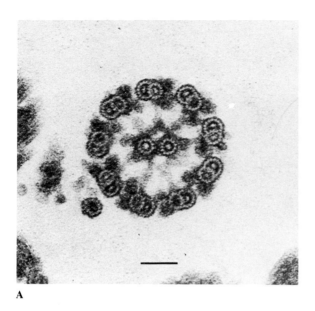

A

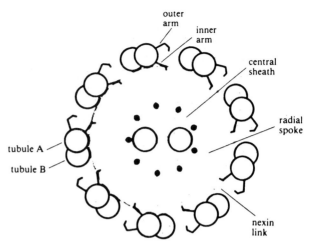

B

Fig. 3-11. Cilia (and flagella). A. Cross section of sea urchin sperm flagella axoneme after fixation with tannic acid, glutaraldehyde, osmium tetroxide. The axoneme is composed of nine outer doublet microtubules and two central singlet microtubules. The white-appearing protofilaments forming the microtubule walls can be seen, as can the dark-staining dynein arms, radial spokes, and central sheath projections (*see adjacent diagram*). *Bar = 50 nm.* (Courtesy of R. W. Linck.) B. Diagram of cross section of a cilium showing microtubule organization and associated structures. See text for detailed explanation.

animals and plants. The microtubules are composed of the protein **tubulin.** Within the axoneme complex are a number of fine, associated structures (Fig. 3-11B). A central sheath encloses the central pair of microtubules and **radial spokes** connect the sheath to the outer nine doublets. These are peripherally connected by links composed of **nexin.** Outer and inner arms extend from each doublet toward the adjacent doublet. At least part of the outer arms is composed of **dynein,** the force-generating enzyme. The mechanism of motility is based on dynein ATPase producing active sliding between the adjacent doublet microtubules. The lengths of the microtubules do not change during bending. Sliding is transformed into bending by the restraint of the radial spokes attached to the central tubules.

Beating of cilia consists of a rapid forward motion, the **effective stroke,** followed by a slower **recovery stroke.** The forward spreading waves of ciliary beating (metachronal rhythm) provides the means by which mucus and particulate matter are moved along the epithelial surface. This action is termed the **mucociliary clearance mechanism.**

A single cell may contain several hundred cilia on its surface. Each cilium arises from a **basal body** (see Fig. 3-9B), which is located in the apical cytoplasm of the cell; in sectional view (vertical plane) at the light microscopic level, these bodies appear as a line of punctate densities just subjacent and parallel to the cell surface. At the electron microscopic level, basal bodies are structurally identical with centrioles, with nine triplets of tubules (see Fig. 3-9D). Indeed, one of the ways in which these bodies develop is from centrioles.

Flagella are singly occurring, extremely long cilia; they are found on some epithelial cells, the most notable of which is the spermatozoon.

Functionally, cilia beat in waves over the surface of the epithelium to move materials across the epithelium on a layer of fluid. Cilia are particularly important in removing inhaled particulate matter from the upper airway passages of the respiratory system and in moving ova through the oviducts following ovulation. They may also be important in the transport of spermatozoa through the ductuli efferentes of the male reproductive tract.

GLYCOCALYX

The glycocalyx is a surface coat that consists of complex carbohydrates in association with either structural proteins embedded in the plasma membrane or proteins present on the membrane surface. Although this glycoprotein encrustation occurs on all surfaces of epithelial cells (lateral and basal surfaces as well; see Fig. 3-9I), it is particularly prominent at the apical surface of certain cells. For example, on the surface of the absorptive cells of the small intestine, an elaborate "fuzz" (**enteric surface coat;** see Fig. 3-9A) is found that contains hydrolytic enzymes, including alkaline phosphatase and various disaccharidases.

Functionally, the surface coat is involved with cellular recognition, adhesion, and binding of various molecules; it may also provide a microenvironment for chemical reactions or may concentrate certain ionic species to be absorbed by the cell.

Specializations of the Lateral Surfaces

JUNCTIONAL COMPLEX

With the light microscope, a darkened area, the **terminal bar,** can be observed at the apical cell boundaries of certain epithelia, especially the intestinal columnar cells (Fig. 3-12). In appropriate sections that are parallel to the surface of the

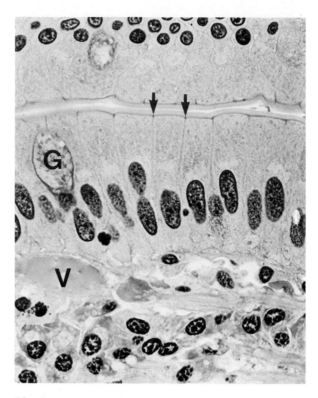

Fig. 3-12. Simple columnar cells of the intestinal villus. Note the border of microvilli at the apical surface. The dense spots at the apical cell boundaries are the terminal bars (*arrows*). Note also the goblet cell (*G*), a unicellular mucous gland. Beneath the epithelium, the connective tissue contains a small blood vessel (*V*) and a number of plasma cells.

epithelium, these terminal bars are seen to be continuous around the entire lateral aspect of the cells (see Fig. 3-9). With the electron microscope, it has been shown that in the areas of terminal bars there are at least three separate structures of specialization where the membranes of adjacent cells make close contacts (junctions). These structures are collectively termed a **junctional complex.**

The first and most apical component of the junctional complex is the **zonula occludens** or **tight junction.** These junctions are belts (zonules) that encompass the entire apical perimeter of the cells. Furthermore, a continuous extracellular space (10—15 nm) between adjacent epithelial cells is "occluded" as the outer leaflets of adjacent cell membranes fuse (Fig. 3-13A; see also Fig. 3-9E) at various junctures; this fusion, of course, results in the obliteration of the intercellular space at these locations. In areas where the occluding type of junction occurs, the fusion of adjacent trilaminar unit membranes results in a single pentalaminar contact. At the electron microscopic level, freeze-fracture preparations reveal an anastomosing network of **junctional fibrils** characteristic of tight junctions (Fig. 3-14). Functionally, the tight junctions serve as permeability seals to prevent, for example, solutes from passing from the outside in (or the inside out) through the epithelial boundary. This property is particularly important in an epithelium like the one that lines the small intestine, where selective absorption can occur only if nondiscriminating intercellular channels are blocked. Tight junctions are also supportive in function, since they maintain a firm attachment between adjacent epithelial cells.

The second component of the junctional complex is the **zonula adherens.** This intermediate junction is located just beneath the zonula occludens (see Figs. 3-9F, 3-13A) and also forms a continuous girdle around the cells. No membrane fusion occurs in these locations, with the result that a small intercellular space (15—20 nm) is present. However, on the cytoplasmic faces of the cell membranes where these junctions occur, numerous filaments are seen embedded in an electron-dense material. These filaments are often continuous with those of the terminal web; or it may be more precise to say that the filaments of the terminal web are anchored in this electron-dense matrix. Functionally, the zonulae adherentes are thought to be regions of cell-to-cell attachment. It has been suggested that this component of the junctional complex more than any other may be responsible for the terminal bar structure seen with the light microscope.

A third component of the junctional complex is the **macula adherens** or **desmosome** (see Fig. 3-13A). In this punctate or spot (**macula** = spot) junction, there is also a slight separation (15—20

nm) of adjacent cell membranes. However, an intermediate line of dense material (see Figs. 3-9G, 3-13B) is usually seen in the intercellular region of this junction. This dark line may represent a condensation or fusion of the cell coats (glycocalyces) in this region. As on the cytoplasmic faces of cell membranes adjacent to zonulae adherentes, a dense plaque of material is found on the inner surface of the cell membranes adjacent to desmosomes (see Fig. 3-9G). Many tonofilaments are also seen embedded in these plaques. Functionally, the macula adherens is considered to be a "spot-weld" type of cell-to-cell attachment.

Desmosomes are not limited in their distribution to the junctional complexes; they are widely found over the lateral surfaces of cells as well as in epithelia where typical junctional complexes do not exist. Likewise, the occluding type of junction may be found without the other components of the junctional complex.

COMMUNICATING JUNCTION

At one time, the specialization known as a **communicating junction** (macula communicans; nexus; gap junction) was thought to be similar to the occluding junction. However, it is now known that communicating junctions are macular-type junctions in which adjacent cell membranes come into very close contact (2 nm) but do not fuse (see Fig. 3-9H). Although maculae communicantes may be sites of cell-to-cell adhesion, functionally they can be considered as synapses between adjacent cells. They have been shown to be areas of low resistance to ionic flow (electrotonic coupling) and are thought to be intimately involved in cell-to-cell communication. See Chapter 2 for additional details.

Specializations of the Basal Surface
BASEMENT MEMBRANE

All epithelia rest on connective tissue. Interposed between an epithelium and the connective tissue is a sheet of material called the **basement membrane.**

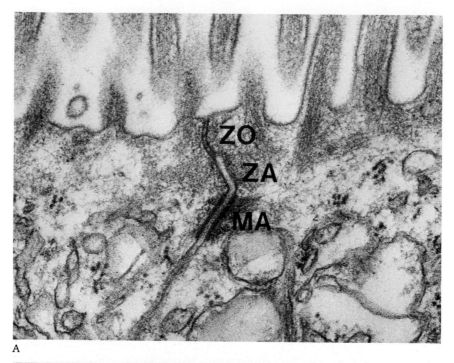

A

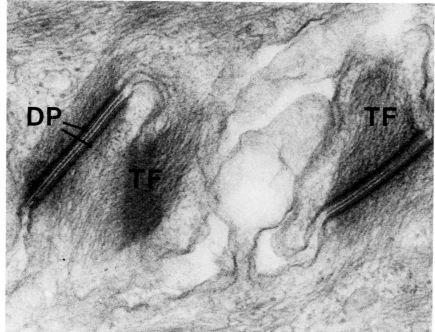

B

Fig. 3-13. A. Junctional complex between adjoining epithelial cells of rat intestine. The elements of the three-part complex usually appear in the following order: an apically located tight or occluding junction, *zonula occludens* (*ZO*), an intermediate junction, *zonula adherens* (*ZA*), and a desmosome, *macula adherens* (*MA*). The term *zonula* signifies that the junction is a belt completely encircling the cell whereas *macula* indicates that the junction is discontinuous (i.e., a discrete spot). The primary function of adhering junctions is to provide cell-to-cell attachment. The continuous occluding junctions form a permeability barrier between the luminal and stromal compartments. Sealing strands (*fibrils*) are visible within the plasma membranes of freeze-fractured tight junctions (see Fig. 3-14). Microvilli project out from the cells' surface. (Courtesy of J. Z. Borysenko.) B. Higher magnification of two desmosomes (macula adherens). Note the intermediate line in the intercellular region and the tonofilaments (*TF*), which are attached to the dense plaques (*DP*) of the desmosome. (From J. Z. Borysenko and J.-P. Revel,

Experimental manipulation of desmosome structure. *Am. J. Anat.* 137:403, 1973. By permission of Wistar Press, Philadelphia.)

Fig. 3-14. Freeze-fracture replica of a tight junction in glandular epithelium of human prostate. The protoplasmic fracture (*PF*) face of the luminal membrane is observed in the upper left-hand part of the illustration. Note cross-fractured microvilli (*MV*). An anastomosing network of junctional fibrilis within the membrane appears as ridges (*R*) on the PF face. In the lower part of the figure, the fracture plane has deviated across the extracellular space to the adjacent glandular cell and reveals the exoplasmic fracture (*EF*) face of its lateral membrane. The network appears as grooves (*G*) on the EF face. The density of intramembranous particles is much greater on the PF face than on the EF face. The granulofibrillar patch (*arrows*) probably represents a small desmosome. (Courtesy of F. B. Merk and P. W. L. Kwan.)

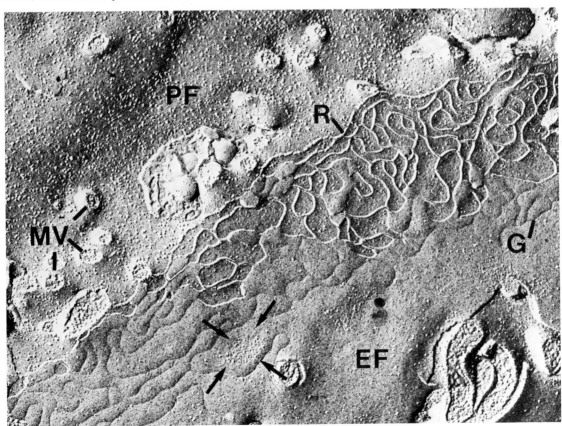

Early studies at the light microscopic level revealed a layer of amorphous material underlying epithelia that was thought to be part of the subjacent connective tissue. Although this membranelike band of material was visible in a variety of preparations, it was best shown with silver techniques or the periodic acid–Schiff (PAS) reaction. Argyrophilia (affinity to silver) of this layer suggested that it might consist of reticular fibers; the positive PAS reaction suggested a carbohydrate component.

Electron microscopic examination of this layer revealed that the basement membrane as seen in the light microscope is really composed of at least two layers or laminae (see Figs. 3-9I, 5-2). The layer closest to the epithelium is called the **basal lamina;** it is composed of glycoprotein and probably accounts for most of the PAS-positivity seen with the light microscope. The layer closest to the connective tissue is called the **reticular lamina;** it is composed of unit collagen fibrils (reticular fibers) embedded in a polysaccharide- and glycoprotein-containing matrix, which no doubt accounts for the argyrophilia and remaining PAS-positivity seen with the light microscope. It is now generally accepted that the basal lamina is elaborated by the epithelium and that the reticular lamina is a product of the subjacent connective tissue. It should be realized that the basement membrane is a composite structure and should not be confused with the basal plasma membrane of the epithelial cells.

Functionally, the basement membrane serves as an underlying support and cushion for epithelia as well as a means of epithelial attachment to subjacent connective tissue. In addition, it acts as a diffusion or filtration barrier; the most dramatic example of this property is seen in the glomerulus of the kidney, where the basement membrane serves as a primary component for ultrafiltration.

HEMIDESMOSOMES

The desmosome can be considered as a bipartite junction in which each of the essentially mirror-image components is formed by adjacent epithelial cells. However, on the basal surfaces of cells that abut on connective tissue, only half of the desmosome is formed (see Fig. 3-9J). These structures are called **hemidesmosomes.** Functionally, these specializations are thought to attach the bases of epithelial cells to the underlying basement membrane.

Specializations of the Cytoskeleton

TONOFILAMENTS (INTERMEDIATE FILAMENTS)

Tonofilaments are cytoplasmic filaments of epithelial cells that are resolved with the electron microscope or with fluorescent antikeratin antibody labeling. However, aggregates of these filaments represent the so-called tonofibrils that are visible with the light microscope without special staining. In stratified squamous epithelia, which are largely protective, the cytoskeleton is composed of an elaborate meshwork of abundant tonofilaments.

Tonofilaments is an old term for the general class of filaments of intermediate size (10 nm). In epithelial cells, intermediate filaments are composed of proteins called **keratins.** These filaments probably serve a supportive function, particularly in dissipating the stresses exerted on desmosomes and hemidesmosomes. Bundles of tonofilaments terminate in these structures (see Figs. 3-9G, J; 3-13B).

TERMINAL WEB

In certain epithelia, especially those with apical appendages, there is a region just below the apical cell border that is devoid of cellular organelles. However, this area does contain a dense accumulation of filaments running parallel to the apical surface (see Figs. 3-9A, 3-10); this margin is called the **terminal web.** Functionally, this web provides support at apical epithelial surfaces and provides an anchorage for apical appendages.

NATIONAL BOARD TYPE QUESTIONS

Select the single best response for each of the following.

1. All of the following are characteristic of surface epithelia, *except:*
   A. They cover all surfaces in the body.
   B. They contain a rich blood supply.
   C. They possess a high capability for regeneration.
   D. They give rise to exocrine glands.
   E. They originate from all three primary germ layers.

2. Which of the following structures contains a simple columnar epithelium?
   A. Blood vessels
   B. Urinary bladder
   C. Ducts of glands
   D. Integument (skin)
   E. Intestines

3. Which of the following is a function of the macula adherens (desmosome)?
   A. Mediates cell-to-cell communication
   B. Forms a permeability seal
   C. Attaches one cell to another
   D. Attaches the cell to the basement membrane
   E. Increases apical surface area

4. The following are criteria for classification of glandular epithelia, *except:*
   A. Number of cells
   B. Nature of secretion
   C. Mode of secretion
   D. Relative complexity of the duct system
   E. Amount of secretion produced

5. Epithelial tissues can be derived from
   A. mesoderm.
   B. ectoderm.
   C. ectoderm and mesoderm.
   D. ectoderm and endoderm.
   E. ectoderm, endoderm, and mesoderm.

Select the response most closely associated with each numbered item.
   A. Cilia
   B. Microvilli
   C. Both
   D. Neither

6. Apical surface specializations
7. Contain contractile elements
8. Involved in absorption
9. Contain tubulin

For the following, select
   A. if only *1, 2, and 3* are correct.
   B. if only *1 and 3* are correct.
   C. if only *2 and 4* are correct.
   D. if only *4* is correct.
   E. if *all* are correct.

10. The basement membrane
    1. is produced in its entirety by the epithelium.
    2. is positive for the PAS-reaction.
    3. contains what is referred to as the "terminal web."
    4. provides basal support for epithelia.

11. Epithelia are specialized to perform which of the following functions?
    1. Protection
    2. Sensory reception
    3. Absorption
    4. Secretion

12. Ciliated pseudostratified columnar epithelium is characteristic of the
    1. esophagus.
    2. duodenum.
    3. parotid gland.
    4. trachea.

ANNOTATED ANSWERS

1. B. Epithelia do not receive a direct blood supply but rely on blood vessels in the underlying connective tissue for their metabolic support.

2. E. Only the intestines contain a simple columnar epithelium. In this case, it is specialized for absorption.

3. C. Desmosomes are numerous at the lateral aspects of cells where they provide cell-to-cell attachments.

4. E. Glandular epithelia are classified according to cell number (e.g., unicellular), nature of the secretion (e.g., mucous), and mode of secretion (e.g., apocrine), but quantity of secretion is not used for this purpose.

5. E. Epithelial tissues can be derived from any of the three embryonic germ layers.

6. C. Both cilia and microvilli are projections from the cell's apical surface, although they perform different functions.

7. B. Only microvilli contain contractile proteins (actin) which interact with myosin in the terminal web. Ciliary motion is produced by active sliding between doublet microtubules.

8. B. Only microvilli serve to amplify the surface area for the process of absorption.

9. A. Only cilia contain the 9 + 2 arrangement of microtubules which are composed of the protein tubulin.

10. C. The basement membrane is rich in carbohydrates and is therefore PAS-positive. Its function is to provide basal support for epithelia.

11. E. Depending on their location and structure, epithelia can perform all of the listed functions.

12. D. Ciliated pseudostratified columnar epithelium is found in the trachea where it provides the "mucociliary clearing mechanism."

BIBLIOGRAPHY

Amsterdam, A., I. Ohad, and M. Schramm. Dynamic changes in the ultrastructure of the acinar cell of the rat parotid gland during the secretory cycle. *J. Cell Biol.* 41:753, 1969.

Borysenko, J. Z., and J.-P. Revel. Experimental manipulation of desmosome structure. *Am. J. Anat.* 137:403, 1973.

Bretcher, A., and K. Weber. Localization of action and microfilament-associated proteins in the microvilli and terminal web of the intestinal brush border by immunofluorescence microscopy. *J. Cell Biol.* 79:839, 1978.

Claude, P., and D. A. Goodenough. Fracture faces of zonulae occludentes from "tight" and "leaky" epithelia. *J. Cell Biol.* 58:390, 1973.

Dodson, J. W., and E. D. Hay. Secretion of collagenous stroma by isolated epithelium grown in vitro. *Exp. Cell Res.* 65:215, 1971.

Drenckhahn, D., and V. Gröschel-Steward. Localization of myosin, actin, and tropomyosin in rat intestinal epithelium: Immunohistochemical studies at the light and electron microscope levels. *J. Cell Biol.* 86:475, 1980.

Farquhar, M. G., and G. E. Palade. Junctional complexes in various epithelia. *J. Cell Biol.* 17:375, 1963.

Fawcett, D. W. Surface specializations of absorbing cells. *J. Histochem. Cytochem.* 13:75, 1965.

Freeman, J. A. Goblet cell fine structure. *Anat. Rec.* 154:121, 1966.

Gibbons, I. R. The Structure and Composition of Cilia. In K. B. Warren (ed.), *Formation and Fate of Cell Organelles.* New York: Academic, 1967. P. 99.

Goodenough, D. A., and J.-P. Revel. A fine structure analysis of intercellular junctions in the mouse liver. *J. Cell Biol.* 45:272, 1970.

Herman, I. M., and T. D. Pollard. Electron microscopic localization of cytoplasmic myosin with ferritin-labeled antibodies. *J. Cell Biol.* 88:346, 1981.

Hirokawa, N., and J. E. Heuser. Quick-freeze, deep-etch visualization of the cytoskeleton surface differentiations of intestinal epithelial cells. *J. Cell Biol.* 91:399, 1981.

Hull, B. E., and L. A. Staehelin. The terminal web: A reevaluation of its structure and function. *J. Cell Biol.* 81:67, 1979.

Ito, S. The surface coat of enteric microvilli. *J. Cell Biol.* 27:475, 1965.

Leblond, C. P., and G. Bennett. Elaboration and Turnover of Cell Coat Glycoproteins. In A. A. Moscona (ed.), *The Cell Surface in Development.* New York: Wiley, 1974. P. 29.

Lentz, T., and J. P. Trinkaus. Differentiation of the junctional complex of surface cells. *J. Cell Biol.* 48:455, 1971.

Linck, R. W. The structure of microtubules. *Ann. N.Y. Acad. Sci.,* 383:98, 1982.

Linck, R. W., et al. Tektin filaments: Chemically unique filaments of sperm flagellar microtubules. *Cell Motility* 1 (Suppl.):127, 1982.

Loewenstein, W. R. Permeability of the Junctional Membrane Channel. In B. R. Brinkley and K. R. Porter (eds.), *International Cell Biology, 1976–1977.* New York: Rockefeller University Press, 1977.

McKeithan, T. W., and J. L. Rosenbaum. Multiple forms of tubulin in the cytoskeletal and flagellar microtubules of *Polytomella. J. Cell Biol.* 91:352, 1981.

McNutt, N. S., and R. S. Weinstein. Membrane ultra-structure at mammalian intercellular junctions. *Prog. Biophys. Mol. Biol.* 26:47, 1973.

Mooseker, M. S. Brush border motility. Microvillar contraction in triton-treated brush borders isolated from intestinal epithelium. *J. Cell Biol.* 71:417, 1976.

Mooseker, M. S., and L. G. Tilney. Organization of an actin filament-membrane complex: Filament polarity and membrane attachment in the microvilli of intestinal cells. *J. Cell Biol.* 67:725, 1975.

Overton, J. Experimental manipulation of desmosome formation. *J. Cell Biol.* 56:636, 1973.

Pierce, G. B., A. R. Midgley, and J. Sri Ram. Histogenesis of basement membrane. *J. Exp. Med.* 117:339, 1963.

Porter, K. R., and M. A. Bonneville. *Fine Structure of Cells and Tissues.* Philadelphia: Lea & Febiger, 1968.

Rodewald, R., S. B. Newman, and M. J. Karnovsky. Contraction of isolated brush borders from the intestinal epithelium. *J. Cell Biol.* 70:541, 1976.

Schaumburg-Lever, G., and W. F. Lever. Secretion from human apocrine glands: An electron microscope study. *J. Invest. Dermatol.* 64:38, 1975.

Simonescu, M., and N. Simonescu. Organization of cell junctions in the peritoneal mesothelium. *J. Cell Biol.* 74:98, 1977.

Simons, K., and S. D. Fuller. Cell surface polarity in epithelia. *Ann. Rev. Cell Biol.* 1:243, 1985.

Staehelin, L. A. Structure and function of intercellular junctions. *Int. Rev. Cytol.* 39:191, 1974.

Staehelin, L. A., and B. E. Hull. Junctions between living cells. *Sci. Am.* 238:140, 1978.

Stephens, R. E. Structural Chemistry of the Axoneme: Evidence for Chemically and Functionally Unique Tubulin Dimers in Outer Fibers. In S. Inoué and R. E. Stephens (eds.), *Molecules and Cell Movement.* New York: Raven Press, 1975. P. 181.

Suzuki, F., and T. Nagano. Development of tight junctions in the caput epididymal epithelium of the mouse. *Dev. Biol.* 63:321, 1978.

Tamarin, A. Myoepithelium of the rat submaxillary gland. *J. Ultrastruct. Res.* 16:320, 1966.

Weinstein, R. S., and N. S. McNutt. Cell junctions. *N. Engl. J. Med.* 286:521, 1972.

4 Blood

Objectives

You will learn the following in this chapter:

How to identify the distinguishing features of the four major types of connective tissues

The composition of blood and the relative proportions of each major component

The usefulness of examining blood microscopically

The three main stages of blood cell development (hemopoiesis)

How to recognize erythrocytes, platelets, and each type of leukocyte in a blood film

The life cycle, the normal aging process, and replacement of erythrocytes

The five types of leukocytes in descending order of incidence and a primary function for each

The mechanisms of blood coagulation and their regulation

Blood is a connective tissue composed of free cells in a fluid interstitium, the plasma. The other connective tissues have some general features in common with blood, in that they maintain cellular populations in an extracellular ground substance. Aside from cellular variability, the main structural difference is that the other connective tissue types possess a variety of extracellular fibers, whereas blood does not have fibers except in the specific instance of blood clot formation. Table 4-1 highlights the distinguishing features of the basic connective tissue types.

Blood is an important homeostatic force that integrates bodily functions. It circulates throughout the body in an enclosed system of channels, propelled by the contraction of the heart, elastic recoil of the large arteries, and movement of muscles, to distribute heat, gases,

nutrients, waste, cells, hormones, antibodies, and other substances to the required regions.

When a blood sample is exposed to air, a clot rapidly forms, trapping the cells in its fibrous matrix. The remaining clear fluid is called **serum.** If clot formation is prevented by heparin or citrate, the blood cells settle freely, composing 45 percent of the total blood volume. The **plasma** composes the remaining 55 percent (Fig. 4-1). Serum, then, is plasma minus the clotting factors when centrifuged. The percentage of packed volume of cellular elements is called the **hematocrit.** Of the usual 45 percent value for normal persons, erythrocytes (red blood cells) compose about 44 percent. The remaining 1 percent comprises leukocytes (white blood cells), which settle loosely in a thin layer on top of the erythrocytes. This layer is often referred to as the **buffy coat.**

A routine examination of whole blood can be a

Table 4-1. Types of Connective Tissue and Their Distinguishing Features

| Type of Connective Tissue | Nature of Interstitium | Cell Types | | Fiber Pattern |
		Free	Fixed	
Blood	Fluid	+	−	None
Connective tissue proper				
Loose	Sol-gel	+	+	Loose
Dense	Sol-gel	Few	+	Dense
Cartilage	Hard gel	−	+	Dense
Bone	Calcified matrix	−	+	Dense

Fig. 4-1. The proportions of the major blood components after centrifugation.

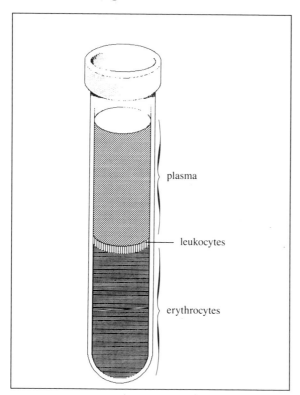

plasma

leukocytes

erythrocytes

valuable diagnostic tool. For example, in patients with anemic conditions the blood has a pale appearance and shows a low hematocrit. High lipid levels give the blood a yellowish hue (lipidemia). Infections usually elevate the leukocyte count in peripheral blood, resulting in larger than normal buffy coats: in some leukemias, the leukocyte layer may be even larger than the erythrocyte layer.

Microscopic examination of blood can reveal alterations in the size and shape of cells, particularly in diseases of the erythrocyte. Furthermore, the determination of the relative proportions of each leukocyte type, called a **differential count,** is extremely valuable not only in diagnosing particular diseases but also in assessing the general health of the patient.

PLASMA

Plasma is a yellowish fluid that acts as a medium for circulating cells and metabolic substances. The fluid constituents of plasma and those of connective tissue proper are closely related in chemical composition and function. Substances are exchanged bidirectionally at the capillary–connective tissue level. The integrative functions of blood largely reflect this intimate relationship.

The primary components of plasma are water, inorganic salts, and a number of proteins, which are classified according to their net charge and resulting migration pattern in an electrical field (electrophoresis; Fig. 4-2).

Albumin is the most abundant plasma protein; its primary function is to maintain the colloid blood pressure so that blood does not lose an excess of fluid to the connective tissues at the capillary level. It is also a carrier of free fatty acids. The globulins are another class of plasma proteins of diverse size and functions. The **gamma (γ) globulins** are of particular interest since they include the circulating antibodies, which play an important role in the immune system. The **beta (β) globulins** are important in the transport of hormones, metal ions, and lipids.

In addition, plasma carries certain particles that are visible microscopically. **Chylomicra** are

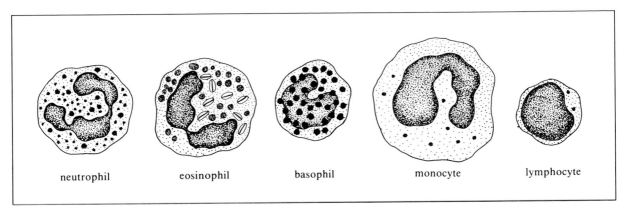

neutrophil　　　eosinophil　　　basophil　　　monocyte　　　lymphocyte

Fig. 4-2. Electrophoretic pattern of normal pooled human serum. The concentrations of the protein fractions are determined from the areas under the respective peaks. The δ-anomaly at the extreme right does not represent another protein fraction. (From Bulletin 2175, American Instrument Co., 1949. Reproduced by permission.)

refractile fatty bodies, which are particularly prominent after a fatty meal. **Hemoconia** are small particles of diverse origin, although most are thought to be fragments of cells.

THE FORMED ELEMENTS

The two broad classes of blood cells are the **erythrocytes** and the **leukocytes.** There are several types of leukocytes, which are classified according to their structural and histochemical features in Romanovsky-stained smears. This method groups the leukocytes into two categories: those with specific granules, the **granulocytes,** and those without specific granules, the **agranulocytes.** These groups are subdivided according to the staining qualities of their cytoplasmic granules and their nuclear configuration, as follows:

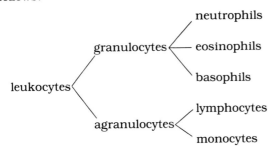

In addition, the blood contains other formed elements, which are not cells but consist of cellular fragments, called **platelets,** which play the major role in the clotting mechanism. Erythrocytes and platelets perform their functions intravascularly, whereas the leukocytes are merely carried by the blood and perform their functions in connective tissue.

Hemopoiesis (Blood Cell Formation)

There are three major stages or periods of hemopoiesis: an embryonic mesoblastic period; a fetal hepatic period; and a fetal, adolescent, and adult myeloid period. In the third week of human embryonic development, yolk sac mesenchymal cells form the stem cells for the blood cell series. Simultaneously, the blood vessels form from the adjacent mesenchyme. During this mesoblastic period of hemopoiesis the earliest hemoglobin-synthesizing cells, **primitive erythroblasts,** are nucleated cells derived from yolk sac stem cells.

By approximately the sixth week of embryonic life the fetal liver serves as the major site of hemopoiesis. Here, erythrocytes, and to a lesser degree granulocytes, develop in small subcapsular foci. Hemopoiesis also occurs in the spleen at about the same time.

As the bones of the fetus develop, the bone marrow becomes more prominent and is established as a major source of blood cells by the end of gestation; it continues as the primary stem cell source throughout adult life. **Medullary hemopoiesis** denotes blood cell formation in the bone marrow, whereas **extramedullary hemopoiesis** denotes blood cell formation in organs and tissues other than bone marrow.

The bone marrow produces the erythrocytes, granulocytes, monocytes, and platelets and supplies stem cells for the lymphocyte subpopulations to the thymus and the other lymphoid organs (see Chap. 10). Whether these cells originate from a single stem cell (monophyletic) or from more than one (polyphyletic) is still somewhat controversial. Recent evidence supports the concept that the various cell lines can originate from the same stem cell. A hemopoietic stem cell is thus defined as a cell capable of differentiating into any of the blood cells as well as maintaining itself by mitotic division. Experimentally, when such a cell is placed in an inductive environment, it will give rise to a large clone of cells; thus, it is referred to as a **colony-forming unit** (CFU). These stem cell colonies, in turn, can give rise to more differentiated colonies, such as those that contain exclusively erythrocyte or granulocyte cell lines.

Once differentiation begins, the erythrocytes and granulocytes go through a series of transformations leading to mature cells, which then leave the bone marrow and enter the circulation. On the other hand, the lymphocytes and monocytes enter the circulation as relatively immature cells, maturing at a later time in other tissues and organs of the body.

Erythrocytes

Mature erythrocytes are anucleate cells shaped like biconcave disks, 8 × 2 μm in dimension (Fig. 4-3B). This shape provides more surface area for gas exchange than a sphere. Erythrocytes are devoid of the usual organelles and maintain no capacity for protein synthesis. Instead, each cell is packed with **hemoglobin,** the iron-containing molecules that bind and carry

Fig. 4-3. Erythrocytes. A. Erythrocytes in various states and profiles. B. Scanning electron micrograph of human erythrocytes. (Courtesy of P.-S. Lin.) Inset: erythrocytes as seen through the light microscope.

A

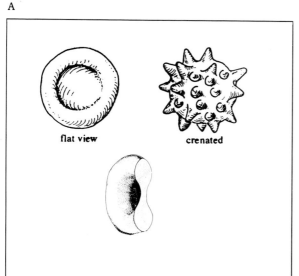

flat view   crenated

B

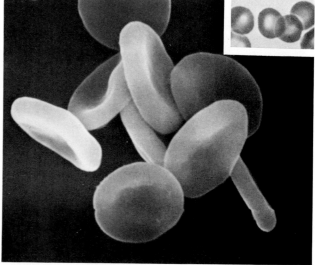

oxygen and carbon dioxide. Hemoglobin is a conjugated protein consisting of four polypeptide chains, each bound to an iron-containing heme group. The structure of the globin chains is genetically determined. A number of inherited disorders in hemoglobin synthesis involve minor amino acid substitutions but nevertheless result in severe physiologic disorders. The best known among these disorders is sickle cell anemia. In this disease, a single amino acid substitution results in less soluble hemoglobin molecules, which cause deformation and rigidity of the erythrocytes. Because of their lack of flexibility, they tend to block capillaries and are prone to lysis. They are also easily trapped and degraded by the phagocytic cells of the spleen, liver, and bone marrow early in the normal erythrocyte life span.

Erythrocytes are normally very flexible but possess no motility of their own. They become cup-shaped when passing through small capillaries and aggregate into stacks, called **rouleaux,** in standing or slow-flowing blood. They can become greatly deformed when passing through small spaces. The subplasmalemmal framework is composed of **spectrin,** which maintains the biconcave shape and provides flexibility.

The tonicity of plasma is 0.9% sodium chloride. Erythrocytes are extremely sensitive to changes in their osmotic environment. In hypertonic solutions, erythrocytes lose water and shrink (**crenation**); in hypotonic solutions, they take in water, swell, and burst (**hemolysis**). The erythrocyte will also undergo hemolysis when antibody to one of its antigens (ABO or Rh factor) interacts with a serum protein, called **complement,** as when two incompatible blood types are mixed.

THE LIFE CYCLE OF ERYTHROCYTES

The life span of an erythrocyte is about 120 days. After a series of division and differentiation steps in bone marrow (**erythropoiesis**), the erythrocytes extrude their nuclei and enter the circulation. Erythropoiesis is regulated by a glycoprotein hormone produced by the kidneys, termed **erythropoietin.** Erythropoietin is released in response to inadequate oxygen in the blood (hypoxia) due to such conditions as hemorrhage, high altitude, or vascular disease. It accelerates erythropoiesis by stimulating both the differentiation of stem cells into erythroblasts and the release of erythrocytes from the bone marrow.

Normal numbers of circulating erythrocytes are maintained by erythropoietin's stimulatory effects on the bone marrow and an adequate supply of dietary iron for the synthesis of hemoglobin. This mechanism provides the means for continuous replacement of senescent erythrocytes. In cases of significant blood loss, this mechanism permits a much more rapid increase in erythrocyte formation, several times greater than the normal turnover rate.

Before release from the bone marrow into the peripheral circulation, erythroblasts go through two distinct morphologic stages that reflect their approaching function in life. First, they acquire substantial numbers of ribosomes for production of enzymes and hemoglobin. This is the stage of the **basophilic erythroblast,** referring to its appearance on the light microscopic level. This stage is followed by a stage in which hemoglobin synthesis has begun and this product is beginning to accumulate in the cytoplasm. In addition, the chromatin condenses as the developmental functions of the nucleus terminate and extrusion of the nucleus is imminent. Now the light microscopic appearance is that of a **polychromatophilic erythroblast.** The nucleus is then extruded, before the erythrocyte's entry into the peripheral circulation. However, in some hemopoietic pathologies, circulating erythroblasts are diagnostic.

Somewhat less than 1 percent of the peripheral erythrocytes exhibit a slight basophilia due to the residual presence of ribosomal RNA. Exposure to supravital stains, such as methylene blue or cresyl violet, causes these organelles to clump, yielding a "reticular" cytoplasmic appearance. Thus, they are called **reticulocytes** (also known as **polychromatophilic erythrocytes**). Reticulocyte counts provide a rough estimate of the rate of erythropoiesis and are used to determine response to treatment of diseases in which erythrocytes are diminished in number. Pernicious anemia is caused by inadequate intestinal absorption of dietary vitamin B_{12} due to insufficient release of gastric intrinsic factor. Vitamin B_{12} is required for maturation of erythrocytes. As a consequence, the erythrocyte count is abnormally low, which is reflected by a commensurate decline in the reticulocyte count. Following parenteral administration of vitamin B_{12}, the reticulocyte count becomes significantly elevated, sometimes to as much as 40 percent of the total erythrocyte count, which reflects an acceleration of erythropoiesis and entry of new erythrocytes into the circulation. The reticulocyte count is always highest during the recovery phase from anemia and gradually declines to normal as the erythrocyte count is restored.

When erythrocytes mature, they lose their capacity for protein synthesis and aerobic metabolism. They derive their energy from glycolysis, most of which is used to maintain hemoglobin in a reduced state and to maintain proper internal ion concentrations by active transport.

Erythrocytes become senescent (old) when they have used up most of the enzymes necessary to maintain adenosine triphosphate (ATP) production. Since they are unable to replace these enzymes, energy-dependent systems such as the calcium pump can no longer be maintained. As the intracellular calcium levels rise, the cell becomes rigid because of calcium cross-linkage with denatured proteins, and it can no longer pass the filtration barriers. In many erythrocyte pathologies, this normal aging process is greatly accelerated so that the cells become prematurely rigid and thus are easily trapped and damaged. For example, in sickle cell anemia, genetically defective hemoglobin polymerizes, distorting the cell shape and allowing abnormal calcium influx (beyond what the calcium pump can handle). This results in rigidity, damage, and death of the cell.

At the end of 120 days of life, the senescent erythrocytes are trapped, engulfed, and degraded by phagocytic cells of the liver, spleen, and bone marrow. Hemoglobin is degraded into bilirubin, while the released iron is complexed with protein and stored as **ferritin** or **hemosiderin** and then reincorporated into the hemoglobin by developing erythrocytes.

Leukocytes

For the most part, leukocytes (white blood cells) are connective tissue cells that use the vascular system for transport from the hemopoietic tissue, the bone marrow, to areas where their services are required. In contrast to erythrocytes, leukocytes are nucleated and motile cells. Their motility allows them to migrate through the walls of small venules (the postcapillary venules) into connective tissue spaces, where they perform phagocytic, immunologic, and related functions.

Leukocytes are active in the repair of tissue damage and in fighting infection. They play a direct role in the inflammatory reactions. **Acute inflammation** is of short duration and primarily involves neutrophils, whereas **chronic inflammation** is of longer duration and involves many of the blood and connective tissue cells. The chronology of events involved in inflammatory responses is summarized in the next chapter, since these reactions occur primarily in the connective tissue proper.

The leukocytes normally constitute about 1 percent of the total blood count. Their number is actually highly variable and may greatly exceed the normal range during acute inflammation. The relative proportions of the various types is fairly constant, as determined by differential counts. Severe alteration (depletion or elevation) of one or more of the leukocyte types may reflect a disease process. The relative numbers and distinguishing features of the different types of leukocytes are summarized in Table 4-2.

THE LIFE CYCLE OF LEUKOCYTES

The granular leukocytes develop in the bone marrow (**myelopoiesis**) and remain in the circulation for only a few days. After performing their functions in the connective tissue, most disintegrate

Table 4-2. Characteristics of Different Types of Leukocytes in Peripheral Blood

Leukocyte Type	% of Total Leukocytes	Cell Diameter (in μm)	Nucleus	Cytoplasmic Granules Specific	Cytoplasmic Granules Nonspecific
Granulocytes					
Neutrophils	60–75	10–12	Several lobes	+	+
Eosinophils	1–3	10–12	Usually two lobes	+	−
Basophils	0.5–1	8–10	S- or U-shaped	+	−
Agranulocytes					
Monocytes	3–8	9–15	Indented or U-shaped	−	+
Lymphocytes	20–40	5–8	Round	−	+

and are phagocytized by macrophages. The total life span of granular leukocytes is 8 to 12 days. Monocytes usually live for several months, while the life span of lymphocytes varies from a few days to several years. Long-lived lymphocytes are regarded as "memory" cells. Senescent leukocytes that remain in the blood are removed from circulation by the phagocytic cells of the liver and spleen.

THE GRANULOCYTES

The granulocytes are categorized according to the affinity of their specific granules for Romanovsky-type stains. Blood smears are prepared on glass slides, allowed to air-dry, fixed in methanol, and then stained with a Romanovsky dye mixture. This mixture contains the ionized dyes eosin −, methylene blue +, and the azures + as well as a number of neutral dyes which stain leukocytes with a variety of rich colors.

Neutrophils

The neutrophils (Fig. 4-4) are the most abundant leukocytes. When they are first released into the blood, their nuclei are unsegmented; thus, they are known as band neutrophils in this immature form. As they mature, their nuclei become increasingly lobular. Most circulating neutrophils are seen as possessing three to five lobes, connected by chromatin strands. A condensed ex-

tension from one of the lobes, in the shape of a drumstick, can be seen in about 3 percent of the neutrophils in the female and represents the inactive X chromosome. Because of the variability in nuclear shape, the neutrophil is often referred to as a **polymorphonuclear leukocyte,** or "poly" for short.

Neutrophils possess two populations of cytoplasmic granules. Small, specific granules that stain with neutral dyes compose the more abundant population (80%). These appear as tiny pink granules, barely visible with the light microscope. These granules contain the antibacterial substances **lactoferrin, lysozyme,** and **cobalamin-binding protein.** The smaller population (20%) consists of nonspecific azurophilic granules that are larger in size and are essentially primary lysosomes containing peroxidase, acid hydrolase, acid phosphatase, and other enzymes involved in antibacterial digestive functions. Like the specific granules, these granules also contain lysozyme.

Neutrophils are chemotactically attracted to areas in which bacteria and other foreign substances are present. Substances known as **chemotactic factors** are generated at the inflammatory site and diffuse into the surrounding tissues. Neutrophils move toward their source in response to the concentration gradient of the chemotactic factors. Many of these factors are liberated from damaged bacteria, although there are also a wide range of host factors, such as

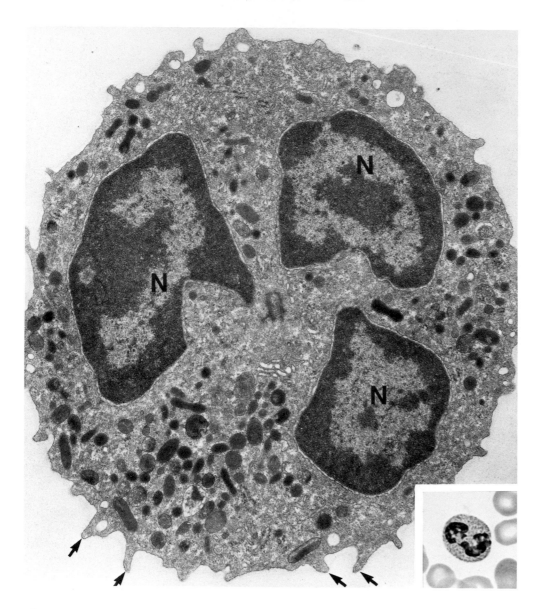

Fig. 4-4. Electron micrograph of a human neutrophil. Note the presence of three lobes of the nucleus (*N*) and numerous cytoplasmic granules of various shapes and sizes. A centriole can be seen in the center of the cell. Short microvilli project from the cell surface (*arrows*). (From A. M. Marmont, E. Damasio, and D. Zucker-Franklin, Neutrophils. In D. Zucker-Franklin et al. (eds.), *Atlas of Blood Cells*, Vol. 1. Milan: Edi Ermes, 1981. By permission of the publisher and D. Zucker-Franklin.) Inset: light micrograph of a neutrophil.

those generated by complement activation and factors released from activated macrophages. Activated platelets and secondary products of coagulation also play a prominent role in neutrophil chemotaxis. Neutrophil phagocytosis of bacteria and other particulate substances is greatly enhanced by certain serum proteins, called **opsonins,** which become attached to the particles. The distal ends of these proteins bind to receptors on the neutrophil membrane, which signals the neutrophil to ingest the particle. Specific antibacterial antibodies of the IgG class and a protein formed by complement activation are very efficient opsonins in this regard.

The presence of neutrophils in histologic section indicates an area of acute inflammation. In these regions, neutrophils phagocytize bacteria in large numbers. The phagosomes fuse with the two types of granules, their enzymes degrading the bacteria. Bacterial killing is also promoted by a process referred to as the **respiratory burst,** in which neutrophils actively metabolize oxygen to produce more bactericidal substances. While fighting infection, they die in large numbers, forming the primary component of pus in an abscess. As they die, new neutrophils are produced. The increased production is seen in the increased number of circulating neutrophils, particularly the band neutrophils.

Eosinophils

Eosinophils (Fig. 4-5) are usually seen with bilobed nuclei and an abundance of orange-red cytoplasmic granules. These granules are known to contain hydrolytic enzymes and peroxidase; in this respect they are typical lysosomes. In addition, they contain a number of other substances that modulate allergic responses and assist in the rejection of parasites.

Eosinophils are present in small numbers in chronic inflammatory reactions. Although they do not phagocytize bacteria and other particulate antigens directly, they avidly phagocytize antigen-antibody complexes, including antibody-coated bacteria. Eosinophils commonly occur in the connective tissues of the respiratory and digestive tracts. Elevated eosinophil numbers are evident in these regions, as well as in peripheral blood during allergic responses (e.g., hay fever and asthma) and parasitic infections. Under these conditions, eosinophils are rapidly mobilized from large reserves in the bone marrow. They are chemotactically attracted to areas where allergic reactions occur. It is generally thought that eosinophils regulate allergic responses by degrading the vasoactive substances—histamine, and leukotrienes produced by basophils and their connective tissue cousins, the mast cells. Eosinophils contain **histaminase** and the enzyme **arylsulphatase,** which degrade histamine and leukotrienes, respectively. The hormone hydrocortisone, which depresses allergic and immune reactions, also causes a marked decline in circulating eosinophils by inhibiting the mobilization of the eosinophil reserve from the bone marrow.

It has recently been established that eosinophils play a central role in the control of certain parasitic diseases, such as **schistosomiasis.** Again, antiparasite antibody potentiates the action of eosinophils. **Major basic protein** (MBP), contained in the crystalloid cores of the granules, is released onto the surface of parasites and promotes antibody-dependent killing of parasites.

Basophils

Basophils (Fig. 4-6) are a rare but distinctive cell type. They usually possess bilobed or U-shaped nuclei, large metachromatic or basophilic granules (1 μm in diameter), and prominent Golgi complexes. The granules contain a number of pharmacologically active mediators and some **glycosaminoglycans.** A strongly anionic, sulfated mucopolysaccharide accounts for the metachromatic staining qualities of the granules. This property, widely attributed to heparin, is actually due to the presence of chondroitin sulfates.

The basophil resembles the connective tissue mast cell in structure and function. Although they are thought to arise from separate precursor cells, the basophil and the mast cell may be con-

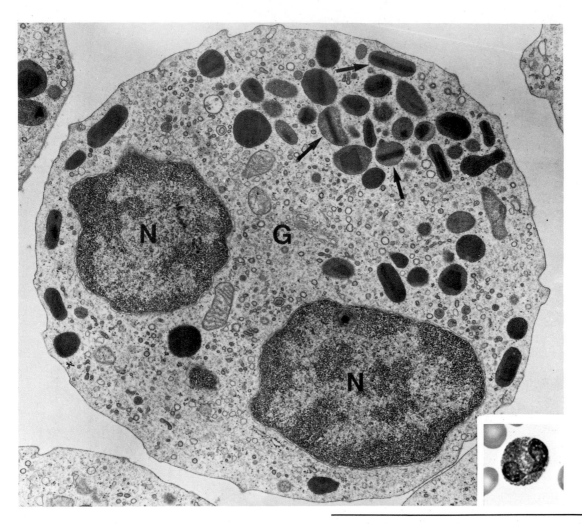

Fig. 4-5. Electron micrograph of a human eosinophil. Both lobes of the nucleus (*N*) can be seen. Most of the granules are polarized at one side of the cell; some contain an electron-dense crystalloid core (*arrows*). Part of the golgi complex (*G*) can be seen in the center of the cell. (Reproduced with permission from D. Zucker-Franklin, Eosinophil Function and Disorders. In G. H. Stollerman et al. (eds.). *Advances in Internal Medicine*, Vol. 19. © 1974 by Year Book Medical Publishers, Inc., Chicago, and with permission of D. Zucker-Franklin.) Inset: light micrograph of an eosinophil.

Fig. 4-6. Basophils. A. An electron micrograph of a human basophil showing four lightly stained lobes of the nucleus (*N*), typical cytoplasmic granules (*arrows*), and aggregated glycogen (*GL*). There is no evidence of granule extrusion. The cell on the right is a lymphocyte. Inset: a light micrograph of a basophil. B. An electron micrograph of a nearly completed degranulating human basophil showing individual granule and granule-membrane extrusion at the cell's perimeter (*black arrows*). These extruded granules and membranes are labeled on their surfaces with cationized ferritin. Only two unaltered granules remain (*white arrows*). (From A. Dvorak et al., Complement-induced degranulation of human basophils. *J. Immunol.* 126:523, 1981. By permission of the Williams & Wilkins Co., Baltimore.)

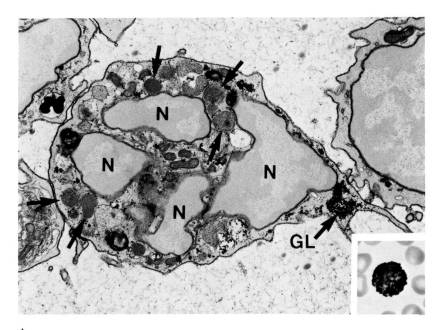

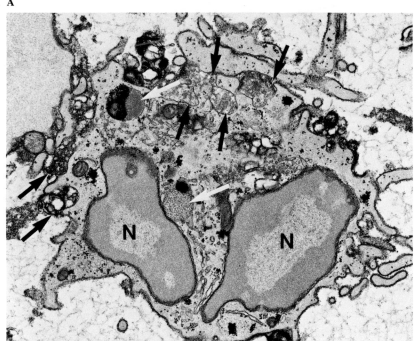

sidered part of the same system. Both are involved in increasing vascular permeability during inflammation and both bind a particular immunoglobulin, IgE, which is produced by plasma cells. In allergic reactions, the allergen (antigen) combines with this immunoglobulin, causing acute degranulation (Fig. 4-6B). The release of histamine and other mediators promotes migration of leukocytes from the circulation into connective tissue and may cause severe local swelling or in extreme cases lead to anaphylactic shock. Additional information on basophil/mast cell mediators is found in the next chapter (see Mast Cells).

THE AGRANULOCYTES

The nongranular leukocytes are often referred to as **mononuclear leukocytes** because of the singular structure of their nuclei. Although they contain no specific granules, they frequently contain a number of azurophilic granules (staining with azure dyes), which are characteristic of primary lysosomes.

Monocytes

Monocytes (Fig. 4-7) are immature macrophages that are in transit to connective tissue. Even

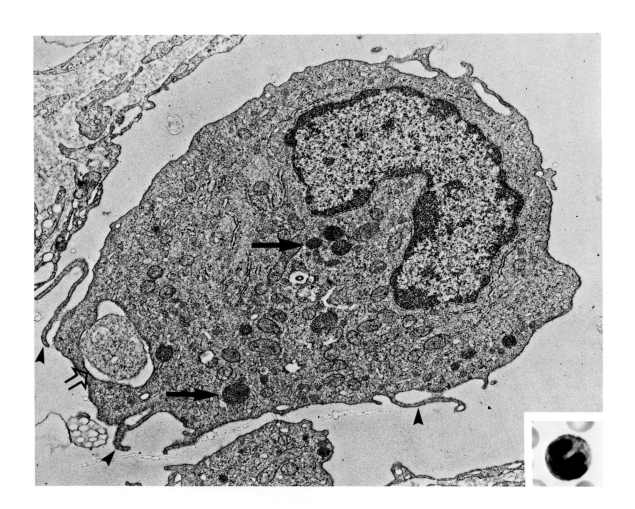

while in circulation, monocytes are highly phagocytic. The monocyte nucleus is usually indented (kidney- or horseshoe-shaped) and rather pale in color. A small number of azurophilic granules containing hydrolytic enzymes are usually present.

Monocytes circulate in the blood for a day or two. Upon entering the connective tissues, they differentiate into macrophages; here they may undergo further division and enzyme synthesis. The macrophages are highly motile, manifesting numerous **pseudopodia,** a characteristic already evident in the monocytes. The structure and functions of tissue macrophages are discussed in the next chapter.

Lymphocytes

Lymphocytes (Fig. 4-8) of various sizes occur in the blood. For convenience, they are arbitrarily categorized according to their size: small (5–8 μm), medium (10–12 μm), and large (14–15 μm). The small lymphocyte is predominant and represents the end cell in lymphocyte differentiation. However, small lymphocytes can recirculate back to the lymphoid organs and upon antigenic stimulation are capable of transforming into large lymphocytes (**blastogenic transformation**). The large lymphocytes (**lymphoblasts**) then divide repeatedly, giving rise to generations of medium, then small lymphocytes, which are identical with the original small lymphocytes in terms

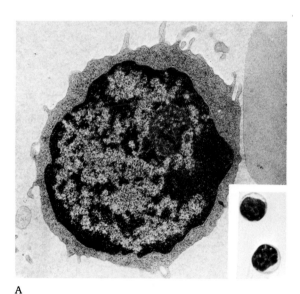

A

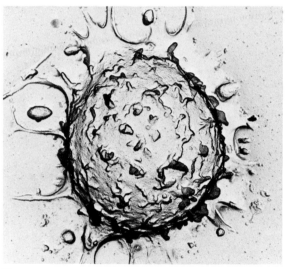

B

◁—————————————————————————

Fig. 4-7. An electron micrograph of a turtle monocyte. In spite of the phylogenetic distance, turtle monocytes closely resemble those of humans. Note the U-shaped nucleus and lysosomes (*arrows*). Although it is an immature macrophage, it already shows evidence of motility, with pseudopodia extending from the surface (*arrowheads*) and phagocytosis (*open arrow*). Inset: light micrograph of a monocyte.

Fig. 4-8. Lymphocytes. A. An electron micrograph of a human small lymphocyte. Note the heterochromatic nucleus, thin rim of cytoplasm filled with ribosomes, and short microvilli. The cell is close to an erythrocyte (*upper right*) (Courtesy of W. Woods and A. Ucci.) Inset: light micrograph of small lymphocytes. B. An elecron micrograph of a surface cast replica of a lymphocyte. The nucleus bulges from the central part of the cell. The cytoplasmic rim is seen as its pseudopodia spread on the glass surface. Short microvilli can be seen projecting from the surface over the nuclear region.

of their specific reactivity with a given antigen. Large lymphocytes are found primarily in the lymphoid organs; medium and small lymphocytes occur in the lymphoid organs and in blood. Large lymphocytes are rarely found in normal peripheral blood.

The nuclei of small lymphocytes are heterochromatic and nearly round, but often slightly indented on one side. The surrounding small rim of cytoplasm is quite basophilic because of the presence of numerous free ribosomes. Occasional azurophilic granules are also present. The nuclei of medium lymphocytes are somewhat less heterochromatic, and the relative cytoplasmic volume is larger. Large lymphocytes are, again, proportionally larger. Their euchromatic nuclei reflect their mitotic potential.

Lymphocytes perform a central function in **immune responses.** Such responses involve antigenic interaction with lymphocyte membrane receptors, interaction of lymphocytes with macrophages and other ancillary cells, transformation and proliferation of lymphocytes, and the synthesis and release of antibodies and chemical mediators by lymphocytes and their close relatives, the plasma cells. Such reactions effectively inactivate and eliminate foreign substances. Lymphocytes and plasma cells are common in sites of chronic inflammation, where their presence is indicative of immunologic involvement.

Lymphocytes are also classified according to life span. Short-lived lymphocytes live only a few days, whereas long-lived lymphocytes may survive months or even years. The latter type are thought to be "memory" cells. Subpopulations of lymphocytes exist, which mature in different lymphoid organs, possess different membrane receptors, and play different roles in the immune system. Additional details on lymphocyte development and function are given in Chapter 10.

Platelets

Although **platelets** have been implicated in pathologic processes such as atherosclerosis, inflammation, and vasospasm, their normal role is to arrest bleeding (**hemostasis**) and to orchestrate the blood clotting mechanism (**thrombosis**).

Platelets (thrombocytes) are the smallest formed elements of blood, being about 2 to 4 μm long and shaped like flattened, convex disks (Fig. 4-9). About one-third of the body's platelets are stored in the spleen. In the circulation they tend to flow in a dispersed state unless activated by various stimuli that initiate the blood clotting mechanism. However, in blood smears they tend to form small clusters, having a natural tendency to adhere to one another.

Platelets are actually cytoplasmic fragments of **megakaryocytes,** very large multilobed cells found in the bone marrow that are derived from the same stem cell as the other myeloid cells. Each megakaryocyte produces about 1,000 to 5,000 platelets. Since platelets are cytoplasmic fragments, they have no nuclei. With the light microscope two regions of the cytoplasm are distinguishable: the **granulomere** and the **hyalomere.** The granulomere is the central zone containing granules that appear purple with conventional blood stains. The granulomere is surrounded by the hyalomere, which is the homogeneous, pale-blue rim of the platelet. In elec-

Fig. 4-9. A light micrograph of platelets as they usually appear in a blood smear. Upon exposure to air, the tiny cell fragments aggregate, which is the initial step in clot formation.

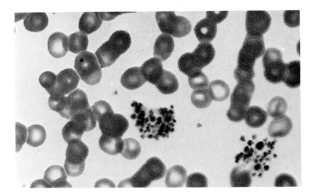

tron micrographs, the hyalomere contains a circumferential bundle of microtubules and some microfilaments. Together these elements of the cytoskeleton probably participate in secretion of platelet substances and coordinate changes in platelet shape that accompany secretion. An activated platelet changes from a flat, convex disk (discocyte) to a rounder shape with conical surface projections (echinocyte) during secretion.

The granulomere contains three types of granules: **dense granules, alpha granules,** and **lysosomes.** Dense granules contain serotonin, ADP, ATP, and calcium. Alpha granules contain platelet-specific proteins such as fibrinogen and other clotting factors involved in the coagulation process.

Hemostasis and thrombosis prevent blood loss and are achieved by several mechanisms. Platelets as well as plasma coagulation proteins and vascular endothelial cells play an integral role in this process. The platelet's normal disk shape is maintained in the circulation except when it is exposed to damaged endothelium or subendothelium. Such exposure triggers a "series of amplifying reactions" initiated by the platelets' (1) adhesion to subendothelial collagen to which they have high affinity, (2) change in shape, and (3) degranulation. A loose **primary hemostatic plug** or **platelet plug** is formed when ADP is released from either platelets or damaged tissues. The secretion of ADP and enzymes causes **thromboxane A** to form in the plasma, which activates other platelets to accumulate, forming the platelet plug. Thromboxane A, like serotonin, is also a potent vasoconstrictor and functions to reduce bleeding from vascular wounds.

Activated substances from platelets, as well as the damaged vascular wall and plasma proteins, initiate the clotting process. Platelets accelerate coagulation reactions due to the binding of the clotting factors to their surface. These factors convert **prothrombin** to **thrombin** on the platelet surface. The resulting thrombin then promotes **primary aggregation** of platelets by recruiting additional platelets from the circulating blood for attachment to those already attached to the vas-

cular wound. Thrombin also stimulates the secretion of substances from the dense and alpha granules regardless of whether platelets are aggregated or not. One of those substances released is ADP which induces a **second wave of aggregation** and stimulates secretion of platelet substances from aggregated platelets. Thrombin, in turn, converts **fibrinogen** to **fibrin,** which polymerizes into a fibrillar network that traps platelets and blood cells. Both prothrombin and fibrinogen are produced by liver cells and secreted into the plasma. The end result of these events is the production of a blood clot or **thrombus,** composed of fibrin, platelets, and trapped blood cells within a constricted vessel, preventing further blood loss from the injured vessel. When the number of platelets is inadequate, a condition known as **thrombocytopenia,** the bleeding time is prolonged.

Platelets also contain microtubules, actin, myosin, mitochondria, and glycogen deposits, which may be involved in clot retraction. **Thrombosthenin** is a platelet substance, similar to the contractile protein actomyosin of muscle, which is responsible for clot retraction—that is, contraction of a loose fibrinogen network into a less porous one that more effectively prevents the loss of blood through the damaged blood vessel wall. Upon vascular regeneration and healing, a plasma protein, **plasminogen,** is converted to the hydrolytic enzyme **plasmin** by **plasminogen activators.** Plasmin dissolves the clot. If the clot becomes loose and travels through the circulation, it is referred to as a **thromboembolus.** This can be life-threatening if the blood supply to a vital organ is obstructed.

Blood clots in the venous and arterial limbs of the circulation are usually quite different in appearance. Venous clots are usually white due to the preponderance of the platelets that often form thrombi in the valves of veins where blood flow is unusually slow. Arterial clots usually have a white head anchored to the platelet adhesion site with a red tail directed downstream consisting of trapped erythrocytes in a fibrin network.

Most of the abnormalities in hemostasis and

thrombosis are attributed to defects in platelet adhesion, aggregation, or secretion, but plasma factors are also crucial. For instance, platelets may not adhere normally to subendothelial connective tissue either as a result of some defect in platelet surface membrane or as a result of a missing plasma factor, such as factor VIII in the case of hemophilia.

NATIONAL BOARD TYPE QUESTIONS

Select the response most closely associated with each numbered item. (The headings may be used once, more than once, or not at all.)

Sites of erythropoiesis during early development:
   A. Bone marrow
   B. Yolk sac
   C. Liver
   D. Lymph nodes
1. Earliest site of erythropoiesis in embryonic development
2. Site of erythropoiesis in the normal adult
3. *Not* a site for erythropoiesis at any time during normal development.

Select the single best response for each of the following:

4. The earliest and most accurate way to assess recovery from anemia is
   A. hematocrit determination.
   B. bone marrow biopsy.
   C. reticulocyte count.
   D. densitometric evaluation of blood color.
   E. determination of clotting time.
5. If a patient is experiencing an allergic reaction in which free antigen-antibody complexes are generated, which formed elements of the blood are expected to be elevated?
   A. Basophils
   B. Erythrocytes
   C. Neutrophils
   D. Eosinophils
   E. Monocytes

Select the response most closely associated with each numbered item.
   A. Neutrophils
   B. Monocytes
   C. Both
   D. Neither

6. Capable of phagocytosis
7. Produce antibodies
8. Derived from bone marrow
9. Prominent in acute inflammation

For the following, select
   A. if only *1, 2, and 3* are correct.
   B. if only *1 and 3* are correct.
   C. if only *2 and 4* are correct.
   D. if only *4* is correct.
   E. if *all* are correct.

10. Subpopulations of lymphocytes are identified by assessment of their
    1. unique surface molecules.
    2. distinct immune functions.
    3. size.
    4. morphology.
11. Eosinophils
    1. possess specific granules containing histamine.
    2. increase in number during parasitic infections.
    3. are derived from megakaryocytes.
    4. usually possess a bilobed nucleus.
12. Aging of erythrocytes is associated with
    1. depletion of enzymes.
    2. failure of calcium pump.
    3. loss of cell flexibility.
    4. loss of ability to divide.

ANNOTATED ANSWERS

1. B. In embryonic development, blood cells first form in the yolk sac islets.
2. A. In the normal adult, erythrocytes are formed in the bone marrow.
3. D. At various stages of development erythrocytes form in the yolk sac, liver, and bone marrow, but *not* in lymph nodes.

4. C. Newly formed erythrocytes, called *reticulocytes*, can be easily counted under the microscope and provide the earliest indication of red cell generation. Ultimately, a rise in hematocrit is indicative of full recovery.

5. D. An elevated eosinophil count is indicative of an allergic reaction, since one of the functions of eosinophils is to phagocytize antigen-antibody complexes.

6. C. Both neutrophils and monocytes are phagocytic cells. However, neutrophils have a primary affinity for bacteria, while monocytes are much less specific.

7. D. Plasma cells and, to some extent, their immediate precursors, B lymphocytes, produce antibodies. Other cell types may interact with antibodies in defense of the body, but they do not produce them.

8. C. Both neutrophils and monocytes are produced in the bone marrow, as are most of the leukocytes.

9. A. Acute inflammation is usually induced by bacteria, and neutrophils are the first to arrive to destroy them.

10. E. Lymphocytes can be categorized according to all of the criteria listed.

11. C. Eosinophils usually possess bilobed nuclei and increase in number when they are involved in rejection of parasites.

12. A. Toward the end of their 120-day life cycle, erythrocytes become depleted of enzymes which run the calcium pump. Subsequent influx of calcium causes cellular rigidity. They lose their ability to divide in maturation, and not in aging.

BIBLIOGRAPHY

Archer, R. K. On the functions of eosinophils in the antigen-antibody reaction. *Br. J. Haematol.* 11:123, 1965.

Bainton, D. F., and M. G. Farquhar. Segregation and packaging of granule enzymes in eosinophilic leukocytes. *J. Cell Biol.* 45:54, 1970.

Bainton, D. F., J. L. Ullyot, and M. G. Farquhar. The development of neutrophilic leukocytes in the human bone marrow: Origin and content of azurophil and specific granules. *J. Exp. Med.* 134:907, 1971.

Barr, R. D., J. Whang-Peng, and S. Perry. Hemopoietic stem cells in human peripheral blood. *Science* 190:284, 1975.

Bessis, M. *Living Blood Cells and Their Ultrastructure.* New York: Springer-Verlag, 1973.

Brass, L., and H. Bensusan. The platelet collagen interaction. *Fed. Proc.* 34:241, 1975.

Chao, F. C., et al. Similarity between platelet contraction and cellular motility during mitosis: Role of platelet microtubules in clot retraction. *J. Cell Sci.* 20:569, 1976.

Cline, M. J. *The White Cell.* Cambridge, Mass.: Harvard University Press, 1975.

Cline, M. J., and D. W. Golde. Cellular interactions in haematopoiesis. *Nature* 277:177, 1979.

Cohn, Z. A. The structure and function of monocytes and macrophages. *Adv. Immunol.* 9:163, 1968.

Daems, W. T. On the fine structure of human neutrophilic leukocyte granules. *J. Ultrastruct. Res.* 24:343, 1968.

Everett, N. B., and W. D. Perkins. Hemopoietic Stem Cell Migration. In A. B. Cairnie, P. K. Lala, and D. G. Osmond (eds.), *Stem Cells of Renewing Cell Populations.* New York: Academic, 1976.

Gowans, J. L. Life span, recirculation, and transformation of lymphocytes. *Int. Rev. Exp. Pathol.* 5:1, 1966.

Graber, S. E., and S. B. Krantz. Erythropoietin and the control of red cell production. *Ann. Rev. Med.* 29:51, 1978.

Hudson, G. Quantitative study of eosinophilic granulocytes. *Semin. Hematol.* 5:166, 1968.

Klebanoff, S. J., and R. A. Clark. *The Neutrophil: Function and Clinical Disorders.* New York: Elsevier, 1978.

McLeod, D. L., M. M. Shreeve, and A. A. Axelrod. Induction of megakaryocyte colonies with platelet formation in vitro. *Nature* 261:492, 1976.

Moffatt, D. J., C. Rosse, and J. M. Yoffey. Identity of the haemopoietic stem cell. *Lancet* 1:547, 1967.

Murphy, P. *The Neutrophil.* New York: Plenum, 1976.

Mustard, J. F., and M. A. Packham. Factors influencing platelet function: Adhesion, release and aggregation. *Pharmacol. Rev.* 22:97, 1970.

Nichols, B. A., and D. F. Bainton. Differentiation of human monocytes in bone marrow and blood: Sequential formation of two granulocyte populations. *Lab. Invest.* 29:27, 1973.

Nichols, B. A., D. F. Bainton, and M. G. Farquhar. Differentiation of monocytes: Origin, nature and fate of their azurophil granules. *J. Exp. Med.* 50:498, 1971.

Nienhuis, A. W., and E. J. Benz. Regulation of hemoglobin synthesis during the development of the red cell. *N. Engl. J. Med.* 297:1318, 1977.

Smith, J. A. Molecular and cellular properties of eosinophils. *Ric. Clin. Lab.* 11:81, 1981.

Spitznagel, J. K., F. G. Dalldorf, and M. S. Leffell. Characterization of azurophil and specific granules from human polymorphonuclear leukocytes. *Lab. Invest.* 30:724, 1974.

Stossel, T. P. How do phagocytes eat? *Ann. Intern. Med.* 89:398, 1978.

Terry, R. W., D. F. Bainton, and M. G. Farquhar. Formation and structure of specific granules in basophilic leukocytes of the guinea pig. *Lab. Invest.* 21:65, 1969.

Volkman, A., and J. H. Gowans. The origin of macrophages from bone marrow in the rat. *Br. J. Exp. Pathol.* 46:62, 1965.

Weiss, J. H. Platelet physiology and abnormalities of platelet function. *N. Engl. J. Med.* 293:531, 1975.

Weiss, L. Histophysiology of bone marrow. *Clin. Orthop.* 52:13, 1967.

Zigmond, S. Chemotaxis by polymorphonuclear leukocytes. *J. Cell Biol.* 77:269, 1978.

Zucker-Franklin, D. The Ultra Structure of Megakaryocytes and Platelets. In A. S. Gordon (ed.), *Regulation of Hematopoiesis.* New York: Appleton-Century-Crofts, 1970. Vol. 2. P. 1533.

Zucker-Franklin, D. Eosinophil Function and Disorders. In G. H. Stollerman, et al. (eds.), *Internal Medicine.* Chicago: Year Book, 1974. Vol. 19. P. 1.

Zucker-Franklin, D., et al. *Atlas of Blood Cells.* Philadelphia: Lea & Febiger, 1981. Vols. 1 and 2.

5 Connective Tissue Proper

Objectives

You will learn the following in this chapter:

How to identify and describe the composition of the three major components of connective tissue proper

The variations in composition and function of the ground substance

The differences in composition and function between collagen, reticular, and elastic fibers

The six major cellular components of connective tissue proper and a primary function for each

The key events involved in inflammation

How to identify the criteria for classification of connective tissues

The major varieties of connective tissues and how structure reflects function in each

---

The connective tissues have a diversity of functions, which are subserved by their three major components: ground substance, fibers, and cells. The proportion of these components is the basis on which the connective tissues are classified (see the last section of this chapter). The cells primarily responsible for manufacture and secretion of the fibrous and amorphous extracellular components (**matrix**) of connective tissue proper are the fibroblasts, which are derived from embryonic mesenchyme. The matrix provides the tissue with its supportive characteristics. Depending on the type of connective tissue, this matrix is composed of a variety of **fibers** and an amorphous viscous gel called the **ground substance.** Blood and connective tissue proper share many common features and are physiologically interdependent. Blood and loose connective tissue, in particular, possess many of the same free cell types, since the work of the blood leukocytes

is performed in connective tissue (e.g., inflammation). The fluid constituents of blood and connective tissue are biochemically related and are in homeostatic balance as well.

THE EXTRACELLULAR COMPONENTS

Ground Substance

The ground substance functions as a molecular sieve, facilitating the diffusion of metabolites between the blood and the tissues while at the same time serving as a physical barrier to prevent the spread of large particles, such as bacteria and other microorganisms. Aside from water and salts, the ground substance of connective tissue proper is composed of glycosaminoglycans, which provide its viscosity. The particular type of glycosaminoglycan varies in different locations,

The most common type is hyaluronic acid, which appears homogeneous and transparent when stained with hematoxylin and eosin (H and E). Other types are sulfated and linked covalently to protein as side chains. Hence, they are generally referred to as **sulfated proteoglycans.** Because they bear a net negative charge, they stain with basic dyes. The four major classes of sulfated glycosaminoglycans are chondroitin sulfate, dermatan sulfate, keratan sulfate, and heparan sulfate. They are distinguished by the chemical structure of their monosaccharide components.

An important property of the connective tissue ground substance is its high viscosity in aqueous solutions. When fluid is injected into the connective tissue, it forms a discrete bleb and remains localized for some time. This property acts as a physical barrier that prevents the spread of bacteria following tissue injury. However, some bacteria are endowed with the ability to produce the enzyme **hyaluronidase,** enabling them to depolymerize hyaluronic acid and thus promote their invasiveness.

In addition to providing structural support and a medium for diffusion of nutrients and gases, glycosaminoglycans exert a direct influence on the surrounding cells, particularly in the course of morphogenesis. Hyaluronic acid commonly accumulates along the mesenchymal cell migration pathways; it is then removed and replaced by sulfated proteoglycans as the tissue continues to differentiate. It has been suggested that a hyaluronate-rich extracellular matrix is suitable for cell migration and proliferation and may prevent precocious differentiation. Specific interactions between the surface receptors of cells and the glycosaminoglycans suggest that the latter may play an important role in the regulation of cellular functions.

There are a number of structural proteins within the ground substance that bind cells to collagen fibers surrounding them. Of these, **fibronectin** has been the most thoroughly investigated. Fibronectin promotes attachment of fibroblasts and other connective tissue cells to collagen and thus can be considered a cell-matrix ligand. In addition, fibronectin plays a role in

other cellular processes such as migration, differentiation, phagocytosis, and chemotaxis. It has also been implicated in directly influencing the cytoskeletal organization of cells, thus altering their shape and presumably modulating their functions. Other structural proteins, namely, **laminin** and **chondronectin,** are more restricted in distribution. Laminin is associated with basement membranes, where it appears to be a specific attachment protein for epithelial cells to type IV collagen, while chondronectin promotes attachment of cartilage cells to collagen. There is good evidence that collagen can interact with cells by means of cell membrane receptors for these structural proteins.

Fibers

Connective tissue fibers provide general support for other tissues. For example, they form a dense supporting framework in the integument; they provide the stroma for parenchymal organs; and they support individual cells, such as muscle or fat cells. Fibers also compose the "connective" structures that bind muscle to bone (tendons) and bone to bone (ligaments). Hollow organs and blood vessels, which expand and contract, contain connective tissue fibers that provide flexibility.

Three types of fibers occur in connective tissues: **collagen, reticular,** and **elastic fibers.** The density, arrangement, and proportion of each type depend on the functional requirement of the tissue. Loose (areolar) connective tissue is the most common type, composed of a sparse network of connective tissue fibers and bundles and significant numbers of fixed and wandering cells. Mesenteries provide good examples of loose connective tissue (Figs. 5-1, 5-2).

COLLAGEN FIBERS

Collagen is present in all types of connective tissues but varies in abundance. Collagen has a breaking point comparable to that of steel, compared on a weight basis. Therefore, the more col-

Fig. 5-1. Whole mount mesentery spread showing collagen (C) bundles, elastic (E) fibers, and cells of the connective tissue; the pale, poorly focused nuclei (*arrows*) belong to mesothelial cells lining both sides of the mesentery. Also note the blood vessels (*open arrows*).

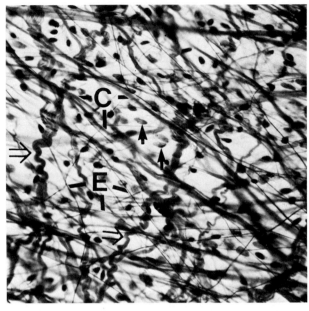

Fig. 5-2. The cells and fibers of connective tissue in a mesentery spread.

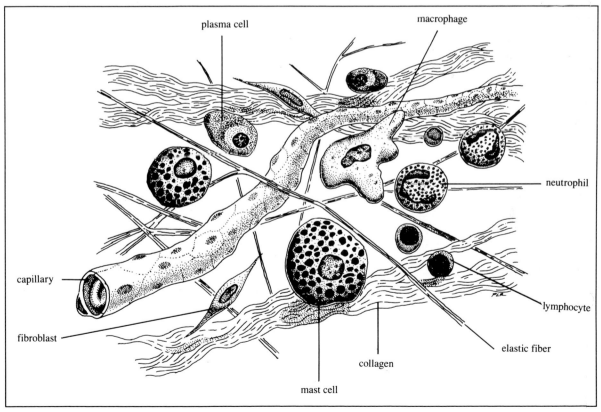

plasma cell

macrophage

neutrophil

capillary

lymphocyte

fibroblast

elastic fiber

collagen

mast cell

lagen is present, the stronger the tissue. Although collagen primarily serves mechanical functions, it plays an important role as a component of basement membranes in the selective permeability of epithelia, particularly vascular permeability.

Collagen is a protein polymer composed of monomeric units, called **tropocollagen,** which are 280 nm long and 1.5 nm wide. The tropocollagen units are arranged in parallel, overlapping by quarter-lengths. This arrangement yields the recurrent 64-nm striations that are characteristic of the collagen fiber (Figs. 5-3, 5-4). Patterns within the tropocollagen also yield several other minor striations.

Most tropocollagen is produced by fibroblasts and released in monomeric form. Polymerization occurs extracellularly. The fibers are readily visible in the light microscope, often reaching several micrometers in diameter. Collagen is produced by chondroblasts and osteoblasts in cartilage and bone, respectively. Collagen of the basal laminae is produced by epithelial cells. Smooth muscle cells also synthesize collagen in some organs.

When collagen is denatured by boiling or chemical treatment, it becomes **gelatin.** Gentler treatment (neutral salt or weak acid solution) gives rise to free tropocollagen units.

Each tropocollagen molecule is composed of three polypeptide chains, called **alpha units,** arranged in a helical configuration. The chains are rich in glycine and proline and contain two amino acids that are not commonly found in other proteins, **hydroxyproline** and **hydroxylysine.** Vitamin C is a cofactor necessary for the enzymatic conversion of proline to hydroxyproline. If vitamin C is not present in sufficient

Fig. 5-3. Collagen microfibrils, fibrils, fibers, and bundles. In collagen bundles, the fibers are bound together by a cementing substance. Under the electron microscope, the microfibrils show periodicity of dark and light bands, which is explained by the arrangement of the rodlike collagen molecules (tropocollagen), each of which measures 280 nm. It is thought that tropocollagen molecules are organized in a stepwise arrangement that produces lacunar and overlapping regions. Lacunar regions contain more stain and appear dark. (From L. C. Junqueira, J. Carneiro, and A. Contropulos, *Basic Histology* [2nd ed.]. Los Altos, Calif.: Lange, 1977. Reproduced with permission.)

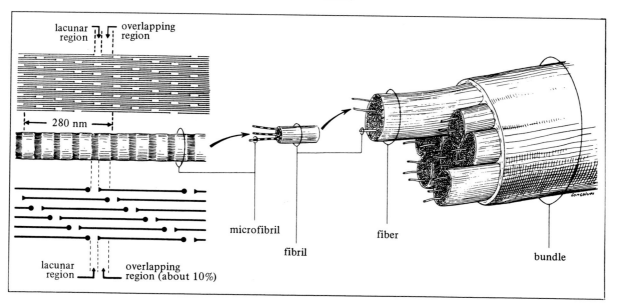

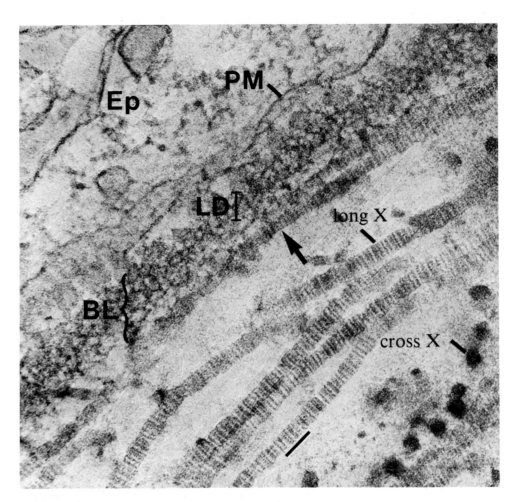

Fig. 5-4. Electron micrograph of a thin section of basal lamina (*BL*) and adjacent collagen fibrils from amphibian skin. The filaments in the lamina densa (*LD*) are small enough (1–2 nm in diameter) to be individual laminin or collagen molecules. They extend from the dense central meshwork to contact the epidermal cell (*Ep*) plasmalemma (*PM*). Collagen fibrils of the reticular lamina in the underlying dermis attach (*arrow*) to the inner part of the basal lamina. Collagen fibrils are cut in cross section (*cross X*) and longitudinal section (*long X*). *Bar = 64 nm.* (Courtesy of E. D. Hay.)

amounts, the deficiency results in a disease known as **scurvy.** Since hydroxyproline is characteristic of collagen, diseases that cause excessive destruction of collagen are revealed clinically by an inordinate amount of hydroxyproline in the urine. Hydroxyproline is involved in hydrogen bonding between polypeptide chains, while hydroxylysine is involved in covalent crosslinking of tropocollagen into bundles of various sizes. Thus both amino acids strengthen collagen molecules. Certain connective tissue diseases are caused by genetic mutations resulting in molecular defects in collagen biosynthesis and turnover. Many of these defects manifest physically as hyperelastic skin, hypermobile joints, skeletal deformities, and poor wound healing. These syndromes are generally attributed to enzymatic defects that prevent the formation of stable cross-links in collagen components.

Collagen from different parts of the body may differ in the amino acid composition of its alpha units. There are at least five molecular types of collagen. Although they do not differ greatly with respect to amino acid content, there are minor but distinct differences in amino acid composition and sequence in their alpha units. **Type I** is the most abundant and widespread collagen type. It is present in nearly all connective tissues. **Type II** is found in cartilage and some tissues of the eye. **Type III** is present in connective tissue components of the skin, cardiovascular system, alimentary tract, and uterus, and is often associated with reticular fibers. **Type IV** is found in basal laminae and is unique in that its molecules are thought to be covalently linked to the glycoproteins, and unlike the others, it lacks periodicity. Various types of epithelial basal laminae may differ in terms of their constituent collagen or glycoprotein composition. **Type V** is present primarily in fetal membranes, but is distributed ubiquitously in adult connective tissues in small amounts.

RETICULAR FIBERS

Reticular fibers are actually thin collagen fibers arranged in delicate networks instead of bundles. They are barely visible with the light microscope, unless stained by silver methods. Areas of developing collagen are initiated as reticular fibers (reticulum). Reticular fibers form a delicate supporting network around individual cells of many tissues and organs, and they constitute the inner stroma of the lymphoid and hemopoietic organs. Fibers of this type also compose the reticular lamina of epithelial basement membranes (see Fig. 5-4). Although it is clear that collagen and reticular fibers are very similar in chemical composition, the distinction is useful histologically in designating fibers of different size and arrangement.

ELASTIC FIBERS

Elastic fibers stretch easily, but they are not as strong as collagen. They break at 150 percent of their original length. Elastic fibers are present in most fibrous connective tissues but are most abundant in tissues that require flexibility, such as the large arteries, the trachea, the framework of the spleen, the skin, and the intervertebral ligaments (ligamenta flava). The thickness, length, and arrangement of elastic fibers vary among different tissues and organs. In large arteries, they form fenestrated sheets or lamellae, while in the mesenteries they form a network between collagen bundles (see Figs. 5-1, 5-2).

Elastic fibers are composed of an amorphous protein called **elastin** and a peripheral microfibrillar component. They are usually less than 1 μm in diameter, exhibit no periodicity, and require specific staining (e.g., resorcin-fuchsin) to be visualized. Like collagen, elastin is rich in glycine and proline; unlike collagen, elastin also has a high content of valine. Elastin also possesses two unique amino acids, desmosine and isodesmosine, which form cross-links between polypeptides in the polymerization of elastin. Fibroblasts and smooth muscle cells synthesize either elastin or the precursor molecules from which the fibers are formed.

CELLS OF CONNECTIVE TISSUE

Both permanent and transient cells inhabit the connective tissues. The cell types and their relative proportions are highly variable and depend largely on fiber density, location, and functional state. Among the permanent cells are **fibroblasts, mesenchymal cells,** and **adipose (fat) cells.** Those of the transient population are the **neutrophils, eosinophils, monocytes,** and **lymphocytes,** which are emigrants from the blood; and **mast cells, plasma cells,** and **macrophages,** which originate from bone marrow—derived precursor cells. Basically, it is convenient to think of the permanent cells as having to do with long-term maintenance of connective tissue, whereas the wandering or transient cells represent short-term events, such as reaction to injury or invasion of microorganisms. Figure 5-2 diagrams the most common connective tissue elements.

Permanent Cells of the Connective Tissue

FIBROBLASTS

Fibroblasts (Fig. 5-5) are widely distributed among the connective tissues. They are long, tapered cells that can assume a variety of shapes depending on the space limitations of their extracellular environment. They are usually found along collagen bundles, where only their thin, flat nuclei are distinguishable. Their appearance

may also vary depending on their state of motility and stage of differentiation, since they are both motile and highly proliferative cells.

Fig. 5-5. Electron micrograph of a thin section showing a group of fibroblasts in a 12-day-old avian cornea. Fibroblasts actively producing collagen have euchromatic nuclei (*N*) and are rich in secretory organelles, such as granular endoplasmic reticulum (*ER*). A centriole (*C*) is also evident. Some collagen fibrils are cut transversely (*cross X*) and others in the longitudinal plane (*long X*). Collagen fibrils are narrow (25 nm in diameter) and arranged in orthogonal layers in all vertebrate corneas. *Bar* = 64 nm. (Courtesy of E. D. Hay.) Inset: light micrograph of a fibroblast in loose connective tissue.

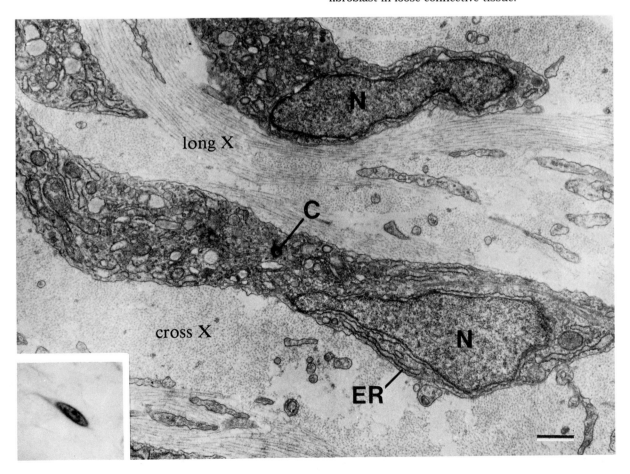

The three types of fibers and the ground substance are produced by fibroblasts. Although several cell types produce collagen, fibroblasts are by far the most widespread and productive. Therefore, fibroblasts possess all the organelles necessary for protein synthesis, including some secretory vesicles. Under certain conditions, particularly during wound healing, they proliferate and become metabolically very active, at which time they resemble smooth muscle cells and may play a role in wound contraction. In most instances fibroblasts do not give rise to other cell types, but apparently they may do so in certain pathologic states.

MESENCHYMAL CELLS

Mesenchymal cells resemble fibroblasts except for their stellate shape, and the two are usually indistinguishable with the light microscope. They are not so widely distributed throughout the connective tissues as are the fibroblasts, and they usually lie in close association with small blood vessels. Thus, they are often referred to as **pericytes** or **perivascular** cells. These cells are not highly differentiated and maintain the developmental multipotentiality of embryonic mesenchymal cells. Mesenchymal cells may develop into other "adult" cell types under certain conditions; it is thought that cells as diverse as mast cells, adipose cells, and even smooth muscle cells may be derived from mesenchymal cells in the adult organism.

ADIPOSE (FAT) CELLS

Adipocytes (Fig. 5-6) are specialized for the synthesis and storage of lipid. They may occur singly but are usually found in groups of varying sizes throughout "loose" connective tissue. In certain areas of the body they may be the predominant cell type. Tissue of this type is often referred to as **adipose tissue.** The individual cells are supported by a delicate reticular network.

Fat cells may alternately accumulate lipid and become depleted. The lipid is stored in a single large droplet (**unilocular**). The droplet may be so

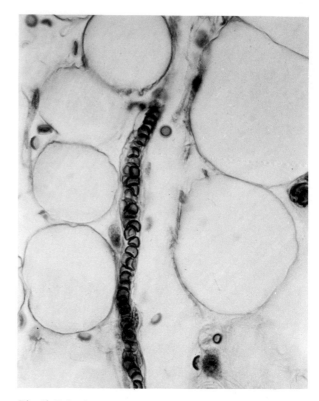

Fig. 5-6. Light micrograph of adipose cells in loose connective tissue. Compare the size of adipocytes with that of erythrocytes in the capillary passing between them.

large that the nucleus appears flattened on one side and is surrounded by only a thin rim of cytoplasm.

The unilocular adipose cell is essentially an enemy storage compartment, which composes the white adipose tissue of humans. Lipid deposition and mobilization are controlled by neuroendocrine secretions and the nutritional state of the organism, although the mechanisms are still poorly understood. However, during both processes adipose cells take on a multilocular appearance and lipid molecules are apparently transported by micropinocytotic vesicles. Adipose cells possess receptors for a number of hormones, including glucagon, ACTH, thyroxine, and others, which are essentially lipolytic (causing lipid breakdown). Insulin inhibits lipolysis and promotes lipogenesis (lipid accumulation).

The size of the adipose tissue mass reflects both the number of adipocytes and their size. Adipose cell precursors proliferate for a limited period postnatally. This process is known as **hyperplastic growth.** Change in the size of adipocytes brought about by lipid accumulation is known as **hypertrophic growth.** Hypertrophic growth (and its reversal) can occur at any time in life. Therefore, both number and size of adipocytes can be influenced postnatally, while influences that occur later in life primarily affect cell size. Loss of adipose tissue mass as a result of caloric restriction is due to a reduction of fat cell size with no reduction in cell number.

As a result of fasting or starvation, adipose cells may be depleted to 3 percent of their normal weight. In some areas, however, such as in the hands and feet and around the eyes and kidneys, the adipose tissue is not depleted but remains permanently to support and cushion these structures.

Multilocular adipose cells are found in some mammals, particularly those that hibernate, and compose the tissue of heat production known as **brown fat.** In humans, this type of fat occurs primarily in the fetus and neonate. The thermogenic properties of brown fat are thought to be induced by the action of norepinephrine and sympathetic innervation. Brown fat cells are also unique in their abundance of mitochondria, which reflects their ability to turn stored energy into heat by interruption of oxidative phosphorylation. The highly vascular nature of brown adipose tissue allows rapid distribution of heat throughout the body.

Transient Cells of Connective Tissue

The transient cells that originate from blood— the granulocytes, monocytes, and lymphocytes— have already been discussed. Their functions are summarized later in this chapter, with respect to their role in inflammation. Mast cells, plasma cells, and macrophages are present in connective tissues and do not normally occur in blood, as such.

MAST CELLS

Mast cells (Fig. 5-7) are widely distributed in the connective tissues, usually in close association with small blood vessels. They are particularly numerous in sites close to the outside environment, such as the dermis of the skin and the lining of the digestive and respiratory tracts. They resemble basophils in that they possess large metachromatic membrane-bound granules. Although the two cells originate from separate bone marrow stem cells, mast cells are often referred to as "connective tissue basophils." However, unlike basophils, which possess multilobed nuclei, mast cell nuclei are unilobed. In addition to their similar appearance, mast cells and basophils contain and secrete similar substances. Both granule-associated and unstored mediators are released in **immediate hypersensitivity reactions** and thus intensify the overall inflammatory reaction. The best known mast cell/basophil mediator is **histamine** which increases vascular permeability and contraction of smooth muscle. Slower contraction of smooth muscle is induced by **leukotrienes** (previously called slow reactive substance of anaphylaxis). In severe allergic reactions, extreme smooth muscle contraction of the bronchioles and pulmonary vessels can be life-threatening. Mast cells and basophils also secrete **eosinophil chemotactic factors, platelet activating factor, prostaglandins,** and a number of enzymes that degrade various connective tissue components. A cell product unique to mast cells and not found in basophils is **heparin,** an anticoagulant that is also involved in lipid metabolism.

Mediator release from mast cells and basophils mainly involves a special class of antibody called IgE. These antibodies are synthesized by plasma cells after exposure to allergens, such as ragweed and pollen, and certain metazoan parasites. These antibodies bind to mast cells and basophils at the Fc domain. Thus mast cells/

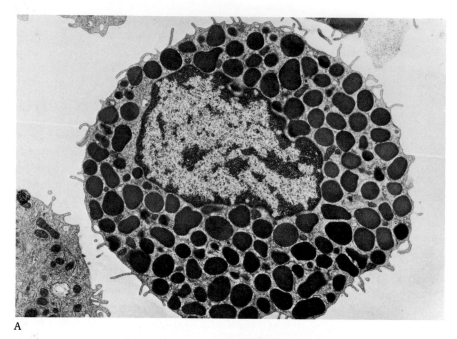

A

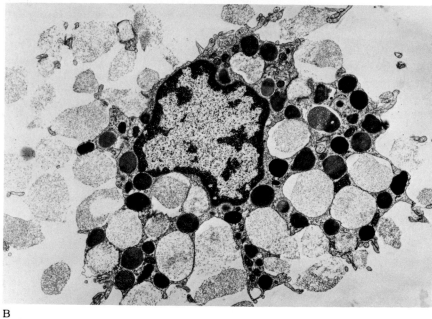

B

Fig. 5-7. Mast cells. A. Electron micrograph of a rat peritoneal mast cell. Note the unlobulated nucleus, the relative uniformity in granule densities, and numerous microvilli. B. Electron micrograph of a de-granulating rat mast cell. The peripheral granules are swollen and show decreased density. Note the intracytoplasmic channels containing numerous pale granules. (Both micrographs courtesy of D. Lagunoff.)

basophils have been shown to have **Fc receptors** on the cell surface. When sensitized hosts are reexposed to the antigen, the antigen binds to the active portion of the IgE molecules (Fab portion). This cross-linking interaction immediately triggers release of mediators. Degranulation is energy-dependent and requires calcium. Ultrastructural studies of the degranulation process show that peripheral granules fuse with the plasma membrane while deeper granules fuse with one another, forming complex channels that connect with the cell surface. Figure 5-7 shows an intact and a partially degranulated mast cell.

LYMPHOCYTES

Lymphocytes perform most of their immunologic functions in connective tissues throughout the body, where they are usually seen in small numbers. They are generally more abundant in the lamina propria (subepithelial connective tissue) of the respiratory tract and the gastrointestinal system. In both instances, these regions are exposed to the outside environment and lymphoid cells protect the epithelium and the underlying tissues against antigenic foreign substances which are inhaled or ingested. Lymphocytes are commonly seen to penetrate and pass throughout epithelia in performance of these functions. Lymphocyte aggregates of conspicuous size can also occur in sites of chronic inflammation (see p. 119). Lymphocytes are discussed in more detail in Chapter 10.

PLASMA CELLS

A certain population of lymphocytes (B cells) differentiate into plasma cells, which are specialized to produce and secrete antibody. The plasma cell is easily distinguishable by its eccentric nucleus, clear juxtanuclear Golgi zone, and intense cytoplasmic basophilia. The nucleus has a characteristic "wheel-spoke" chromatin pattern (Fig. 5-8). The extensive, often distended, lamellar rough endoplasmic reticulum and prominent Golgi apparatus are indicative of the plasma cell's role in immunoglobulin production (Fig. 5-9).

Fig. 5-8. Light micrograph of loose connective tissue. A capillary (C) is surrounded by connective tissue cells. Among them are a number of well-differentiated plasma cells (*arrows*).

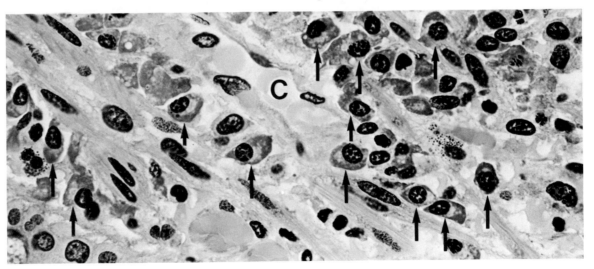

Plasma cells are rarely found in blood. They are widely dispersed throughout the connective tissues, being most numerous in the connective tissues of the digestive and respiratory tracts. Like lymphocytes, they are concentrated in the lymphoid organs as well. Plasma cells are derived from antigen-stimulated small lymphocytes that have undergone blastogenesis and differentiation. The plasma cell is an end cell, incapable of further differentiation. Its life span is about 2 weeks. Although lymphocytes are motile, plasma cells are rather sedentary. For further information on plasma cells and antibody production, see Chapter 10.

Fig. 5-9. Electron micrograph of an immature plasma cell. Although its chromatin pattern is still uncharacteristic of the mature plasma cell nucleus, the rough endoplasmic reticulum is well developed and already occupies most of the cytoplasm. (Courtesy of J. André-Schwartz.)

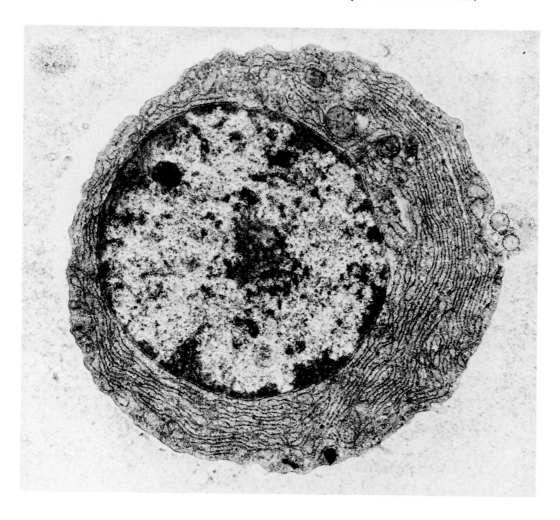

MACROPHAGES

Macrophages are long-lived highly motile, avidly phagocytic connective tissue cells that are derived from monocytes (bone marrow origin). Their capacity for phagocytosis and pinocytosis is marked by numerous lysosomes, vacuoles, and residual bodies. Macrophages may assume many shapes, depending on their levels of activity. The surfaces of mature and active macrophages are thrown into numerous folds. Long pseudopodia extend out in ameboid movement.

Sessile macrophages are difficult to identify with the light microscope, but active cells are characterized by their irregular shape, acidophilic cytoplasm, and the usual presence of residual bodies (Fig. 5-10). Macrophages are capable of phagocytizing large particles, even other cells (Fig. 5-11).

Masses of foreign material in connective tissue that are too large to be phagocytized by individual macrophages, such as a splinter, induce the formation of **foreign body giant cells.** These multinucleated cells are derived from the fusion of monocytes and macrophages. They are large enough to wall off or enclose a mass of foreign matter and thus isolate it from the surrounding tissue. These isolated structures may eventually be extruded, or they can remain at the tissue site for a long time. Unlike their macrophage precursors, foreign body giant cells are not actively phagocytic.

Phagocytosis involves discrimination between self and nonself, and is termed **phagocytic recognition.** Most inert particles are ingested without the help of specific recognition factors from the serum. Such nonspecific phagocytosis is particularly common in the lung, where alveolar macrophages clear the airways of various environmental materials and industrial pollutants (see Chap. 12, Fig. 12-17).

More specific interactions may be involved in the phagocytosis of microorganisms. For example, macrophages recognize certain carbohydrate residues on the surfaces of microbes. Even more specificity is rendered to macrophages by **opsonins,** various serum proteins that first coat

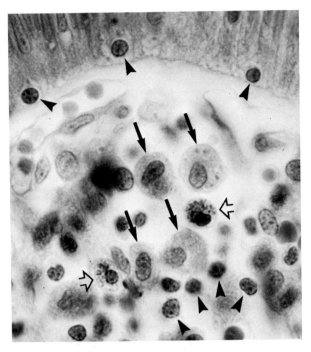

Fig. 5-10. Light micrograph of free cells in the sub-epithelial connective tissue of the small intestine. Note the large, immature macrophages (*arrows*) with only a few residual bodies; and smaller, mature macrophages (*open arrows*) with numerous residual bodies. Lymphocytes (*arrowheads*) are present both in the connective tissue and in the epithelium.

the microbial or foreign cell surface. The main opsonins are IgM and IgG serum immunoglobulins and derivatives of the third component of complement, C3. These particle-bound opsonins are recognized by specific Fc and C3 receptors on the macrophage surface, which promote attachment to and phagocytosis of the foreign material. In this way, opsonins provide a much greater degree of specificity than nonimmunologic phagocytosis.

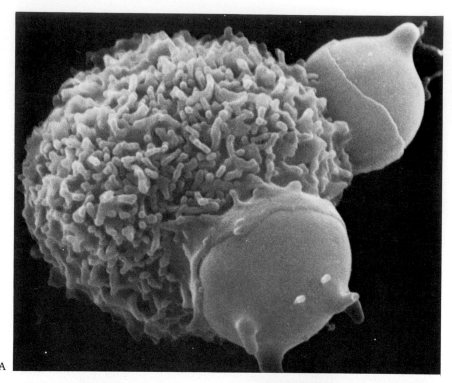

A

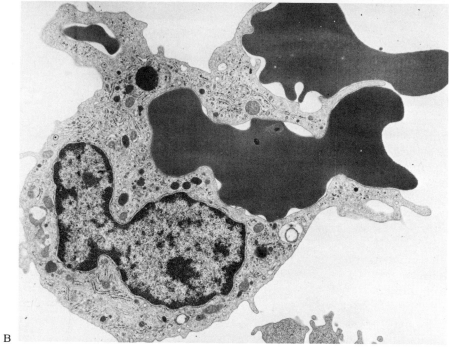

B

Fig. 5-11. Macrophages. A. Scanning electron micrograph of a mouse macrophage in the process of ingesting aldehyde-treated erythrocytes. The macrophage membrane extends as a collar over the erythrocytes. Numerous microvilli project from the macrophage surface. (Courtesy of J.-P. Revel.) B. Transmission electron micrograph of a human macrophage ingesting erythrocytes. Note the nucleus, segments of rough endoplasmic reticulum, and variety of lysosomes. (Courtesy of D. Zucker-Franklin.)

◁————————————————————▷

Macrophages also phagocytize damaged cells and extracellular matrix. This recognition is probably mediated by the glycoprotein **fibronectin,** which has a high affinity for damaged tissues. This fibronectin serves as a nonspecific opsonin for damaged tissues in inflammation and the process of normal morphogenesis.

The postengulfment events of phagocytosis are described in detail in Chapter 2.

Macrophages also play a direct role in both humoral and cell-mediated immune responses. This role generally involves antigen trapping and processing, presentation of antigens to lymphocytes, and the production of immunoregulatory substances. How macrophages present antigens to lymphocytes is not known precisely. However, physical contact between the two cells is required for lymphocyte activation. Lymphocyte proliferation, in turn, is driven by macrophage-soluble proteins, the best known being **interleukin 1.** Macrophages also produce a variety of other factors that either enhance or inhibit specific immune functions.

As a secretory cell, the macrophage produces not only immunoregulatory substances, but also a vast array of other products that reflect the cell's tremendous versatility. Among these substances are enzymes such as the **lysosomal hydrolases; neutral proteinases,** such as plasminogen activator, collagenese, and elastase; **arginase;** and the ubiquitous antimicrobial substance **lysozyme.** In addition, macrophages produce several proteins of the **complement** system, the antiviral substance **interferon,** a variety of

growth factors and **mitogenic proteins** that regulate proliferation and activity of many different cell types, *endogenous pyrogen*, which is an important mediator of fever, the lipids, **prostaglandins,** and **leukotrienes,** which act as mediators of inflammation, **hydrogen peroxide** and **free radicals of oxygen,** which play a role in destruction of microbes and foreign cells, and others.

THE RETICULOENDOTHELIAL SYSTEM

In addition to connective tissue macrophages, phagocytosis occurs in a variety of cells distributed throughout the body. These cells differ in appearance and bear different names in different organs. This "macrophage system" includes reticular and endothelial lining cells of certain organs and has, therefore, been termed the **reticuloendothelial system.** The cells of this system include blood **monocytes,** fixed and free **macrophages** of connective tissue, **alveolar** (lung) **macrophages, reticular cells** of the lymphoid organs (spleen and lymph nodes) and bone marrow, **Kupffer cells** of the liver, and the **microglia** of the central nervous system. More recently, this system has been redefined in more precise terms and renamed the **mononuclear phagocyte system** (MPS). Minimum criteria for inclusion are similar morphology, bone marrow origin, and a high level of phagocytic activity mediated or enhanced by antibody.

INFLAMMATION

The functional aspects of blood leukocytes and free connective tissue cells can be summarized by outlining the key events that occur in inflammation. Inflammation is a dynamic process centered around small blood vessels, particularly the postcapillary venules and the surrounding connective tissue.

In response to injury or invasion of microorganisms, blood leukocytes are chemotactically attracted to the affected site. Release of histamine by basophils and mast cells causes vasodilation (redness), allowing the leukocytes to migrate into the connective tissue in large numbers. Leakage of plasma into the connective tissue results in edema (swelling). The first cells to arrive are the neutrophils, which avidly phagocytize microorganisms. Monocytes, macrophages, and lymphocytes appear later in varying proportions, depending on the stage and duration of the inflammatory reaction. Plasma cells and eosinophils may appear in chronic inflammation where there is immunologic involvement. Macrophages appear after the neutrophils in acute inflammation, persist throughout chronic inflammation, and perform the clean-up chores after the reaction subsides. In response to foreign bodies and to certain bacterial infections, macrophages fuse to form multinucleated giant cells that surround and isolate the affected region.

CLASSIFICATION OF CONNECTIVE TISSUES

The separation of connective tissue into categories is not clear-cut. As in all systems, the classification represents a continuum of types from which examples are chosen as representative. Sometimes a connective tissue falls squarely between two representative categories.

Embryonic Connective Tissues

1. **Mesenchymal connective tissue** (Fig. 5-12A) fills the spaces between developing organs

Fig. 5-12. Developing connective tissue. A. Fetal connective tissue developing from mesenchyme. The stellate mesenchymal cells have produced fine collagen fibers around themselves. B. "Mucous" connective tissue of the umbilical cord. Here the cells have differentiated into fibroblasts. The collagenous stroma is also quite well developed.

A

B

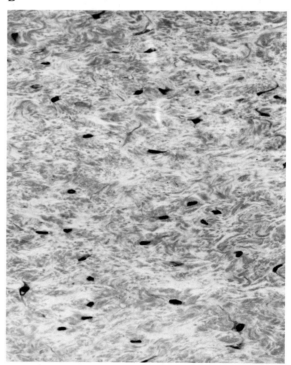

and is largely composed of stellate mesenchymal cells and a fluid ground substance. The mesenchymal cells are multipotential and can give rise to fibroblasts, chondroblasts, osteoblasts, muscle cells, blood cells, fat cells, or endothelial cells. As development proceeds, the formation of various fiber types and the relationship of fibers to cell types yield an adult connective tissue that is specialized for a particular function.

2. **Mucous connective tissue** (Fig. 5-12B) is similar to mesenchymal connective tissue except that it contains some collagen fibers and a more viscous ground substance. This type of tissue is typified by the umbilical cord, where it is termed **Wharton's jelly.**

Mature Connective Tissues

The mature connective tissues are categorized according to: (1) the relative density of collagen fibers (loose vs. dense), which represent the most common connective tissue types; (2) the predominant cell type, particularly when there are many cells and few fibers; and (3) the predominant fiber type other than collagen. These connective tissue types are usually highly specialized and restricted to a few locations. The following represent the most common types of mature connective tissues.

1. **Loose (areolar) tissue** is the prototypical connective tissue that supports most epithelia and composes the stroma of many organs, forming **septa** that separate organs into lobes and provide support and means of passage for blood vessels and nerves. It also comprises subcutaneous tissue (superficial fascia) and most of the deep fascia. Loose connective tissue has an abundance of cells and ground substance, but has relatively sparse fiber development. Here the fibers form a meshwork that houses the various cell types (Fig. 5-13).

2. **Dense (fibrous) connective tissue** differs from the loose variety in having a greater proportion of fibers, fewer cells, and less ground substance. There are two types of dense tissue, which vary according to the arrangement

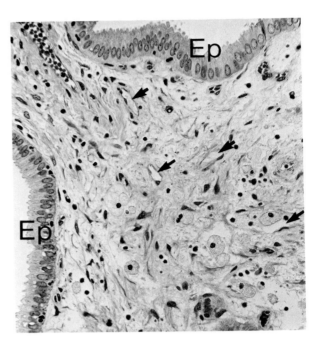

Fig. 5-13. Loose (areolar) connective tissue of the gallbladder. Note the simple columnar epithelial lining (*Ep*). The underlying connective tissue is rather cellular and contains a number of small vessels (*arrows*).

of the component fibers. The **irregular type** is characterized by a thick, random weave of collagen fibers with very few cells (Fig. 5-14A). Those cells that are present are 95 percent fibroblasts. Sample locations include the dermis, capsules of organs, and sheaths of tendons and nerves. In the **regular type,** the fibers are arranged in parallel according to a definite plan that reflects the mechanical requirements of the tissue (Fig. 5-14B). The few fibroblasts found here are very elongate, conforming to the minimum space left between the tightly packed fibers. This arrangement results in a flexible tissue with great resistance to pulling forces. This tissue, therefore, is found where strong connections are required, as between bone and muscle (tendon)

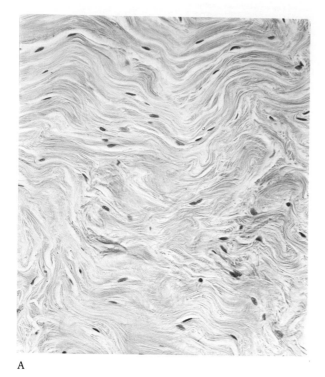

A

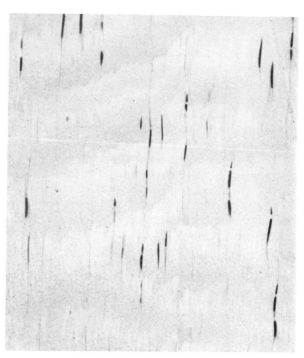

B

Fig. 5-14. Dense collagenous connective tissue. A. Dense irregular connective tissue. Note the irregular arrangement of the collagen bundles. Most of the cells are fibroblasts, scattered throughout the connective tissue. B. Dense regular connective tissue (tendon). Note the parallel arrangement of the collagen bundles. Fibroblasts are seen squeezed between the bundles.

and from bone to bone (ligament). It also occurs in the cornea, where the orthogonal arrangement of collagen layers is both strong and optically clear.

3. **Adipose tissue** is loose connective tissue in which the predominant cell type is the adipocyte or fat cell. It functions as an energy reserve in times of fasting, provides insulation against heat loss through the skin, and provides a protective padding for delicate organs.

4. **Reticular connective tissue** is a loose connective tissue, composed primarily of a delicate network of reticular fibers and associated closely with reticular cells, which maintain the fibers and in some instances perform phagocytic functions. A reticular fiber network composes the inner stroma of most solid organs and serves as a support for all epithelial tissues and for individual muscle and adipose cells. A well-developed reticular connective tissue composes the inner stroma of lymphoid organs, such as the spleen and lymph nodes, as well as the hemopoietic tissues of the bone marrow. The "reticular" cells of lymphoid organs are highly phagocytic and are thought to be involved in antigen processing (see Chap. 10 for further details).

5. **Elastic connective tissue** is characterized by a preponderance of elastic fibers that compose the connective tissue between the vertebrae

(ligamenta flava) as well as the suspensory ligament of the penis. Elastic fibers are an important component of certain cartilages that require much flexibility (elastic cartilage) and of the walls of large arteries that tolerate constant expansion from the force of blood moving through them.

NATIONAL BOARD TYPE QUESTIONS

Select the single best response for each of the following.

1. All of the following can be considered "connective tissues," *except*:
   A. Blood
   B. Muscle
   C. Cartilage
   D. Tendon
   E. Bone
2. Reticular laminae are produced by
   A. fibroblasts.
   B. epithelial cells.
   C. macrophages.
   D. mast cells.
   E. none of the above.
3. The most abundant component of dense connective tissue are
   A. calcium salts.
   B. lipids.
   C. glycosaminoglycans.
   D. nucleic acids.
   E. collagen.
4. The periodicity of collagen fibrils is attributed to
   A. helical configuration of alpha units.
   B. presence of glycine and proline.
   C. quarter-length overlapping of tropocollagen units.
   D. presence of contractile elements.
   E. cross-links between collagen fibrils.

Select the response most closely associated with each numbered item. (The headings may be used once, more than once, or not at all.)
   A. Histamine
   B. Hyaluronic acid
   C. Immunoglobulin
   D. Lysozyme
   E. Prothrombin

5. Fibroblast
6. Mast cell
7. Macrophage
8. Plasma cell

For the following, select
   A. if only *1, 2, and 3* are correct.
   B. if only *1 and 3* are correct.
   C. if only *2 and 4* are correct.
   D. if only *4* is correct.
   E. if *all* are correct.

9. Connective tissue proper can be classified according to the
   1. relative density of fibers.
   2. predominant cell type.
   3. predominant fiber type.
   4. composition of adjacent tissues.
10. Mesenchymal cells are direct precursors of
   1. fibroblasts.
   2. plasma cells.
   3. adipose cells.
   4. macrophages.
11. Elastin is a major component of which of the following?
   1. Plasma
   2. Basement membrane
   3. Tendon
   4. Aorta
12. Which of the following is (are) functions of connective tissue ground substance?
   1. Medium for diffusion of gases and nutrients
   2. Barrier for bacterial spread
   3. Lubricant
   4. Structural strength

ANNOTATED ANSWERS

1. B. The "connective tissues" are rich in extracellular components. Only muscle does not meet this criterion; contractile elements are intracellular.
2. A. Reticular laminae are components of basement membranes, which are composed of reticular fibers (collagen units), which are in turn synthesized by fibroblasts.
3. E. The term "dense" refers to the relative abundance of collagen fibers.
4. C. The periodicity of collagen fibrils (seen only with the electron microscope) is due to quarter-length overlap of tropocollagen units. Although A, B, and E are characteristics of collagen, they do not contribute to its periodicity.
5. B. In addition to producing connective tissue fibers, fibroblasts produce the ground substance, the most common variety being hyaluronic acid.
6. A. The mast cell produces histamine, the substance responsible for inducing vascular permeability. Hence mast cells are often found in close proximity to blood vessels, particularly the postcapillary venules.
7. D. Macrophages produce many enzymes and antimicrobial substances. One such substance is lysozyme, which is also produced by neutrophils.
8. C. Plasma cells produce antibodies that are secreted into the tissue fluids. Antibodies are found in the gamma globulin fraction of plasma and are often referred to as immunoglobulins.
9. A. Connective tissue proper is classified by relative number of fibers (loose; dense), predominant fiber type (elastic; reticular), and cell type (adipose; mesenchymal). Composition of adjacent tissues is irrelevant for this purpose.
10. B. Fibroblasts and adipose cells are permanent residents of connective tissues and therefore are derived directly from mesenchyme. In contrast, other cells migrate from other sites and pass through intermediate stages of differentiation. Plasma cells are derived from lymphocytes, and macrophages from monocytes.
11. D. Elastin is the protein that composes the elastic fibers and laminae. These structures are highly stretchable, allowing the aorta to accommodate a volume of blood on ventricular contraction and to dampen its flow on recoil.
12. A. Ground substance is viscous and so provides lubrication and a medium for metabolic exchanges with blood capillaries. It also serves as a barrier against the spread of large particles, including bacteria. Fibers provide the structural component of the extracellular matrix.

BIBLIOGRAPHY

Allison, A. C., P. Davis, and S. de Petris. Role of contractile microfilaments in macrophage movement and endocytosis. *Nature* 232:153, 1971.

Austen, K. F. Reaction mechanisms in the release of mediators of immediate hypersensitivity from human lung tissue. *Fed Proc.* 33:2256, 1974.

Bornstein, P. The biosynthesis of collagen. *Ann. Rev. Biochem.* 143:567, 1974.

Burwen, S. J., and B. H. Satir. Plasma membrane folds on the mast cell surface and their relationship to secretory activity. *J. Cell Biol.* 74:690, 1977.

Carpenter, J. C., A. Perrelet, and L. Orci. Morphological changes of the adipose cell membrane during lipolysis. *J. Cell Biol.* 72:104, 1977.

Carr, I. *The Macrophage. A Review of Ultrastructure and Function.* New York: Academic, 1973.

Church, R. L., S. E. Pfeiffer, and M. L. Tanzer. Collagen biosynthesis: Synthesis and secretion of a high molecular weight collagen precursor (procollagen). *Proc. Natl. Acad. Sci. U.S.A.* 68:2638, 1971.

Doyle, B. B., et al. Collagen polymorphism: Its origin in the amino acid sequence. *J. Mol. Biol.* 91:79, 1975.

Fain, J. N. Insulin as an activator of cyclic AMP accumulation in rat fat cells. *J. Cyclic Nucleotide Res.* 1:359, 1975.

Gay, S., and E. J. Miller. *Collagen in the Physiology and Pathology of Connective Tissue.* Stuttgart: Gustav Fisher, 1978.

Gordon, S., and Z. A. Cohn. The macrophage. *Int. Rev. Cytol.* 36:171, 1973.

Gottle, L., et al. The ultrastructural organization of elastin. *J. Ultrastruct. Res.* 46:23, 1974.

Gross, J. Collagen biology: Structure, degradation, and disease. *Harvey Lect.* 68:351, 1974.

Gross, J., et al. Mode of Action and Regulation of Tissue Collagens. In D. E. Woolley and J. M. Evanson (eds.), *Collagenase in Normal and Pathological Connective Tissues.* New York: Wiley, 1980. P. 11.

Hall, D. A. *The Aging of Connective Tissue.* New York: Academic, 1976.

Hascall, V. C. Proteoglycans: Structure and Function. In V. Ginsberg (ed.), *Biology of Carbohydrates.* New York: Wiley, 1981. Vol. 1. P. 1.

Hausberger, F. X. Influence of nutritional state on size and number of fat cells. *Z. Zellforsch. Mikrosk. Anat.* 64:13, 1964.

Hay, E. D. (ed.). *Cell Biology of Extracellular Matrix.* New York: Plenum, 1981.

Heathcote, J. G., and M. E. Grant. The molecular organization of basement membranes. *Int. Rev. Connect. Tissue Res.* 9:191, 1981.

Huber, H., and J. H. Fudenberg. The interactions of monocytes and macrophages with immunoglobulins and complement. *Semin. Hematol.* 3:160, 1970.

Jarrett, L., and R. M. Smith. Ultrastructural localization of insulin receptors on adipocytes. *Proc. Natl. Acad. Sci. U.S.A.* 72:3526, 1975.

Jayson, M. I. V., and J. B. Weiss (eds.). *Collagen in Health and Disease.* London: Churchill Livingstone, 1981.

Kono, T., and F. W. Barhan. The relationship between the insulin-binding capacity of fat cells and the cellular response to insulin. *J. Biol. Chem.* 246:6210, 1971.

Kulonen, E., and J. Pikkarainen (eds.). *Biology of the Fibroblast.* New York: Academic, 1973.

Lagunoff, D. Contributions of electron microscopy to the study of mast cells. *J. Invest. Dermatol.* 58:296, 1972.

Leduc, E. J., S. Avrameas, and M. Bouteille. Ultrastructural localization of antibody in differentiating plasma cells. *J. Exp. Med.* 127:109, 1968.

Levy, M. H., and E. F. Wheelock. The role of macrophages in defense against neoplastic disease. *Adv. Cancer Res.* 20:131, 1974.

Mathews, M. B. *Connective Tissue, Macromolecular Structure and Evolution.* Heidelberg: Springer-Verlag, 1975.

Napolitano, L. The differentiation of white adipose cells. *J. Cell Biol.* 18:663, 1963.

Nelson, D. S. (ed.). *Immunobiology of the Macrophage.* New York: Academic, 1976.

Page, R. C., P. Davies, and A. C. Allison. The macrophage as a secretory cell. *Int. Rev. Cytol.* 52:119, 1978.

Ross, R. The elastic fiber. A review. *J. Histochem. Cytochem.* 21:199, 1973.

Ross, R., and P. Bornstein. Elastic fibers in the body. *Sci. Am.* 224:44, 1971.

Slavin, B. G. The cytophysiology of mammalian adipose cells. *Int. Rev. Cytol.* 33:297, 1972.

Snodgrass, M. J. Ultrastructural distinction between reticular and collagenous fibers with an ammoniacal silver stain. *Anat. Rec.* 187:191, 1977.

Steer, H. W. Mast cells of the human stomach. *J. Anat.* 121:385, 1976.

Steinman, R. M., and Z. A. Cohn. The Metabolism and Physiology of the Mononuclear Phagocytes. In B. W. Zweifach, L. Grant, and R. T. McCluskey (eds.), *The Inflammatory Process.* New York: Academic, 1974. P. 449.

Stossel, T. P. Phagocytosis: Recognition and ingestion. *Semin. Hematol.* 12:83, 1975.

Toole, B. P. Hyaluronate and hyaluronidase in morphogenesis and differentiation. *Am. Zool.* 13:1061, 1973.

Unanue, R. R., and J. C. Cerotti. The function of macrophages in the immune response. *Semin. Hematol.* 7:225, 1970.

Veis, A., and A. G. Brownell. Collagen biosynthesis. *Crit. Rev. Biochem.* 2:417, 1975.

Von der Mark, K. Localization of collagen types in tissues. *Int. Rev. Connect. Tissue Res.* 9:265, 1981.

6 Cartilage and Bone

Objectives

You will learn the following in this chapter:

Histologic features distinguishing the three basic types of cartilage: hyaline cartilage, elastic cartilage, and fibrocartilage

Biochemical basis of staining differences distinguishing cartilage matrix and bone matrix

Histology of mature bone tissue (compact and spongy) and of bone organs

Mechanisms of endochondral and intramembranous bone formation

Role of osteoclastic bone resorption and osteocytic osteolysis in calcium homeostasis

Histology of bone fracture repair

As pointed out in Chapter 4, the connective tissues are made up of cellular elements and intercellular materials. However, unlike the epithelial tissues, for example, they have a much greater abundance of the intercellular constituents, which consist of fibers and a hydrated embedding substance. In the supportive connective tissues these constituents take on varying degrees of rigidity and thus function not only to provide support and attachment for tissues and organs, but also to provide structural support for the body.

The two general types of supportive connective tissue are cartilage and bone.

CARTILAGE
General Features

Cartilage is a highly resilient form of connective tissue, providing strength and support in areas of the body that also require varying degrees of flexibility. The cells of mature cartilage are called chondrocytes (Fig. 6-1); they are responsible for the production of the fibers and ground substance, which together with water combine to form a hydrated, amorphous gel called the **matrix.** It is the extracellular matrix with its embedded fibers that not only gives cartilage its resiliency, but also allows it to bear weight and to achieve considerable tensile strength.

All types of cartilage develop directly or indirectly from mesenchyme. During early chondrogenesis, newly proliferating chondroblasts form precartilage. However, after chondroblasts synthesize and secrete enough matrix components they become completely surrounded by matrix and are then referred to as chondrocytes. The space in this matrix occupied by each chondrocyte is a **lacuna** (hole). In histologic preparations, these cells shrink away from surrounding matrix

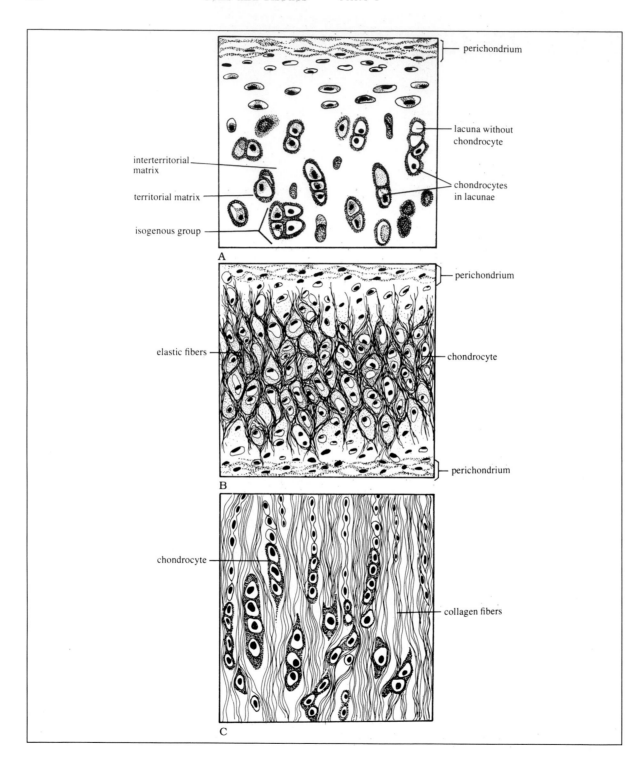

perichondrium

lacuna without
chondrocyte

interterritorial
matrix

chondrocytes
in lacunae

territorial matrix

isogenous group

A

perichondrium

elastic fibers

chondrocyte

perichondrium

B

chondrocyte

collagen fibers

C

Fig. 6-1. The histologic appearance of the three varieties of cartilage. A = hyaline cartilage; B = elastic cartilage; C = fibrocartilage.

and reveal the small lacunae in which they reside (Fig. 6-1A). The cells in these preparations have a basophilic cytoplasm and, due to the effects of shrinkage, an irregular cell border. With the electron microscope the shrinkage has been shown to be artifactual, because the potential space of the lacuna is completely filled by the chondrocyte. In electron micrographs, chondrocytes possess an extensive rough endoplasmic reticulum (RER), a well-developed Golgi apparatus, and numerous vesicles in various stages of discharge at the cell surface. These vesicles contain material with approximately the same density as the extracellular matrix. In resting cartilage, the protein secretory apparatus of the chondrocytes is less prominent.

The cartilage matrix is characterized as basophilic because of its affinity for histologic dyes that are basic or cationic; it also exhibits metachromasia when stained with toluidine blue. Chemically, the principal constituents of the ground substance are proteoglycans, which consist of protein and complex carbohydrates (glycosaminoglycans) such as the chondroitin sulfates. The highly acidic sulfate moieties that bind cationic dyes account for the basophilic and metachromatic staining properties of the matrix. The carbohydrate component also causes the matrix to be positive acid-Schiff (PAS)-positive. Based on the intensity of matrix staining with basic dyes, two regions are distinguished. Immediately surrounding the chondrocyte is a "capsule" of strongly basophilic matrix; elsewhere between cells or cell groups the matrix is less basophilic. These areas are termed the **territorial matrix** and **interterritorial matrix,** respectively (see Fig. 6-1A). The basis for this distinction is probably due to a greater concentration of glycosaminoglycans immediately around the cells and therefore a greater concentration of acidic

groups. Embedded in the matrix are either collagen or elastic fibers.

Except for the bearing surfaces of cartilage in joint cavities, cartilage is covered externally by a firm layer of specialized dense connective tissue called the **perichondrium** (Fib. 6-1A, B). This structure consists of an outer layer that is mostly fibrous and an inner layer that is more cellular with chondrogenic potential.

Developmentally, cartilage arises from mesenchyme, like other connective tissues. Growth of cartilage occurs by two mechanisms: **appositional** and **interstitial.** In appositional growth, cells located in the chondrogenic inner layer of the perichondrium differentiate into chondrocytes. The newly formed cartilage cells produce fibers and ground substance that are apposed to the existing cartilage and increase its mass. In interstitial growth, chondrocytes deep in the cartilage divide by mitosis and elaborate new matrix to expand the cartilage from within. Daughter cells from these mitotic divisions tend to remain in small clusters of elliptical cells called **isogenous groups** (Fig. 6-1A); they represent the descendants of a single chondrocyte.

Cartilage has no vasculature, lymphatic network, or innervation of its own. Chondrocytes are nourished by diffusion of oxygen and nutrients through the matrix from blood vessels located in surrounding connective tissues. However, vessels may pass through cartilage in "tunnels" without supplying it directly.

Regeneration of cartilage probably occurs in young cartilage only; in the adult, damage to cartilage results in a connective tissue scar. With age certain cartilages have a tendency to calcify. Since this process prevents diffusion of nutrients through the matrix, the chondrocytes die.

Types of Cartilage

Based on the amount of fibers and ground substance and the type of fibers, three varieties of cartilage are distinguished: **hyaline cartilage, elastic cartilage,** and **fibrocartilage** (see Fig. 6-1).

HYALINE CARTILAGE

Hyaline cartilage (see Fig. 6-1A) is the most wide-spread and characteristic form of cartilage. It is called **hyaline (hyalos** = glass) because of its glassy, whitish-blue appearance in the fresh state. It forms the majority of the temporary skeleton in mammalian embryos; in adults it is found in the nasal septum, larynx, trachea, and bronchi of the respiratory system, on the articulating surfaces of bones, and on the ventral ends of the ribs where they attach to the sternum. Chondroblasts of hyaline cartilage are derived directly from mesenchyme. Its abundant ground substance contains delicate collagen fibrils. In fresh and routine histologic preparations the matrix appears homogeneous, partly as a result of the similar refractive indices of the ground substances and collagen fibrils and partly because the basophilic ground substance is abundant enough to mask the acidophilic collagen embedded in it (Fig. 6-2). The collagen is type II and lacks the 640-Å periodicity. In addition to collagen the matrix contains proteoglycans with covalently bound chondroitin sulfates and keratan sulfate. The perimeter of developing and mature hyaline cartilage is bounded by a perichondrium. Since hyaline cartilage matrix tends to become rigid with age due to impregnation by calcium, interstitial growth is progressively lost. This infiltration of calcium also retards normal diffusion of nutrients causing necrosis. Further growth is purely appositional from undifferentiated cells of the chondrogenic layer of the perichondrium. Even this appositional growth is diminished in mature hyaline cartilage as evidenced by the fibrous connective tissue scar that forms from the perichondrium of a fractured cartilage.

Functionally, hyaline cartilage provides flexible support (e.g., in the respiratory passageways) and bearing surfaces in the joints. Because of its flexibility and ability to grow rapidly, it provides an excellent supporting framework for the developing embryo; in later stages it provides the mechanism by which long bones grow in length.

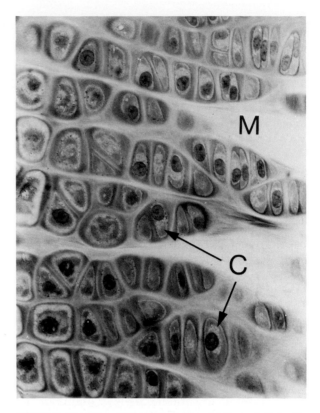

Fig. 6-2. Hyaline cartilage from the epiphyseal disk of a growing long bone. The chondrocytes (*C*) occupy lacunae in the cartilage matrix (*M*). The collagen is only faintly visible, being masked by amorphous components of the cartilage matrix. The territorial matrix forms a darker staining rim around the perimeter of each lacuna.

ELASTIC CARTILAGE

Elastic cartilage (see Fig. 6-1B) is considered to be a modification of hyaline cartilage. However, its chondrocytes are derived from fibroblasts rather than directly from mesenchyme. In the fresh state it has a yellowish color. It is found supporting the external ear, the auditory and eustachian tubes, the epiglottis, and part of the larynx (cuneiform and corniculate cartilages). Its sparse ground substance is extensively infiltrated with elastic fibers, the property for which it is named. The apparently randomly oriented fibers can be seen in routine histologic preparations but are seen to best advantage in sections treated with elastic stains. The fibers are least abundant just subjacent to the perichondrium but nevertheless extend into this layer. They are most abundant in the territorial matrix immediately surrounding the chondrocytes within the center of a piece of cartilage (Figs. 6-3, 6-4).

Functionally, elastic cartilage provides an extremely flexible support.

Fig. 6-3. Elastic cartilage. Chondrocytes (*C*) are locked within lacunae. Elastic fibers (*E*) radiate out in all directions.

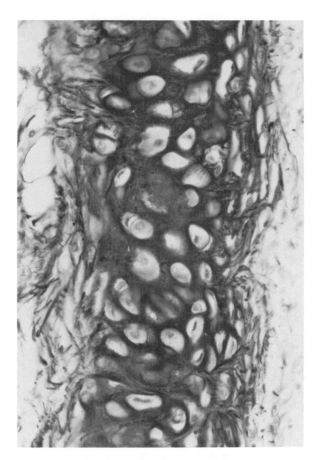

Fig. 6-4. Section of elastic cartilage within the epiglottis stained to demonstrate elastic fibers. Some of the coarser fibers extend into the perichondrium to the left and right in the photo. The chondrocytes, though poorly preserved, occupy the central area. Their lacuna are the lighter oval areas within the surrounding darker matrix.

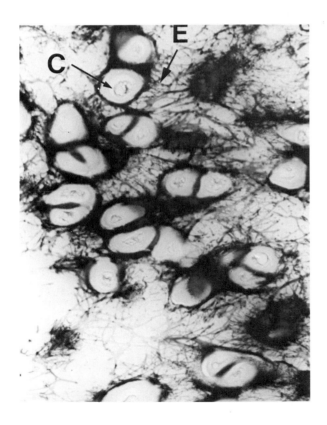

FIBROCARTILAGE

Fibrocartilage (see Fig. 6-1C) is a combination of hyaline cartilage and dense regular connective tissue. It is found in the intervertebral disks, the symphysis pubis, and in certain tendinous insertions. Its extremely sparse ground substance is heavily infiltrated with dense collagen fibers that are arranged in approximately parallel bundles. This relative preponderance of cationic collagen relative to ground substance explains the acidophilic staining properties of fibrocartilage compared to other types of cartilage. The cells are located between the fibrous elements and are often aligned in rows. In fibrocartilage a distinct perichondrium is lacking; chondrocytes arise from existing fibroblasts. The dense bundles of collagen are easily seen in routine histologic preparations.

Functionally, fibrocartilage combines the stress-bearing properties of cartilage and tendon/ligament for a firm but not rigid support. These properties are particularly advantageous in the intervertebral disks of the spinal column.

Repair of damaged cartilage, regardless of the type of cartilage, occurs by the formation of fibrocartilage.

BONE TISSUE AND BONE ORGANS

From structural, functional, and developmental points of view, it is pedagogically advantageous to consider bone as consisting of **bone tissue** and **bone organs.** Therefore, in this summary the distinction between "bone" as tissue and "bones" as organs is made. Bone tissue is the mineralized supportive connective tissue that forms the framework of bone organs, which in turn provide the supporting framework for the body.

Bone Organs

Bone organs (Fig. 6-5) are the structural and protective components of the axial and appendicular skeleton. They support the body and limbs, protect internal organs of the cranial, thoracic, and pelvic regions, secure the skeletal muscles for movement and locomotion, and house the adult hemopoietic tissues in their internal spaces. As organs, bones consist of bone tissue, external and internal investments of connective tissue, tendinous insertions, ligamentous attachments, vessels, nerves, and the bone marrow, which consists of blood-forming elements or adipose de-

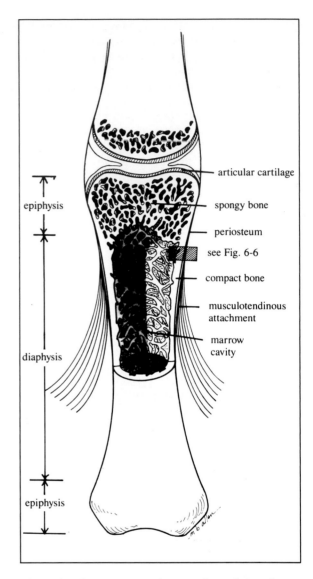

Fig. 6-5. A bone organ and some of its relationships.

pots. Additionally, in certain bone organs that move in relation to others, specializations of their surfaces for **articulation** occur.

Bone tissue (see the following section), like other connective and supportive tissue, consists of cells, fibers, and ground substance. However, in bone tissue the matrix with embedded fibers is impregnated with inorganic salts; this mineralization gives bone organs their special rigidity. Morphologically, bone tissue is organized in two ways. When the tissue forms a compact solid mass with relatively few intervening spaces, it is known as **compact bone;** when the tissue forms a three-dimensional network of intercommunicated osseous projections called **trabeculae,** with many intervening spaces, it is known as **spongy, trabecular,** or **cancellous bone** (Fig. 6-6). In general, compact bone forms the outer supportive "shell" for bone organs, while the spongy variety forms an anastomosing internal framework. These two arrangements are often referred to as **cortical bone** and **medullary bone,** respectively. Their organizational relationship is seen to best advantage in the long bones of the appendicular portion of the skeleton. Here in a bone organ such as the femur, compact bone forms the cor-

tex of the long cylindrical shaft called the **diaphysis** and the cortices of the variably shaped ends called the **epiphyses** (see Figs. 6-5, 6-6), while spongy bone normally forms an internal supporting framework at each end. The hollow diaphyseal core is called the **medullary cavity;** it is in direct communication with the cancellous spaces at each end, and together they contain the bone marrow. Hemopoietic tissue develops from undifferentiated cells within the marrow cavity. In the adult two types of bone marrow are present: an actively hemopoietic **red marrow** and an

Fig. 6-6. A human femur dried and stripped of its organic constituents such as tendons, periosteum, marrow, and epiphyseal cartilage. It has been sectioned lengthwise to reveal the spongy (cancellous) bone within the epiphyseal-diaphyseal junction. The large arrow indicates the bony union established between epiphysis and diaphysis after the cartilaginous epiphyseal disk was obliterated. C = compact bone forming the cortex or shaft of the bone.

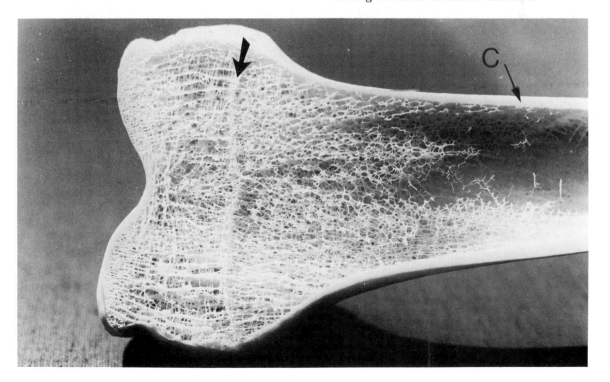

inactive, fat-infiltrated **yellow marrow.** Red marrow is found in the sternum, ribs, vertebrae, and pelvis in the adult. In addition, hemopoietic red marrow is found within the epiphysis while in the adult the diaphyseal marrow cavity is filled primarily with fat.

Normally bone organs are covered externally by a layer of specialized dense connective tissue called the **periosteum** (see Figs. 6-5, 6-13). Like the perichondrium, this structure consists of an outer vascularized layer that is mostly fibrous or capsulelike and an inner layer that is more cellular. The latter possesses osteogenic potential. A functional periosteum is absent in certain regions such as articulating surfaces and places where tendons or ligaments are attached; in these areas the osteogenic potential is also absent. Lining the bony surfaces of the medullary spaces as well as the spaces in cortical bone traversed by blood vessels is a layer of flattened connective tissue cells that also possesses osteogenic potential; this layer is called the **endosteum.** In the bones of the skull, the periosteum is called the **pericranium,** and the **dura mater** fuses to the periosteum. In adults the dura exhibits a limited osteogenic potential. Functionally, these areas of osteogenic potential are of great importance for bone remodeling and fracture repair.

Tendons and ligaments attach to bones by way of the periosteum. The periosteum in turn is attached to underlying bone tissue by dense collagen fibers extending from its outer fibrous layer into the mineralized bone matrix in a plane that is approximately perpendicular to the bone surface. During bone growth collagen fibers from tendons become anchored deeper in the newly deposited bone. These fibers of attachment are called **Sharpey's fibers.**

Blood vessels are associated with bones in patterns that vary according to the shape of the organs. In typical long bones, the vascular supply is from vessels that penetrate the shaft and marrow through a foramen called the **nutrient canal,** from vessels in the periosteum that penetrate the cortex, and from vessels that enter the epiphyses. Nerves may accompany these vessels.

Enclosed within fluid-filled joint cavities, the articular surfaces of bone organs are covered with caps of hyaline cartilage. These bearing surfaces lack a perichondrium.

Bone Tissue

Bone is a highly specialized, hard connective tissue of complex structure and function. Like cartilage, it consists of cells and an intercellular matrix of fibers and ground substance. However, certain of the cellular constituents in bone induce a mineralization of the soft matrix, which gives this supportive tissue a hardness and strength not possible in cartilage. Also in contrast to cartilage, the bone matrix has a high degree of structural organization, especially with respect to the packing of collagen fibers. These properties enable bone to withstand and recover from tension and compression and to perform its mechanical work with a minimum of material and weight. Thus, bone is an ideal tissue for supportive and protective skeletal functions.

In addition, bone is a metabolically active tissue. Throughout life it is continuously being remodeled by resorption of old bone and deposition of new bone. These antagonistic processes are involved in bone development, growth, and fracture repair. They respond to mechanical stress by reorganizing bone to bear weight more efficiently. Bone tissue also participates in a vital metabolic role as a reservoir for minerals, particularly calcium and phosphorus, which fulfill homeostatic needs. Therefore, bone is a dynamic and plastic tissue that responds to a variety of metabolic and mechanical stimuli.

CONSTITUENTS OF BONE TISSUE MATRIX

Bone matrix is a mineralized organic matrix. The mineral salts that constitute approximately 60 percent of bone volume account for its hardness and rigidity and serve as a reservoir from which the body may extract calcium for other uses. Although bone primarily contains calcium, phosphate, carbonate, and citrate, other minerals such as sodium, magnesium, and fluoride occur in bone as well. Small amounts of harmful radioactive minerals that may occur in the environment can become incorporated into bone also. The predominant form of bone mineral is a calcium phosphate salt similar to hydroxyapatite $(Ca_{10}[PO_4]_6[OH]_2)$.

The hydrated organic components of bone matrix account for approximately 40 percent of its volume. Collagen composes 95 percent of this organic material; the amorphous ground substance accounts for only 5 percent of it. Although the ground substance consists of some chondroitin-4-sulfate and keratan sulfate, most of its proteoglycans lack the acidic sulfate groups so common in cartilage matrix. Compared with cartilage matrix, which is basophilic because of its high content of acidic sulfated ground substance, decalcified bone is acidophilic because of its abundant acidophilic collagen content and relatively small amounts of acidic ground substance. In histologic sections containing both bone and cartilage, this staining differential facilitates the distinction between the two where other morphologic clues may be absent.

CELLULAR CONSTITUENTS OF BONE TISSUE

In developing as well as adult bone tissue, four types of cells are recognized. **osteogenic cells, osteoblasts, osteocytes,** and **osteoclasts.**

Osteogenic Cells (Osteoprogenitor Cells)

Osteogenic cells are pluripotential stem cells derived from mesenchyme. Under appropriate conditions these cells can proliferate and differentiate into chondroblasts or osteoblasts. In poorly vascularized areas where oxygen tension is low, these stem cells preferentially differentiate into chondroblasts, which deposit a cartilaginous matrix. In more vascularized areas where oxygen tension is sufficient, these same stem cells preferentially differentiate into osteoblasts, which secrete a bone matrix that subsequently

ossifies into rigid bone tissue. Osteogenic cells participate not only in the development of bone but also in the repair of bone fractures because they retain their pluripotential capacity even in the adult to develop into the cells that function in the reconstruction of a bone, that is, chondroblasts and osteoblasts.

In mature bone osteogenic cells form the cellular layer of the periosteum and constitute the single layer of cells (endosteum) that covers the bony surfaces within the marrow cavity and lines all blood vessel–containing channels (Volkmann's canals and haversian canals) within the bone organ. Histologically, they are flat, inconspicuous cells with a pale-staining, elongate nucleus and sparse eosinophilic cytoplasm.

Osteogenic cells have also been implicated in establishing the appropriate microenvironment for attracting colony forming units (CFUs) and promoting their proliferation and differentiation into myeloid cells, which initiate myelopoiesis in the marrow cavity (see Chap. 4).

Osteoblasts

Osteoblasts differentiate from osteogenic stem cells, secrete organic components of the bone matrix, and participate indirectly in its subsequent calcification. Newly deposited organic bone matrix is called **osteoid (prebone)** prior to its mineralization and, unlike calcified bone matrix, is undetectable in x-rays. Once osteoblasts become isolated in the rigid bony matrix that they deposit around themselves, their morphology changes in specific ways, and they are then classified as osteocytes.

In histologic section, osteoblasts are frequently seen with one side deployed against a bony surface that they are in the process of constructing, but within which they have not yet become incarcerated (Fig. 6-7). Osteoblasts usually appear as plump, polygonal cells, with an intensely basophilic cytoplasm and a large negative image of the Golgi complex (Fig. 6-8). In electron micrographs, osteoblasts display a well-developed RER and Golgi apparatus. Both features are typical of active secretory cells. Thus many secretory vesi-

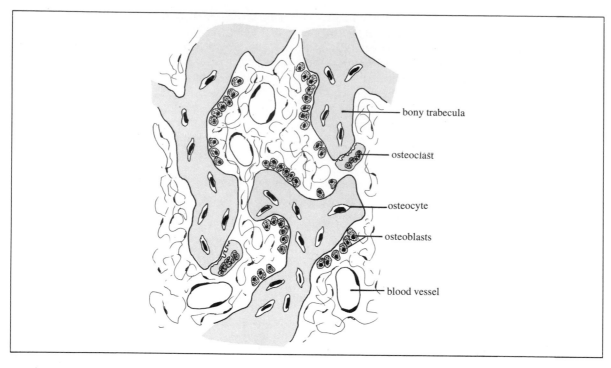

bony trabecula

osteoclast

osteocyte

osteoblasts

blood vessel

Fig. 6-7. Bone tissue formation against an existing surface.

Fig. 6-8. Numerous osteoblasts (*Ob*) apposed to the surfaces of two spicules of bone (*B*). The negative images of Golgi bodies are conspicuous in each osteoblast. *O* = osteocyte.

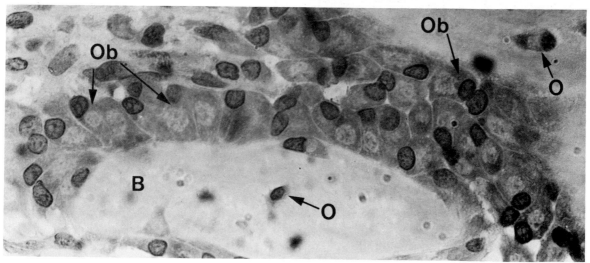

cles are present within these cells, which contain organic components of bone matrix to be secreted by exocytosis—that is, procollagen and the amorphous components of bones' ground substance. In addition, small vesicles (30–100 nm in diameter) are released into the extracellular space. They are called **matrix vesicles** and are derived from the plasmalemma of the osteoblasts. Matrix vesicles contain alkaline phosphatase, which liberates phosphate ions from organic phosphate compounds by enzymatic hydrolysis. This is a significant event in the calcification of osteoid since it provides adequate amounts of inorganic phosphate for precipitation of calcium ions. The phospholipids of the vesicle membrane attract and bind calcium ions, which facilitate this process. The result is the formation of crystals resembling hydroxyapatite. Diseases such as rickets and osteomalacia, which interfere with this process, result in bone characterized by excessive amounts of osteoid with weak weight-bearing properties.

Osteoblasts and osteocytes, unlike the osteogenic stem cells of their origin, are postmitotic. This fact becomes significant during the repair of fractured bone, as will be discussed.

Osteocytes

Osteocytes are the principal cells of bone tissue. Like chondrocytes, they are incarcerated in their surrounding matrix and are located in potential spaces called **lacunae** (see Figs. 6-8, 6-15). However, mineralized bone matrix is not freely diffusible to oxygen and nutrients as is the matrix of cartilage. Therefore, to prevent their own death, osteocytes are connected with one another by cytoplasmic processes that penetrate the bony matrix through small canals called **canaliculi,** which open near blood vessels often contained within haversian canals (see Fig. 6-15). Morphologically, osteocytes have an appearance similar to osteoblasts. However, the electron microscope reveals that the RER and Golgi apparatus are less prominent, especially in osteocytes located in deeper, older regions of bone tissue. This morphologic distinction is expected, since osteocytes

that maintain bone are metabolically less active than osteoblasts that initially form bone. Fine structural studies have also shown that gap junctions (maculae communicantes) are present at points of contact between osteocytic processes in the canaliculi, and the processes themselves are surrounded by a nonmineralized intralacunar matrix.

Osteoclasts

The preponderance of evidence now indicates that **osteoclasts** differentiate from circulating monocytes. This concept replaces the previous assumption that osteoclasts were derivatives of osteogenic cells.

Osteoclasts are responsible for degrading bone matrix at sites where bone will be remodeled. Remodeling takes place during normal development and growth of bones, during maintenance of mature bone, and during repair of bone fractures. The precise role that the osteoclast performs in each of these events is described in following sections. However, in general, remodeling involves the coordinated catabolic action of osteoclasts, which break down bone matrix (**osteoclastic resorption**), and the anabolic action of osteoblasts, which deposit bone matrix. During bone growth there is a net surplus of bone deposited by osteoblasts. On the other hand, with advancing age, osteoclastic resorption progressively outpaces bone deposition, which results in **osteoporosis** in the elderly.

Osteoclasts are most frequently located against the surfaces of bone, where they exert their resorptive activity. They are commonly located in shallow depressions of bone (**resorption bays, Howship's lacunae**), which they have excavated (Fig. 6-9). The osteoclast is a multinucleated giant cell, often containing 30 or more round nuclei contributed by the fusion of monocytes. Their cytoplasm is acidophilic to about the same extent as the bone tissue to which they are apposed. This staining similarity often requires some concentrated scrutiny in initial attempts to identify and locate osteoclasts. Osteoclasts also resemble megakaryocytes. However, the latter

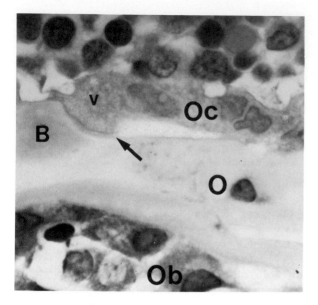

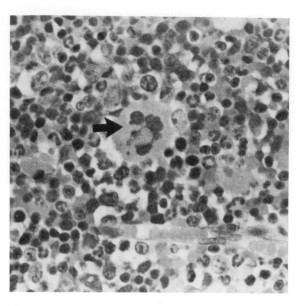

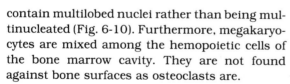

Fig. 6-9. An osteoclast (*Oc*) eroding away the surface of a spicule of bone (*B*). The arrow indicates the site along which the ruffled border is apposed. Just internal to the ruffled border is a foamy-appearing vacuolated area (*v*) within the osteoclast. This osteoclast shows only four of its nuclei in this section. Also note an osteocyte (*O*) and a row of osteoblasts (*Ob*) at the other side of the bony spicule.

Fig. 6-10. Section through the bone marrow showing a megakaryocyte (*arrow*). The multilobed character of its nucleus is evident. The cell occupies an area among many smaller hemopoietic cells.

contain multilobed nuclei rather than being multinucleated (Fig. 6-10). Furthermore, megakaryocytes are mixed among the hemopoietic cells of the bone marrow cavity. They are not found against bone surfaces as osteoclasts are.

The nuclei of the osteoclast are usually located away from the bony surface to which its cytoplasm is apposed. In histologic section, the cytoplasm contiguous to the bony surface is organized into an elaborate **ruffled border,** which in electron micrographs appears as an array of irregular villuslike projections of the cytoplasm abutting on the bony surface (Figs. 6-9, 6-11, 6-12). Electron microscopy also reveals an area lacking villuslike structures, called the **clear zone,** which surrounds the ruffled border and is

also apposed to the bony surface. The clear zone contains many actin microfilaments that may be involved in anchoring the osteoclast to the bony surface. Subjacent to the ruffled border in light micrographs is a foamy-appearing area that in electron micrographs consists of numerous vacuoles and expanded extensions of the intervillous spaces near the base of the ruffled border (see Fig. 6-9).

Osteoclastic resorption of bone matrix proceeds in two stages: the initial dissolution of minerals and the subsequent enzymatic degradation of collagen. Demineralization of bone occurs as a result of localized acidification. Experimental evidence strongly suggests that osteoclasts may excrete one or more acids that increase the solubility of bone mineral salts along the ruffled border. However, the details of this mechanism are not clear. The collagenous component of the matrix is degraded by the action of

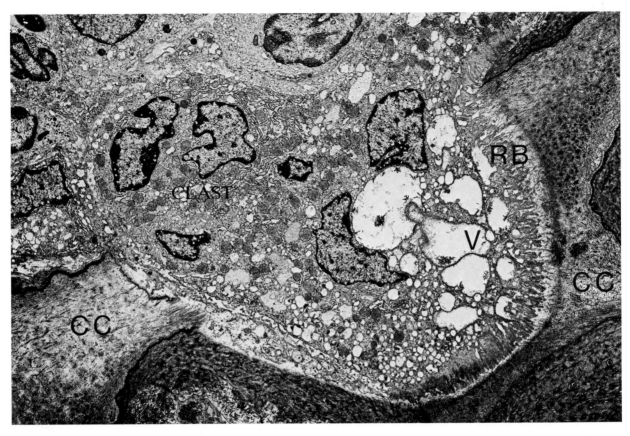

Fig. 6-11. An electron micrograph of an active osteoclast (*CLAST*) resorbing an area of calcified cartilage (*CC*). The ruffled border (*RB*) is apposed to an eroded surface of calcified cartilage. Subjacent to the ruffled border are numerous vacuoles (*V*) of various sizes, some of which are expended extensions of the intervillous spaces at the base of the ruffled border. (From M. E. Holtrop and G. J. King, The ultrastructure of the osteoclast and its functional implications. *Clin. Orthop. Rel. Res.* 123:177, 1977. With permission of J. B. Lippincott Co., Philadelphia.)

acid hydrolases presumably secreted at the base of the intervillus spaces. Exposed collagen fibrils projecting from the demineralized bone surface occupy intervillous spaces of the ruffled border where these enzymes are released. Although osteoclastic resorption of bone is essentially an extracellular activity, there is some evidence that osteoclasts may occasionally phagocytize bits of bone matrix, which are processed by lysosomes within the osteoclast.

In addition to its participation in bone remodeling, the osteoclast mobilizes calcium from its bony reservoir (the skeleton) and makes it available to the bloodstream, where calcium titer is rigorously maintained within a narrow range by the antagonistic action of two hormones: **calcitonin** and **parathyroid hormone.** Calcitonin reduces osteoclastic resorption while parathyroid hormone accelerates it. The influence of these two hormones on the osteoclast is directly evi-

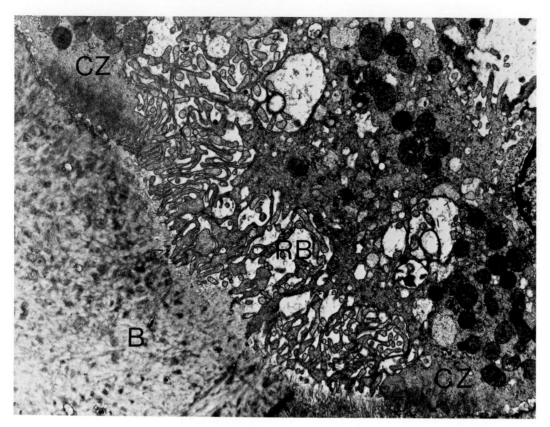

Fig. 6-12. An electron micrograph of an active osteoclast exhibiting a ruffled border (*RB*) and clear zone (*CZ*) apposed to a surface of bone (*B*). (From M. E. Holtrop and G. J. King, The ultrastructure of the osteoclast and its functional implications. *Clin. Orthop. Rel. Res.* 123:177, 1977. With permission of J. B. Lippincott Co., Philadelphia.)

dent in that parathyroid hormone stimulates development and activity of the ruffled border and clear zone while calcitonin diminishes the size of the ruffled border and clear zone.

Bone calcium is also mobilized by **osteocytic osteolysis,** a significantly different mechanism attributed to osteocytes (to be discussed later in this chapter).

ARRANGEMENT OF THE CONSTITUENTS

It has already been stated that bone tissue is organized morphologically into compact and spongy varieties. Macroscopically, this organization represents "dense" and "loose" arrangements of bone tissue, respectively. Microscopically, however, it reflects complex structural and functional relationships of cells, extracellular materials, and blood supply. To study these relationships and the arrangement of various bone constituents with the light microscope, two types of bone preparations have traditionally been made. Since bone mineral does not treat the normal implements of microtomy kindly, or vice versa, whereas the organic constituents usually do, it became obvious that the bone mineral had to be removed prior to cutting the tissue into thin sections for examination. Due to the fact that bone salts are soluble in acid, pieces of bone tissue or organs are so treated following fixation and prior to routine histologic preparation. In these **decalcified bone preparations** (Figs. 6-13, 6-14), the final product is thus a section of bone tissue that contains only organic materials such as cells, matrix, and blood vessels. In the other type of preparation, pieces of bone are cleaned and dried, sawed into relatively thin pieces, and

then ground between grinding stones to the appropriate thinness for histologic examination. In these **ground bone preparations** (Fig. 6-15) only the bone mineral remains. All cellular and most organic materials are absent; their former locations are represented histologically as blackened spaces caused by entrapped air.

Spongy bone has a relatively simple structure; it consists of an interconnected network of bony plates or bars with many intervening spaces (see Fig. 6-6). These plates or bars are composed of microscopic layers of bone tissue called **lamellae.** The laminated arrangement is a result of the appositional nature of bone tissue formation. In true lamellae the collagen fibers are oriented in parallel arrays. The parallel orientation of collagen in one lamella is arranged at a 90-degree angle with respect to collagen orientation in the adjacent lamellae. This provides greater bone strength. Located among the lamellae are the lacunae with their enclosed osteocytes. Radiat-

Fig. 6-13. A cross section through compact bone forming the shaft of a long bone, decalcified. Most of the haversian canals (*HC*) are cross-sectioned with tiny osteoblasts occupying orbits around them. Several cement lines within the outer (*O*) and inner (*I*) circumferential lamellae are evident. Skeletal muscle (*M*) inserts into the periosteum (*P*) covering the outer surface of the bone. A grazing section through a Volkmann's canal (*V*) is visible also. The marrow cavity (*MC*) is on the right.

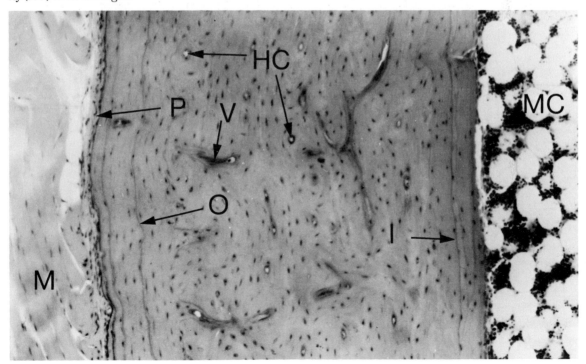

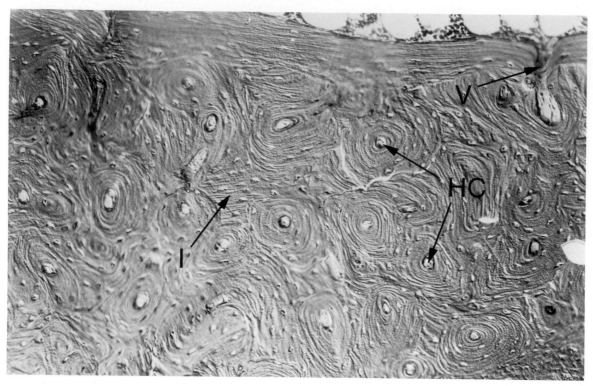

Fig. 6-14. A cross section of decalcified bone as in Figure 6-11 but viewed with Nomarski optics to provide an appreciation of the multiple haversian lamellae surrounding each haversian canal (*HC*). A Volkmann's canal (*V*) can be seen penetrating the inner circumferential lamellae and opening into the marrow cavity. Patches of older bone are evident also as interstitial lamellae (*I*).

ing between the lacunae and to the surface of the bony projections are the canaliculi. The blood supply for cancellous bone cells depends on capillaries that occupy the intervening marrow spaces. Nourishment of osteocytes occurs by diffusion through the canaliculi from these spaces.

Compact bone (see Fig. 6-6) is much more complex in its microscopic organization. Its arrangement reflects the ability of this variety of bone tissue to attain considerable thickness and yet to maintain its cells in close proximity to blood vessels. Three patterns of lamellar organization are seen in compact bone.

Haversian lamellae (see Figs. 6-13, 6-14, 6-15) are the most prominent lamellar arrangement and form the primary units of compact bone structure, called the **osteons** or **haversian systems.** These units consist of lamellae arranged concentrically around a central haversian canal. Haversian canals contain blood vessels, nerves, and some connective tissue; the canals are lined with cells of osteogenic potential (osteoprogenitor cells). Likewise, lacunar osteocytes are arranged concentrically in the osteons with their canaliculi radiating toward the **haversian canals** (see Fig. 6-15). The haversian systems are longitudinally arranged in the cortex of long bones. In some regions haversian canals freely anastomose with each other; in other regions adjacent haversian canals are connected with each other, the

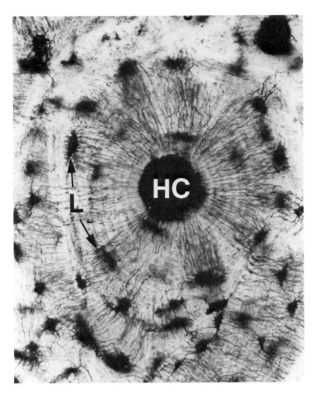

Fig. 6-15. Osteon from a ground section of compact bone. The canaliculi are the dark slender lines connecting the lacunae (*L*) to one another and to the central haversian canal (*HC*).

external bone surface, or the marrow cavity by channels that run approximately perpendicular to their planes. These channels are **not** surrounded by concentric lamellae and are called **Volkmann's canals** (see Fig. 6-13). Volkmann's canals contain branches of blood vessels traveling within haversian canals.

Interstitial lamellae (see Figs. 6-14, 6-15) are fragments of laminated bone tissue that are packed between the roughly cylindrical osteons. They represent remnants of older, partially resorbed and remodeled osteons. The boundaries between osteons and interstitial lamellae are marked by **cement lines.**

Circumferential lamellae are circular lamellae

that form the external and internal lamination of cortical bone. Their orientation is approximately perpendicular to that of the haversian lamellae. Outer circumferential lamellae occur beneath the periosteum, while inner circumferential lamellae occur adjacent to the endosteum (see Figs. 6-13, 6-14). Sharpey's fibers from tendons and ligaments are anchored in the outer circumferential lamellae.

OSTEOCYTIC OSTEOLYSIS

Osteolysis is a process of deep-seated bone resorption that is centered around the activity of old osteocytes and is therefore referred to as osteocytic osteolysis. In haversian systems or trabeculae of spongy bone, the most superficial, recently trapped osteocytes are relatively large and resemble osteoblasts; histochemical studies demonstrate that they also contain alkaline phosphatase. Away from the appositional surfaces (i.e., deeper within the osteons or trabeculae), the older osteocytes are smaller and show no alkaline phosphatase activity. In contrast, the oldest osteocytes in the deepest portions of osteons or trabeculae and their surrounding bony matrix are characterized by a number of marked changes: (1) osteocytes and their lacunae are larger; (2) the lacunar rims and adjacent matrix exhibit metachromasia when stained with toluidine blue; (3) alkaline phosphatase activity reappears in the cytoplasm of osteocytes and in the adjacent matrix; (4) microradiographic studies show a loss of bone mineral surrounding the osteocytes in ground bone preparations; (5) alpharadiography demonstrates a loss of organic matrix surrounding the osteocytes in decalcified bone preparations; and (6) polarized light microscopy demonstrates the degradation of the collagen fraction of the matrix.

The metachromatic staining reaction of the perilacunar matrix reflects a degradation or hydrolysis of the proteoglycans to form acidic glycosaminoglycans that possess sulfate or carboxyl groups. The presence of these moieties provides the electronegative charges responsible for toluidine blue metachromasia. In addition, in routine preparations areas of matrix hydrolysis are basophilic. These staining properties provide easy and reliable histologic methods for the demonstration of osteocytic osteolysis.

The highly ordered nature of collagen enables it to rotate the plane of polarized light. This property is called **birefringence** and is easily demonstrated using polarizing optics. In areas where the osteolytic process is occurring, there is a loss of birefringence resulting from the degradation of collagen. This loss coincides with areas of matrix metachromasia and basophilia. Degradation of collagen and ground substance is effected by proteolytic enzymes manufactured by resorbing osteocytes.

A primary aim of bone resorption in the adult is the maintenance of proper plasma calcium levels. The functional significance of osteocytic osteolysis is that it occurs in the oldest, deepest, most mineralized portions of bone tissue; these calcium-rich reservoirs are therefore made accessible to the body through the action of the osteocyte. Osteoclasia is usually concerned with the resorption of superficial bone tissue that is less mineralized. It is also important in the removal of bone that has been altered in some way, for example, in areas undergoing extensive osteolysis or in fracture sites.

Development of Bone Tissue and Bone Organs

Osseous development or **osteogenesis** is a complex process consisting of cellular migration, differentiation and modulation, and extracellular deposition of organic matrix and mineralization; the complexity of this process invariably creates difficulties for the beginning student. To circumvent some of these problems it is important to consider osteogenesis in two contexts: the formation of bone **tissue** (cells and intercellular mineralized matrix), and the formation of bone **organs** (e.g., bone tissue, periosteum, blood vessels). With a knowledge of bone tissue formation, one can reduce the complexities of bone organ

development to a sequence of predictable and understandable events.

DEVELOPMENT OF BONE TISSUE

Like other connective tissues, bone is mesenchymal in origin. Except for a transient period in the developing embryo in sites where mainly the so-called membrane bones develop, bone tissue normally forms in only one way: **by apposition against a preexisting surface through the action of osteoblasts.** This process is biphasic. First, osteoblasts produce and secrete unmineralized matrix called **preosseous tissue** or **osteoid,** which consists of ground substance and collagen. Subsequently, mineralization of the matrix occurs.

Formation of Bone Tissue without a Preexisting Surface

As a transitory event in early embryonic life, some bone tissue develops in sites where no existing surfaces are present. These sites correspond to areas where the **initiation** of the "membrane" bones in the head region occurs and where the **initiation** of the bone collar surrounding "cartilage models" occurs. In these areas mesenchyme proliferates to form a highly vascular connective tissue. Certain mesenchymal cells differentiate into osteoblasts which elaborate fibers and ground substance. Subsequently, this osteoid becomes mineralized, entrapping the cells in lacunae, which are now called osteocytes. The result, of course, is bone tissue. Further growth occurs appositionally. However, true lamellae are not present because the fibrils of collagen are deposited in a random fashion by the cells. This type of primitive bone tissue with osteocytes embedded in a nonlamellated, mineralized matrix is called **woven bone** or **primary bone.** It must be emphasized that this mechanism of bone tissue formation is one of initiation only. Once the small slivers of bony material called **spicules** are formed, a surface is present and bone tissue formation proceeds by the normal mechanism **against an existing surface.**

Formation of Bone Tissue against an Existing Surface

This method of bone tissue formation occurs on surfaces provided by either calcified cartilage or bone. When such a surface is present, pluripotential connective tissue (mesenchymal) cells called **osteoprogenitor cells** round up and position themselves against this mineralized surface (see Figs. 6-7, 6-8). These cells, which exhibit intense basophilia and possess all of the cytologic machinery necessary for protein synthesis, are called osteoblasts at this point. They elaborate ground substance and lay down collagen fibrils that are generally oriented with respect to the existing surface. Mineralization of this osteoid entraps the osteoblasts (at which point they are called osteocytes) and provides a "new" surface. Replenishment of osteoblasts for the new surface is accomplished by continued differentiation of osteoblasts from osteoprogenitor cells. Continued deposition and mineralization of osteoid results in the formation of bony matrix and entrapment of cells in their own matrix. This process repeats itself as bone is built. Mineralization of osteoid into rigid matrix means that interstitial growth cannot take place. Therefore, **the growth of all bone tissue takes place only by apposition to a surface.** As the bony spicules grow to form larger beams of tissue called **trabeculae** and partially fuse, an anastomosing network of spongy bone tissue results. All bone tissue forms first as spongy bone; compact bone is formed later as the intervening spaces are filled in with more bone tissue.

DEVELOPMENT OF BONE ORGANS

Bone organs develop in the embryo by replacement of **performed** connective tissue models. Two mechanisms of development are traditionally described. If the preformed model is composed of primitive connective tissue (mesenchyme), the mechanism of bone organ formation is termed **intramembranous ossification;** if the preformed model is composed of hyaline cartilage, the mechanism is termed **intracartilaginous** or **endochondral ossification.** The various aspects of bone organ development include formation of a periosteum; establishment of the vasculature; migration and modulation of osteoprogenitor cells to become osteoblasts; formation of bone tissue; apposition and resorption of bone tissue; and development of marrow cavities, tendinous insertions, and ligamentous attachments.

Development of Bone Organs in Mesenchyme: Intramembranous Ossification

The bone organs formed by intramembranous ossification are called **membrane bones** or **mesenchymal bones.** They include the frontal and parietal, and part of the temporal and occipital bones that form the calvaria of the skull; part of the mandible; the facial bones; and the clavicles. The models that are first formed are "membranes" of highly vascularized mesenchymal tissue from which osteoblasts differentiate. Development of these organs is initiated by the formation of bone tissue without a preexisting surface, as described earlier; continued development is completely by appositional growth against existing surfaces. The result is woven bone in a spongy arrangement. As the trabeculae thicken with the deposition of more matrix and the deployment of additional osteoblasts the intervening vascular spaces become smaller, and the woven bone appears lamellar. However, the collagen is randomly oriented so that the bone formed is still of the woven variety. Lamellar bone forms only after woven bone is remodeled, when the collagen becomes highly ordered. The mesenchyme surrounding the developing bone organ condenses and becomes the periosteum, which provides the cells needed for appositional growth.

In areas destined to become compact bone, the blood vessels within intertrabecular spaces become encased completely during continuing apposition of bone against trabecular surfaces, until the trabecular arrangement is replaced by typical haversian systems.

Development of Bone Organs in Hyaline Cartilage: Endochondral Ossification

The bone organs formed by endochondral ossification are called **cartilage bones** or **endochondral bones.** They include the majority of the bone organs of the axial portion of the skeleton and all the bone organs of the appendicular portion. This mechanism of development is characterized by the formation of mesenchymally derived hyaline cartilage models. For instance, the vertebral bones are preceded by a condensation of mesenchyme in which chondrification centers arise to form a cartilaginous vertebral precursor. This cartilage anlage is remodeled into a larger bony replica. This transformation process is called **endochondral bone formation.** The typical formation of a long bone of an appendage is used here to demonstrate the processes of the endochondral mechanism (Fig. 6-16).

At an appropriate point in intrauterine life in an area of the cartilage model that corresponds to the future diaphysis, cartilage cells hypertrophy (Fig. 6-16A), their lacunae enlarge, and the surrounding matrix calcifies (Fig. 6-16B). Since little metabolic exchange can occur through the mineralized matrix, the chondrocytes degenerate and die. Simultaneously, the vascularized perichondrium that surrounds this portion of the developing bone organ becomes osteogenic; it can therefore now be called the periosteum. Cellular elements in this region modulate and become osteoblasts. The osteoblasts then lay down a thin sheet of bone tissue around the circumference of the model in its midportion, which is termed the **bone collar** (see Fig. 6-16B). The mechanism by which this periosteal band of bone tissue forms is identical with that previously described in sites where no existing surfaces are present. Some authors refer to bone collar formation as a

Fig. 6-16. Some major events in the formation of a long bone organ by endochondral ossification. A. Hyaline cartilage model; hypertrophy of central chondrocytes. B. Hypertrophied chondrocytes begin to die due to initiation of matrix calcification; formation of the bone collar. C. Invasion of blood vessels and pluripotential osteoprogenitor cells; resorption of calcified cartilage matrix to form exposed surfaces for bone tissue apposition in primary center of ossification. D. Growth of bone organ and formation of marrow cavity through cartilage proliferation at epiphyseal ends, bone tissue apposition at calcified cartilage surfaces, and resorption in diaphyseal cavity; initiation of secondary center of ossification above; elongation of bone collar. E. Further growth of bone organ; formation and development of secondary ossification center above, leaving cartilaginous epiphyseal plate separating epiphysis from diaphysis; appearance of additional secondary center of ossification below simultaneously with appearance of the secondary center above; growth in girth of bone organ by concomitant bone tissue apposition on outer diaphyseal surface and resorption from inner surface. Black, calcified cartilage; black arborizations, blood vessels; parallel diagonal lines, bone tissue.

form of intramembranous ossification, where the "membrane" is the periosteum.

While the bone collar is forming, vascular tufts that are collectively called the **periosteal** or **mesenchymal bud** invade and erode the calcified cartilage in the interior of the model (Fig. 6-16C). Carried inward with this bud are some cells that become osteoblasts; others give rise to blood-forming cells. The osteoblasts lay down bone tissue on the surfaces of the remaining calcified cartilage by the mechanism of formation of bone tissue against an existing surface, as already described. Histologically, the resulting trabeculae have a heterogeneous appearance due to staining differences of their calcified cartilage "cores" and bone tissue surfaces; in contrast, the trabeculae of the bone collar, which are composed only of bone tissue, have a homogeneous appearance. These areas of initial bone tissue formation in the developing bone organ are collectively termed

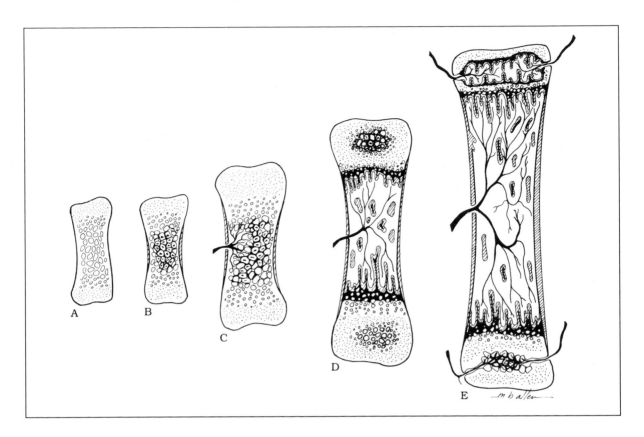

the **primary center of ossification.** The intervening spaces between diaphyseal trabeculae become the primitive marrow cavity and contain developing blood cells.

Subsequent to the formation of the primary ossification center in the midportion of the diaphysis, the adjacent cartilage toward both future epiphyses undergoes similar chondrocyte and matrix changes (Fig. 6-16D,E). However, in these regions the process becomes much more ordered. The chondrocytes become arranged in parallel, longitudinal columns and undergo their changes in a linear fashion from epiphyses to diaphysis; that is to say, identifiable zones of change occur along the columnar axes. From the epiphyseal regions toward the diaphysis, the zones are as follows: (1) zone of resting or reserve cartilage; (2) zone of proliferating cartilage; (3)

zone of maturing and hypertrophying cartilage; and (4) zone of calcifying cartilage. Collectively, these cartilaginous zones make up what is later called the **epiphyseal plate** (Fig. 6-17). The orientation of these cartilage columns not only provides for the formation of bone tissue at their diaphyseal ends, but also, and more importantly, provides the morphologic arrangement for the growth of the bone organ in **length.**

The zone of resting cartilage consists of small, flattened chondrocytes that are held in reserve until new proliferating cells for growth are required. The zone of proliferating cartilage contains flattened cells that divide mitotically only in the longitudinal axis to increase the length of the columns and therefore the length of the bone organ. In the zone of hypertrophying cartilage, the cells and lacunae enlarge and begin their regres-

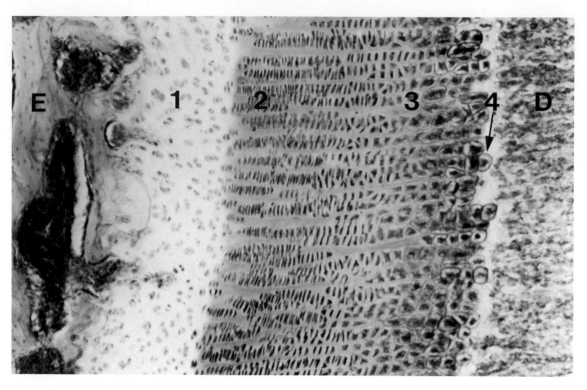

Fig. 6-17. Epiphyseal plate area showing the zones of hyaline cartilage in the plate. A portion of epiphyseal bone (E) is visible to the left. *1* = resting zone of cartilage; *2* = proliferating zone of cartilage characterized by stacks of flattened chondrocytes; *3* = maturing cartilage characterized by hypertrophy of chondrocytes; *4* = zone of calcifying cartilage characterized by only a few chondrocytes and bits of eroded cartilage matrix. Abutting diaphysis (D) contains advancing capillaries and developing bony trabeculae.

sive changes. In the zone of calcifying cartilage, the matrix mineralizes and the chondrocytes die. Once calcification begins, blood vessels from the diaphyseal center invade and erode the mineralized ends of the columns (see Figs. 6-16E, 6-17); they carry with them cells that become osteoblasts. As before, the osteoblasts deposit bone tissue on remnants of the calcified cartilage; therefore, extensions of bone tissue resembling

stalactites appear at the bases of the cartilage columns. The histologic picture of this region shows slender irregularly shaped spicules of basophilic cartilage matrix with a thin veneer of acidophilic bone matrix deposited against its surfaces. As the epiphyses begin to "move" (i.e., grow) away from the diaphysis by proliferative events in the epiphyseal growth plate, osteoclasts appear on these basal bony trabeculae and begin to resorb the bone tissue. This resorption of calcified cartilage and bone tissue by osteoclasts with a concomitant proliferation of cartilage essentially maintains a constant thickness of the growth plate and also provides for the enlargement of the subjacent marrow cavity.

The epiphyseal plate can be likened to a series of coin stacks of specified height. In a simplified explanation, if a number of coins are added to the top of the stacks (proliferation) and an equal number are removed from the bottom (calcification and resorption), the height of the stack is maintained but the stack is spatially displaced. In effect, this is the function of the epiphyseal plate and the mechanism by which bone organs grow in length. This analogy breaks down, however, when one realizes that the "coins" in the epiphyseal plate are different or at least in different stages. It must be understood that each zone undergoes the complete sequence from proliferation to calcification, albeit in a staggered fashion. One should also remember that any histologic section represents a stationary time frame in the cycle of dynamic cells or tissues. In the case of cartilage columns of the epiphyseal plate, the apparent spatial organization reflects ongoing temporal changes in each zone. For example, the zone of calcification at the time the bone organ was histologically prepared was the zone of hypertrophy in a previous time frame, and so on. It is this sequence of temporal changes in each zone *and* the spatial arrangement of several zones in sequential stagger that allow the bone organ not only to grow in length, but also to grow in a continuous fashion.

The proliferation of chondroblasts in the epiphyseal plate is stimulated by somatomedin and thyroid hormone. As these hormonal influences subside with the attainment of adult size, the proliferation of chondroblasts ceases. This allows the advancing osteoclasts to degrade the remaining calcified cartilage of the epiphyseal plate, and the bony union of epiphysis and diaphysis is accomplished. With the bony replacement of the epiphyseal disk, growth in length of bone ceases. The bony union of the epiphysis with the diaphysis occurs at different times in different bones. In an adolescent the epiphysis of the lesser trochanter is not yet united with the shaft of the femur. Consequently these particular disks are weak and vulnerable to fracture (avulsions) in adolescents.

Meanwhile, back at the periosteum the bone collar elongates so that it encircles the entire bone organ (see Fig. 6-16C,D,E). Furthermore, new osteoblasts arise from osteoprogenitor cells in the periosteum and deposit bone tissue on ex-

isting bony surfaces appositionally. Successive layers of appositional bone provide the means by which the bone organ grows in **girth.** To maintain the thickness of the developing shaft and to increase the latitude of the marrow cavity, osteoclasts effect resorption from the medullary surfaces.

At birth, the long bone organs usually have cartilaginous epiphyses and a bony diaphysis. After birth, **secondary centers of ossification** occur in the epiphyses by a mechanism similar to the one that occurred earlier in the midportion of the diaphysis (see Fig. 6-16D,E). Formation of spongy bone tissue spreads centrifugally and thus eventually leaves cartilage only on the external surfaces of the epiphyses as the **articular cartilages** and at the diaphyseo-epiphyseal junction as the definitive **epiphyseal plate** (see Fig. 6-16E). The latter is a joint of sorts in that it binds bone to bone and is called a **synchrondrosis.** When the bone organ reaches full size at maturity and the cartilage of the epiphyseal plate is used up, a bony fusion results, which can be considered a synostosis. The events that take place in the epiphyseal plate resulting in a lengthening of the diaphysis also occur, albeit more randomly, in the articular cartilages. This process effectively increases the size of the epiphyses proportionately to the rest of the bone organ. However, in the adult the articular cartilages remain and serve as the bearing surfaces in the hinged, movable joints called **diarthroses.** Furthermore, remodeled spongy bone is maintained in the epiphyses, and the intervening marrow spaces are continuous with the large marrow (medullary) cavity of the diaphysis (see Figs. 6-5, 6-6).

All bone tissue formed initially in the development of bone organs is in the form of woven bone because of the random orientation of the collagen fibers. True lamellar bone (secondary bone) with collagen in parallel arrays is formed later only through remodeling of woven bone by the combined actions of osteoclasts and osteoblasts. For example, in humans lamellar bone forming true haversian systems occurs in the shafts of long bones only after the age of 1 year. This internal reorganization of primary compact bone to form the adult haversian systems is called **secondary bone formation.** Higher orders of bone tissue formation continue throughout life due to a continuous remodeling process.

This summary is at best a superficial description of the formation of bone organs. In most instances, there are either more or fewer centers of ossification than the one diaphyseal center and two epiphyseal centers discussed here. The number can range up to and including seven or more secondary centers of ossification, since condyles and tuberosities commonly have individual ossification centers. In these cases, the articular cartilages fulfill the growth functions.

Blood Supply to Bones

The vascular system of bones is best appreciated now that the role of the periosteal buds in bone development has been described. The periosteal buds that supply the developing diaphysis, metaphysis, and epiphysis become the nutrient, metaphyseal, and epiphyseal arteries, respectively, of a mature bone. The blood supply to cortical bone in the shaft of a long bone is provided by cortical branches of nutrient, metaphyseal, and epiphyseal arteries located in the marrow cavity. Arterioles from these marrow arteries enter Volkmann's canals and branch along with capillaries into the haversian canals. Oxygen and nutrients diffuse through canaliculi to reach osteocytes within the osteon. Marrow arteries also flood sinusoidal capillaries within the marrow to support metabolic needs of marrow tissue. Venous drainage exits through nutrient veins found in Volkmann's canals.

It should be appreciated that the nutrient and metaphyseal arterioles do not anastomose with the epiphyseal vessels. During development the growth plate is supplied with oxygen by epiphyseal vessels since calcification of cartilage along the diaphyseal side of the growth plate prevents adequate diffusion to the epiphysis.

Lymphatics occur in the periosteum but not in the cortex or marrow.

Joints

Joints are assemblies of connective tissue which bind bones together and determine the relative mobility of one bone to another bone. Joints may allow considerable mobility, various degrees of mobility, or restricted mobility.

Generally the least mobile joints are the **synarthroses.** There are three subtypes classified according to the type of intervening connective tissue connecting bones. A collagenous or elastic union forms a **syndesmosis;** a cartilage union forms a **synchondrosis;** a bony union forms a **synostosis.**

Two examples of syndesmoses are the cranial sutures and the ligamenta flava of the vertebral column. The cranial sutures unite the flat bones of the skull. The intervening connective tissue is mostly collagen which can be quite extensive in the newborn, forming the fontanelles. Growth of the flat cranial bones occurs by the intramembranous process as appositional growth along the free edges of the bone involved in the joint expands the bony vault and allows for growth of the brain to occur. The collagenous joint is gradually obliterated as ossification continues until by middle age the sutures have been replaced by bone to become synostoses (see below). The ligamenta flava are elastic ligaments connecting the lamina of adjacent vertebral arches.

The most common synchondrosis is represented by the epiphyseal growth plate joining the epiphyses and diaphysis of developing bones prior to its replacement by the ossification process. Another hyaline cartilage synchondrosis is the spheno-occipital joint in the base of the skull which allows for bone growth adequate to accommodate the increasing size of the brain in the young. Synchondroses are also formed by fibrocartilage as in the anterior intervertebral joints. In these cases the ends of opposing bones are each encased in articular hyaline cartilages, which are joined to each other by a circumferential fibrocartilage called the **annulus fibrosus.** Enclosed within the fibrocartilage is the nucleus pulposus, which is a gelatinous mass confined in place by the surrounding annulus fibrosus. This type of joint not only binds the vertebrae together but absorbs force sustained along the vertical axis of the spinal column. Another example of a synchondrosis constructed of fibrocartilage is the pubic symphysis.

Diarthroses are the highly mobile joints located between the articular cartilages of long bones, in the temporomandibular joint, in the zygapophyseal joints between the articular processes of vertebral arches, in the sacroiliac, and in most of the sternocostal joints. This type of joint is enclosed by a collagenous capsule that is continuous with the periosteum of the involved bones. The interior of the capsule is lined by a synovial membrane which encloses a fluid-filled synovial cavity. The weight-bearing surfaces of the opposing articular cartilages is bathed in synovial fluid since the articular surface of the cartilage is devoid of synovial membrane. The synovial fluid reduces friction between the weight-bearing articular cartilages. There is usually a flat interarticular cartilage between the articular cartilages within the joint cavity which also bears weight and reduces friction. Some joints, however, like the temporomandibular joint and most of the sternocostal joints, have an interarticular ligament instead of an interarticular cartilage. Part of the joint capsule is reinforced by tendons from muscles which originate from or insert onto one or both bones near the joint. However, other areas of the capsule are incomplete and allow small pouches of the synovial membrane to project through. These pouches are termed **bursae.** They reduce friction of overlying muscle and tendon movements which slide along the surface of the joint while operating the joint. The synovial membrane is one to three cells thick. The connective tissue supporting these cells is highly vascularized. An ultrafiltrate escaping from these capillaries crosses the cell lining of the synovial membrane to form part of the synovial fluid along with mucous secretions from synovial lining cells.

Abnormalities of Bone Formation

Any disease process that interferes with secretion of organic matrix or with calcification of osteoid significantly alters bone formation. The following paragraphs are brief descriptions of bone formation abnormalities.

Scurvy is caused by inadequate amounts of dietary vitamin C (ascorbic acid), which results in reduced hydroxylation of proline and lysine. The resulting impairment of collagen cross-linking reduces secretion of collagen and formation of osteoid. Although osteoid deposition is reduced, calcification of existing osteoid is completed. In fact remaining osteoid is usually hypercalcified. Nevertheless, if scurvy occurs during bone development, resulting bones are narrower and weaker as a result of diminished osteoid available for normal growth.

Rickets caused by vitamin D deficiency is the result of inadequate calcium and phosphorous absorption by the gastrointestinal tract. Consequently, osteoid is inadequately calcified resulting in weak bones. Inability to bear weight causes the bowing of the legs characteristic of children with rickets. Another critical consequence is impaired calcification of the epiphyseal disk during bone development, which causes immediate deformations in growing bones that are especially prominent along the ribs. In adults the effects of vitamin D deficiency are less pronounced and result in **osteomalacia.** During osteomalacia the normal turnover and maintenance of bone matrix is impaired due to insufficient calcification of new osteoid.

Osteoporosis is a common condition of aging. In this case the osteoclastic resorption of bone matrix exceeds the diminishing rate of bone matrix deposition.

Acromegaly is a condition caused by excessive release of growth hormone (somatotropin). The resulting production of somatomedin by the liver causes disproportionate subperiosteal bone growth. Excessive release of somatomedin before ossification of the epiphyseal growth plate causes gigantism. However, acromegaly is the result of excess somatomedin after these growth plates have been ossified. The new bone is deposited by appositional growth from the periosteum conferring an unusual thickness to bones of the hands, feet, and mandible plus all membrane bones.

Healing of Bone Fractures

A bone fracture involves not only bone matrix but also the nutrient blood vessels and periosteum. As a result of damage to these blood vessels, a blood clot forms at the fracture site and the blood supply to the osteocytes is interrupted there. These osteocytes will die due to insufficient blood supply, but their connection with Volkmann's canals and the anastomosing network of the haversian system will limit the extent of cell death to a short zone nearest the fracture plane.

The first sign of healing is the formation of new soft tissue around the perimeter of broken bone fragments (**external callus**) and between them (**internal callus**). Almost immediately, osteogenic cells differentiate from the cellular layer of the periosteum and to a lesser extent from the endosteum. The rate of differentiation is so high that it produces a palpable thickening of the periosteum. Growth of the osteogenic cells in the external callus proceeds at a faster rate than its vascularization. Hence, many of these osteogenic cells differentiate into chondroblasts, which deposit hyaline cartilage in the callus. Deeper in the callus, bone begins to form from osteoblasts derived from osteogenic cells as a result of an improved blood supply. As the callus grows around the two ends of fractured bone, mostly through interstitial growth of new cartilage, fusion of the callus weakly unites the broken ends. Following this event the cartilage is replaced exactly as it is during endochondral bone formation. The cartilage matrix calcifies, chondrocytes die, and cancellous bone is deposited by osteoblasts upon calcified cartilaginous surfaces. This cancellous bone is constructed mostly in the external callus and within the marrow cavity. As in normal bone development, it represents a tempo-rary support that will be remodeled by the action of osteoclasts and osteoblasts into the compact bone of the cortical shaft.

NATIONAL BOARD TYPE QUESTIONS

For the following, select
    A. if only *1, 2, and 3* are correct.
    B. if only *1 and 3* are correct.
    C. if only *2 and 4* are correct.
    D. if only *4* is correct.
    E. if *all* are correct.

1. Which of the following statements about bone collagen is (are) true?
   1. Osteoclasts are incapable of dismantling the collagenous component of bone matrix.
   2. Osteoblasts are responsible for the synthesis of the collagenous component of bone matrix.
   3. The collagen fibers within adjacent concentric lamellae surrounding a Haversian canal are oriented in the same direction.
   4. Sharpey's fibers are composed of collagen derived from the periosteum and inserting tendons and ligaments.
2. Which of the following characteristics is (are) common to all three types of cartilage?
   1. Both appositional and interstitial growth
   2. Basophilic matrix
   3. Lack both a blood supply and lymphatic drainage
   4. Form a template for the formation of endochondral bone
3. Which of the following statements regarding the stages of endochondral bone growth is (are) true?
   1. A periosteal bud invades a calcified, hyaline cartilage template.
   2. The bone collar replaces a cartilage template.

3. Growth in length is the result of proliferation of cartilage in the epiphyseal plate.
4. Examples of bones formed exclusively by this mechanism are the frontal, parietal, and occipital bones.

4. Regarding hyaline cartilage:
   1. Calcification of its matrix occurs progressively with age, often contributing to the death of chondrocytes.
   2. Fractures of this type of cartilage are repaired in the adult primarily by the perichondrium.
   3. Its basophilic matrix is due to the presence of acidic, sulfated chondroitins.
   4. It lacks a perichondrium.

5. Which of the following statements regarding osteoclasts is (are) true?
   1. Osteoclasts are multinucleated.
   2. Parathyroid hormone reduces the development and activity of the ruffled border of osteoclasts.
   3. Local acidification caused by osteoclasts causes dissolution of minerals from bone matrix.
   4. Osteoclasts have basophilic cytoplasm.

6. Which of the following statements about bone is (are) true?
   1. Rickets and osteomalacia are characterized by abnormally low amounts of osteoid.
   2. Osteoporosis is a decrease in bone mass caused by a higher rate of osteoclastic resorption compared to bone formation by osteoblasts.
   3. Acromegaly is due to growth of the epiphyseal disk caused by excess release of growth hormone.
   4. The histologic appearance of mature bone tissue is essentially identical in bones formed by intramembranous vs. endochondral mechanisms.

7. Bone canaliculi
   1. interconnect lacunae within a Haversian system (osteon).
   2. contain cytoplasmic processes of osteocytes.

3. interconnect the innermost lacunae of an osteon to their haversian canal.
4. contain capillaries.

8. Which of the following tissues will have an acidophilic matrix?
   1. Hyaline cartilage
   2. Fibrocartilage
   3. Elastic cartilage
   4. Decalcified bone

9. Which of the following statements regarding the epiphyseal plate in a growing long bone is (are) true?
   1. Proliferation of its chondrocytes is accelerated by somatomedin.
   2. Growth in length of a bone is terminated the moment the epiphyseal plate is obliterated by the ossification process.
   3. Interstitial growth is prominent within the epiphyseal plate.
   4. Fibrocartilage is the major component of the epiphyseal plate.

10. Which of the following statements regarding the organization of bone is (are) true?
    1. Newly deposited unmineralized bone matrix is termed osteoid and is difficult to detect in x-rays.
    2. Woven bone contains highly organized collagen arranged into lamellae.
    3. Volkmann's canals do not have concentric lamellae surrounding them.
    4. In an adult long bone, cancellous bone is present in equal quantity in the epiphysis and diaphysis.

11. Fibrocartilage is located in which of the following?
    1. Certain tendinous insertions
    2. Eustachian tube
    3. Intervertebral disk
    4. Epiglottis

12. Which of the following statements regarding bone tissue abnormalities is (are) true?
    1. Rickets caused by vitamin D deficiency is characterized by impaired calcification of the epiphyseal disk.
    2. Osteomalacia is characterized by excessive calcification of osteoid.

3. Acromegaly is the result of excessive deposition of subperiosteal bone.
4. Scurvy is characterized by excessive osteoid deposition.

ANNOTATED ANSWERS

1. C. For further discussion, refer to Osteoclasts on page 137.
2. B. Fibrocartilage exhibits primarily an acidophilic matrix because the collagen is present in greater proportion than the basophilic ground substance. Only hyaline cartilage forms a template for bone formation.
3. B. The flat bones of the skull are formed by intramembranous ossification as well as the bony collar of endochondral bones.
4. A. Hyaline cartilage is surrounded by perichondrium except at the articulating surfaces within synovial joints.
5. B. Parathyroid hormone increases osteoclastic resorption, which is characterized by the increased development and activity of the ruffled border.
6. C. Acromegaly occurs after the epiphyseal disc has been replaced by bone.
7. A. Capillaries do not extend beyond the haversian canals.
8. C. See question 2. Decalcification of bone exposes the acidophilic collagen component.
9. A. In a growing bone there may be some fibrocartilage from a tendinous insertion anchored in the lateral surface of the epiphyseal plate, which itself is composed of hyaline cartilage.
10. B. Collagen is deposited in a random orientation in woven bone. In an adult long bone, the cancellous bone in the diaphysis has been resorbed away by osteoclasts leaving it primarily in the epiphysis.
11. B. The eustachian tube and epiglottis are formed of elastic cartilage.
12. B. For further discussion, refer to Abnormalities of Bone Formation on page 151.

BIBLIOGRAPHY

Anderson, H. C. Calcification of rachitic cartilage to study matrix vesicle function. *Fed. Proc.* 35:147, 1976.

Anderson, H. C. Matrix Vesicles of Cartilage and Bone. In G. H. Bourne (ed.). *The Biochemistry and Physiology of Bone* (2nd ed.). New York: Academic, 1976. Vol. 4, p. 135.

Barer, M., and J. Jowsey. Bone formation and resorption in normal human ribs. *Clin. Orthop.* 52:241, 1967.

Bassett, C. A. L., and I. Herrmann. Influence of oxygen concentration and mechanical factors on differentiation of connective tissues in vitro. *Nature* 190:460, 1961.

Bélanger, L. F. Osteocytic osteolysis. *Calcif. Tissue Res.* 4:1, 1969.

Bernard, G. W., and D. C. Pease. An electron microscope study of initial intramembranous osteogenesis. *Am. J. Anat.* 125:271, 1969.

Büring, K. On the origin of cells in heterotopic bone formation. *Clin. Orthop.* 110:293, 1975.

Cameron, D. A. The Ultrastructure of Bone. In G. H. Bourne (ed.), *The Biochemistry and Physiology of Bone* (2nd ed.). New York: Academic, 1972. Vol. 1, p. 191.

Decker, J. D. An electron microscope investigation of osteogenesis in the embryonic chick. *Am. J. Anat.* 118:591, 1966.

Doty, S. B. Morphological evidence of gap junctions between bone cells. *Calcif. Tissue Int.* 33:509, 1981.

Doty, S. B., and B. H. Schofield. Electron microscope localization of hydrolytic enzymes in osteoclasts. *Histochem. J.* 4:245, 1972.

Fischman, D. A., and E. D. Hay. Origin of osteoclasts from mononuclear leukocytes in regenerating newt limbs. *Anat. Rec.* 143:329, 1962.

Frost, H. M. Tetracycline-based histological analysis of bone remodeling. *Calcif. Tissue Res.* 3:211, 1969.

Gonzales, F., and M. J. Karnovsky. Electron microscopy of osteoclasts in healing fractures of rat bone. *J. Biophys. Biochem. Cytol.* 9:299, 1961.

Göthlin, G., and J. L. E. Ericsson. The osteoclast. *Clin. Orthop.* 120:201, 1976.

Hall, B. K. The origin and fate of osteoclasts. *Anat. Rec.* 183:1, 1975.

Ham, A. W., and S. Gordon. The origin of bone that forms in association with cancellous chips transplanted into muscle. *Br. J. Plastic Surg.* 5:154, 1952.

Holtrop, M. E. The ultrastructure of bone. *Ann. Clin. Lab. Sci.* 5:264, 1975.

Holtrop, M. E., and G. J. King. The ultrastructure of

the osteoclast and its functional implications. *Clin. Orthop.* 123:177, 1977.

Irving, M. H. The blood supply of the growth cartilage in young rats. *J. Anat.* 98:631, 1964.

Jande, S. S. Effects of parathormone on osteocytes and their surrounding bone matrix. An electron microscopic study. *Z. Zellforsch. Mikrosk. Anat.* 130:463, 1972.

Leblond, C. P., and M. Weinstock. Radioautographic Studies of Bone Formation. In G. H. Bourne (ed.), *The Biochemistry and Physiology of Bone* (2nd ed.). New York: Academic, 1971. Vol. 3, p. 181.

Owen, M. Cellular dynamics of bone. In G. H. Bourne (ed.), *The Biochemistry and Physiology of Bone* (2nd ed.). New York: Academic, 1971. Vol. 3, p. 271.

Pritchard, J. J. The Osteoblast. In G. H. Bourne (ed.), *The Biochemistry and Physiology of Bone* (2nd ed.). New York: Academic, 1972. Vol. 1, p. 21.

Rasmussen, H., and P. Bordier. The cellular basis of metabolic bone disease. *N. Engl. J. Med.* 289:25, 1973.

Salter, R. B., and W. R. Harris. Injuries involving the epiphyseal plate. *J. Bone Joint Surg.* 45:587, 1963.

Schenk, R., and H. Willenegger. Morphological findings in primary fracture healing. *Symp. Biol. Hung.* 7:75, 1967.

Tenenbaum, H. C., and J. N. M. Heersche. Differentiation of osteoblasts and formation of mineralized bone in vitro. *Calcif. Tissue Int.* 34:76, 1982.

Tonna, E. A., and E. P. Cronkite. The periosteum: Autoradiographic studies on cellular proliferation and transformation, utilizing tritiated thymidine. *Clin. Orthop.* 30:218, 1963.

Trueta, J., and M. H. M. Harrison. The normal vascular anatomy of the femoral head in adult man. *J. Bone Joint Surg.* 35:442, 1953.

Urist, M. R. Bone: Formation by autoinduction. *Science* 150:893, 1965.

7 Muscle

Objectives

You will learn the following in this chapter:

Histologic organization of the three main types of muscle tissue: skeletal, cardiac, and smooth muscle

Ultrastructural elements of the muscle cell participating in muscle contraction and relaxation

The neuromuscular junction

The organization of neuromuscular spindles and Golgi tendon organs in regulation of length and tension of skeletal muscles

Muscle regeneration

The functional cellular unit of muscle tissue is the muscle cell (**myofiber**), which synthesizes and maintains a group of proteins responsible for the contractile character of this tissue. Three broad categories of muscle tissue are recognized, based on distinctive functional and structural features: **skeletal, cardiac,** and **smooth muscle.** Skeletal and cardiac muscle are collectively referred to as striated, because the intracellular arrangement of their contractile protein filaments generates an alternating series of transverse bands along the fiber when viewed with the light microscope in longitudinal section (Fig. 7-1). Smooth muscle derives its name from its lack of striations, resulting from its less ordered array of contractile protein filaments (see Fig. 7-18).

SKELETAL MUSCLE

Because skeletal muscle is attached to the bony skeleton, it is primarily involved in the initiation of body movement and locomotion. However, other examples of skeletal muscle include the muscles of facial expression, which are anchored in underlying bone and inserted into the dermis of the skin, and the skeletal muscle component of the upper esophagus.

Muscle cells are long, cylindrically shaped cells arranged in parallel with one another and aligned within the long axis of muscle. The longest cells extend the entire length of a muscle from its origin to its tendinous insertion, but shorter ones are more common.

The extension of a tendon's collagen fibers into the body of a muscle increases the anchoring surface area for the attachment of muscle fibers. The collagen fibers become distributed in different patterns characteristic of a given muscle, establishing a specific musculotendinous geometry tailored to the gross function of that muscle. Consequently, the tendon may continue through the muscle as a single, grossly visible structure, as several complex branches, or as a diffuse net-

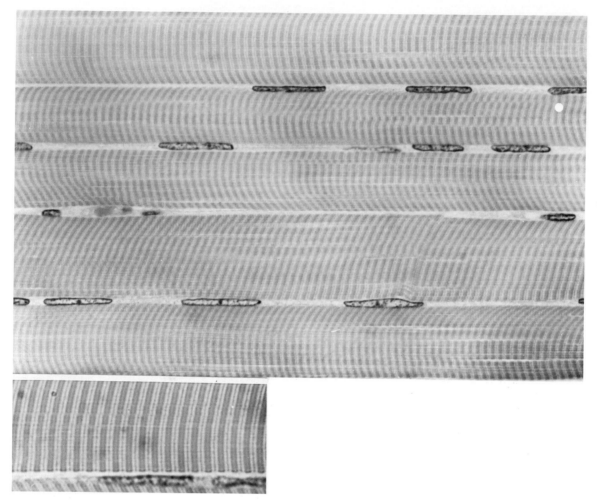

Fig. 7-1. Longitudinal section of human skeletal muscle showing five cells (muscle fibers) crossing the picture. Note the peripheral location of their nuclei and the cross striations. *Lower left:* A higher magnification showing the dark-staining A band, the light staining I band, and the Z line bisecting the I band.

work visible only by microscope. These various patterns of musculotendinous geometry are structural vectors that direct the force generated by muscle contraction to the point of tendinous insertion.

Three levels of connective tissue organization confer structural integrity to a muscle during contraction: the **epimysium, perimysium,** and **endomysium.** The external surface of a skeletal muscle is surrounded by the **epimysium,** a dense connective tissue sheath consisting of collagen and fibroblasts. The epimysium binds the muscle together and is continuous with the tendons by which muscles insert into bony prominences of the skeleton. The epimysium is synonymous with the deep fascia. Within the muscle, adjacent muscle fibers are gathered into bundles or **fascicles** by the **perimysium.** Individual myofibers within each fascicle are invested by reticular fibers (**endomysium**). Internal to the reticular fiber investment, each muscle fiber is further circumscribed by an **external lamina** similar in composition and appearance to the basal lamina underlying epithelia.

Skeletal muscle develops from **myoblasts**—round, noncontractile cells with single, centrally located nuclei. Myoblasts differentiate from fields of mesenchyme in various parts of the embryo. Hence, the trunk musculature is formed from myotomal mesenchyme; limb musculature is formed from mesenchyme of somatic mesoderm; and facial muscles, muscles of mastication, and muscles of the pharynx and larynx are derivatives of branchial arch mesenchyme.

During the course of development myoblasts fuse with one another to form increasingly longer multinucleate myotubes that eventually elongate into mature myofibers. The myotubes synthesize contractile proteins and exhibit contractile properties coincident with the establishment of innervation. The recruitment of individual myoblasts into a single myofiber explains how skeletal muscle fibers come to contain as many as 50 to 100 nuclei each. The nuclei of mature cells become peripherally located subjacent to the plasmalemma (**sarcolemma**) (see Fig. 7-1).

The major contractile proteins of skeletal muscle are **myosin** and **actin,** which occur as parallel filaments within the horizontal axis of the cell. Myosin forms **thick filaments** (10–12 nm) and actin forms **thin filaments** (5 nm). They are arranged in parallel bundles or **myofibrils,** which are oriented in the long axis of the fiber (see Fig. 7-5). Each myofibril is circumscribed by a sleeve of endoplasmic reticulum known as the **sarcoplasmic reticulum** (SR), which is specialized for regulating the intracellular calcium available to myofibrils during contraction and relaxation of muscle. Long mitochondria are located between and parallel to myofibrils. The myosin and actin filaments form alternating regions along the

myofibril. These filaments interdigitate slightly in the relaxed state and extensively during muscle contraction, when they interact and slide past each other actively to shorten the cell (Fig. 7-2). The shortest contractile segments of each myofibril are the **sarcomeres,** which are linearly repeating units of the myofibril (see Figs. 7-2, 7-5). The sarcomere is composed of a central array of myosin filaments that are 1.5 μm long, which interdigitate at both ends with actin filaments that are 1 μm long. The actin filaments insert into an essentially rigid transverse structure called the **Z disk** or **line,** which defines the limits of each sarcomere. Since the actin and myosin filaments interdigitate slightly in the uncontracted state, the length of a relaxed sarcomere is less than 2.5 μm. Contracted sarcomeres are 2 μm or less in length. The combined shortening of all sarcomeres along the myofibril represents the total distance a muscle shortens during contraction.

The sarcomeres from neighboring myofibrils are in perfect alignment, so that the thick filaments of adjacent myofibrils form a dense transverse striation called the **A band.** The aligned thin filaments form a less dense transverse striation referred to as the **I band.** These alternating A and I bands impart the striated appearance to longitudinally sectioned muscle. They are termed **anisotropic** (A) and **isotropic** (I), in reference to their refractile characteristics when viewed with polarized light microscopy. The alignment of A and I bands in one myofibril with A and I bands of adjacent myofibrils is apparently due to a system of **intermediate filaments** (composed of the proteins **desmin** and **vimentin**) that interconnect Z disks of adjacent myofibrils (see Fig. 7-1). During muscle contraction the thin filaments from each I band slide past the thick filaments as they migrate into the A band (see Fig. 7-2). The result is shortening of the sarcomere, with the Z disks moving toward the A band. A fully contracted sarcomere does not have visible I bands, since the thin filaments have migrated completely into the A band where they interdigitate with thick filaments (see Fig. 7-2). The filaments themselves do not change

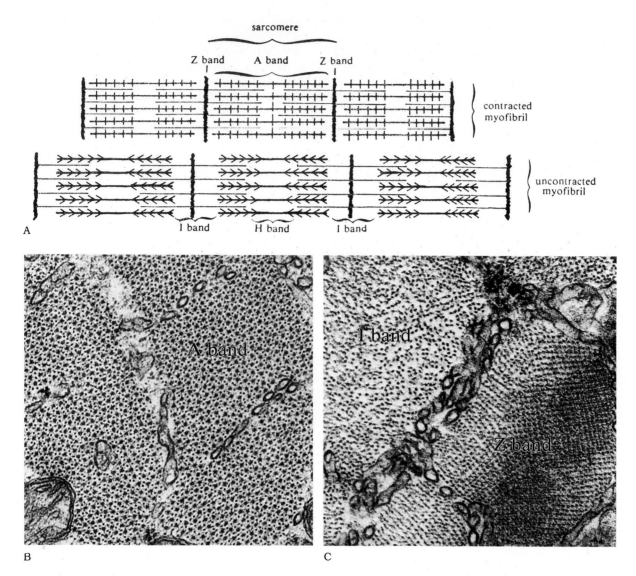

A

B

C

Fig. 7-2. A. Portions of contracted and uncontracted myofibrils. A sarcomere is the distance between successive Z lines. During contraction the I bands, H bands, and sarcomeres shorten in width. B. High magnification electron micrograph of a cross-section through the A band in the region where the thick filaments (myosin) and thin filaments (actin) interdigitate. C. High-magnification electron micrograph of a cross-section through the I band and Z line area.

length during contraction. The H band is the central area of the A band not occupied by actin filaments in the relaxed sarcomere. However, as the actin filaments invade both ends of the A band during contraction, the width of the H bands diminishes accordingly (see Fig. 7-2). The H band also includes a bare zone where no myosin cross-bridges occur.

Even in a relaxed sarcomere there is a certain amount of overlap of thick and thin filaments in the region referred to as the **A-I junction.** Cross-sectional views through this region of the A band reveal a hexagonal array of thick and thin filaments interdigitating with one another (see Fig. 7-2). It is within the A-I junction that sliding of filaments begins during initiation of muscle contraction. Electron microscopy has been an important tool in elucidating the macromolecular events occurring in the A-I junction during contraction. In this junction, flexible cross-bridges (myosin heads) of heavy meromyosin (HMM) extending away from the thick myosin filaments engage the actin filaments and forcefully pull the thin filaments into the A band region (Fig. 7-3; see also Fig. 7-2). This is an energy-dependent process requiring the hydrolysis of adenosine triphosphate (ATP), and the cross-bridges are sites of myosin adenosine triphosphatase (ATPase) activity. In the presence of elevated calcium, myosin ATPase is activated, ATP is hydrolyzed, and the cross-bridges pull the thin filaments into the A band where they interdigitate with the thick myosin filaments, resulting in the simultaneous contraction of all the sarcomeres of each myofibril.

Intracellular Control of Muscle Contraction

In mammalian muscle the actin filament stimulates myosin ATPase activity, but its ability to do so is regulated by the **troponin-tropomyosin system,** which confers calcium dependency on actin and myosin interaction. The actin filament is actually a double helix of globular actin monomers arranged around a long filamentous protein

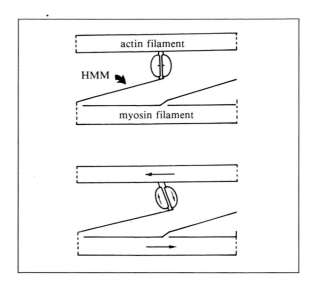

Fig. 7-3. The movement of myosin cross-bridges relative to the myosin backbone during contraction. The part of the myosin molecule having ATPase activity resides on the end of the flexible portion (*HMM*), which can move away from the myosin filament proper to engage the actin filament during contraction. (From H. E. Huxley, The mechanism of muscular contraction. *Science* 164:1356, 1969. Copyright 1969 by the American Association for the Advancement of Science. Reproduced with permission.)

called **tropomyosin** (Fig. 7-4). Associated with periodic intervals along the helix is a regulating protein called **troponin,** which exerts a conformational constraint on the actin filament through its influence on tropomyosin. This conformation sterically masks the myosin cross-bridge binding sites along the actin filament and prevents engagement of myosin cross-bridges. The inhibition of actin-myosin interaction is reversed in the presence of calcium ion elevation ($> 10^{-6}$M). The calcium ions bind to troponin, which then allows conformational changes in the actin filament that are conducive to myosin engagement.

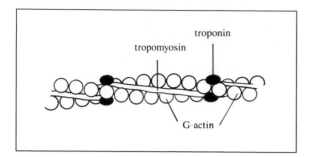

Fig. 7-4. Globular actin monomers (G-actin), troponin, and the tropomyosin filament in their relative positions forming the helical thin filament of the I band. (After S. Ebashi, M. Endo, and I. Ohtsuki, Control of muscle contraction. *Q. Rev. Biophys.* 2:351, 1969. Reproduced with permission.)

Fig. 7-5. Thin section of skeletal muscle as it might appear with electron microscopy. Proceeding from the plasmalemma (*sarcolemma*) inward are the sarcoplasmic reticulum (*SR*), the sarcomere of a myofibril, a mitochondrion separating adjacent myofibrils, and a sarcomere with its associated sarcoplasmic reticulum. The arrows indicate points along the plasmalemma where T tubules invaginate the fiber at the A-I junction of sarcomeres. The terminal cisterns (*TC*) of the SR are associated with the T tubules through short junctional feet, forming the triad where excitation-contraction coupling occurs.

Since calcium plays such an essential role during muscle contraction, its concentration within the cytoplasm must be precisely controlled. This control is exerted by the SR, which cycles calcium between the cytoplasmic compartment, where it activates the myofibrils during contraction, and the SR compartment, where calcium is sequestered during relaxation. Calcium is released from the SR for muscle contraction and retrieved in order for muscle to relax. The cue for release of calcium from the SR is depolarization of the sarcolemma caused by release of neurotransmitter from the innervating nerve terminal. Depolarization spreads into the interior of the muscle fiber along transverse invaginations of the sarcolemma (**T tubules**), which occur at the A-I junction in mammalian skeletal muscle. At each of these points, dilated sacs of the SR (**terminal cisterns**) are closely apposed to the T tubules (Figs. 7-5, 7-6, 7-7). **Junctional feet** spanning the gap between SR membrane and T tubule membrane are believed to convey some information from the depolarized T tubule to the

SR, triggering the release of calcium ions (Figs. 7-7, 7-8). The exact mechanism is not understood, but the structural association between T tubule and terminal cisterns on each side (**triad**) is critical for coupling depolarization of sarcolemma with calcium-mediated contraction of myofibrils. This triad is therefore the site of **excitation-contraction coupling** in skeletal muscle.

Motor Innervation of Skeletal Muscle

The terminal axon of a motor neuron (**alpha motor neuron**) branches into smaller axons, each of which forms a synapse with one myofiber. The family of myofibers innervated by the axons of a single motor neuron is termed a **motor unit.** The nerve cell body of the alpha motor neuron is located in the anterior gray horn of the spinal cord.

The **neuromuscular junction (motor end plate)** is the site of neuromuscular transmission (Fig. 7-9; see also Fig. 8-3). It includes the axon terminal and a specialized region of the sarcolemma called the **sole plate.** The sole plate is a highly convoluted region of the sarcolemma with two levels of organization: (1) The **primary synaptic cleft** or **trough** is a depression in the sar-

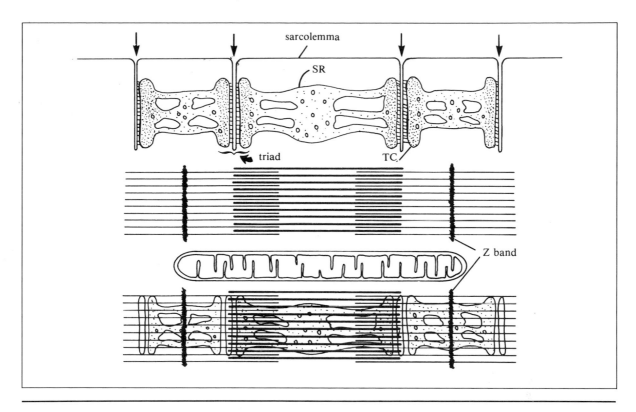

Fig. 7-6. Electron micrograph of skeletal muscle cell near its surface. S = sarcolemma; TT = transverse tubule; TC = terminal cistern of sarcoplasmic reticulum; LT = longitudinal tubule of sarcoplasmic reticulum. Arrow indicates origin of a transverse tubule with the sarcolemma. During muscle contraction, calcium is released from the terminal cisterns; during relaxation calcium is sequestered by the longitudinal tubules of the sarcoplasmic reticulum.

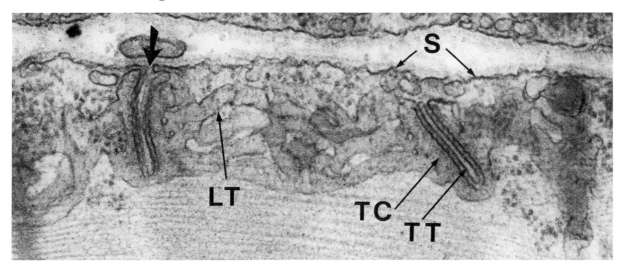

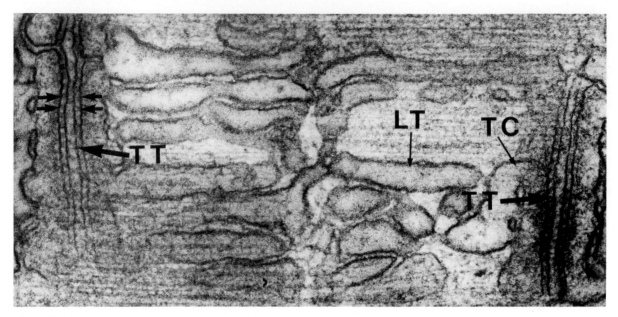

Fig. 7-7. High-magnification electron micrograph showing the location of junctional feet (*arrows*) linking the transverse tubules (*TT*) with the terminal cistern (*TC*). *LT* = longitudinal tubule.

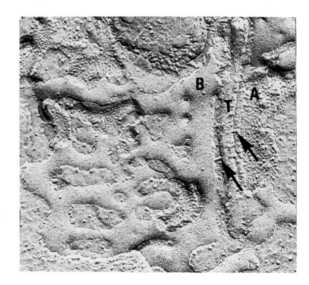

Fig. 7-8. This is a portion of a freeze-fractured skeletal muscle cell. The fracture plane passes through the triad exposing the outer or cytoplasmic leaflet (*A*) and the inner or luminal leaflet (*B*) of the sarcoplasmic reticulum. The particles on the cytoplasmic leaflet are believed to be the calcium, magnesium-ATPase that pumps calcium ions between the cytoplasm and the sarcoplasmic reticulum. The transverse tubule (*T*) is visible between the terminal cisterns. Arrows indicate the junctional feet spanning the gap between T-tubule and terminal cistern. (From T. Beringer, A freeze-fracture study of sarcoplasmic reticulum from fast and slow muscle of the mouse. *Anat. Rec.* 184:647, 1976.)

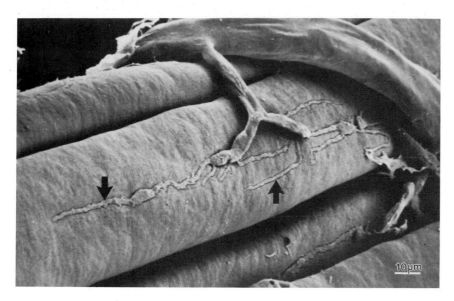

Fig. 7-9. A scanning electron micrograph of the myoneural junction. The arrows show the axonal branches terminating at the motor endplate of a skeletal muscle cell. Notice that the axon terminals rest in shallow depressions in the surface of the muscle cell surface. These shallow depressions are the primary synaptic cleft. (From J. Desaki and Y. Uehara, The overall morphology of neuromuscular junctions as revealed by scanning electron microscopy. *J. Neurocytol.* 10:101, 1981.)

colemma occupied by the innervating axon (see Fig. 7-9); (2) the **secondary synaptic clefts** are highly infolded areas of the primary cleft (Fig. 7-10). The sarcolemma at these locations houses membrane molecules involved in neuromuscular transmission. The **acetylcholine receptor** is located on the outer lips of the secondary clefts, while **acetylcholinesterase** is deployed along the inner aspect of the secondary clefts. An intervening **external lamina** maintains the structural integrity of the junction. The postsynaptic area or **subneural apparatus** includes not only the sole plate but also a localized concentration of muscle cell nuclei located in the underlying cytoplasm.

Nonmyelinating Schwann cells invest the neuromuscular junction.

Skeletal muscle is dependent on an intact, functioning nerve supply for adequate development beyond the myotube stage as well as for maintenance of the myofiber in mature muscle. If the innervation to a muscle fiber is surgically interrupted, the muscle will undergo a complex series of degenerative changes characterized immediately by loss of neurally evoked contraction (paralysis), and followed by muscular atrophy signaled by dismantling of the myofibrils. If the regenerating nerve can reestablish functional neuromuscular contact with the denervated muscle, the muscle will return to its normal functional state. Over a longer period of time, however, denervated muscle atrophies, disintegrates, and is replaced by connective tissue.

The differentiation of muscle to the multinucleate myotube stage is independent of neural control; this stands in striking contrast to the profound effects exerted on the subsequent development of muscle by innervating neurons. Nerve-induced modifications of mammalian

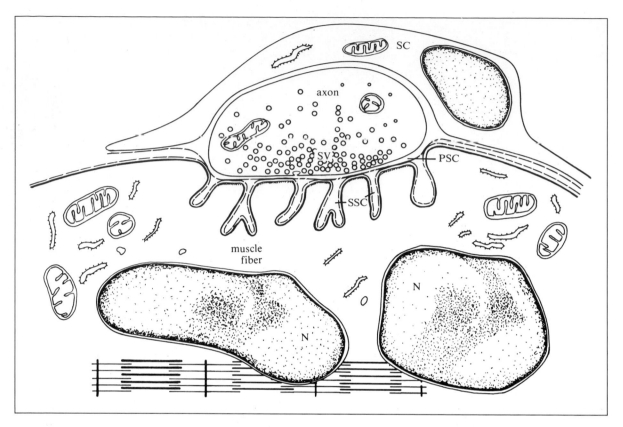

Fig. 7-10. Motor end plate of skeletal muscle, showing axon terminal of alpha motor neuron (*axon*); synaptic vesicles (*SV*); primary synaptic cleft (*PSC*); secondary synaptic clefts (*SSC*); nonmyelinating Schwann cell (*SC*); concentration of muscle cell nuclei (*N*) in the sole plate. Also examine Figure 8-2.

muscle serve to divide it into at least two broad physiologic categories that develop soon after birth: **fast-twitch** and **slow-twitch muscle.** Innervation acts, therefore, as a cue to elicit from muscle a coordinated variety of functional and structural characteristics that were potentially present as a result of muscle differentiation concluded prior to withdrawal from the cell cycle and fusion into myotubes.

Fast-twitch muscle contracts and relaxes more rapidly than slow-twitch muscle. The primary basis for this distinction rests in the direct relation between the intrinsic speed of shortening of a sarcomere and the myosin ATPase activity of the myosin cross-bridges, which is greater in fast-twitch muscle. The relative oxidative and glycolytic enzymatic properties further distinguish these fiber types, slow-twitch muscles being oxidative and fast-twitch muscles primarily glycolytic, although the latter type also includes a subgroup displaying a combination of glycolytic and oxidative properties. This difference in metabolic properties is reflected in the higher content of mitochondria in slow-twitch as opposed to fast-twitch muscle. As a corollary to this, fast-twitch muscle, which is more dependent on the less efficient anaerobic glycolysis for production of ATP, fatigues more easily than slow-twitch muscle. The greater relative volume of SR in fast-twitch muscle reflects the ability of this type of muscle to relax more rapidly than slow-twitch muscle.

All muscle fibers innervated by the same nerve (motor units) exhibit common contractile characteristics, so that a single axon branches to innervate all fast-twitch or all slow-twitch fibers exclusively. However, since any given muscle has a mixture of motor units, very few muscles of the body are homogeneous for any one fiber type.

The different fiber types can be identified by histochemical procedures for myosin ATPase and for oxidative and glycolytic enzymes. The distinction is important in the diagnosis of several neuromuscular disorders that may be identified by their relative and selective effects on particular fiber types.

Sensory Innervation of Skeletal Muscle

Sensory nerves to muscle consist of numerous unmyelinated fibers and a few myelinated fibers that innervate the perimuscular connective tissue. Some of these nerves from tendons and joints provide proprioceptive information to the cerebrum. Others originate from neuromuscular spindles and neurotendinous organs (of Golgi) and are involved in neural reflex arcs that adjust tension and length of skeletal muscles.

Neuromuscular Spindles

Neuromuscular spindles are stretch receptors located within skeletal muscles. They are found primarily in slow contracting extensor muscles involved in the maintenance of posture against gravitational forces and in muscles where very fine movements are exhibited, such as muscles of the hand and the extraocular muscles. They monitor static (fixed) and dynamic (changing) aspects of muscle length and respond to passive increases in muscle length through a nervous reflex arc (**stretch reflex** or **myotatic reflex**) that

provokes contraction within the regular muscle fibers. The resulting contraction resists excessive stretching that may injure the muscle. The stretch reflex is mediated by a sensory nerve leading from the spindle to the spinal cord, where it synapses with the alpha motor neuron innervating the skeletal muscle.

Human neuromuscular spindles are composed of three to 12 specialized striated muscle fibers called **intrafusal fibers** because they are encapsulated by perimysial connective tissue and situated within the belly of skeletal muscles. Each spindle is 2 to 5 mm long and has a parallel orientation with surrounding regular muscle fibers (**extrafusal fibers**). There are two morphologic types of intrafusal fibers within each spindle, a few **nuclear bag fibers** and a large number of **nuclear chain fibers.** Nuclear bag fibers are larger in diameter and contain round nuclei aggregated in the noncontractile central (equatorial) portion, which is flanked by myofibrils at each of its contractile polar ends. Nuclear chain fibers are smaller in diameter and have numerous elongate nuclei arranged in a single row surrounded by myofibrils.

Two types of **sensory** nerves innervate intrafusal fibers making them sensitive to passive stretch: **primary fibers** (Ia), which are heavily myelinated and fast conducting, and **secondary fibers** (II), which are unmyelinated and slow-conducting (Fig. 7-11). Primary endings innervate the equatorial region of nuclear bag and nuclear chain fibers and terminate in an **annulospiral** configuration on intrafusal fibers. Secondary endings innervate the juxtaequatorial regions but are most prominent on nuclear chain fibers and terminate in **multibranched (flowerspray)** configurations on intrafusal fibers (see Fig. 7-11). Both types of sensory fiber respond to static and dynamic conditions of extrafusal muscle length. Since intrafusal fibers have common connective tissue attachments with the extrafusal fibers, stretching a muscle such as the quadriceps by tapping the patellar tendon also stretches its neuromuscular spindles, provoking sensory discharge. Both primary and secondary

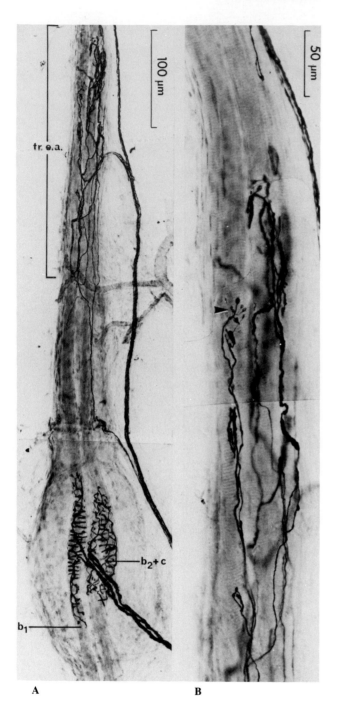

Fig. 7-11. Innervation pattern of neuromuscular spindle from cat peroneus brevis muscle. Nerves are densely stained with silver. A. The equatorial region is at the lower part of the figure and part of one pole is at the upper part of the figure. The course of all three intrafusal muscle fibers can be followed from the equatorial region to the pole region although they are only faintly visible: b_1 = bag$_1$ fiber; b_2 = bag$_2$ fiber; c = chain fiber. A primary afferent nerve ending is plainly visible as an annulospiral terminal on the bag$_1$ fiber. A gamma nerve is conspicuous in its course toward the pole or trail ending area (*tr. e. a.*), which is shown at higher magnification in B. B. The arrowhead indicates the terminal of a gamma neuron upon the bag$_1$ fiber. (From D. Barker et al., Studies of the Histochemistry, Ultrastructure, Motor Innervation and Regeneration of Mammalian Intrafusal Muscle Fibers. In S. Homma (ed.), *Understanding the Stretch Reflex, Progress in Brain Research.* Amsterdam: Elsevier, 1976. Vol. 44, p. 82.)

sensory nerves to the spinal cord form monosynaptic junctions with alpha motor neurons, causing contraction of extrafusal fibers within that muscle (agonist) and its synergists but inhibiting contraction of antagonist muscles. The contraction of extrafusal fibers allows the stretched intrafusal fibers to shorten and cease their afferent discharge to alpha motor neurons in the spinal cord. The nervous reflex arc to the agonist muscle is a monosynaptic one; the nervous arc to the antagonist muscle involves two synapses with an interneuron interposed between the sensory and alpha motor neuron. Primary sensory nerves respond to both the degree and rate of stretch and elicit a quick, brief contraction; secondary nerves respond to degree of stretch only and elicit a more sustained contracture.

Intrafusal fibers also receive **motor** innervation from **fusimotor nerves** (**gamma neurons**), which alter the sensitivity of the spindle to stretch by regulating contraction of myofibrils within the polar regions of intrafusal fibers. Fusimotor nerves terminate at various points along the fiber from the juxtaequatorial to polar regions (see Fig. 7-11). When intrafusal myofibrils contract, the primary and secondary sensory endings to the equatorial and juxtaequatorial regions are stretched, thereby reducing their threshold for sensory discharge. When these sensory nerves are stretched beyond this threshold, the stretch reflex is triggered. Gamma neurons continuously coordinate the length of intrafusal fibers with voluntary contraction and relaxation of extrafusal muscle so that the spindle will be sensitive to passive stretch at many lengths assumed by extrafusal fibers.

Three types of intrafusal fiber are distinguished based on their reaction speed to changes in muscle length, what condition of muscle lengthening they respond to (static or dynamic), and gamma innervation. Two different nuclear bag fibers exist: a **slow-contracting bag fiber** (bag$_1$), which responds to dynamic conditions of muscle stretch, and a **fast-contracting bag fiber** (bag$_2$), which responds to static conditions of muscle length. These two types of bag fibers have independent gamma innervations. Nuclear chain fibers are fast-contracting fibers that respond to static conditions of muscle length and often share the same gamma innervation with fast-contracting bag fibers.

In certain muscle diseases where neuromuscular spindles fail to develop and in diseases of the alpha motor neuron (**lower motor neuron disease**), the stretch reflex is impaired or abolished.

Golgi Tendon Organs

Golgi tendon organs are encapsulated sensory nerves that are present within tendons near the musculotendinous junctions. Unlike neuromuscular spindles, they are oriented in series with extrafusal muscle fibers and monitor increases in muscle tension rather than length. The tendon organs reduce muscle tension during excessive muscle contraction. The discharge frequency of Golgi tendon organs increases with increasing tension on the muscle.

The Golgi tendon organ consists of unmyelinated nerve endings encapsulated by endoneurial connective tissue and enmeshed among the collagen fibers of the tendon. It is believed that muscle tension is transferred to the tendon, causing the collagen fibers to compress the nerve ending, stimulating it to generate sensory impulses traveling back to the spinal cord. Within the spinal cord the sensory nerves synapse with an internuncial neuron, which inhibits alpha motor neurons to the same muscle (agonist) and augments them to the antagonist muscle.

Injury and Regeneration of Skeletal Muscle

Muscle necrosis commonly results from several types of injuries including denervation, severe localized edema and hemorrhage, traumatic injuries resulting in muscle tears, and ischemia due to arterial occlusion. Subsequent muscle regeneration arises from a population of satellite cells, which resides between the plasmalemma of the damaged muscle cell and its basal lamina. The number of satellite cells is usually 1 to 5 percent of the nuclear population within adult muscle. Satellite nuclei are distinguished from these intrinsic muscle cell nuclei by being more heterochromatic and by their cytoplasm lacking myofibrils.

During embryonic development myogenic stem cells divide, producing myoblasts that fuse into myotubes and enlarge into mature muscle fibers. These developmental events are repeated during regeneration of injured muscle. Initially, satellite cells proliferate to produce a daughter cell pool of myoblasts and more satellite cells. The fusion of myoblasts into myotubes occurs within the basal lamina of the original damaged fiber. Revascularization at this time is essential for continued regeneration. Reinnervation of the developing myotube is essential to sustain continued growth and maturation.

The retention of an undamaged basal lamina is essential for directing growth and reestablishing properly aligned muscle. Severe damage to the basal lamina or to the endomysial and perimysial connective tissue investments may provoke collagen fibrosis, resulting in disorientation of regenerated muscle fibers and defective muscle function.

Although excessive amounts of necrotic tissue in some severe muscle injuries may result in bacterial infection or crippling fibrosis that requires surgical intervention, it should be appreciated that surgical excision of necrotic muscle inadvertently removes the satellite cells that are required for complete muscle regeneration. Nuclei from within the damaged fibers are postmitotic and, although they may be incorporated into a regenerating fiber, are incapable of proliferating or producing a de novo population of muscle fibers to replace necrotic muscle.

Satellite cells are not present in cardiac or smooth muscle.

CARDIAC MUSCLE

Cardiac muscle fibers share many structural similarities with skeletal muscle but with certain significant modifications, to be discussed here. Cardiac fibers are either **mononucleate** or **binucleate,** with the nuclei being centrally located. They are smaller than skeletal muscle fibers and frequently branch. They are arranged to form the curved contractile walls of the heart and therefore take tortuous courses in and out of the plane of section, making cardiac muscle appear more complex in histologic section. Their ends are attached to other myocardial fibers and to the connective tissue skeleton of the heart. The connection of one myocardial cell to another occurs at the **intercalated disk,** a prominent cross striation that distinguishes cardiac muscle from skeletal muscle in longitudinal section (Fig. 7-12).

The myofibril structure of cardiac muscle is similar to that of skeletal muscle. However, the SR associated with the myofibrils is less well developed, since cardiac muscle depends on the influx of extracellular calcium to a greater degree than does skeletal muscle during contraction. T tubules are less frequent, occurring only at the Z lines of each sarcomere; this indicates that the spread of depolarizing current into the interior of cardiac muscle is less efficient than in skeletal muscle, where T tubules occur at each A-I junction (two per sarcomere). The junctional areas

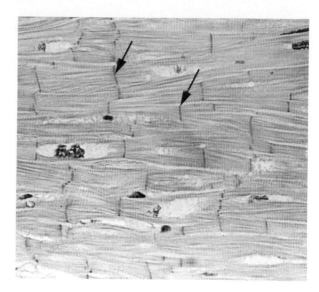

Fig. 7-12. Longitudinal section of cardiac muscle. Most of the transverse striations are faint except for the intercalated disks, which are the pronounced striations (*arrows*).

between T tubules and the terminal cisterns of the SR are also less extensive and occur as **diads,** with only one terminal cistern adjoining a T tubule at any one level, rather than as triads. The SR also forms frequent diadlike relations with the sarcolemma, analogous to those formed with the T tubules for excitation-contraction coupling (Fig. 7-13).

The ends of the myocardial cells are joined together by specialized regions of their sarcolemmas known as **intercalated disks,** which confer structural integrity to the myocardium and subserve electrical coupling between cardiac muscle cells (see Fig. 7-13). With the light microscope, intercalated disks appear as dense bands running in a stepwise transverse direction across the fiber. Electron microscopy reveals that the intercalated disk consists of three structurally distinct regions: (1) the **macula adherens** (desmosome), (2) the **fascia adherens,** and (3) the **gap junction** (see Fig. 7-13). The macula adher-

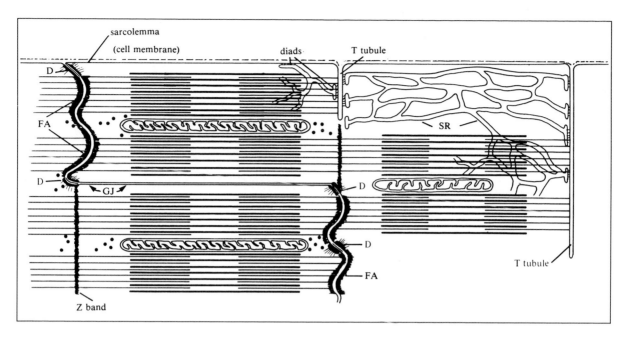

Fig. 7-13. A thin section through cardiac muscle as it might appear with electron microscopy. Portions of two cardiac muscle fibers are depicted in the area where their plasmalemmas associate to form the intercalated disk. Desmosomes (*D*) provide structural integrity to the disk. Thin filaments insert into the fascia adherens (*FA*). The gap junctions (*GJ*) are located in the horizontal part of the disk. The disk occurs where a Z band would have been. T tubules occur at the Z lines. The sarcoplasmic reticulum (*SR*) forms a sleeve around the myofibrils, but here it is depicted alone to show its pattern more clearly.

ens provides a means of spot attachment between fibers, maintaining the structural integrity of cardiac muscle during contraction. The fascia adherens is the site of insertion of actin filaments from myofibrils onto the sarcolemma (Fig. 7-14). Gap junctions are sites of low resistance for the passage of ionic currents from fiber to fiber within the heart. In this way cardiac muscle fibers are electrically coupled so that a neurally evoked depolarizing current initiating contraction may spread throughout the myocardium from cell to cell without each fiber requiring innervation. Gap junctions become uncoupled under conditions of cardiac ischemia, causing cessation of the heartbeat. The gap junctions occur on the top of each "step" or longitudinally oriented part of the disk, while the macula adherens and fascia adherens form the transverse portions of the disk (Figs. 7-15, 7-16).

Specialized Cardiac Muscle Fibers

The cardiac conduction system consists of several specialized muscle fibers responsible for distributing the impulse for contraction throughout the heart. It includes **nodal fibers** in the **sinoatrial** (S-A) and **atrioventricular** (A-V) **nodes,** and **Purkinje fibers** in the **atrioventricular bundle of His.** The impulse for contraction is generated first in a specialized region of the atrium called the S-A node, a focal aggregation of smaller specialized muscle fibers that exhibit inherent con-

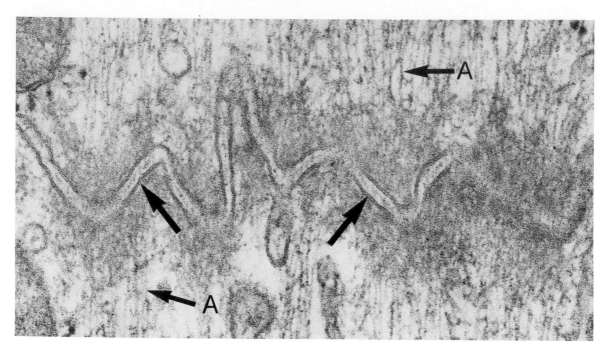

Fig. 7-14. Intercalated disk from mouse ventricle. Shown is the fascia adherens region (*arrows*) which has numerous actin filaments (*A*) anchored in the subsarcolemmal opaque material. × 110,000. (From M. S. Forbes and N. Sperelakis, Intercalated disks of mammalian heart: A review of structure and function, *Tissue and Cell* 17:605, 1985. Reproduced with permission from Longman Group.)

tractile rhythmicity due to their ability to depolarize spontaneously. Since these nodal fibers depolarize at a faster rate than the regular myocardial fibers which they drive, they are commonly called **pacemaker fibers.** Depolarization initiated by S-A nodal fibers spreads by gap junctions throughout the regular atrial musculature to reach the A-V node. Nodal fibers in both nodes are smaller than regular cardiac muscle fibers and have fewer myofibrils.

Purkinje fibers are specialized conduction fibers that constitute a grossly dissectable atrioventricular bundle extending from the A-V node through the subendocardium of the interventricular septum toward the apex of the heart, where its branches enter the right and left ventricles. Here they terminate on regular cardiac musculature in the papillary muscles and in the adjacent myocardium. This ensures that ventricular contraction begins at the apex of the heart for complete evacuation of blood from the ventricles. An injury to this conduction system interferes with the synchronous beating of the heart. Purkinje fibers are long fibers attaining greater girth than the surrounding cardiac muscle cells of the ventricles, but since they are specialized for conduction rather than contraction, they lack T tubules and contain few myofibrils. This paucity of myofibrils is apparent in histologic section. Wispy myofibrils occupy a peripheral location in the cell surrounding a large amount of poorly stained cytoplasm, making them easily distinguishable from regular cardiac muscle cells (Fig. 7-17).

Purkinje fibers are not connected to one another by typical intercalated disks, but desmo-

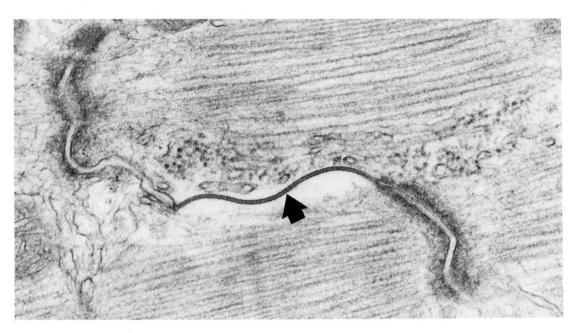

Fig. 7-15. Intercalated disk from mouse atrium. A gap junction (*arrow*) forms the longitudinal segment of the intercalated disk. ×61,500. (From M. S. Forbes and N. Sperelakis, Intercalated discs of mammalian heart: A review of structure and function, *Tissue and Cell* 17:605, 1985. Reproduced with permission from Longman Group.)

Fig. 7-16. Freeze-fracture replica of longitudinal segment of intercalated disk from mouse ventricle. The fracture plane passes through the sarcolemma of the lower cell exposing two gap junctions (*arrows*) before fracturing through the cytoplasm of the upper cell. ×71,000. (From M. S. Forbes and N. Sperelakis, Intercalated discs of mammalian heart: A review of structure and function, *Tissue and Cell* 17:605, 1985. Reproduced with permission from Longman Group.)

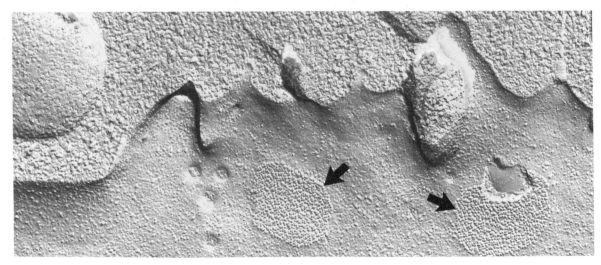

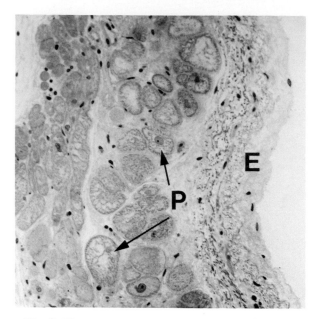

Fig. 7-17. Purkinje fibers (*P*) in the subendocardium of the human heart. *E* = endocardium.

somes and gap junctions are scattered along their apposing cell membranes. Although specialized fibers occupying the S-A and A-V nodes confer an inherent rhythmic contractility to the heart independent of innervation, the rate of firing of **nodal fibers** can be altered by the autonomic nerves that innervate them. Parasympathetic nerves from the vagus slow the heart rate, whereas sympathetic nerves accelerate it. Vagal axons synapse with postganglionic nerves within the myocardium; these nerves distribute mostly to nodal fibers of the S-A and A-V nodes. Postganglionic sympathetic nerves issue from the cervical and upper thoracic ganglia and distribute to the nodal fibers and conduction system. Innervation of regular unspecialized cardiac fibers appears to be mostly sympathetic.

Innervation

Cardiac neuromuscular junctions differ from those of skeletal muscle in that no postsynaptic motor endplate region is present on the sarcolemma. Along the length of the nerve, unmyelinated portions containing synaptic vesicles simply approach the sarcolemma with an intervening gap of 100 nm or less. The nerve continues, forming numerous junctions with other fibers. This type of innervation is called **innervation en passant.**

Surgical denervation of the heart removes the basis by which the autonomic nervous system adjusts the heart rate, but the heart will continue to beat at an intrinsic baseline rate established by the nodal fibers of the S-A node.

SMOOTH MUSCLE

Visceral musculature is composed almost exclusively of the smooth variety, the only exception other than cardiac muscle being the occurrence of some skeletal muscle in the upper portion of the esophagus. Smooth muscle fibers may occur singly, as in the lamina propria of the intestinal villi, but most commonly they are organized into sheets of closely apposed fibers. These sheets or layers of smooth muscle form the muscular walls of the alimentary canal and the ducts of its associated exocrine glands, of respiratory passages, urinary and genital ducts, blood vessels, and the larger lymphatics. The arrector pili muscles, which elevate hairs from the surface of the skin, are also smooth muscle. Myoepithelial cells are similar to smooth muscle cells but are ectodermal in origin, as opposed to the mesodermal origin of all other muscle. Myoepithelial cells are associated with the secretory alveoli of the mammary, salivary, sweat, and lacrimal glands. Other ectodermally derived smooth muscle is found in the dermis of the skin, the nipple, prepuce, glans penis, and scrotum; it also composes the intrinsic muscles of the eye (ciliary sphincter and dilator pupillary muscles). Smooth muscle cells are generally small fibers (20–50 μm long). However, they range in length from about 20 μm in vascular walls to nearly 500 μm in the pregnant uterus.

Smooth muscle cells are small fusiform fibers with a single elongate centrally located nucleus containing several nucleoli (Fig. 7-18). In longitudinal section the nuclei often exhibit a corrugated shape described as "corkscrew"; this occurs as a result of fixation during the contracted state. Otherwise the nuclei have smooth contours with blunt or rounded ends. When arranged in sheets, regions of contracted and uncontracted smooth muscle can be encountered in a single plane of section. The fibers are packed in a staggered fashion, with the thickest nucleated central portion of one fiber apposed to the thin, tapered processes of adjacent muscle fibers. When cross-sectioned, this organization of smooth muscle fibers produces round cellular

profiles of variable diameter. The smaller-diameter profiles are planes of section through the tapered ends of the cells, and the larger-diameter profiles are planes of section through the central portion of the cell, which contains the nucleus (see Fig. 7-18). Electron microscopy reveals that mitochondria, a pair of centrioles, free ribosomes, rough endoplasmic reticulum, and a Golgi body reside in the conical cytoplasm at each nuclear pole.

Smooth muscle tissue is associated with small amounts of collagen and elastic fibers with scattered fibroblasts. Individual smooth muscle fibers are supported by reticular fibers, and closely apposed to the cell surface is an external lamina similar in composition and appearance to the basal lamina underlying epithelium. Desmosomes are occasionally found for cell-to-cell contact.

Actin and myosin, the two major contractile proteins of skeletal muscle, are also present in smooth muscle and form the thin and thick filaments seen with the electron microscope (see Fig. 7-19). These filaments are not organized into myofibrils, however, and therefore no striations are visible at the light microscopic level (see Fig. 7-18). Their three-dimensional organization within the cell cannot be easily appreciated, even

Fig. 7-18. Longitudinally sectioned smooth muscle cells in the wall of the human intestine. There is a single nucleus occupying the central thick portion of each cell. Smooth muscle cells are tapered away from the central nucleated part (*arrow*). Notice the absence of striations, which are so evident in skeletal and cardiac muscle.

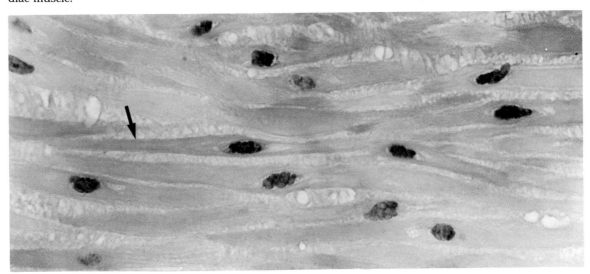

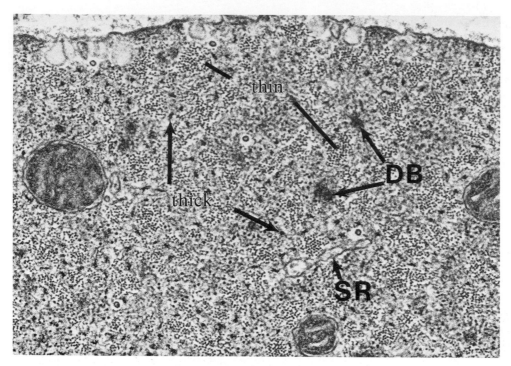

Fig. 7-19. Electron micrograph of a cross-sectioned smooth muscle cell. Thin filaments (*thin*) of actin occur in bundles; thick filaments (*thick*) of myosin occur singly and are evenly distributed. *DB* = dense bodies. Sarcoplasmic reticulum (*SR*) is sparse. (From P. Cooke, A filamentous cytoskeleton in vertebrate smooth muscle fibers. *J. Cell Biol.* 68:539, 1976. Reproduced by copyright permission of The Rockefeller University Press.)

from sections prepared for electron microscopy. Furthermore, the apparent liability of thick filaments in the absence of calcium complicates the interpretation of myofilament organization and cooperation during contraction. There is some evidence that thick myofilaments exist in a disaggregated or molecularly dispersed state in relaxed smooth muscle and that they aggregate into discrete filaments only with excitation-contraction coupling, when intracellular calcium

levels are higher. Nevertheless, evidence indicates that the sliding filament mechanism of muscle contraction does operate during smooth muscle contraction.

In addition to the thick and thin filaments, a network of intermediate filaments (10 nm) exists. Intermediate-sized filaments are anchored to fusiform, amorphous **dense bodies** distributed throughout the cell as well as to dense bodies associated with the sarcolemma. This intermediate filament–dense body network is believed to represent an intracellular cytoskeleton (Fig. 7-20). The dense bodies also serve as attachment points for actin filaments. The distribution of the intermediate filaments and dense bodies changes with different lengths of smooth muscle fibers. In unstretched fibers the intermediate filament–dense body network is uniformly distributed throughout the cytoplasm. In stretched fibers the intermediate filament–dense body network becomes consolidated in the center of the muscle fiber (see Fig. 7-20).

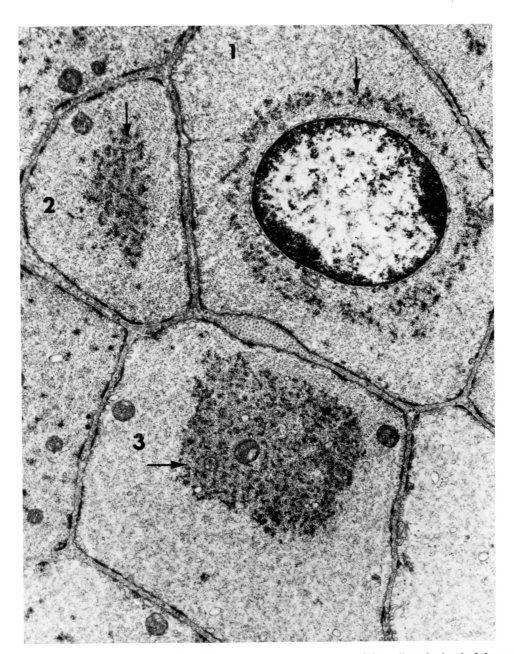

Fig. 7-20. Electron micrograph of three cross-sectioned smooth muscle cells at low magnification. These cells have been treated to dissolve the thin filaments. They were then stretched to demonstrate the change in distribution of dense bodies (*arrows*) within the cell at three different levels: (*1*) in the middle of the cell at the level of the nucleus, (*2*) at one end or pole of the cell, and (*3*) between the pole and nucleus of the cell. (From P. Cooke, A filamentous cytoskeleton in vertebrate smooth muscle fibers. *J. Cell Biol.* 68:539, 1976. Reproduced by copyright permission of The Rockefeller University Press.)

No T tubules occur in smooth muscle cells, probably because these cells are small enough in diameter so that ionic currents generated across the sarcolemma are sufficient to initiate the slowly developing tension that is characteristic of smooth muscle contraction.

The SR is deployed subjacent to the sarcolemma in the form of longitudinal tubular elements. Electron-opaque material spans a 10-nm gap between SR and sarcolemma, a structural arrangement that is probably the site of excitation-contraction coupling of smooth muscle analogous to the triad of skeletal muscle and the diads of cardiac muscle.

Smooth muscle is innervated by unmyelinated postganglionic nerves of the sympathetic and parasympathetic divisions of the autonomic nervous system. Depending on the relative receptivity of smooth muscle in various locations of the body, nervous influences from these two divisions of the autonomic nerves will cause contraction or relaxation. For instance, sympathetic nerves cause relaxation of intestinal and bronchial smooth muscle, whereas they cause contraction of vascular smooth muscle in many other locations. Innervating axons of smooth muscle fibers are not associated with elaborate postsynaptic specializations of the sarcolemma as in skeletal muscle motor end plates; instead the nerve fiber simply comes in close proximity to the smooth muscle cell where innervation occurs. Smooth muscle fibers are electronically coupled to one another by gap junctions so that a neurally evoked depolarizing current may spread from an innervated fiber to neighboring uninnervated smooth muscle fibers.

Contraction of smooth muscle may be neurally or hormonally evoked, but smooth muscle in certain locations exhibits spontaneous contractile rhythmicity similar to that of cardiac muscle. Mechanical stretch is also capable of eliciting smooth muscle contraction, as in the urinary bladder.

NATIONAL BOARD TYPE QUESTIONS

For the following, select
   A. if only *1, 2, and 3* are correct.
   B. if only *1 and 3* are correct.
   C. if only *2 and 4* are correct.
   D. if only *4* is correct.
   E. if *all* are correct.

1. Which of the following statements regarding intrafusal fibers is (are) correct?
   1. Nuclear bag fibers contain a row of elongate nuclei.
   2. Afferent nerves innervate the equatorial regions of both nuclear chain and nuclear bag fibers.
   3. Gamma nerves terminate as annulospiral endings on intrafusal fibers.
   4. Gamma nerves alter the sensitivity of spindles to stretch by regulating myofibril contraction within the polar regions of intrafusal fibers.

2. Which of the following statements regarding a motor unit is (are) correct?
   1. The nerve cell body is located in the anterior gray horn of the spinal cord.
   2. A single motor unit contains a mixture of fast-twitch and slow-twitch muscle fibers.
   3. All muscle cells of a single motor unit are innervated by axon branches of the same alpha motor neuron.
   4. Skeletal muscles are composed exclusively of either all slow-twitch motor units or all fast-twitch motor units.

3. During the normal contraction of a sarcomere the
   1. I band narrows as actin filaments invade the A band.
   2. H band narrows as actin filaments invade the A band.
   3. Z disks move closer together as the sarcomere contracts.
   4. A band narrows as the sarcomere contracts.

4. Which of the following are insertion points for actin filaments?
   1. Fascia adherens of the intercalated disk
   2. Dense bodies within smooth muscle cells
   3. Z disks of skeletal muscle
   4. Desmosomes of the intercalated disk

5. Neuromuscular spindles
   1. are located in tendons.
   2. consist of intrafusal fibers enclosed within perimysial connective tissue.
   3. are in series with regular extrafusal fibers.
   4. participate in a stretch reflex via a sensory neuron that synapses with an alpha motor neuron.

6. Which of the following statements regarding transverse tubules is (are) correct?
   1. Transverse tubules are absent from smooth muscle cells and Purkinje fibers.
   2. The lumen of transverse tubules is continuous with the extracellular space.
   3. The transverse tubular membrane is continuous with the sarcolemma.
   4. Neurally provoked depolarization of the sarcolemma is conducted along the transverse tubular network.

7. Which of the following events is (are) associated with contraction as opposed to relaxation of skeletal muscle?
   1. Calcium binds to myosin ATPase on the heavy meromyosin cross-bridges.
   2. Calcium binds to troponin, triggering exposure of myosin binding sites along the actin filament.
   3. Calcium is released from the terminal cisterns of sarcoplasmic reticulum.
   4. Calcium is sequestered by the longitudinal elements of sarcoplasmic reticulum.

8. During prolonged cardiac ischemia, which components of the intercalated disk become uncoupled?
   1. Desmosomes
   2. Fascia adherens
   3. Zonula adherens
   4. Communicating junctions (gap junctions)

9. The sarcoplasmic reticulum
   1. forms a sleeve around myofibrils in skeletal and cardiac muscle cells.
   2. is more extensively developed in regular cardiac muscle than in skeletal muscle cells.
   3. forms triads with the transverse tubular system in skeletal and cardiac muscle cells.
   4. forms triads with the transverse tubules in smooth muscle cells.

ANNOTATED ANSWERS

1. C. For further discussion, refer to Neuromuscular Spindles on page 167.

2. B.

3. A. Although the thick filaments composing the A band engage in dynamic activities involving myosin-actin interaction, they do not change in length during muscle contraction.

4. A. Tonofilaments insert into desmosomes.

5. C. For further discussion, refer to Neuromuscular Spindles on page 167.

6. E. Since T tubules are extensions of the plasmalemma and conduct depolarizing impulses, they are not required on small cells such as smooth muscle or on noncontractile Purkinje fibers.

7. A. Retrieval of cytoplasmic calcium by the longitudinal elements of the sarcoplasmic reticulum causes relaxation.

8. D. Uncoupling of gap junctions during ischemia disrupts the depolarizing current between muscle cells.

9. B. Contraction of regular cardiac muscle fibers depends on some extracellular calcium and therefore does not require as well-developed sarcoplasmic reticulum as skeletal muscle. There are no T tubules in smooth muscle.

BIBLIOGRAPHY

Allbrook, D. Skeletal muscle regeneration. *Muscle Nerve* 4:234, 1981.

Barker, D., et al. Studies of the Histochemistry, Ultrastructure, Motor Innervation, and Regeneration of Mammalian Intrafusal Muscle Fibers. In S. Homma (ed.), *Understanding the Stretch Reflex, Progress in Brain Research.* Amsterdam: Elsevier, 1976. Vol. 44, p. 67.

Beringer, T. A freeze-fracture study of sarcoplasmic reticulum from fast and slow muscle of the mouse. *Anat. Rec.* 184:647, 1976.

Boyd, I. A. The Mechanical Properties of Dynamic Nuclear Bag Fibres, Static Nuclear Bag Fibres and Nuclear Chain Fibres in Isolated Cat Muscle Spindles. In S. Homma (ed.), *Understanding the Stretch Reflex, Progress in Brain Research.* Amsterdam: Elsevier, 1976. vol. 44, p. 33.

Bray, D. F., and D. G. Rayns. A comparative freeze-etch study of the sarcoplasmic reticulum of avian fast and slow muscle fibers. *J. Ultrastruct. Res.* 57:251, 1976.

Buchthal, F., and H. Schmalbruch. Motor unit of mammalian muscle. *Physiol. Rev.* 60:9, 1980.

Burke, R. E., D. N. Levine, and F. E. Zajac III. Mammalian motor units: Physiological-histochemical correlation in three types of cat gastrocnemius. *Science* 174:709, 1971.

Constantin, L. L., C. Franzini-Armstrong, and R. J. Podolsky. Localization of calcium accumulating structures in striated muscle. *Science* 147:158, 1965.

Cooke, P. A filamentous cytoskeleton in vertebrate smooth muscle fibers. *J. Cell Biol.* 68:539, 1976.

Cooke, P., and F. S. Fay. Correlation between fiber length, ultrastructure, and the length-tension relationship of mammalian smooth muscle. *J. Cell Biol.* 52:105, 1972.

Devine, C. E., A. V. Somlyo, and A. P. Somlyo, Sarcoplasmic reticulum and excitation-contraction coupling in mammalian smooth muscles. *J. Cell Biol.* 52:690, 1972.

Fawcett, D. W., and N. S. McNutt. The ultrastructure of the cat myocardium I. Ventricular papillary muscle. *J. Cell Biol.* 42:1, 1969.

Fay, F. S., and P. H. Cooke. Reversible disaggregation of myofilaments in vertebrate smooth muscle. *J. Cell Biol.* 56:399, 1973.

Forbes, M. S., and N. Sperelakis. Intercalated discs of mammalian heart: A review of structure and function. *Tissue Cell* 17:605, 1985.

Fozzard, H. A. Heart: Excitation-contraction coupling. *Ann. Rev. Physiol.* 39:201, 1977.

Franzini-Armstrong, C. Studies of the triad. I. Structure of the junction in frog twitch fibers. *J. Cell Biol.* 47:488, 1970.

Gauthier, G. F., and H. A. Padykula. Cytological studies of fiber types in skeletal muscle: A comparative study of the mammalian diaphragm. *J. Cell Biol.* 28:333, 1966.

Granger, B. L., and E. Lazarides. The existence of an insoluble Z-disc scaffold in chicken skeletal muscle. *Cell* 15:1253, 1978.

Hanson, J., and H. E. Huxley. The structural basis of contraction in striated muscle. *Symp. Soc. Exp. Biol.* 9:228, 1955.

Huxley, H. E. The mechanism of muscular contraction. *Science* 164:1356, 1969.

Kelly, D. E., and M. A. Cahill. Filamentous and matrix components of skeletal muscle Z-discs. *Anat. Rec.* 172:623, 1972.

Kelly, D. E., and A. M. Kuda. Subunits of the triadic junction in fast skeletal muscle as revealed by freeze-fracture. *J. Ultrastruct. Res.* 68:220, 1979.

Kucera, J., and K. Dorovini-Zis. Types of human intrafusal muscle fibers. *Muscle Nerve* 2:437, 1979.

Luff, A. R., and H. L. Atwood. Changes in the sarcoplasmic reticulum and transverse tubular system of fast and slow skeletal muscles of the mouse during postnatal development. *J. Cell Biol.* 51:369, 1971.

McCallister, L. P., and R. Hadek. Transmission electron microscopy and stereo ultrastructure of the T system in frog skeletal muscle. *J. Ultrastruct. Res.* 33:360, 1970.

McNutt, N. S., and D. W. Fawcett. The ultrastructure of the cat myocardium: II. Atrial muscle. *J. Cell Biol.* 42:46, 1969.

Ovalle, W. K., Jr. Fine structure of rat intrafusal muscle fibers: The equatorial region. *J. Cell Biol.* 52:382, 1972.

Padykula, H. A., and G. F. Gauthier. The ultrastructure of the neuromuscular junctions of mammalian red, white, and intermediate skeletal muscle fibers. *J. Cell Biol.* 46:27, 1970.

Page, S. G. A comparison of the fine structure of frog slow and twitch muscle fibers. *J. Cell Biol.* 26:477, 1965.

Peachey, L. D. The sarcoplasmic reticulum and transverse tubules of the frog's sartorius. *J. Cell Biol.* 25:209, 1965.

Pepe, F. A. Structure of muscle filaments from immunohistochemical and ultrastructural studies. *J. Histochem. Cytochem.* 23:543, 1975.

Sjostrand, F. S., E. Andersson-Cedergren, and M. M. Dewey. The ultrastructure of the intercalated discs of frog, mouse, and guinea pig cardiac muscle. *J. Ultrastruct. Res.* 1:271, 1958.

Small, J. V., and A. Sobieszek. The contractile apparatus of smooth muscle. *Int. Rev. Cytol.* 64:241, 1980.

Somlyo, A. V. Bridging structures spanning the junctional gap at the triad of skeletal muscle. *J. Cell Biol.* 80:743, 1979.

Somlyo, A. P., and A. V. Somlyo. Vascular smooth muscle. I. Normal structure, pathology, biochemistry, and biophysics. *Pharmacol. Rev.* 20:197, 1968.

Sommer, J. R., and E. A. Johnson. Cardiac muscle: A comparative study of Purkinje fibers and ventricular fibers. *J. Cell Biol.* 36:497, 1968.

Sommer, J. R., and R. A. Waugh. The ultrastructure of the mammalian cardiac muscle with special emphasis on the tubular membrane systems. *Am. J. Pathol.* 82:191, 1976.

Swash, M., and K. P. Fox. Muscle spindle innervation in man. *J. Anat.* 112:61, 1972.

Thaemert, J. C. Ultrastructural interrelationships of nerve processes and smooth muscle cells in three dimensions. *J. Cell Biol.* 28:37, 1966.

Truex, R. C., and W. M. Copenhaver. Histology of the moderator band in man and other mammals, with special reference to the conduction system. *Am. J. Anat.* 80:173, 1947.

8 Nerve

The **neuron** is the structural and functional cellular unit of the nervous system. It displays two highly developed physiologic properties: **irritability,** which is the capacity to generate nervous impulses in response to various stimuli, and **conductivity,** the ability to transmit these impulses along its cellular processes. Both of these properties are essential for communicating information in the form of nervous impulses between the central nervous system (brain and spinal cord) and other parts of the body.

Peripheral nerves, those emanating from the spinal cord and cranium, initiate specific responses from cells they contact or innervate, such as muscle contraction or cell secretion. The actions of peripheral nerves are in turn integrated and coordinated by neurons of the central nervous system.

Nervous tissue includes not only a wide variety of neurons but also a class of nonneuronal cells with which they are associated: the **Schwann** **cells** of the peripheral nervous system and the **glial cells** of the central nervous system.

THE NEURON OR NERVE CELL

The neuron is composed of three integral parts (Fig. 8-1): (1) the **nerve cell body (perikaryon),** which contains the nucleus; (2) one or more **dendrites,** the receptive processes of the neuron that respond to stimuli and conduct impulses toward the perikaryon; and (3) a single **axon,** which arises from the cell body or occasionally from the dendrite and conducts impulses away from the perikaryon.

Neurons are classified according to the number of processes originating from the cell body and comprise three major groups: **unipolar, bipolar,** and **multipolar neurons.** Unipolar neurons have a single process. They are most common in the developing nervous system of the embryo prior to becoming bipolar and multipolar neurons. In the

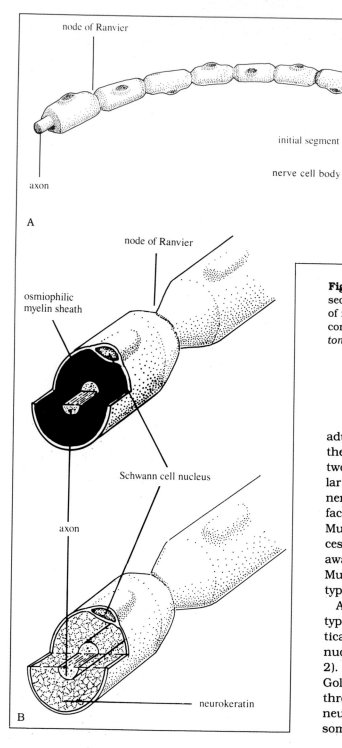

node of Ranvier

axon hillock

initial segment

nerve cell body

dendrites

A

node of Ranvier

osmiophilic myelin sheath

Schwann cell nucleus

axon

neurokeratin

B

Fig. 8-1. *A.* Neuron with myelinated axon. *B.* Cross-sectional profiles depict light microscopic appearance of myelin sheath after osmium fixation (top) and after conventional paraffin embedding procedures (*bottom*).

adult a special type of unipolar neuron occurs in the sensory ganglia. Bipolar neurons consist of two processes, one axon and one dendrite. Bipolar neurons are not common but they are prominent in a few specialized tissues, such as the olfactory mucosa, the retina, and the inner ear. Multipolar neurons consist of more than two processes, a single axon (which may branch further away from the cell body) and multiple dendrites. Multipolar neurons are by far the most common type of neuron.

Although the nerve cell body among different types of neurons varies in shape, it characteristically contains a large spherical, euchromatic nucleus with a very prominent nucleolus (Fig. 8-2). Neurons have a well-developed perinuclear Golgi complex, and mitochondria are present throughout the cytoplasm. Even though adult neurons are incapable of cell division, centrosomes may be found in neurons that have non-

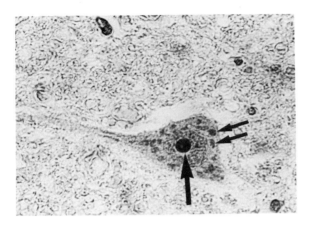

Fig. 8-2. A section through the cell body of an alpha motor neuron in the ventral grey horn of the spinal cord. The cytoplasm contains basophilic densities known as Nissl bodies which represent clusters of rough endoplasmic reticulum (*small arrows*). The nucleolus is large and conspicuous (*large arrow*).

motile cilia, such as those in the bipolar neurons of the olfactory epithelium. Mitochondria are present throughout the neuron.

Neurofibrils, which are responsible for the argyrophilic staining properties of nerve cells, are long threadlike structures distributed throughout the neuron that are visible with the light microscope when stained in this fashion. The electron microscope reveals that neurofibrils are bundles of much smaller **neurofilaments** 10 nm in diameter.

Although smooth endoplasmic reticulum is distributed throughout the neuron, **rough endoplasmic reticulum** (RER) is confined to the nerve cell body and dendrites. With the light microscope, RER is visible in the cell body as coarse clumps of basophilic material (Nissl substance) (see Fig. 8-2). The axon and **axon hillock,** a conical portion of the cell body where the axon originates, are devoid of RER. Consequently, the axon is heavily dependent on proteins synthesized in the cell body because it is incapable of protein synthesis itself. These proteins are actively conveyed from their site of synthesis in the cell body

throughout the length of the axon by a process called **axoplasmic transport** (see later section). Axoplasmic transport is known to involve **microtubules,** since drugs which bind to or disperse microtubules interfere with axoplasmic transport. Microtubules are present throughout the entire neuron. Understanding the dependency of the axon on the synthetic machinery of the cell body is a prerequisite to understanding the events that occur during the regeneration of the axon after injury.

Structure of the Synapse

The structural and functional link between the axon of one neuron and the dendrite of another neuron is a simple kind of **synapse** where **synaptic transmission** occurs. During synaptic transmission, a nerve impulse from the axon of one neuron initiates a nerve impulse in the dendrite of another neuron. In peripheral nerves, which have chemical synapses, a chemical neurotransmitter is involved in the physiologic events of synaptic transmission. The neurotransmitter is released from the axon into the synaptic cleft on the arrival of the depolarizing nerve impulse. The neurotransmitter diffuses across the 25-nm synaptic cleft that separates the axon (presynaptic membrane) from the dendrite (postsynaptic membrane) and depolarizes the dendritic membrane, generating a nerve impulse that is propagated along the dendrite of the second neuron. This simple kind of synapse is termed **axodendritic.** However, synapses also occur between two axons, between two dendrites, and between axon and nerve cell body. Synapses also occur between an axon and muscle cells and also between axons and secretory epithelium.

Within the axon terminal are **synaptic vesicles**—spherical, membrane-bound structures containing neurotransmitter (Fig. 8-3). During synaptic transmission these vesicles fuse to the axon membrane and rupture, releasing transmitter molecules by exocytosis into the synaptic cleft. The presence of these vesicles on only one side of the synapse (i.e., presynaptic terminal) explains why a neuron participating in a **chemi-**

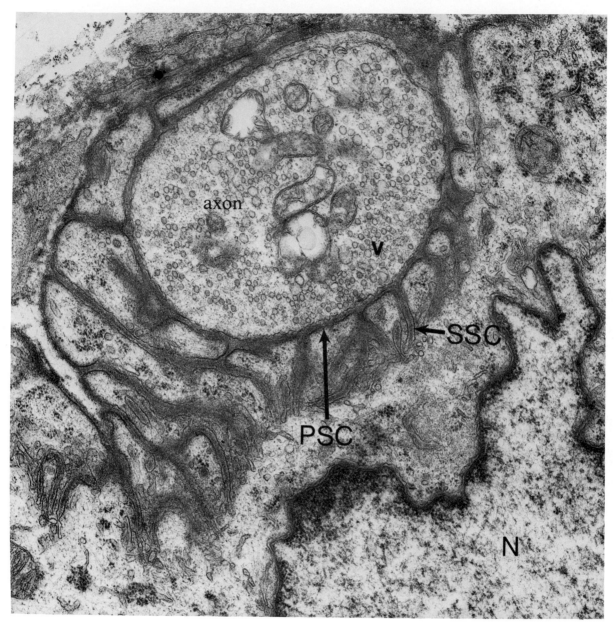

Fig. 8-3. Electron micrograph of a neuromuscular synapse. Numerous synaptic vesicles (v) occur within the axon terminal. N = muscle cell nucleus; PSC = primary synaptic cleft; SSC = secondary synaptic cleft.

cal synapse conducts impulses in only one direction across the synapse (structural and functional asymmetry). Two examples of chemical synapses are the neuromuscular junctions of skeletal muscle, where acetylcholine is the transmitter, and the great majority of axodendritic synapses, where the transmitter may be acetylcholine, norepinephrine, or one of several other chemical transmitters. Synaptic vesicles are not always located at the axon terminal but wherever synaptic transmission takes place. For instance, synaptic vesicles are deployed at multiple sites along an axon participating in **en passant** synapses with cardiac and smooth muscle.

In addition to the chemical synapse, which occurs extensively in both peripheral and central nervous systems, there is another type of synapse called an *electrical synapse,* which occurs predominantly in the central nervous system. The electrical synapse is composed of a gap junction, which structurally and electrically couples the presynaptic and postsynaptic membranes. This type of synapse allows bidirectional conduction across the synapse, and depolarization is mediated directly by ionic current instead of chemical transmitters so synaptic vesicles are not present.

Role of the Axolemma in Synaptic Transmission

The plasmalemma of the axon (axolemma), like that of the muscle cell, is an electrogenic membrane. Because of its ability to partition ions within the axon from those outside the axon, a net negative charge is established inside the axon (−90 mV) with respect to the extracellular space. This net negative charge is referred to as the **resting membrane potential** (RMP). The RMP results from the ability of ionic pumps in the axolemma to pump cations, mostly sodium, out of the axon. When a nerve is stimulated, sodium enters the axon and the RMP is reduced to a threshold potential (−60 mV) beyond which the axon initiates an **action potential.** During the action potential, the axolemma is further de-

polarized by an increase in its permeability to all cations. This rapid ionic influx is propagated along the axon to its synaptic termination. In the particular instance of a chemical synapse, the local influx of calcium ions specifically triggers the release of neurotransmitter from synaptic vesicles into the synaptic cleft by exocytosis (see Fig. 8-3). After diffusing across the cleft, the neurotransmitter induces depolarization of another neuron, muscle cell, or epithelial cell. An immediate reversal of sodium flux is initiated to terminate the action potential and hyperpolarize the axon membrane sufficiently to reestablish the RMP.

Synapses may be **excitatory** or **inhibitory,** depending on whether the transmitter depolarizes or hyperpolarizes the postsynaptic neuron with respect to its threshold potential for firing. This action is a function of the various specific neurotransmitters and the type of receptor in the postsynaptic membrane.

Inclusions

Fat droplets and pigments are among the inclusions found in nerve cells. The pigments are the golden-brown **lipofuscin** found abundantly in ganglionic neurons and the brownish-black **melanin** found abundantly in certain nerves of the central nervous system.

Glycogen particles are present in embryonic neurons only. The absence of glycogen in the adult neuron underscores its dependency on the oxidative metabolism, its limited anaerobic capacity, and therefore its vulnerability during even short periods of anoxia.

NERVE SHEATHS

All axons of peripheral neurons (and some dendrites) are circumscribed by a single layer of Schwann cells arranged in sequence along the length of the axon (see Fig. 8-1). These cells constitute the **sheath of Schwann** and are derived from neural crest cells. The sheath of Schwann is occasionally referred to as the **neurilemma.**

Schwann cells assist the axon, which they invest in several ways. They insulate axons from one another; they influence the conduction velocity of nervous impulses transmitted along the axon; and they participate in events associated with regeneration of injured axons. An axon is ensheathed by either of two types of Schwann cell configurations: **myelinated** or **unmyelinated.**

Unmyelinated axons are the slowly conducting axons. In this configuration, several axons are usually associated with each Schwann cell of the sheath, each axon occupying a separate concave recess in the Schwann cell surface (Fig. 8-4).

In the myelinated configuration, Schwann cells are associated with a single axon exclusively. Schwann cells of myelinated axons are formed into broad cytoplasmic sheets that are coiled around the axon (Fig. 8-5). These coils are so tightly wound that cytoplasm is present only within the innermost and outermost revolutions of the Schwann cell. The outermost revolution contains most of the cytoplasm, including the nucleus. The cytoplasm is so completely excluded from the middle or intervening revolutions that the cytoplasmic surfaces of the plasmalemma are in contact, apparently fused. When sectioned and viewed with the electron microscope, these fused cytoplasmic surfaces of plasmalemma appear as a **major dense line** (3 nm wide) coiled around the axon (Fig. 8-6). This major dense line is interrupted at staggered intervals by a narrow channel of cytoplasm connecting the innermost and outermost revolutions of the Schwann cell. These are the **Schmidt-Lanterman clefts.** Alternating with the major dense line is a less dense **intraperiod line** (2 nm wide) formed by close apposition of the external surfaces of adjacent revolutions of plasmalemma. Consequently, the **myelin sheath** is constructed of concentric revolutions of Schwann cell plasmalemma (see Figs. 8-5, 8-6). Since the Schwann cell plasmalemma has an unusually high lipid-to-protein ratio, the properties of the myelin sheath are dictated by its lipid components. Specifically, the higher electrical resistance, lower capacitance, and hydrophobic nature of lipids in Schwann cell plasmalemma relative to axolemma serve to insulate axons. Furthermore, these lipid properties of the myelin sheath are responsible for higher conduction velocities of myelinated axons compared with unmyelinated axons.

Since the myelin sheath consists entirely of cell membrane, its composition is mostly lipoprotein. Therefore, in conventional paraffin embedding procedures using organic solvents for dehy-

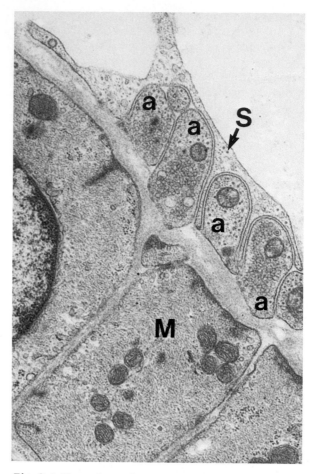

Fig. 8-4. Unmyelinated axons innervating smooth muscle cells (*M*). Several axons (*a*) occupy recesses in the cytoplasm of a single Schwann cell (*S*). Small synaptic vesicles are visible in three of the axons.

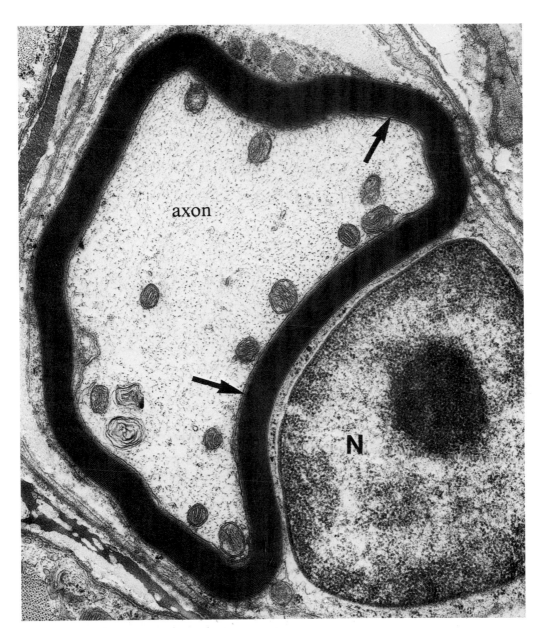

Fig. 8-5. Electron micrograph of a myelinated axon.
Arrows point to the myelin sheath. *N* = Schwann cell
nucleus.

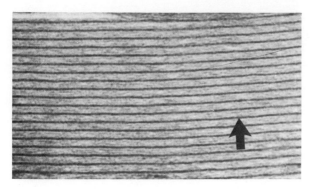

Fig. 8-6. Higher magnification of myelin sheath. Arrow indicates major dense line; intraperiod lines alternate with the dense lines.

dration, the lipid components are dissolved away, resulting in poor preservation of the myelin sheath. A proteinaceous residue called **neurokeratin** is left behind, which forms a network around the axon. Consequently, the light microscopic appearance of myelinated axons prepared in this manner, cross-sectioned, and stained with hematoxylin and eosin is usually a dot (representing the axon) surrounded by a translucent halo (representing the leached-out myelin) with a variable but often lacy-appearing neurokeratin network within (Fig. 8-1, 8-7). The myelin sheath can be preserved by osmium tetroxide fixation, in which case it appears black due to the deposition of reduced osmium (see Figs. 8-1, 8-8).

In myelinated axons fixed with osmium, periodic indentations along the sheath of Schwann are visible with the light microscope, indicating the lateral limits of adjacent Schwann cells deployed along the axon. These indentations are the **nodes of Ranvier** where a minute portion of the axolemma is exposed to the extracellular space (see Fig. 8-1). Since the axon between nodes is insulated by myelin, the nerve impulse is forced to jump from node to node, a phenomenon called **saltatory conduction** (from

L. **saltare,** to leap). This results in a faster conduction velocity than that observed along unmyelinated axons where the depolarizing ionic current is propagated along the complete length of axon. Consequently, demyelinating diseases reduce conduction velocity along affected nerves, which can be measured clinically. A short length of axon remains bare of Schwann sheath where it originates from the axon hillock. This is the **initial segment** where the action potential is generated (see Fig. 8-1). When an axon branches, it does so at the nodes.

Examples of myelinated neurons are the alpha motor neurons (axon only) innervating skeletal muscle and the dendrites of certain somatic afferent neurons. With the exception of these sensory neurons, dendrites generally have no Schwann sheath. In the central nervous system a different cell, the **oligodendrocyte,** is responsible for myelination of axons. Unlike myelinating Schwann cells, oligodendrocytes send out multiple processes that contribute myelin sheaths to several axons simultaneously instead of to a single axon.

At birth the myelin sheaths are virtually complete in the peripheral nervous system but during growth of the newborn, myelination must continue in order to keep pace with lengthening axons. In the central nervous system, including the spinal cord, myelination is still incomplete at birth.

CONNECTIVE TISSUE INVESTMENTS

All peripheral nerves, both myelinated and unmyelinated, are arranged into three levels of organization by connective tissue sheaths (Fig. 8-9). The outermost connective tissue investment, enclosing an entire nerve trunk, is the **epineurium.** It is composed of irregularly arranged collagenous and elastic fibers and fibroblasts. The epineurium extends into the nerve trunk, separating groups of axons into fascicles. The epineurium can be followed back to the spinal cord where it is continuous with the dura mater.

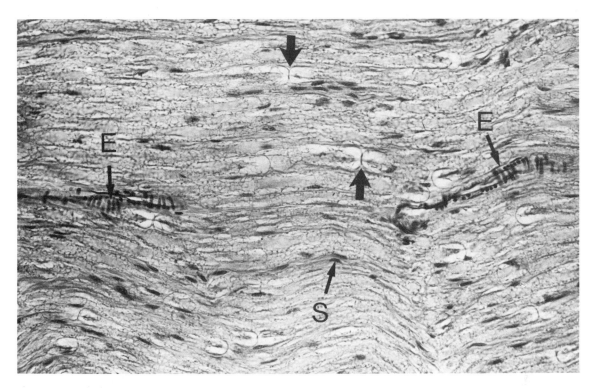

Fig. 8-7. A conventionally prepared section through a large myelinated nerve. The myelin sheath is poorly preserved because osmium was not used during fixation. Subsequent dehydration leached out the lipids from the myelin. The resulting neurokeratin produces a chaotic pattern that obscures the view. However, at several points the nodes of Ranvier (*unlabeled arrows*) are apparent and a short segment of axon can be discerned at these points. The elongate nuclei oriented with the long axis of the axons belong to Schwann cells (S). The closely arranged elongated nuclei oriented 90 degrees with respect to the long axis of the axons belong to endothelial cells (E) lining a capillary travelling within the nerve trunk.

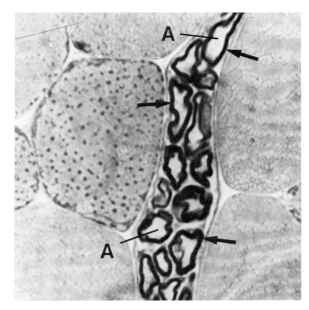

Fig. 8-8. Myelinated axons coursing through a field of skeletal muscle. The myelin sheath has been preserved with glutaraldehyde and blackened by impregnation with osmium. Myelin sheaths are indicated by arrows; A = axons.

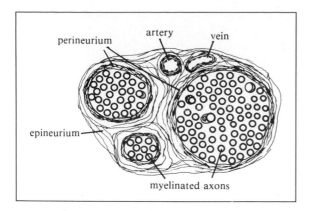

Fig. 8-9. Connective tissue investments of several nerve fascicles. The endoneurium that surrounds each myelinated axon is not indicated.

These individual fascicles are further ensheathed by another connective tissue investment called the **perineurium,** whose internal aspect is delineated by a continuous sheet of flat epithelial cells (**perineurial epithelium**) supported by a basal lamina. The **endoneurium** is the innermost connective tissue sheath, surrounding individual axons within the fascicle, and is separated from the sheath of Schwann by a basal lamina.

HISTOLOGIC APPEARANCE

In longitudinal section of hematoxylin and eosin–stained nerve, the axons are visible as pale, eosinophilic, linear structures that are somewhat camouflaged by the associated neurokeratin network and therefore not easily distinguished. Most visible are the abundant, dark, basophilic Schwann cell nuclei, whose long axes are oriented with the long axis of the nerve. A few fibroblast nuclei are also present. The whole nerve usually presents an undulating or wavy appearance in longitudinal section, probably due to the presence of elastic fibers in the epineurium.

Most nerves that are encountered in histologic section of other tissues or organs will appear as relatively small singular fascicles circumscribed by a perineurium.

BLOOD SUPPLY

Nerves are profusely vascularized with longitudinally oriented, anastomosing blood vessels. Arterioles run through the epineurial and perineurial connective tissue, and a capillary network pervades the endoneurium.

AXOPLASMIC TRANSPORT

Axoplasmic transport refers to the process by which molecular substances and organelles are conveyed along the axon. Three major types of transport have been recognized according to their direction and speed of transport: **fast anterograde** (300–400 mm/day), **slow anterograde** (1–5 mm/day), and **fast retrograde** (300–400 mm/day).

Both the fast anterograde and fast retrograde systems transport the vesicular components of the axoplasm. Therefore, synaptic vesicles as well as various proteins are assembled in the cell body and transported in the anterograde direction. Autoradiographic evidence indicates that newly synthesized proteins within the endoplasmic reticulum are carried by transport vesicles to the Golgi apparatus before entering the axon. It is proposed that Golgi-derived vesicles then fuse with the axonal **smooth endoplasmic reticulum** (SER), accounting for membrane flow or transport of the SER into the axon. In the retrograde direction, multivesicular bodies and lamellar bodies are transported from the axon terminal (in addition to some constituents collected from the extracellular space) to the cell body, where they may interact with lysosomes. Mitochondria are transported in both directions at this speed. Localized anoxia arrests both fast anterograde and fast retrograde mechanisms of transport, since they are heavily dependent on oxidative metabolism.

The slow anterograde component of axonal transport carries the cytoskeletal proteins, which comprise microtubules, neurofilaments, and microfilaments plus the bulk of the cytoplasmic matrix. Although microtubules move at the slow rate, they are known to be involved in the underlying mechanism of fast transport since fast transport is blocked by microtubule-binding drugs. In addition, actin and myosin may cooperate with microtubules during transport, but many details remain to be clarified. Although microtubules and possibly neurofilaments and microfilaments may all be involved in the fast transport of vesicular elements, they grow into the axon at the slow rate, which also corresponds to the rate at which axons grow during normal development and during regeneration following injury.

DEGENERATION AND REGENERATION OF PERIPHERAL NERVES

Although compression and section injuries to the axons of peripheral nerves do not generally result in the death of the neuron, several degenerative changes occur in the axon distal to the site of injury, proximal to the site of injury, and in the nerve cell body itself. These changes are followed by regeneration of the axon by multiple sprouting from its proximal stump.

Within several minutes after an axon is crushed or severed, both the axon and its myelin sheath distal to the site of injury begin to disintegrate (**anterograde** or **wallerian degeneration**). Almost immediately, the myelin lamellae are loosened at the intraperiod line, beginning first in the paranodal area, which appears under the light microscope as a retraction of the myelin sheath from the nodes, and the Schmidt-Lanterman clefts become dilated (Fig. 8-10A). This process spreads distally from the injury eventually to involve the entire axon within 36 hours. Next, the myelin begins to subdivide adjacent to the swollen Schmidt-Lanterman clefts and at the nodes to form ovoid segments (**myelin ovoids**) (Fig. 8-10B,C). The myelin ovoids contain segments of axon that have fragmented at the level of the nodes and near the dilated Schmidt-Lanterman incisures. Schwann cells, however, remain healthy, proliferate, and remove disintegrating axonal and myelin debris by phagocytosis. Schwann cells also lay down several layers of basal lamina, thus establishing a tunnel to guide regenerating axonal sprouts from the proximal stump back to their original synaptic contacts.

Degeneration of the proximal stump of a severed axon is usually not severe, sometimes involving only one or two internodes from the site of injury (**retrograde degeneration**). The extent of degeneration depends on the proximity of the injury to the cell body. If the axon is damaged close enough to the cell body, the complete neuron may die. Once retrograde degeneration ceases, regeneration may begin from the proximal segment of the axon.

Within a few days after injury to the axon, several characteristic changes occur in the cell body. It becomes swollen, and its nucleus develops a more prominent nucleolus and becomes displaced to an eccentric position within the cell body. The Nissl substance gradually disperses, remaining intact only at the cell periphery (**chromatolysis**). These cell body responses are more severe with increasing proximity of injury to the cell body. Axonal injuries close to the synapse provoke limited cell body response, while axonal injury very close to the cell body causes death of the neuron. These responses are most striking in alpha motor neurons, where the nucleus is normally centrally located and the Nissl substance is prominent. In other neurons, such as the ganglion cells, the response is less striking either because the nucleus may normally occupy an eccentric position or because the Nissl substance is not normally prominent.

Hypertrophy of the nucleolus and replacement of RER by nonmembrane-bound polyribosomes are signals that the neuron is increasing its synthetic capacity in order to support growth of the regenerating axon. The growth of the regenerating axon (1–5 mm/day) reflects the rate of slow

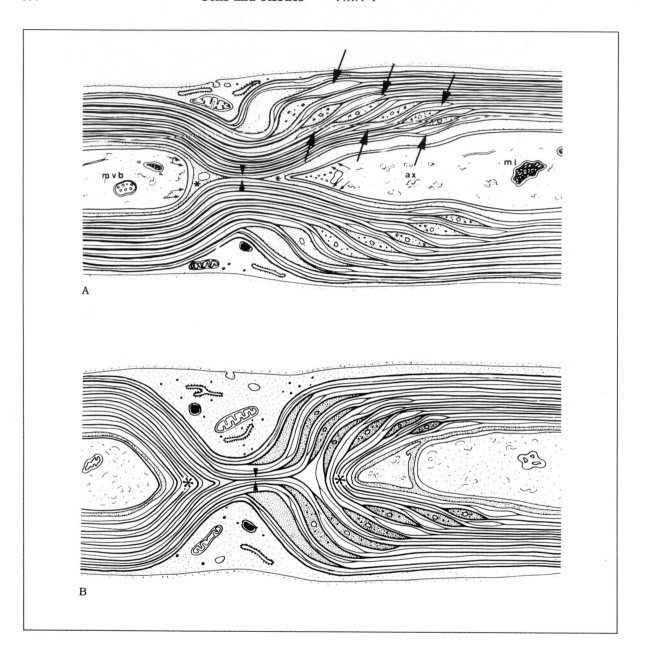

A

B

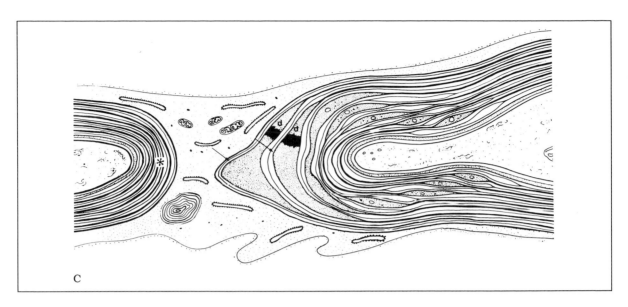

C

Fig. 8-10. Schmidt-Lanterman incisures during
changes following nerve crush. A. At 24 hours after
crush the axon collapses opposite the incisure with
maximum narrowing opposite the wide end of site of
future cleavage. At this site the axoplasm has seg-
mented (*double arrows*). Inner Schwann cell cytoplasm fuses across the fiber (*asterisks*) while the innermost lamellae become apposed (*arrowheads*). ax
= axoplasm; ml = major dense line; mvb = multivesicular body. B. At 24 to 36 hours after crush, inner myelin lamellae (*asterisks*) have fused across the
fiber while the outer lamellae are still apposed (*arrowheads*). C. At 36 hours after crush a transverse cleavage separates ovoids. End of ovoid at right contains
an intact incisure, while the adjacent ovoid has no
incisure. On the left the myelin lamellae (*asterisk*)
have been retracted into the ovoid while at the right
some lamellae (*arrows*) are still widely separated from
ovoid and are connected to one another by desmo-
somelike bands (*d*). (From M. N. Ghabriel and
G. Allt, The role of Schmidt-Lanterman incisures in
wallerian degeneration: II. An electron microscopic
study. *Acta Neuropath. Berl.* 48:95, 1979.)

axoplasmic transport, which involves assembly of the axoplasmic cytoskeletal elements such as microtubules, neurofilaments, and microfilaments and their growth into the lengthening axon. Once axon regeneration is complete and the original synaptic contacts are reestablished, chromatolysis is reversed.

GENERAL ORGANIZATION OF THE SPINAL CORD AND OUTFLOW OF PERIPHERAL NERVES

The nervous system is conveniently divided into two parts: the **central nervous system** (CNS), which includes the brain and spinal cord, and the **peripheral nervous system** (PNS), which includes the nerves emanating from the spinal cord and cranium that distribute to other areas of the body.

The **spinal cord** is the final common pathway for conveying motor commands from the brain to the rest of the body and for funneling peripheral sensory information back to the brain. Nerves enter and leave the spinal cord at regular intervals along its length, with sensory and motor nerves initially following separate routes. Sensory nerves enter the cord through the **dorsal roots;** motor nerves emerge from the cord through the **ventral roots.** At a short distance from the cord these two roots join to form mixed spinal nerves carrying both sensory and motor nerve fibers (see Fig. 8-11). Small branches of these nerves are among those observed in histologic sections of the tissues and organs.

The spinal cord itself is organized into distinct **white** and **gray areas.** The gray part of the cord is a roughly H-shaped central region housing mostly nerve cell bodies and their dendrites. This central gray area is surrounded by white matter arranged into **dorsal, lateral,** and **ventral columns,** which are composed of descending and ascending myelinated nerves connecting various levels of the spinal cord (Fig. 8-11). The white color is imparted to these columns by the presence of myelin. The columns also contain a few unmyelinated fibers, but no nerve cell bodies or dendrites.

The arms on the H-shaped gray region are designated as **ventral** and **dorsal gray horns.** The dorsal horn is essentially a sensory area (afferent) and the ventral horn a motor area (efferent). The ventral gray horn contains the nerve cell bodies of multipolar alpha motor neurons (**somatic efferent**), whose myelinated axons exit the cord along the ventral root to innervate skeletal muscle.

Sensory nerves enter the cord along the dorsal root, but their nerve cell bodies are located within an expansion of the dorsal root called the **dorsal root ganglion** or **cranial-spinal ganglion** (Fig. 8-11). **Ganglion** is a term designating a collection of nerve cell bodies outside the CNS. The dorsal root ganglion contains sensory nerve cell bodies, each with a single process that divides into a myelinated dendrite that distributes to some peripheral area of the body and an axon that enters the dorsal gray horn of the spinal cord through the dorsal root. Within the cord these sensory neurons synapse with other sensory neurons whose cell bodies are within the dorsal horn. These secondary sensory neurons then give rise to axons that enter the white matter and form the ascending and descending sensory tracts running through the dorsal column and connecting segments of the cord to one another or to higher centers of the brain.

Autonomic Nervous System

A small enlargement at the juncture of the ventral and dorsal horns called the **intermediolateral gray** houses preganglionic nerve cell bodies of the autonomic nervous system, whose axons flow out from the cord along the ventral roots (see Fig. 8-11). The autonomic part of the peripheral nervous system (**visceral efferent**) operates without the intervention of conscious thought. It innervates mostly smooth and cardiac musculature, as well as some secretory epithelium. Autonomic nerves consist of two neurons arranged in sequence, extending from the inter-

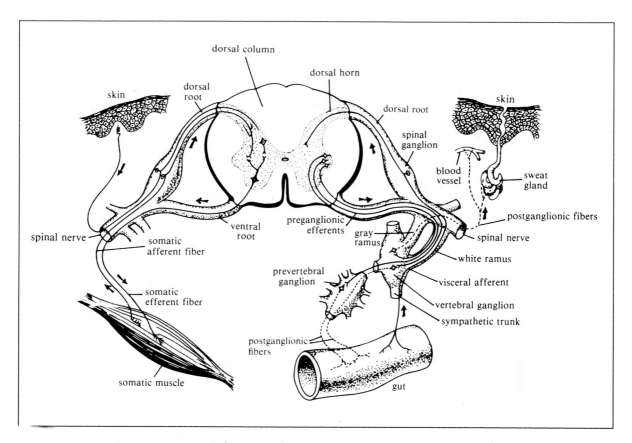

Fig. 8-11. Cross-sectional diagram of the spinal cord illustrating nervous connections with the peripheral nervous system. (After W. M. Copenhaver, R. P. Bunge, and M. B. Bunge (eds.), *Bailey's Textbook of Histology* [16th ed.]. Baltimore: Williams & Wilkins, 1971. Reproduced with permission.)

mediolateral gray of the spinal cord to the structure they innervate. This arrangement requires an intervening **autonomic ganglion** where synapses occur between the two neurons. The first neuron whose cell body is in the intermediolateral gray is the **preganglionic neuron,** whose axon innervates the cell body of the **postganglionic neuron** within the ganglion. The axon of the postganglionic neuron extends from the ganglion and establishes synaptic contact

with smooth or cardiac musculature or secretory epithelium. The smooth musculature could be in various locations, including the walls of blood vessels, the ducts of endocrine organs, or the walls of the digestive tract.

Preganglionic fibers are lightly myelinated, whereas postganglionic axons are usually unmyelinated.

The autonomic nervous system comprises **sympathetic** and **parasympathetic** divisions, which have coordinated and generally antagonistic effects on the structures that they dually innervate. Parasympathetic nerves issue from the brain stem and spinal cord (craniosacral segment); sympathetic nerves issue from the **thoracolumbar** segments of the spinal cord.

Parasympathetic ganglia (terminal ganglia) are generally located near or within the structures that are innervated by their postganglionic fibers. This is not the case, however, for **sympathetic ganglia.** Most sympathetic ganglia (vertebral ganglia) are connected to one another in two long **sympathetic trunks** running parallel to the spinal cord along its ventrolateral aspect (see Fig. 8-11). The other important sympathetic ganglia are not part of the sympathetic trunk; these are the **collateral sympathetic ganglia** (prevertebral ganglia), which are part of nerve plexuses such as the celiac plexus in the abdomen.

Sympathetic preganglionic fibers pass from the spinal nerves through short **white communicating rami** to the sympathetic trunk, where they synapse with a postganglionic neuron that returns to the spinal nerve through a **gray communicating ramus.** Preganglionic axons destined to synapse with a postganglionic neuron with collateral sympathetic ganglia follow the white communicating ramus but pass directly through the sympathetic trunk to their destination.

Histology of the Ganglia

All ganglia are contained within a connective tissue capsule that is continuous with the epineurial and perineurial connective tissue of the nerve processes entering or emerging from the ganglion.

Within the ganglion each nerve cell body is enveloped by a single layer of ovoid **satellite cells** (Fig. 8-12). Since the satellite cells separate the nerve cell body from capillaries within the ganglion, it is expected that they may play some regulatory role in metabolic exchange between the perikaryon and its blood supply. The satellite cell layer around the cell body is continuous with the Schwann sheath of the axon extending away from the cell body. Satellite cells are derivatives of neural crest tissue, as are Schwann cells.

External to the satellite cells is a basal lamina and external to that a **connective tissue capsule** composed of collagen and fibroblasts (often referred to as **capsule cells;** see Fig. 8-12). The connective tissue capsule of each nerve cell body is continuous with the endoneurium of its axon.

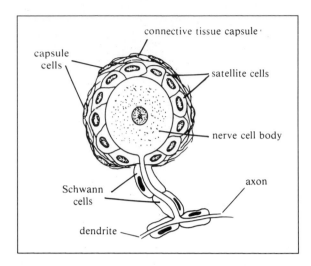

Fig. 8-12. Nerve cell body of spinal ganglion (sensory ganglion). Note that the single process extending from the cell body divides into two processes. One is an axon going to the spinal cord; and the other is a dendrite arriving from some peripheral sensory terminal.

Nerve fibers from the craniospinal and autonomic ganglia are part of the peripheral nervous system.

CRANIOSPINAL OR DORSAL ROOT GANGLIA (SENSORY GANGLIA)

Nerve cell bodies within dorsal root ganglia are ovoid in shape with centrally located nuclei. These cell bodies occupy a peripheral location within the ganglia near the capsule while their nerve fibers travel within the central core of the ganglion. These nerve cells are unipolar neurons. They are sometimes referred to as pseudounipolar because a single unmyelinated process extends away from the cell body and branches into an axon and dendrite (see Fig. 8-12). The axon is myelinated and enters the spinal cord, while the myelinated dendrite distributes peripherally to terminate as a sensory receptor in the skin (**somatic afferent terminal**) or in a visceral organ (**visceral afferent terminal**). Consequently, there are no synapses in dorsal root ganglia. The skin area innervated by dendrites from a single posterior root is a **dermatome.**

The dendrites terminate as **free nerve endings** (**unencapsulated**), which are receptive to sensations of temperature, pressure, or pain, and as **encapsulated endings,** which are mechanoreceptors for sensation of touch and pressure (more details later in this chapter).

AUTONOMIC GANGLIA

Both parasympathetic and sympathetic ganglia contain **multipolar neurons** with a single unmyelinated postganglionic axon. In contrast to sensory neurons, the nucleus occupies an eccentric position within the cell body (Fig. 8-13). The central versus eccentric location of the nucleus

Fig. 8-13. Nerve cell bodies within an autonomic ganglion. Note the eccentric position of the nuclei within the cell bodies (*arrow*). The small heterochromatic nuclei surrounding these cell bodies belong mostly to the satellite cells. Although these nerve cell bodies in autonomic ganglia are multipolar, it is usually not evident in section.

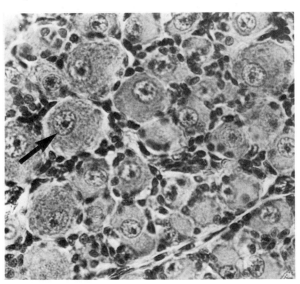

within the cell body is a good criterion for distinguishing craniospinal ganglia from autonomic ganglia. Autonomic ganglia contain synapses between preganglionic axons and the postganglionic neuron.

CEREBELLUM AND CEREBRUM

The complicated neural connections of the cerebellum and cerebrum are more appropriately handled in a text of neuroanatomy, but the general histologic features of the cerebral cortex and cerebellar cortex will be discussed here.

Cerebellar Cortex

The cerebellum is concerned primarily with coordination and refinement of skeletal muscle activity, maintenance of equilibrium (body position in space), and muscle tone. The cerebellum influences muscular activity; it does not initiate it. Most of its influences are exerted indirectly on the spinal cord.

The **cerebellar cortex** is histologically a trilaminar structure. It consists of an outer **molecular layer,** an inner **granular layer,** and a **Purkinje cell layer** separating the two (Figs. 8-14, 8-15).

In section, the Purkinje cell layer consists of a single row of Purkinje cells whose cell bodies are located on the outer surfaces of the granular layer (Fig. 8-16). The Purkinje cell has a flask-shaped cell body with a central vesicular nucleus. In the cytoplasm, a concentric arrangement of Nissl bodies surrounds the nucleus. In conventionally prepared sections, the cell body with its nucleus and the Nissl bodies are the only cellular features easily observed (see Figs. 8-15, 8-16). The axon and dendrites are not easily demonstrated with conventional histologic techniques. However, with silver staining techniques and electron microscopy, it is known that an apical dendrite ascends into the molecular layer, where it arborizes into a profusely branching dendritic tree (see Fig. 8-15). The dendrites are arranged in a single geometric plane oriented at right angles to the long axis of the folia. A myelinated axon issues from the Purkinje cell base, penetrating

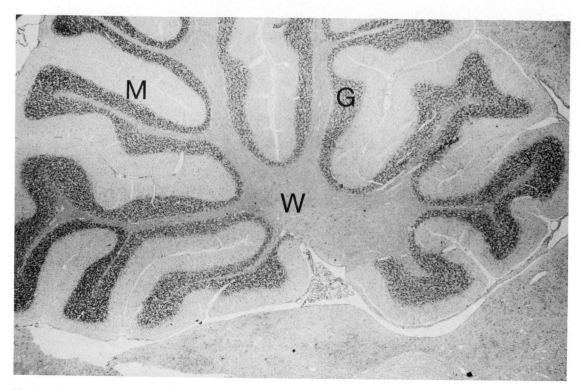

Fig. 8-14. A section of cerebellum seen at low magnification demonstrating the trilaminar cortex. *M* = molecular layer, *G* = granular layer, *W* = white matter. The Purkinje cell layer is seen at a higher magnification in figure 8-16.

Fig. 8-15. Cerebellar cortex. *Left:* after hematoxylin and eosin staining; *right:* after silver impregnation.

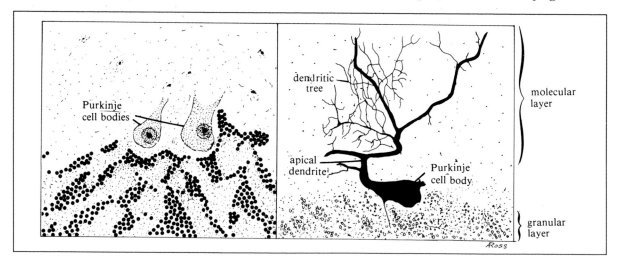

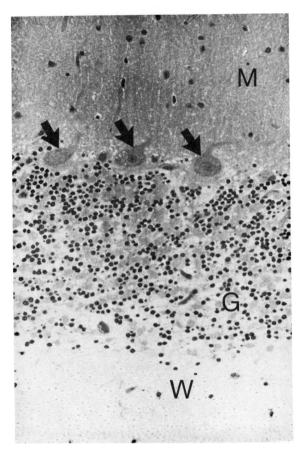

Fig. 8-16. Higher magnification of cerebellar cortex showing cell bodies of three Purkinje fibers (*unlabelled arrows*) forming the Purkinje layer. Above the Purkinje cell layer is the molecular layer (*M*); below it is the granular layer (*G*) with its numerous small nuclei. Myelinated axons from Purkinje cells form the white matter (*W*) below the granular layer.

the granular layer before entering the underlying white matter. This Purkinje cell axon is the exclusive, final pathway leading from the cerebellar cortex through which cerebellar influences are exerted.

The granular layer consists of a large population of **granule cells** of extremely high packing density. With conventional stains, the thin cytoplasmic rims and cell processes are not revealed. The granule cell nuclei stain well, giving this layer the appearance of being composed exclusively of nuclei (see Fig. 8-16). The granule cells have short dendrites and send an unmyelinated axon into the molecular layer where it bifurcates, both branches running parallel to the long axis of the folia. These long parallel fibers run transversely through the plane occupied by the Purkinje cell dendrites and establish multiple synapses with them.

The molecular layer itself contains two cell types (basket and stellate) but consists mostly of dendritic arborizations and unmyelinated axons. As a result, it stains poorly with hematoxylin and eosin or with Weigert's myelin stain.

Cerebral Cortex

The cerebral cortex is responsible for analyzing the sensory information arriving from remote parts of the body, for initiating muscular activity, and for learning, memory, and association of diverse types of information. Of the three major nerve cell types found in the cerebral cortex (stellate, fusiform, and pyramidal), the **pyramidal cell** is the most characteristic, not only because of its enormous numbers but also because of its unique triangular-shaped cell body (Fig. 8-17). This cell has a large vesicular nucleus surrounded by considerable Nissl material. An **apical dendrite** extends toward the surface of the brain and an axon emerges from the base of the triangular cell body, penetrating the deeper layers of the cortex or entering the medullary white matter. The pyramidal cell axon is the principal path of output from the cerebral cortex.

The pyramidal cells are of various sizes, the largest being the giant pyramidal cells of Betz in the area of the brain where motor activity is initiated. The various nerve cell bodies of the cortex are arranged in layers; generally, six major layers of nerve cells are recognized. The pyramidal cells are contained mostly in layers II, III, V, and VI. Each layer is characterized by the size of the py-

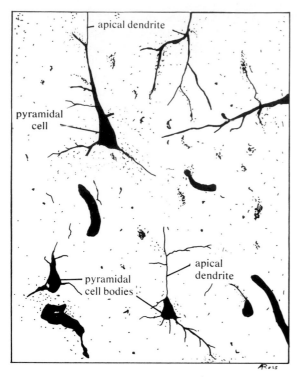

Fig. 8-17. Pyramidal cells from cerebral cortex after silver impregnation.

ramidal cells and their degree of dendritic and axonal branching.

The Nissl stain demonstrates the nerve cell bodies and their relative organization into a laminar cortex, while the Golgi silver stain reveals, in addition, many of the larger dendritic and axonal processes (see Fig. 8-17). The Weigert stain for myelin shows the distribution of myelinated fibers within the cortex.

Neuroglia

Neuroglial cells are supporting cells within the CNS that perform functions similar to those of the Schwann cells of the peripheral nervous sys-tem. They include the **astrocyte,** the **oligoden-drocyte,** and **microglia.**

Two types of stellate-shaped astrocytes are rec-ognized, but they are believed to be modulations of the same cell. **Fibrous astrocytes** are found principally in white matter; **protoplasmic astro-cytes** are located predominantly in gray matter. Fibrous astrocytes have several long cytoplasmic processes that branch infrequently. Protoplas-mic astrocytes have shorter, more branched cyto-plasmic processes that are profusely embellished with many fine secondary projections. Both have oval, euchromatic nuclei but their cytoplasmic processes are demonstrated only after certain metallic stains. In electron micrographs the cyto-plasm is replete with **glial filaments** (microfila-ments similar to the neurofilaments in neurons). Bundles of these glial filaments extend through-out the cell and into most of its cytoplasmic pro-cesses as fibrils visible with the light microscope after staining with gold or silver.

Great numbers of astrocytic processes are in-terposed between nerve cells and the surface of the CNS and between nerve cells and blood ves-sels entering or leaving the CNS. An array of as-trocytic foot processes (dilated terminals of as-trocyte cytoplasmic processes) form the **glia limitans** just beneath the pia mater, the inner-most connective tissue investment of the CNS. The only intervening structure between the glia limitans and pia mater is a basal lamina derived from the embryonic neuroepithelium that sur-rounds the entire brain and spinal cord. Other foot processes of the same astrocytes extend in the other direction, where they contact nerve cells or their processes. A dense array of astro-cytic feet is also applied against blood vessels en-tering the brain and is present throughout their entire vascular course within the CNS. Although the purpose of these astrocytes is unclear, the idea that they constitute part of the blood-brain barrier has been thoroughly refuted.

When areas of nervous tissue are destroyed by physical injury or pathologic causes, astrocytes are capable of proliferating and clearing the area of nerve cell debris by phagocytosis; they may even form scars.

The oligodendrocyte is the myelinating cell of the CNS. Unlike its homologue in the peripheral nervous system, the Schwann cell, the oligodendrocyte has several processes that form the internodal myelin for several axons at a time. Oligodendrocytes are similar in appearance to the astrocyte but with significantly fewer processes and a more heterochromatic nucleus. In electron micrographs, their cytoplasm contains abundant microtubules.

Microglia remain controversial since their origin remains unclear. Among various claims microglia have been assigned a mesodermal origin but the exact cell of origin has not been identified with certainty. However, it is generally appreciated that microglia are not derived from the neuroepithelium as are the other glial cells. It has been claimed that they hypertrophy during inflammation of brain tissue and function as macrophages. Although difficult to identify with the electron microscope, in the light microscope microglia are small cells with deeply staining, elongate nuclei and a few short, irregular cytoplasmic processes best exhibited with the silver carbonate stain of Hortega.

Ependyma

Ependymal cells are derivatives of the embryonic neuroepithelium, which in the adult constitutes a relatively continuous epithelial lining for the ventricles of the brain and the central canal of the spinal cord. The ependyma is only a single cell thick, varying from cuboidal to columnar depending on location.

The ependyma is also a component of the **choroid plexus,** which produces most of the cerebrospinal fluid. During embryonic development of the neural tube, choroid plexuses are formed when the ependymal lining and pia mater come into contact at the attenuated roof plate of the neural tube. Consequently, choroidal capillaries become sandwiched between the ependyma and pia mater, forming the choroid plexus at its adult location within the four ventricles of the brain. Cerebrospinal fluid is formed when an ultrafil-

trate of the plasma, having escaped from fenestrated choroidal capillaries, is secreted by ependymal cells into the ventricles. Unlike ependymal cells lining the ventricles elsewhere, the ependymal cells of the choroid plexus are joined together by occluding junctions that prevent the entry of proteins into the cerebrospinal fluid. In addition, ependymal cells not part of the choroid plexus have cilia, which assist movement of the cerebrospinal fluid.

NEURON DEGENERATION IN THE CENTRAL NERVOUS SYSTEM

In contrast with the ability of peripheral nerves to regenerate successfully after traumatic injury, nerves totally intrinsic to the CNS fail to regenerate. After a central axon is severely injured or severed, oligodendrocytes fail to proliferate or to assist regeneration of the axon as do Schwann cells of the peripheral nervous system. Instead of constructing a tunnel of basal laminae to guide regenerating axonal sprouts, oligodendrocytes simply die (secondary demyelination). Their subsequent replacement by a dense astrocytic scar effectively blocks regenerative sprouting of the injured axon. Laboratory experiments demonstrate that central neurons possess the ability to regenerate, but the failure of oligodendrocytes to assist in this process seems to be the major factor preventing successful reestablishment of neural connections.

Comparison of Afferent and Efferent Nerve Endings

Efferent nerve endings are axon terminals in synaptic contact with muscle and secretory epithelial cells, where they provoke contraction or secretion, respectively. Their morphology at neuromuscular junctions has already been described.

Afferent nerve endings are dendritic terminals that act as sensory receptors. These nerve endings are capable of transducing various sensory stimuli such as temperature, touch, pressure, and pain into nerve impulses that are conducted back to the CNS for perception and analysis. The afferent fibers of neuromuscular spindles and neurotendinous organs of Golgi have already been described. Other afferent fibers are involved in the senses of hearing, sight, smell, and taste and are discussed in more detail in subsequent chapters. Generally, however, the more common afferent nerve endings are grouped into two morphologic categories: **free nerve endings** and **encapsulated nerve endings.**

Free nerve endings are the bare ends of unmyelinated dendrites and possess no Schwann cell investment at their termini. Although morphologically indistinguishable, this category includes nerves that are receptive to temperature, pain, or pressure.

Encapsulated nerve endings occur at the terminals of myelinated dendrites but have an unmyelinated ending that is encapsulated by a continuation of the endoneurium or perineurium. Endings of this type occur mostly, but not exclusively, in the skin. Of these, the **pacinian corpuscles** (Fig. 8-18) and **Meissner's corpuscles** are the most prominent (see Chap. 13 for details).

NATIONAL BOARD TYPE QUESTIONS

For the following, select
- A. if only *1, 2, and 3* are correct.
- B. if only *1 and 3* are correct.
- C. if only *2 and 4* are correct.
- D. if only *4* is correct.
- E. if *all* are correct.

1. The myelin sheath
   1. consists of lipid contributed by concentric revolutions of Schwann cell plasmalemma.
   2. is most well developed around postganglionic axons.
   3. is well developed along axons with high conduction velocity.
   4. is a component of the perineurium.
2. Which of the following statements regarding axoplasmic transport is (are) true?
   1. Axoplasmic transport is necessitated by the absence of ribosomes in the axon.
   2. Fast axoplasmic transport operates at 300 to 400 mm/day.
   3. Slow axoplasmic transport operates at 1 to 5 mm/day.
   4. Slow axoplasmic transport operates at the same rate as the growth of microtubules into the axon.
3. The initial segment of a peripheral neuron
   1. has no myelin sheath.
   2. has no Schwann sheath.
   3. is the site where an action potential is generated.
   4. contains rough endoplasmic reticulum.

Fig. 8-18. Pacinian corpuscle in the cat pancreas. The axon (*arrow*) is surrounded by multiple concentric extensions of the endoneurium and perineurium. The pacinian corpuscle is an example of an encapsulated nerve ending.

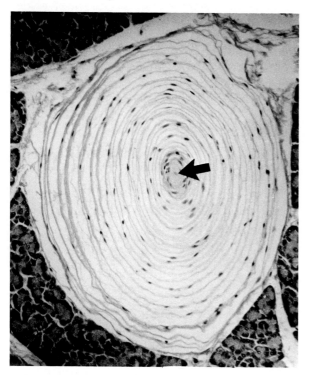

4. Which of the following statements regarding myelin is (are) true?
   1. The axons of alpha motor neurons innervating skeletal muscle are heavily myelinated.
   2. The myelin sheath is the major component of encapsulated nerve endings.
   3. Demyelinating diseases cause a reduction in nerve conduction velocity along affected neurons.
   4. In the central nervous system, an oligodendrocyte contributes myelin to one axon in the same manner as Schwann cells.
5. During degeneration and regeneration of an injured peripheral axon,
   1. retrograde degeneration inevitably involves the entire axon proximal to the site of injury.
   2. distal to the injury myelin begins to retract from the nodes of Ranvier and to break up into segments.
   3. the rough endoplasmic reticulum remains unaffected in the cell body.
   4. Schwann cells construct a tunnel of basal lamina to guide regenerating axonal sprouts back to original synaptic contacts.
6. Nerve cell bodies of
   1. autonomic neurons are located within the intermediolateral gray of the spinal cord.
   2. alpha motor neurons are located in the ventral gray horn of the spinal cord.
   3. postganglionic neurons are located within autonomic ganglia.
   4. Purkinje cells are located within the granular layer of the cerebellum.
7. Which of the following statements regarding autonomic ganglia (visceromotor) is (are) true?
   1. They contain synapses between preganglionic axons and postganglionic nerve cells.
   2. They contain unipolar nerve cell bodies.
   3. They each have a connective tissue capsule which is continuous with the epineurium of nerves emerging from the ganglia.
   4. Their nerve cell bodies have no satellite cells associated with them.
8. Which of the following statements regarding the connective tissue investments of nerves is (are) true?
   1. The epineurium is devoid of elastic fibers.
   2. The epineurium is continuous with the dura mater at the spinal cord.
   3. The epineurium and perineurium lack arterioles.
   4. A continuous epithelium forms the innermost boundary of the epineurium.
9. Protoplasmic astrocytes
   1. are located primarily in gray matter.
   2. have foot processes that form the glia limitans next to the pia mater.
   3. extend foot processes against the blood vessels of the central nervous system.
   4. contribute myelin to axons of the central nervous system.

ANNOTATED ANSWERS

1. B. For further discussion, refer to Nerve Sheaths on page 187.
2. E.
3. A. It is necessary that the initial segment be devoid of any sheath. Its axolemma must be exposed to facilitate ionic currents associated with the initiation of the nerve impulse.
4. B. Encapsulated nerve endings are devoid of myelin sheaths but rather have specialized extensions of the endoneurium and perineurium. Each oligodendrocyte contributes myelin to several axons.
5. C. Retrograde degeneration is more severe with injuries closer to the cell body and minor at a greater disance. Dispersal of Nissl substance always accompanies any damage to the axon.

6. A. Only the myelinated axon of the Purkinje cell passes through the granular layer on its path to the underlying white matter.
7. B. Unipolar neuron cell bodies are contained within sensory ganglia in the mature nervous system.
8. C. The epineurium and perineurium are well vascularized.
9. A. Oligodendrocytes are the myelinating cells in the central nervous system.

BIBLIOGRAPHY

Balin, R. H. M., and P. K. Thomas. Changes at the nodes of Ranvier during wallerian degeneration: An electron microscope study. *Acta Neuropathol.* 14:237, 1969.

Baumgarten, H. G., A.-F. Holstein, and C. Owman. Auerbach's plexus of mammals and man: Electron microscopic identification of three different types of neuronal processes in myenteric ganglia of the large intestine from rhesus monkeys, guinea pigs and man. *Z. Zellforsch. Mikrosk. Anat.* 106:376, 1970.

Cajal, R. S. In R. M. May (ed.), *Degeneration and Regeneration of the Nervous System.* New York: Hafner, 1959, Vols. 1 and 2.

Cajal, S., and Y. Ramon. *Histologie de Système Nerveux de l'Homme et des Vertébrés.* Madrid: Consejo Superior de Investigaciones Científicas, 1952, 1955. Vols. 1, 2.

Coggeshall, R. A fine structural analysis of the myelin sheath in rat spinal roots. *Anat. Rec.* 194:201, 1979.

Droz, B. Protein metabolism in nerve cells. *Int. Rev. Cytol.* 25:363, 1969.

Ghabriel, M. N., and G. Allt. The role of Schmidt-Lanterman incisures in wallerian degeneration. I. A quantitative teased fibre study. *Acta Neuropathol.* (Berl.) 48:83, 1979.

Ghabriel, M. N., and G. Allt. The role of Schmidt-Lanterman incisures in wallerian degeneration: II. An electron microscopic study. *Acta Neuropathol.* (Berl.) 48:95, 1979.

Grafstein, B., and D. S. Forman. Intracellular transport in neurons. *Physiol. Rev.* 60:1167, 1980.

Helén, P., and A. Hervonen. Nerve endings in human sympathetic ganglia. *Am. J. Anat.* 162:119, 1981.

Heuser, J. E., et al. Synaptic vesicle exocytosis captured by quick freezing and correlated with quantal transmitter release. *J. Cell Biol.* 81:275, 1979.

Hirano, A., and H. M. Dembitzer. The transverse bands as a means of access to the periaxonal space of the central myelinated nerve fiber. *J. Ultrastruct. Res.* 28:141, 169.

Hubbard, J. I. (ed.). *The Peripheral Nervous System.* New York: Plenum, 1974.

Jones, E. G., and W. M. Cowan. The Peripheral Terminations of Nerve Fibers. In L. Weiss and R. O. Greep (eds.), *Histology* (4th ed.). New York: McGraw-Hill, 1977. P. 339.

Katz, B. *Nerve, Muscle, and Synapse.* New York: McGraw-Hill, 1966.

LaVail, J. H., and M. M. La Vail. The retrograde intraaxonal transport of horseradish peroxidase in the chick visual system: A light and electron microscopic study. *J. Comp. Neurol.* 157:303, 1974.

Lee, J. C. Electron microscopy of wallerian degeneration. *J. Comp. Neurol.* 120:65, 1963.

Morell, P., and W. T. Norton. Myelin. *Sci. Am.* 242:88, 1980.

Moore, R. Y. Regeneration in the Mammalian Nervous System. In H. L. Leffert (ed.) *Growth Regulation by Ion Fluxes. Ann. N.Y. Acad. Sci.* 339:102, 1980.

Ochs, S. Systems of material transport in nerve fibers (axoplasmic transport) related to nerve function and trophic control. *Ann. N.Y. Acad. Sci.* 228:202, 1974.

Ohmi, S. Electron microscopic study on wallerian degeneration of the peripheral nerve. *Z. Zellforsch. Mikrosk. Anat.* 54:39, 1961.

Pappas, G. D., and S. G. Waxman. Synaptic Fine Structure—Morphological Correlates of Chemical and Electronic Transmission. In G. D. Pappas and D. P. Purpura (eds.), *Structure and Function of Synapses.* New York: Raven, 1972. P. 1.

Patsalos, P. N., M. E. Bell, and R. C. Wiggins. Pattern of myelin breakdown during sciatic nerve wallerian degeneration: Reversal of the order of assembly. *J. Cell Biol.* 87:1, 1980.

Peters, A. Further observations on the structure of myelin sheaths in the central nervous system. *J. Cell Biol.* 20:281, 1964.

Peters, A., S. L. Palay, and H. F. Webster. *The Fine Structure of the Nervous System.* New York: Hoeber, 1970.

Price, D. L., and K. R. Porter. The response of ventral horn neurons to axonal transection. *J. Cell Biol.* 53:24, 1972.

Robertson, J. D. The ultrastructure of adult vertebrate peripheral myelinated nerve fibers in relation to myelinogenesis. *J. Biophys. Biochem. Cytol.* 1:271, 1955.

Shanthaveerappa, T. R., and G. H. Bourne. New observations on the structure of the pacinian corpuscle and its relation to the perineural epithelium of peripheral nerves. *Am. J. Anat.* 112:97, 1963.

Teichberg, S., and E. Holtzman. Axonal agranular reticulum and synaptic vesicles in cultured embryonic chick sympathetic neurons. *J. Cell Biol.* 57:88, 1973.

Tsukita, S., and H. Ishikawa. The movement of membranous organelles in axons: Electron microscopic identification of anterogradely and retrogradely transported organelles. *J. Cell Biol.* 84:513, 1980.

Webster, H. de F. The relationship between Schmidt-Lantermann incisures and myelin segmentation during wallerian degeneration. *Ann. N.Y. Acad. Sci.* 122:29, 1965.

Weiss, P., and H. B. Hiscoe. Experiments on the mechanisms of nerve growth. *J. Exp. Zool.* 107:315, 1948.

Williams, P. L., and S. M. Hall. Prolonged in vivo observations of normal peripheral nerve fibers and their acute reactions to crush and deliberate trauma. *J. Anat.* 108:397, 1971.

II Organ Systems

⑨ Organology

Objectives

You will learn the following in this chapter:

How to identify the tissue constituents which all tubular organs have in common and describe how they are arranged in relation to one another

The distinguishing features of the four basic types of surface membranes

How to distinguish a serosa from an adventitia

The components of the framework or stroma of compact organs and how they support the parenchyma

How the arrangement of the blood supply in tubular organs compares with that in compact organs

Three locations where glands which secrete their contents into the lumina of tubular organs may appear

---

An organ is an orderly arrangement of tissues into a functional unit. For the most part, organs are composed of several different tissue types, constructed according to two basic patterns: (1) tubular or hollow organs, and (2) compact or parenchymal organs

TUBULAR ORGANS

From an embryologic standpoint, the body may be considered as a large cylindrical tube containing many internal tubes, such as the **digestive** tract, **vascular** channels, **respiratory** passages, **urinary** and **genital** tubes, and so forth. Each system, although modified for various functions, is structurally similar to the others in that they are all composed of layers of tissue superimposed on one another in a given order.

Most tubes have internal and external surfaces composed of epithelium. Between these surfaces are alternating layers of connective tissue and muscle. If one thinks of the body as a large tube, the abdominal wall would be a good example of such an arrangement of tissues. It consists of an outer epithelial layer, stratified squamous-keratinized epithelium; a connective tissue layer (loose connective tissue and fascia); a muscle layer (skeletal), followed by more layers of connective tissue and muscle; and finally, an inner epithelial layer, simple squamous epithelium (mesothelium). These layers are grossly separable into definite cleavage planes, since certain layers of the wall adhere more closely to one another than do other layers. Figure 9-1 illustrates the layering pattern and cleavage planes, which separate the body wall into three coats or **tunics.** The digestive tract, for the most part, is similarly arranged and can also be separated into three tunics (Figs. 9-2, 9-3).

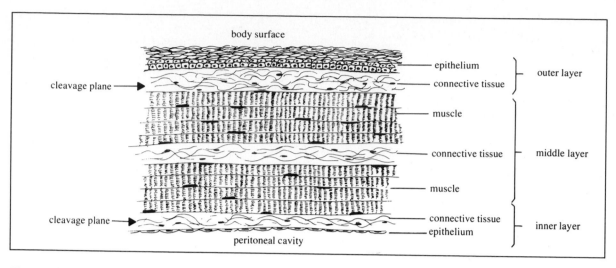

Fig. 9-1. Layer pattern of the abdominal wall. The three major layers are easily separated at the cleavage planes in the gross specimen.

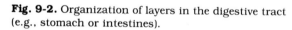

Fig. 9-2. Organization of layers in the digestive tract (e.g., stomach or intestines).

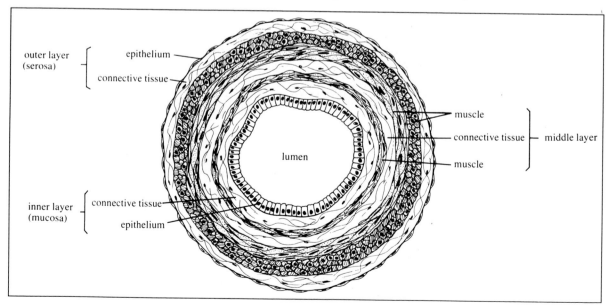

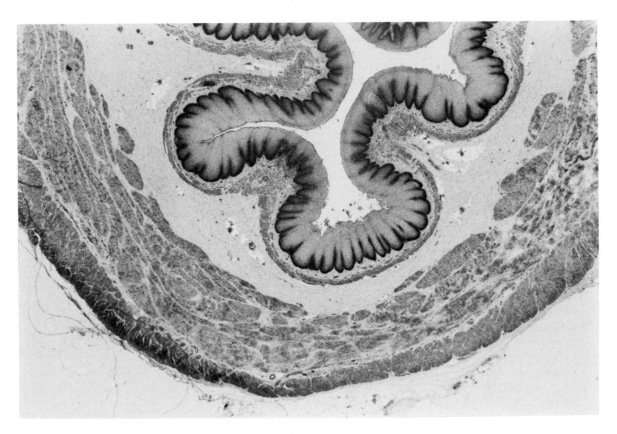

Fig. 9-3. Light micrograph of partial cross section of the esophagus. Note that the epithelium is stratified squamous. The thin underlying layer is connective tissue, followed by smooth muscle, connective tissue, smooth muscle and outer connective tissue (adventitia). See Figure 9-2 for orientation.

These two illustrations have corresponding layers of similar classes of tissue. For example, in the body wall, the outer epithelium is stratified squamous-keratinized, the muscle is skeletal; in the digestive tract, the outer epithelium is simple squamous (mesothelium), the muscle is smooth; and so on.

Thus, a tubular organ has three coats: (1) an inner coat, consisting of epithelium and the underlying connective tissue; (2) a middle coat, consisting of alternating layers of muscle and connective tissue; and (3) an external coat, consisting of connective tissue and epithelium. Other tubular organs are variants of this basic structure. The variants generally reflect specialization of function and are discussed in detail with each organ system.

Surface Membranes

A lining epithelium with its underlying connective tissue (inner or outer tunic) is easily separable from the rest of the organ and is generally referred to as a **surface membrane.** The nature of the surface membrane represents the most important functional variable in tubular organs. There are four basic types of surface membranes:

1. Cutaneous membrane (skin): forms a dry external covering of body wall that is protective in nature.
2. Mucous membrane: the inner lining of all internal tubes opening to the outside environment; a moist membrane, usually lubricated by a mucous secretion produced by glands in the epithelium (goblet cells) or in the underlying connective tissue (e.g., digestive and respiratory systems). The internal lining of the urinary and genital systems are also considered to be mucous membranes, since they are internal tubes with external openings. The urinary mucous membrane is bathed by urine and the genital mucous membrane by specialized secretions of the reproductive system. These modifications correlate with specialized conditions.
3. Serous membrane: the lining of body cavities (peritoneum, pleura, pericardium) and their reflections over viscera within these cavities. Thus serous membranes form the outer lining of organs suspended in these cavities. This is a moist membrane, bathed by serous fluid that originates from blood plasma. The epithelium of the serous membrane is a thin simple squamous epithelium called **mesothelium,** which allows passage of fluid and other substances between the body cavities and the blood and lymphatic vessels.
4. Vascular membrane: the inner lining of blood vessels (including the heart) and lymphatics. It is a moist membrane, lubricated by blood or lymph. The epithelium is a simple squamous variety called **endothelium.**

The outer coat of a tubular organ suspended in a body cavity is a serous membrane usually referred to as **serosa.** Examples of such organs are the stomach and the heart. If the organ is not suspended in a body cavity, but passes retroperitoneally, for example, it does not have an outer membrane; its outer coat is composed of connective tissue that blends into the surrounding connective tissue and is called **adventitia.** Examples of such organs are the esophagus and the trachea. A mucous membrane is often referred to as a **mucosa.**

The blood supply to a tubular organ comes from the outer aspect of the tube, penetrating the outer coat vertically and giving off lateral branches in the connective tissue layers that course parallel to the layers. These lateral branches in turn give off vertical branches, course through the next layer (muscle), and branch again in the connective tissue in parallel fashion, as illustrated in Figure 9-4. Veins and nerves generally follow the path of arteries. The small branches of the vascular system anastomose freely in the connective tissue layers. Thus, in case of a vascular occlusion, this anastomosing network assures adequate collateral circulation, preventing loss of blood supply to any part of the organ. The vascular system is discussed in more detail in Chapter 11.

Fig. 9-4. Vascularization of hollow organs.

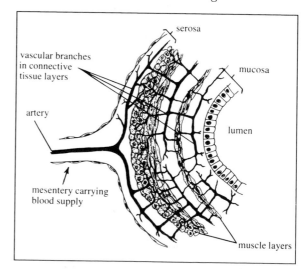

COMPACT ORGANS

Compact organs are recognized grossly by their localized solid form. They vary in shape and size. The compact organs may be very large, such as the liver, or very small, such as a lymph node. Regardless of shape, size, or embryonic origin, compact organs have a common pattern.

Compact organs have an extensive connective tissue **framework** or **stroma.** They are usually surrounded by a dense connective tissue **capsule.** If the organ is suspended in a body cavity, it is covered by a serous membrane. On one side of the organ there is a thicker area of connective tissue that penetrates into the organ somewhat; this area may be indented or notched and is called the **hilus.** From the capsule, strands of connective tissue called **trabeculae** or **septa** ex-tend into the organ, some of which join with the connective tissue at the hilus. In certain instances the trabecular connective tissue is relatively abundant and divides the organ into complete compartments called **lobules.** Throughout the remaining area of the organ (between the capsule, trabeculae, and hilus) is found a delicate interlacing network of reticular fibers. These diffuse fibers form the framework for the **parenchyma** (Figs. 9-5, 9-6).

Fig. 9-5. Light micrograph of a salivary gland. A thin capsule (C) surrounds the organ. Connective tissue septa (S) separate the organ into lobules containing the parenchyma. Centrally, an enlarged area of connective tissue (arrows) contains blood vessels (filled with blood) and ducts (clear lumens). These structures are close to the hilus of the organ, which is out of the plane of section.

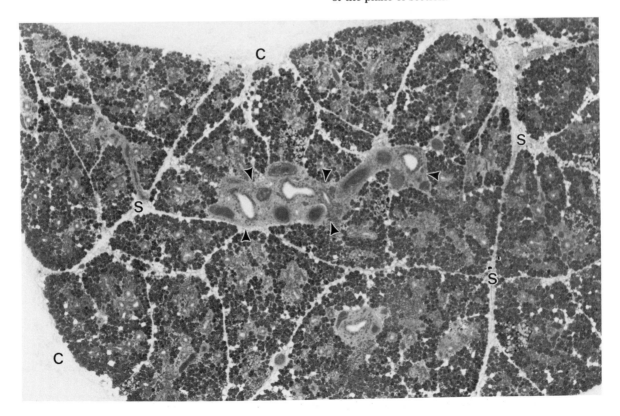

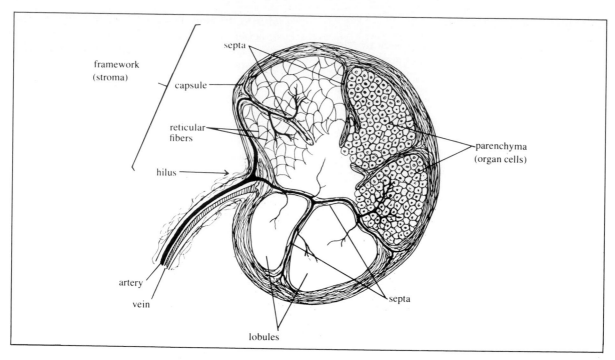

Fig. 9-6. Organization of compact organs. At upper left is the framework; at right, the parenchyma; and at lower left, lobulation of the organ when the septa are continuous and complete.

The parenchyma is the predominant functional tissue of the organ; it occurs in masses, cords, strands, or small tubules, depending on the organ. In the liver, for example, the hepatocytes are arranged in cords, whereas in the kidney the cells of the nephrons are arranged in small tubules. The parenchymal cells may be uniformly arranged (the same throughout the organ), or they may be separated into a subcapsular region known as the **cortex** and a deeper or more central region known as the **medulla.** In the latter case, the cortical and medullary areas usually represent different functional regions of the organ.

The larger compound glands with duct systems (exocrine glands) constitute distinct compact organs, although they are usually not independent either morphologically or functionally, but are intimately associated with the other organs (e.g., salivary glands with the oral cavity; pancreas with the duodenum). The smaller compound glands and simple glands lie within the walls of the tubular organs and therefore are not considered distinct solid organs, but part of the mucous membrane of the tubular parent organ. The endocrine glands also include those that represent distinct solid organs, such as the pituitary and thyroid, and those which form parts of other organs, such as the pancreatic islets and the corpus luteum of the ovary.

The blood supply of compact organs usually follows a definite pattern. The supplying artery enters the hilus and branches repeatedly in the connective tissue trabeculae. At certain points small arteries leave the trabeculae and extend into the parenchyma, where they give off capillary branches. Veins and nerves generally follow the route of the arteries (see Fig. 9-6).

The generalized patterns of tubular and compact organs should be visualized in the study of each organ system. When this has been done, all that remains to be learned in each organ system are the departures from the general pattern and the cytologic details, which, of course, reflect the function of the organ.

NATIONAL BOARD TYPE QUESTIONS

Select the single best response for each of the following.

1. The inner linings of tubular organs which open to the outside are referred to as
   A. basement membranes.
   B. cutaneous membranes.
   C. mucous membranes.
   D. serous membranes.
   E. vascular membranes.
2. Parenchymal cells of compact organs are usually physically supported by
   A. blood vessels.
   B. collagen fibers.
   C. elastic fibers.
   D. reticular fibers.
   E. smooth muscle cells.

For the following, select
   A. if only *1, 2, and 3* are correct.
   B. if only *1 and 3* are correct.
   C. if only *2 and 4* are correct.
   D. if only *4* is correct.
   E. if *all* are correct.

3. Which of the following tubular organs contain(s) a serosa or serous membrane?
   1. Colon
   2. Heart
   3. Stomach
   4. Trachea

4. Which of the following is (are) characteristic of the hilus?
   1. It is continuous with the capsule of organs.
   2. It is found in both tubular and compact organs.
   3. It contains blood vessels.
   4. It is composed of parenchymal cells.
5. Which of the following compact organs is (are) attached to tubular organs in the adult?
   1. Pituitary
   2. Pancreas
   3. Thyroid
   4. Salivary glands

ANNOTATED ANSWERS

1. C. Inner membranes of tubular organs which open to the outside are moist membranes that are usually lubricated by mucous secretions and are therefore called mucous membranes.
2. D. Reticular fibers provide a delicate network of support for parenchymal cells, while coarser, primarily collagenous structures provide support for the entire organ (capsule and septa).
3. A. The colon, heart, and stomach are suspended in body cavities and therefore are covered on the outside by serous membranes. The trachea is not and therefore has an adventitia.
4. B. The hilus is a thickening of connective tissue on one side of compact organs. It is continuous with the capsule and provides the entry point for blood vessels and nerves.
5. C. The pancreas and the salivary glands are solid organs whose secretions are conducted via ducts to the gastrointestinal tract. Although the pituitary and thyroid are derived from the embryonic foregut, they lose these attachments and secrete directly into the blood.

10 Lymphoid System

Objectives

You will learn the following in this chapter:

The stages of development and maturation of the immune system

How to identify the functional differences between the primary and secondary lymphoid organs

The differences between cell-mediated and humoral immunity

Some of the major lymphokines produced by T cells and the role they play in immunity

The major classes of immunoglobulins and the two characteristics which make each distinct

The distinguishing features of diffuse and nodular lymphoid tissue

How to identify the distinguishing features of the thymus and describe the microenvironment in which T cells mature

What is meant by the term "bursa-equivalent"

The major structural-functional similarities and differences between lymph nodes, the spleen, and the gut-associated lymphoid tissues

The cellular mechanisms involved in the immune response

The primary functions of the lymphoid organs are protective or immunologic in nature. These organs are the source of **immunocompetent cells,** which have the capacity to react with and neutralize foreign substances (**antigens**) to which the body may be exposed. Whether these substances are pathogens, such as bacteria and viruses, or endogenous abnormal constituents, such as those found in tumors, the body can normally eliminate whatever antigen it is presented with. Lymphocytes, plasma cells, and macrophages perform direct immunologic functions that effectively neutralize these antigens. Other cells, such as reticular cells and granular leukocytes, perform more specialized ancillary functions in certain types of immunologic reactions.

These cells and their precursors form the primary cellular populations of the lymphoid organs, although the term **lymphoid cells** is usually limited to lymphocytes and their close relatives, the plasma cells. The cellular population of any lymphoid organ is highly variable and largely reflects the organ's functional role in the development of the immune system or its state of immune reactivity. The term **lymphoid system** includes not only the cells within distinct lymphoid organs but also the widely distributed lymphoid cells found in the peripheral circulation and in loose connective and epithelial tissues. The term **immune system** includes lymphoid cells and accessory cells, such as macrophages, and their secretory products.

DEVELOPMENTAL OVERVIEW

The ontogeny of immunity consists of an orderly development of lymphoid cells and organs that culminates in immunologic maturation about the time of birth, when most antigens are first encountered (Fig. 10-1). The origin of stem cells for the lymphoid cell series can be traced to the mesenchymally derived cells of the yolk sac islands, in early embryonic development. Soon thereafter, the vasculature becomes confluent and these multipotential cells migrate to other temporary depots, such as the liver and spleen, where they proliferate and differentiate along the various leukocyte lines. Later, the bone marrow becomes the predominant source of stem cells (called **hemocytoblasts**) from which lymphoid cells are derived. The bone marrow persists as a stem cell source even in adult life. In late fetal development, many stem cells migrate from the bone marrow (or more generally, from the stem cell compartment) to populate the primary or central lymphoid organs. Within the microenvironments of central lymphoid organs, epithelially derived cells induce the immigrant stem cells to proliferate and differentiate into immunocompetent lymphocytes.

There are two **primary lymphoid organs** among the endothermic (warm-blooded) vertebrates. Phylogenically, these organs are most distinct in terms of structure and function in the avian class (birds). The **thymus** is derived from the embryonic foregut and is the microenvironment in which **T lymphocytes** (thymus-derived cells) mature. The other organ is also derived from the gut (cloaca) and is called the **bursa of Fabricius;** here the stem cells are induced to mature into **B lymphocytes** (bursa-derived cells). Although all mammals possess a thymus, the site of B cell development has been attributed to a more diffuse system called the **bursa-equivalent,** which may involve the gut-associated lymphoid tissue (e.g., the appendix and Peyer's patches), the liver, or the bone marrow itself, depending on the species or the stage of development, or both.

Shortly after birth, cells from the central lymphoid organs (T and B cells) migrate to the **sec-**ondary or **peripheral lymphoid organs:** the lymph nodes, spleen, and the gut-associated lymphoid tissue. Here the T and B cell populations inhabit fairly distinct "zones," ready for their first encounter with antigens.

TYPES OF IMMUNITY

T and B lymphocytes are morphologically similar but functionally distinct. T cells are primarily involved in **cell-mediated (cellular) immunity,** whereas B cells and their immediate derivatives, the plasma cells, are primarily involved in **humoral immunity.**

In cell-mediated immunity, activated T lymphocytes (**effector T cells**) eliminate antigens such as foreign cells either by attacking them directly or by releasing a variety of nonspecific substances in their presence, called **lymphokines.** One of these chemical mediators causes lysis of foreign cells and is therefore called **lymphotoxin.** Another, known as **blastogenic factor,** induces proliferation of nonsensitized lymphocytes. Still others, too numerous to name, attract (**chemotaxis**) and activate macrophages and various granulocytes, which assist the lymphocytes in eliminating antigens (Table 10-1).

The primary distinguishing feature of cell-mediated immunity is that specifically sensitized lymphocytes seek out the antigen. Contact with the antigen is required to trigger the reaction; therefore, the reaction is localized. Two examples of cell-mediated immune responses are the rejection of a foreign (histoincompatible) transplant and the reaction to a chemical sensitizing agent, such as tuberculin. Both elicit a localized delayed hypersensitivity reaction.

Among the effector T cells are several varieties that can be distinguished by unique cell surface molecules and by the specialized effector functions that they perform. For example, some effector T cells have an affinity for destroying tumor cells, while others preferentially fight infections. T cells also function as regulators of immune responsiveness. One subpopulation capable of enhancing the immune response comprises **helper**

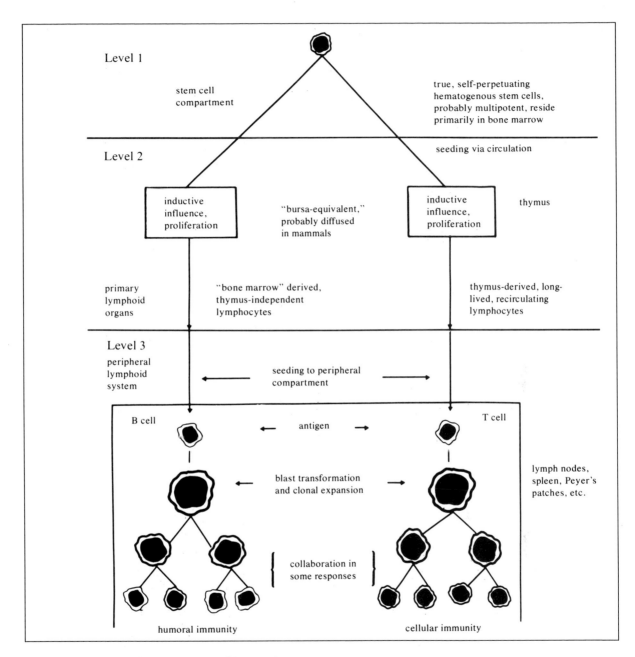

Fig. 10-1. Overview of the three main functional compartments of the lymphoid system. (From G. Nossal and G. Ada, *Antigens, Lymphoid Cells and the Immune Response.* New York: Academic, 1971. Reproduced with permission.)

Table 10-1. Some of the Better-Known Lymphokines (Products of Activated T Cells)

Mediators affecting macrophages
  Migration-inhibitory factor
  Macrophage-activating factor
  Chemotactic factor

Mediators affecting granular leukocytes
  Migration-inhibitory factor
  Histamine-releasing factor
  Chemotactic factors

Mediators affecting lymphocytes
  Blastogenic (mitogenic) factor
  Factors affecting antibody production

Factors affecting other cell types
  Cytotoxic factors (lymphotoxin)
  Growth-inhibitory factors
  Interferon
  Immunoglobulin-binding factor

Source: Modified from R. E. Rocklin. Mediators of Cellular Immunity. In H. H. Fudenberg et al. (eds.), *Basic and Clinical Immunology.* Los Altos, Calif.: Lange, 1980.

T cells; another capable of inhibiting the immune response comprises **suppressor T cells.** Like other lymphocyte subpopulations, these can be distinguished functionally and by their unique surface molecules.

In humoral immunity, activated B lymphocytes and plasma cells secrete specific antibodies that circulate, combine with antigens as they are encountered, and form inactive complexes. Many particulate and soluble antigens are handled in this way. The distinguishing feature of humoral immunity is that lymphocyte contact with antigen is not required in order to destroy or inactivate the antigen. Instead, following sensitization specific antibodies are secreted by the cells and are distributed throughout the body fluids. In this case, the secretory products themselves seek out the antigen. Antibodies are proteins found in the globulin fraction of plasma. They are generally referred to as **immunoglobulins** (Ig), of which there are five different classes. Each of the immunoglobulin types has a distinctive "backbone" structure.

Immunoglobulin G (IgG) is the predominant type found in serum. IgG antibodies have a high affinity for antigens and thus are very effective in neutralizing bacterial toxins and viruses, especially during a secondary response. However, IgG is rather ineffective in activating complement.

IgM is often referred to as a macroglobulin because of its high molecular weight. The IgM molecule is a polymer composed of five subunits, each resembling IgG in its general organization. IgM is produced early in the primary response and activates complement efficiently. Therefore, IgM is very effective as a cytolytic agent (lysis of foreign cells). IgM also plays a prominent role in antigen agglutination and opsonization.

IgA occurs in two forms. Serum IgA is a monomer, resembling IgG. The functions of serum IgA have not been well elucidated. The dimeric form of IgA appears in seromucous secretions such as saliva, tears, colostrum, and secretions of the pulmonary and digestive systems. The dimeric molecule is stabilized against proteolysis by combining with another protein, called the secretory piece, which is synthesized by epithelial cells. Since this form of IgA is found in secretory products, it is referred to as **secretory IgA** or sIgA. Secretory IgA plays an important role in protecting the surfaces that are exposed to the external environment against penetration of microorganisms.

IgE is found in very low concentrations in the serum. Most of the IgE in the body is bound to basophils and mast cells, where it induces release of histamine and other mediators, particularly in certain allergic reactions. IgE is also thought to play an important role in the elimination of parasites (more on this in Chap. 5).

IgD is found in only trace amounts in the serum and is uniquely susceptible to proteolytic degradation. It is the main immunoglobulin found on the surface of lymphocytes in the newborn. In the adult, IgD and IgM are found on the surface of B lymphocytes. The interaction of these immunoglobulin receptors is thought to play a role in lymphocyte activation.

Although certain types of antigens elicit either cell-mediated or humoral immunity, many immune responses require the cooperative efforts of T and B lymphocytes. Helper and suppressor T cells play a direct role in regulation of the humoral as well as the cell-mediated immune response.

The developmental sequence leading to the two types of immunity is summarized in Figure 10-1.

LYMPHOID (LYMPHATIC) TISSUE

The term **lymphoid tissue** refers to the parenchyma of lymphoid organs and loose connective tissues throughout the body in which lymphoid cells are the predominant cellular population. The connective tissue framework in these regions usually consists of fine reticular fibers and reticular cells, sometimes referred to as **reticulum** or **reticular meshwork.** Lymphoid tissue is usually described in terms of the relative densities of lymphoid cell aggregates. **Diffuse lymphatic tissue** refers to rather loose aggregates, whereas **nodular lymphatic tissue** represents a denser, more highly organized form. A **nodule** usually consists of dense lymphoid tissue with a light central region, called the **germinal center,** and a darker, more peripheral cap or corona. The germinal center, especially when active, contains many large lymphocytes or lym-

phoblasts (euchromatic nuclei), whereas the periphery of the nodule consists of small, tightly packed lymphocytes (heterochromatic nuclei) (Fig. 10-2).

The stroma of the primary lymphoid organs (thymus and bursa) contains no reticular fibers. The stellate reticular cells are epithelial in origin and are nonphagocytic. Cells of this population are thought to provide the inductive effect on incoming bone marrow stem cells. In the primary lymphoid organs, the parenchyma can be described as diffuse lymphoid tissue, although it is not uniform in lymphocyte density. There are no nodules in the primary lymphoid organs.

In contrast, the secondary lymphoid organs are composed of a stroma that is rich in reticular fibers. The reticular cells are mesenchymally derived, and most of them are highly phagocytic. Other reticular cells perform different functions, such as synthesis of reticular fibers and antigen trapping. The parenchyma is composed of both diffuse and nodular lymphoid tissue. The areas of diffuse lymphoid tissue are predominantly populated by T cells, whereas the nodules are composed primarily of B cells.

THE PRIMARY (CENTRAL) LYMPHOID ORGANS
The Thymus

The thymus develops from an epithelial anlage of the third branchial pouch and migrates caudally

Fig. 10-2. Diffuse and nodular lymphoid tissue.

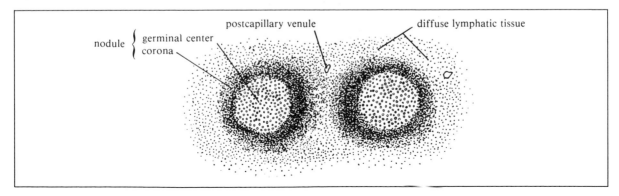

and medially. When fully developed, the thymus is a paired organ located in the midline of the superior mediastinum, beneath the upper part of the sternum. It attains its greatest relative weight and is most highly developed about the time of birth. It is the generator of T lymphocytes.

STROMA

The thymus is surrounded by a thin connective tissue capsule. Septa extend in from the capsule, separating the thymus into partial lobules. Smaller septa extend into each lobule from the main septa (Fig. 10-3). Although reticular fibers are absent, stellate-shaped cells, often referred to as **epithelial-reticular cells,** are attached to one

another by desmosomes and form a delicate inner framework (Fig. 10-4). The epithelial-reticular cells are highly branched and are derived from endoderm. Their epithelial origin reflects the fact that they are secretory cells producing a variety of peptide hormones, most of which regulate T cell development and maturation. Unlike reticular cells of secondary lymphoid organs, epithelial-reticular cells of the thymus are not phagocytic.

——————————————————————————▷

Fig. 10-4. A portion of a thymic lobule. The capsule and septae are composed primarily of collagen fibers and contain some small blood vessels. The cortex is heavily infiltrated with lymphocytes, supported by a network of stellate epithelial-reticular cells. The medulla is composed of more tightly packed epithelial cells and fewer lymphocytes. It also contains thymic corpuscles, consisting of concentrically arranged epithelial cells. (From L. Weiss, *Cells and Tissues of the Immune System.* Englewood Cliffs, N.J.: Prentice-Hall, 1972. Reproduced by permission.)

Fig. 10-3. A light micrograph of the human thymus, preinvolution. Connective tissue septa divide the thymus into lobules. Each lobule has a distinct outer cortex (*C*) and central medulla (*M*). Small septa penetrate into the cortex.

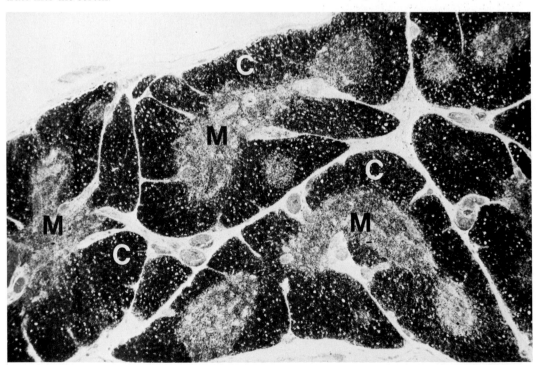

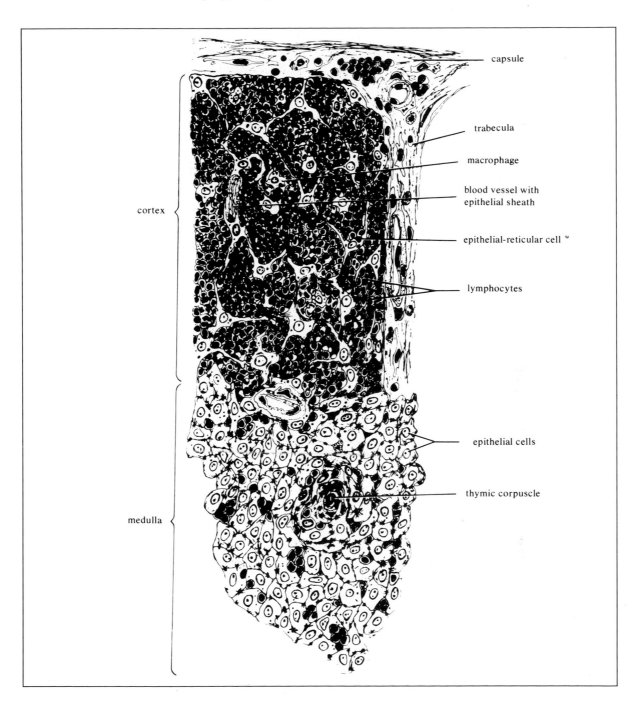

capsule

trabecula

macrophage

blood vessel with
epithelial sheath

epithelial-reticular cell

lymphocytes

cortex

epithelial cells

thymic corpuscle

medulla

PARENCHYMA

The parenchyma within each lobule is separated into a peripheral **cortex** and a central **medulla.** Since the lobules are incomplete, the medulla is continuous between adjacent lobules (see Fig. 10-3). The cortex is primarily composed of aggregated lymphocytes (thymocytes). The medulla is lighter in appearance, since there are fewer lymphocytes but more epithelial-reticular cells (with euchromatic nuclei) in this region. Scattered throughout the medulla are other cells resembling epithelium that are concentrically arranged into "thymic corpuscles"; their function is unknown (Fig. 10-5; see also Fig. 10-4). Macrophages are present in significant numbers, particularly in the medulla. Mast cells, plasma cells, and granular leukocytes may also be found in small numbers.

Fig. 10-5. Light micrograph of the thymic medulla. Note the thymic corpuscles (*asterisks*), surrounded by epithelial cells with pale euchromatic nuclei (*arrows*) and lymphocytes with dark heterochromatic nuclei.

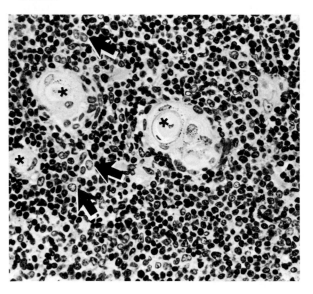

BLOOD SUPPLY

The blood supply to the thymus consists of small vessels that penetrate the capsule, ramify in the interlobular connective tissue, and enter the parenchyma, coursing along the corticomedullary zone. Capillaries extend from the arteries in this region to the cortex, where they anastomose extensively with one another. The capillaries drain into the postcapillary venules and veins in the medulla. Lymphoid cells migrate in or out of the thymus through the postcapillary venules. The capillaries of the cortex, however, are impervious to cells and macromolecules; thus, antigens cannot enter the cortex directly, and those that enter the medulla are rapidly phagocytized by macrophages before the antigens can diffuse into the cortex. This phenomenon is the basis of the concept known as the **blood-thymus barrier.**

FUNCTIONAL ASPECTS

The cortex of the thymus of a neonate shows extensive proliferative activity of lymphocytes. The lymphocytes undergoing **blastogenesis** are randomly distributed throughout the cortex. The lymphocyte proliferation is driven by hormonelike inductive substances that are produced by the epithelially derived cells. This process does not involve antigenic stimulation. In fact, antigens are prevented from entering this region because of the presence of the blood-thymus barrier. Concomitant with lymphocyte proliferation is extensive lymphocyte death and phagocytosis of dead cells by macrophages; the significance of this event has not been elucidated (Fig. 10-6).

Over ten hormonelike factors have been isolated from the thymus or blood that are reputed to cause transformation of bone marrow stem cells (prothymocytes or pre-T cells) into mature T cells. Three of these factors have been well characterized: **serum thymus factor, thymopoietin,** and **thymosin.** Each is a small protein capable of inducing T cell maturation, either in appearance of cell surface molecules characteristic of immunocompetent T cells or in performance of im-

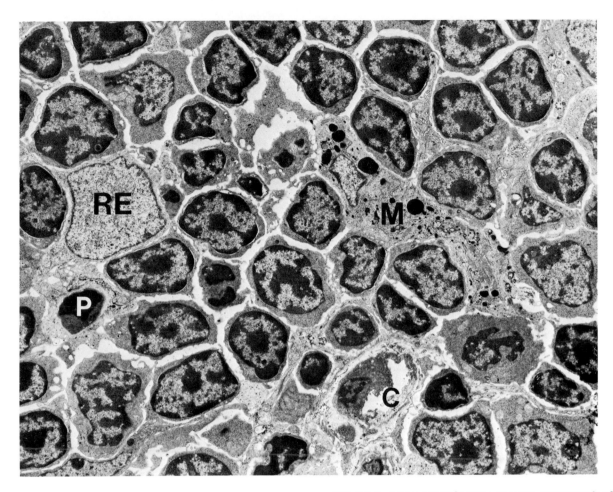

Fig. 10-6. A low-magnification electron micrograph of thymic cortex. Most of the cells are lymphocytes of various sizes. The large lymphocytes (lymphoblasts) have prominent nucleoli and more euchromatin compared with small lymphocytes. Also note the lightly stained nucleus of a reticuloepithelial cell (*RE*), the macrophage (*M*) with numerous residual bodies, a capillary (*C*), and a dead lymphocyte with a pyknotic nucleus (*P*). (Courtesy of J. André-Schwartz.)

mune functions. The mechanism of hormone action involves elevations of intracellular cyclic AMP (cAMP) in precursor cells. Exogenous cAMP and other agents known to elevate intracellular cAMP, such as isoproterenol and epinephrine, mimic the action of thymic hormones.

The functional importance of the thymus in immunologic maturation has been clearly demonstrated in thymectomy experiments on neonatal animals. Thymectomized animals are unable to populate the peripheral lymphoid organs with immunocompetent T cells and usually succumb to infection. A thymic implant or injection of autologous T cells will usually restore cell-mediated immunity.

At puberty, the thymus begins to undergo **involution,** which is probably mediated by adrenocortical and sex hormones. The lymphocyte population becomes greatly depleted and is replaced largely by adipose tissue. The thymic corpuscles become greatly enlarged. In the mature individual, immunocompetence has been established and the thymus plays a less significant role. In instances of severe peripheral lymphoid organ damage, the thymus can repopulate these organs even in adult life. The gradual, age-related involution of the thymus is termed **age involution.** However, more rapid thymic involution, referred to as **accidental involution,** can occur at any time in life as a result of severe stress, prolonged disease, ionizing radiation, and dietary deficiencies. Although this process can lead to significant immunodeficiency, it can be reversed by removal of stressful stimuli, disease cure, or improved diet, as the case may be.

T lymphocytes can be distinguished from other lymphoid cells by the fact that they possess unique cell surface molecules not present on other cells. T cells are generally long-lived and migrate extensively between the blood and the secondary lymphoid organs.

The Bursa-Equivalent

The bursa of Fabricius is an avian central lymphoid organ, a generator of B lymphocytes. Histologically, the bursa is similar to the thymus. It is more completely lobulated, however, with each lobule clearly separated into cortex and medulla. Bursectomized chicks do not develop the capacity to produce humoral antibodies, although cell-mediated immunity remains intact. In mammals, an equivalent developmental system exists, possibly in the gut-associated lymphoid tissue or in even more diffuse microenvironments associated with epithelia. In humans, there is no concrete evidence that points to any given organ as a bursa-equivalent. The existence of such a system is implied from a B cell deficiency disease called **agammaglobulinemia,** in which no humoral immunity develops. B lymphocytes (and plasma cells) are distinguished by the presence of **membrane-bound immunoglobulins** on their surface that serve as receptors for antigens.

THE SECONDARY (PERIPHERAL) LYMPHOID ORGANS

The peripheral lymphoid organs, particularly the lymph nodes and spleen, are not well developed before birth. Shortly after birth, however, they become heavily populated by both T and B lymphocytes, and their development parallels the establishment of immunocompetence.

The cellular kinetics of immune mechanisms involving secondary lymphoid organs include antigen trapping; stimulation, proliferation, and differentiation of lymphocytes; migration of these cells to other depots in the body; and production of antibodies or lymphokines. Variations in the primary pattern depend on the species, nature of the antigen, and the dose and route of administration. All immune mechanisms are characterized by specificity, diversity, and memory.

Lymph Nodes

Lymph nodes are small encapsulated organs through which lymph flows. They are most prominent in the inguinal and axillary regions but are found throughout the body in small groups, associated with the regional lymphatic drainage. Their intimate association with lymphatic vessels reflects their function as **lymph filters.** Lymph-borne antigens are trapped by lymph nodes. Antigenic stimulation is followed by the appropriate immune response.

STROMA

The lymph node is covered by a dense connective tissue capsule. Trabeculae extend into the organ from the capsule. **Afferent lymphatics** penetrate the capsule and become confluent with the system of sinuses within the node. At the concave aspect of the organ is a thick region of connective tissue called the **hilus;** the blood supply to the node and the **efferent lymphatics** are located here. The inner stroma is composed of a delicate network of reticular fibers and reticular cells, many of which are phagocytic and are involved in antigen trapping (Figs. 10-7, 10-8).

PARENCHYMA

The parenchyma of the lymph node is composed of lymphoid tissue organized into an outer cortex and an inner medulla. The cortex is composed

of nodules with distinct germinal centers, surrounded by diffuse lymphoid tissue (the **paracortical region**). The medulla is composed of lymphoid cells organized into strands, called **medullary cords.** An occasional nodule may be present in the medulla. Macrophages are usually found in and around medullary cords in large numbers (Fig. 10-9; see also Figs. 10-7, 10-8).

LYMPHATIC SINUSES

Lymph that enters the lymph node through the **afferent lymphatics** passes through the organ by way of a system of sinuses along the capsule (**subcapsular** or **marginal sinuses**), trabecular (**cortical sinuses**), and medullary cords (**medullary sinuses**) (Fig. 10-10; see also Fig. 10-9). Lymph also flows through the diffuse lymphatic

Fig. 10-7. A lymph node. On the right is the stroma, on the left the parenchyma. The blood supply and lymphatics are shown in the central portion.

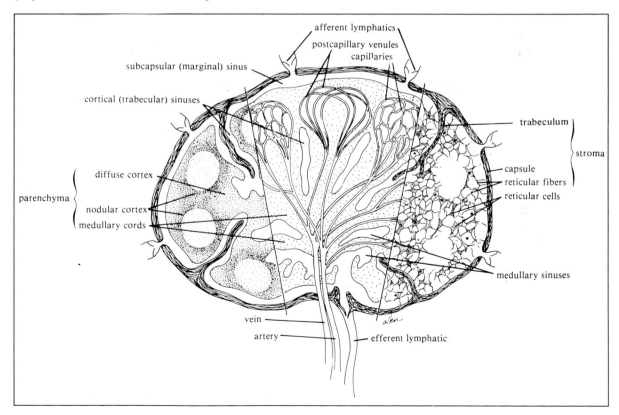

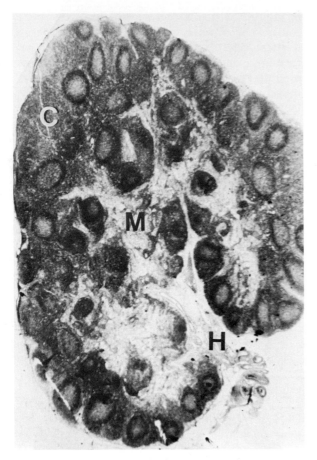

Fig. 10-8. A low-magnification light micrograph of a lymph node. Numerous nodules are seen in the cortex (*C*). The more central medulla (*M*) is directly associated with the hilus (*H*), which contains a number of blood and lymphatic vessels.

tissue, but at a slower rate. The framework of the sinus walls is composed of a reticular fiber meshwork. The sinuses are lined with two types of cells: macrophages and nonphagocytic endothelial cells. Unlike the lining cells of blood and lymphatic vessels, which are continuous, those lining the sinuses of the lymph node are discontinuous so that their walls are freely permeable to wandering cells. The lymph finally exits the lymph node through the **efferent lymphatics** at

the hilus (see Fig. 10-7). Ultimately, most of the lymphatics drain into large collecting lymphatic vessels, which bring the lymph directly into the venous circulation (in the neck region).

BLOOD SUPPLY

Arteries enter the lymph node at the hilus and pass through the trabeculae to the medullary cords and finally to the cortical lymphatic tissue, where they supply small capillaries to the diffuse cortex and around the germinal centers of the nodules (see Fig. 10-7). Postcapillary venules, located in the diffuse cortex, are a special pathway by which lymphocytes in the blood can enter the lymph nodes directly (lymphocyte recirculation).

FUNCTIONAL ASPECTS

The diffuse cortex (paracortical region) of the lymph node is populated predominantly by T lymphocytes. The nodules are B lymphocytic zones (Fig. 10-11). Neonatal thymectomy or bursectomy (in birds) results in the underdevelopment of the corresponding zones within the lymph node. Likewise, antigens that induce cell-mediated immunity (e.g., skin transplant) stimulate proliferation of T lymphocytes in the diffuse cortex, whereas humoral immunity is associated with enlargement of the nodular cortex, particularly the germinal centers (Fig. 10-12).

Lymph-borne antigens from connective tissue regions of the body are transported by the afferent lymphatic vessels to regional lymph nodes, where they induce immune reactivity. The mechanisms of antigen trapping and the cellular kinetics of humoral immunity are briefly as follows: Both soluble and particulate antigens are extensively phagocytized by macrophages and phagocytic reticular cells. Other more specialized reticular cells, called **dendritic cells,** are found in nodules where they trap and maintain antigen in nondegraded form on their plasma membranes. It is thought that this phenomenon is associated with antigenic stimulation of B lymphocytes, which proliferate in the germinal centers, espe-

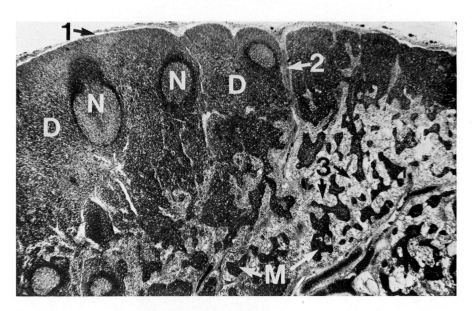

Fig. 10-9. A light micrograph of part of a lymph node. The upper portion is the cortex, composed of diffuse (*D*) and nodular (*N*) lymphoid tissue. At the lower right is the medulla, composed of anastomosing medullary cords (*M*). Note the system of lymphatic sinuses within the node: the subcapsular (or marginal) sinus (*1*), a trabecular (or cortical) sinus (*2*), and the medullary sinuses (*3*).

Fig. 10-10. A light micrograph of a lymph node injected with colloidal carbon but unstained. The lymphatic sinuses are filled with the carbon, illustrating the pathway of lymph flow; the subcapsular sinus (*1*), trabecular sinuses (*2*), and medullary sinuses (*3*). The nodules in the cortex remain relatively free of carbon. See Figure 10-9 for orientation.

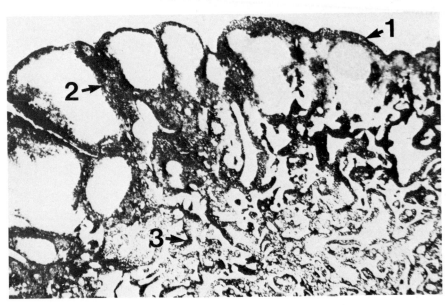

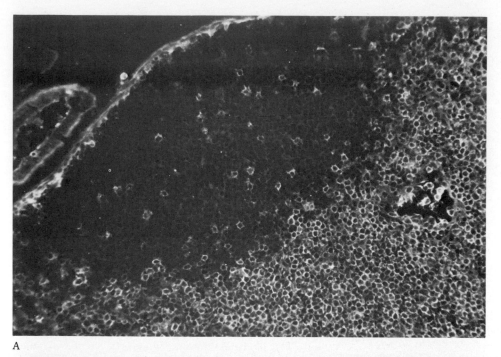

A

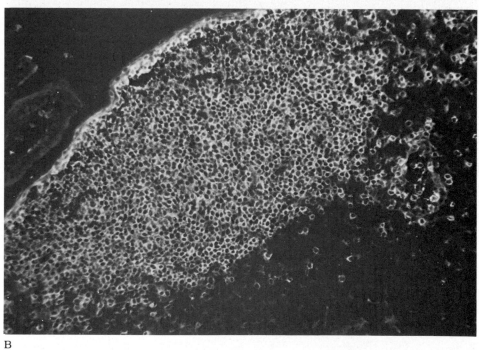

B

Fig. 10-11. Lymph node of a mouse. Distribution of T and B lymphocytes as revealed by fluorescence immunocytochemistry. The T and B cells are specifically stained in these frozen sections by antibodies to the surface markers of T and B cells, respectively. A. The lymphatic nodules in the cortex are largely unstained, while the deep cortex is deeply stained, indicating it as the site of concentration of T lymphocytes. B. The cells of the lymphatic nodules are deeply stained, indicating that B lymphocytes are concentrated there. (From I. L. Weissman, Development and distribution of Ig-bearing cells in mice. *Trans. Rev.* 24:159, 1975. © 1975 Munksgaard International Publishers Ltd., Copenhagen, Denmark.)

cially in a strong immune reaction. During a peak humoral immune response, plasma cells, which differentiate from stimulated B cells, can be found in the medullary cords in large numbers. Many lymphoid cells enter the lymphatic sinuses and leave the node by way of the efferent lymphatics, migrating to other peripheral lymphoid organs and to connective tissue spaces around the body, particularly the lamina propria of the small intestine. Some cells, particularly the long-lived "memory cells," are known to recirculate back to lymph nodes through the postcapillary venules of the diffuse cortex.

Fig. 10-12. A light micrograph of a nodule with a prominent germinal center in the outer cortex of a lymph node, adjacent to the subcapsular sinus (S). The germinal center (GC) is a locus of B cell proliferation and therefore contains many lymphoblasts. It stains more lightly than the corona around it, which contains numerous small lymphocytes. Note the reticular fibers (*arrow*) at the outer edge of the nodule and the fibrous connective tissue capsule (C).

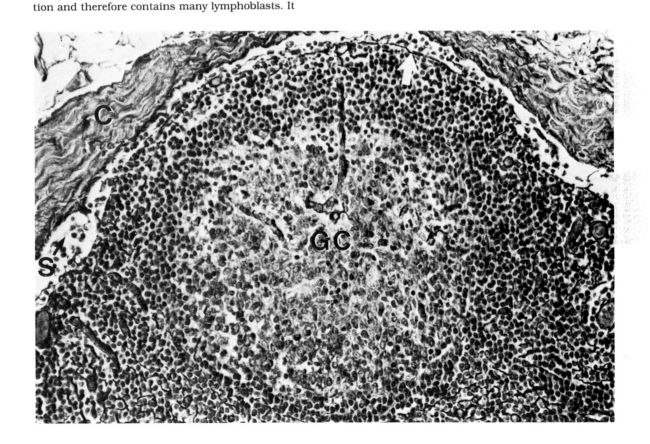

The Spleen

The spleen is the largest lymphoid organ of the body. It is located in the abdominal cavity, beneath the diaphragm and behind the stomach. The spleen is interposed in the systemic circulation and acts, in a general sense, as a blood filter. Besides being a source of immunocompetent cells, it has several nonimmunologic functions. In fetal life, the spleen functions temporarily as a hemopoietic organ. In addition, it acts as an elastic reservoir for blood in many mammals, but in humans it plays a much smaller role in the regulation of circulating blood volume. The filtration mechanism of the spleen effectively traps senescent (aged) blood cells as well as bloodborne antigens; aged erythrocytes and leukocytes are degraded and disposed of. As in the lymph nodes, antigenic stimulation is followed by the appropriate immune response by lymphoid cells of the parenchyma.

STROMA

The spleen is encapsulated by a thick layer of dense, irregular connective tissue. Since the organ is suspended in the abdominal cavity, it is covered by a serous membrane. Branching trabeculae extend into the organ from the capsule. The connective tissue composing the capsule and trabeculae contains a significant component of elastic fibers and smooth muscle, reflecting the organ's "elastic" quality. The blood supply enters the organ through a thick connective tissue hilus. The inner framework around which the parenchyma and the venous sinuses are organized is composed of a network of reticular fibers and reticular cells (Fig. 10-13).

PARENCHYMA

The parenchyma of the spleen is composed of lymphoid tissue, referred to as the **splenic pulp.** Freshly cut sections show what is appropriately described as "islands" of white pulp in a "sea" of red pulp. The white pulp is composed of diffuse and nodular lymphoid tissue, while the reddish appearance of the red pulp reflects the predominance of erythrocytes in the blood that fills these areas (Figs. 10-14, 10-15).

The white pulp is organized around the arteries of the parenchyma. Diffuse lymphoid tissue forms a cuff around the arterial branches, composing the **periarterial lymphocyte sheath (PALS).** Nodular lymphoid tissue extends from the sheath at regular intervals. The parenchyma of the red pulp is composed of diffuse lymphoid tissue organized in cords, which is highly infiltrated with blood cells (Fig. 10-16). The red pulp cords are surrounded by anastomosing **venous sinuses.** Between the red and white pulp are poorly defined regions called the **marginal zones,** which receive much of the blood entering the spleen. These zones are important in antigen trapping and distribution of incoming cells (see Figs. 10-13, 10-14).

BLOOD SUPPLY

The organization of the spleen can be best understood when the blood supply of the organ is considered (see Fig. 10-13). The **splenic artery** enters the hilus and branches in the trabeculae (**trabecular arteries**). As the arteries pass from the trabeculae and enter the parenchyma, the adventitia layer is largely replaced by a dense network of reticular fibers that are highly infiltrated with lymphocytes. The arteries are referred to here as **central arteries,** while the cuff of lymphocytes surrounding them is known as the periarterial lymphocyte sheath. Associated with the sheath are occasional nodules with prominent germinal centers. Central arteries supply many small capillaries to the area surrounding the periarterial lymphocyte sheaths, the marginal zones. The central arteries finally terminate in the red pulp as highly branched small vessels termed **penicilli.** The lining cells of the venous sinuses are discontinuous and present little barrier to cell movement between the red pulp cords and the sinuses. The sinuses themselves anastomose freely and are drained by **red pulp veins,** which, in turn, join the **trabecular veins.** The

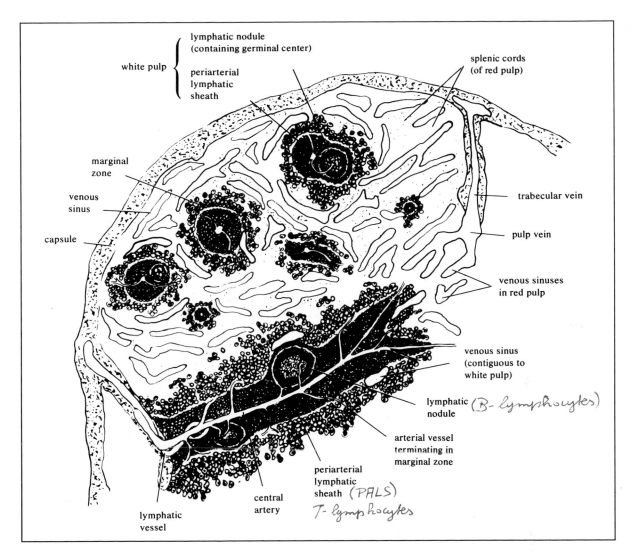

Fig. 10-13. The organization of the human spleen. The white pulp has two components: periarterial lymphocyte sheaths and nodules. The white pulp is surrounded by the marginal zone. The remainder of the tissue depicted is the red pulp, which consists primarily of splenic sinuses separated by splenic cords. The pattern of blood flow is as follows. A trabecular artery enters the white pulp and becomes the central artery. The central artery passes through white pulp and gives rise to many branches; a few end within white pulp while some supply the nodule. Most terminate at the periphery of the white pulp, emptying in or near the marginal zone. Other arterial vessels ter- minate in real pulp cords. The sinuses drain into pulp veins, which, in turn, drain into trabecular veins. A sinus may abut the white pulp and receive lymphocytes or other free cells that migrate from white pulp across its wall and into its lumen. (From L. Weiss and M. Tavossoli, Anatomical hazards to passage of erythrocytes through the spleen. *Semin. Hematol.* 7:372, 1970. By permission.)

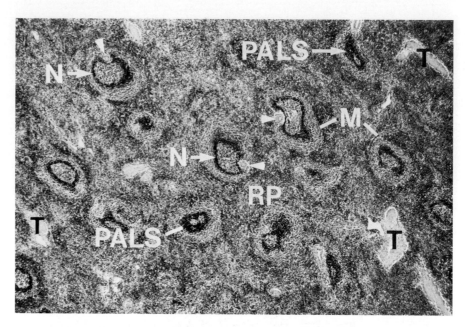

Fig. 10-14. A low-magnification light micrograph of the human spleen. The parenchyma consists of "islands" of white pulp in a "sea" of red pulp (*RP*). The white pulp is composed of periarterial lymphocyte sheaths (*PALS*) and nodules (*N*) with prominent germinal centers. The white pulp is surrounded by the marginal zone (*M*) and is associated with small arteries (*arrowheads*). Bits of trabecular (*T*) connective tissue are also seen.

splenic vein finally exits the organ at the hilus, entering the portal system of veins. The lymphatic drainage of the spleen is present but poorly defined. Unlike the lymphatics of the lymph node, those of the spleen are not of major functional significance.

FUNCTIONAL ASPECTS

The dense reticular meshwork in the marginal zones and red pulp cords (where capillaries from the central arteries terminate) functions as an effective trap for antigens and senescent blood cells. These regions contain large numbers of macrophages and phagocytic reticular cells that remove and degrade trapped cells and particles. Senescent cells apparently lose much of their flexibility, becoming easily damaged and unable to pass through the reticular meshwork. The lining cells of the sinuses are nonphagocytic.

As an effector organ in immunity, the spleen has much in common with the lymph nodes. The diffuse lymphoid tissue (the periarterial lympho-

Fig. 10-15. Low-power electron micrograph of human spleen, including portions of both white and red pulp. The central artery (*CA*) with branch (*arrow*) is surrounded by the periarterial lymphocyte sheath (*PALS*) composed primarily of small lymphocytes and a few lymphoblasts (*arrows*). Other arterial branches (*A*) are seen passing through the white pulp. These terminate as capillaries (*C*) in the marginal zone (*MZ*), where many reticular cells (*arrowheads*) are found. The adjacent red pulp is composed of red pulp cords (*RPC*) and sinuses (*S*). (From J. A. G. Rhodin, *An Atlas of Histology*, New York: Oxford University Press, 1974.)

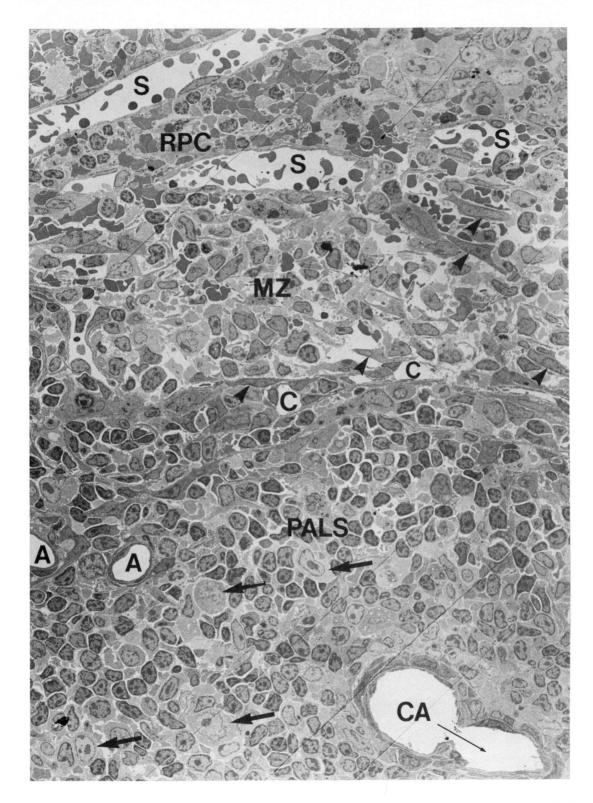

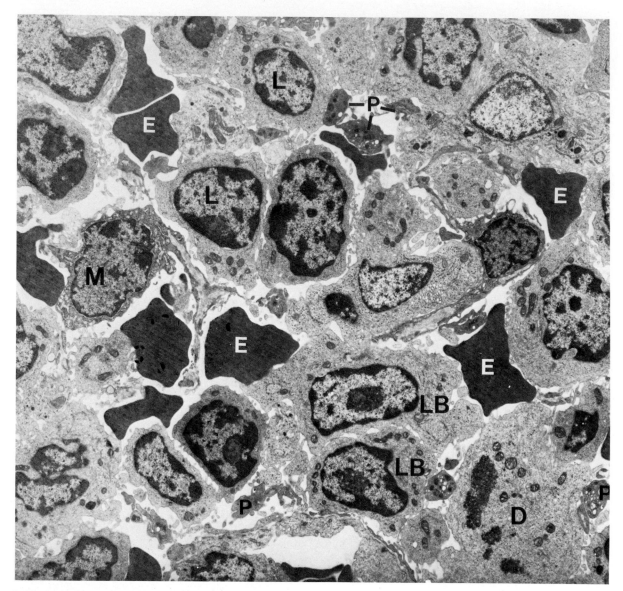

Fig. 10-16. An electron micrograph of the splenic red pulp of a mouse. Seen here are a number of lymphoblasts (*LB*) and smaller lymphocytes (*L*). Erythrocytes (*E*) and platelets (*P*) are also present in significant numbers. Note a macrophage (*M*) crawling in a sinus and a lymphocyte dividing (*D*). Its chromosomes are visible. (Courtesy of J. André-Schwartz.)

cyte sheath) is populated predominantly by T cells, as is shown by both neonatal thymectomy and induction of cell-mediated immunity. Similarly, the nodules are B cell zones involved primarily in humoral immunity. Again, the cellular mechanisms involved in cell-mediated immunity are not well understood. In a humoral immune response, bloodborne antigens are first trapped in the red pulp cords and marginal zones, where they are phagocytized by macrophages. Shortly thereafter, the antigen is found in association with the plasma membranes of dendritic reticular cells within the nodules. The subsequent cellular events are similar to those described in the lymph node, namely, enlargement of germinal centers due to proliferation of B cells, plasma cell maturation and accumulation in red pulp cords, and migration of lymphoid cells to other peripheral lymphoid organs and connective tissue regions of the body.

The Gut-Associated Lymphoid Tissues

The lamina propria of the digestive and respiratory tracts is often considered a lymphoid tissue, since this subepithelial layer has a rather reticular stroma and contains large numbers of lymphoid cells. Most plasma cells in this layer secrete an antibody (IgA) that is especially effective in preventing bacteria and viruses from penetrating the overlying epithelium. At different levels of the alimentary canal, the lamina propria is greatly enlarged by the presence of more highly organized lymphoid tissue. This tissue forms the tonsils, Peyer's patches, the appendix, and solitary nodules that are scattered throughout the entire tract but are particularly numerous in the colon. Together, they are called the **gut-associated lymphoid tissues (GALT).**

As already discussed, these organs, either as a whole or individually, may represent the bursa-equivalent, at least in some mammalian species. However, if this is so they must function as such only briefly, since they develop and function as peripheral lymphoid organs, beginning shortly after birth. These organs maintain a close associ-

ation with an epithelial surface (which itself is highly infiltrated with lymphocytes), and they too are composed of diffuse and nodular lymphoid tissue that represents T and B cell zones, respectively. Likewise, cellular proliferation is antigen-driven, especially by ingested antigens. Cells recirculate through postcapillary venules in the diffuse lymphoid tissue.

The epithelium associated with the lymphoid follicles (nodules) is histologically distinct from the surrounding epithelium and is referred to as **follicular epithelium.** This specialized epithelium is modified so as to enhance uptake of luminal particles and microorganisms by providing a localized decrease in the epithelial barrier. In this way the underlying lymphocytes and macrophages are stimulated to mount an immune response. The follicular epithelium varies histologically in accordance with the surrounding epithelial characteristics at various levels of the gastrointestinal tract. It is particularly well developed over the nodules of the Peyer's patches located in the walls of the ileum (to be discussed later in this chapter).

THE TONSILS

The tonsils form a ring of lymphoid tissue around the throat entrance. They consist of the paired **palatine** and **lingual tonsils** and the single **pharyngeal tonsil.** The features distinguishing these types being of only minor importance, we will briefly discuss their common features instead.

Since tonsils are composed of lymphoid tissue in the lamina propria of the mouth and pharynx, they are closely associated with the lining epithelium. The epithelial type depends on the location; the epithelium is stratified squamous in the palatine and lingual tonsils, pseudostratified in the pharyngeal tonsil. The epithelium is highly infolded, forming deep crypts (Fig. 10-17). Deep in the lamina propria, a scanty capsule with projections of trabeculae toward the epithelium may be seen. A number of small glands are located in this region, their ducts opening into the bases of the crypts. Skeletal muscle is located just be-

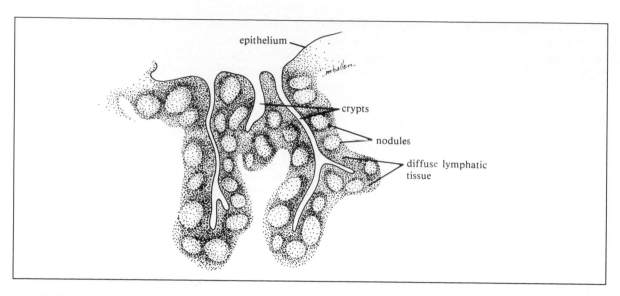

Fig. 10-17. A tonsil, showing the relation between the epithelium and the lymphatic tissue.

neath the glands. Reticular fibers and associated cells form the inner framework for housing the lymphoid tissue.

The lymphoid tissue of tonsils contains nodules with unusually large germinal centers surrounded by diffuse lymphoid aggregates, much like the cortex of the lymph node. The nodules are usually not so symmetric as those of most lymph nodes and the spleen. Small lymphocyte aggregates form "caps" on germinal centers, which are oriented toward the epithelium, and many cells infiltrate the epithelium itself (Fig. 10-18). Pyknotic lymphoid cells are commonly found in saliva. These features are also common to other gut-associated lymphoid structures.

PEYER'S PATCHES

Structures that are histologically similar to tonsils are found in the ileum of the small intestine. Solitary nodules, commonly found throughout the alimentary canal, are aggregated into groups called **Peyer's patches** or simply **aggregated nodules.** These aggregates, numbering 30 to 40, are usually confined to the lamina propria, but some larger aggregates may extend into the underlying layers and bulge into the lumen, flattening the villi above them. The nodules are interspersed with areas of diffuse lymphoid tissue (Fig. 10-19).

The follicular epithelium associated with the nodules is highly specialized. These are areas where no villus projections occur. While most of the constituent cells are the typical columnar cells with closely packed microvilli, others are unique attenuated cells that form thin cytoplasmic bridges between adjacent columnar cells. These cells actively trap antigens from the gut lumen and present them to the cells of the lymphoid nodules below. Lymphocytes and macrophages can frequently be seen in close association with these cells, forming what may be called **intraepithelial lymphoid nests** (Fig. 10-20).

THE APPENDIX

The appendix is a blind evagination of the cecum, at the proximal end of the colon. Its lamina propria is composed almost entirely of lym-

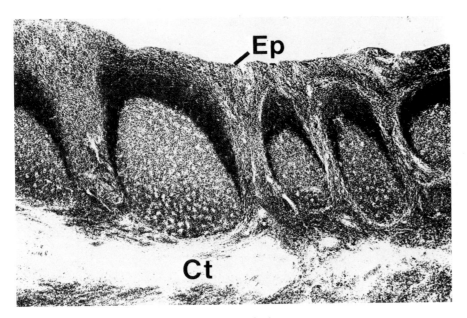

Fig. 10-18. A light micrograph of a portion of a human palatine tonsil. Note that the nodules have large germinal centers and dense "caps" of small lymphocytes facing the epithelium (*Ep*). The epithelium is also highly infiltrated with lymphocytes and difficult to distinguish. Beneath the nodules is some dense connective tissue (*Ct*).

Fig. 10-19. Part of a Peyer's patch. The lymphoid tissue is located within the wall of the ileum, occupying both the lamina propria and the submucosa.

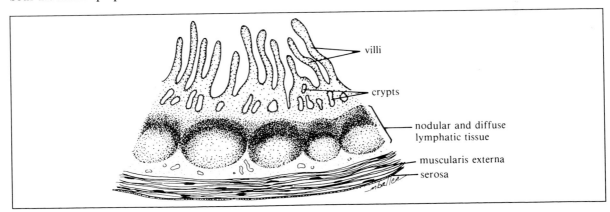

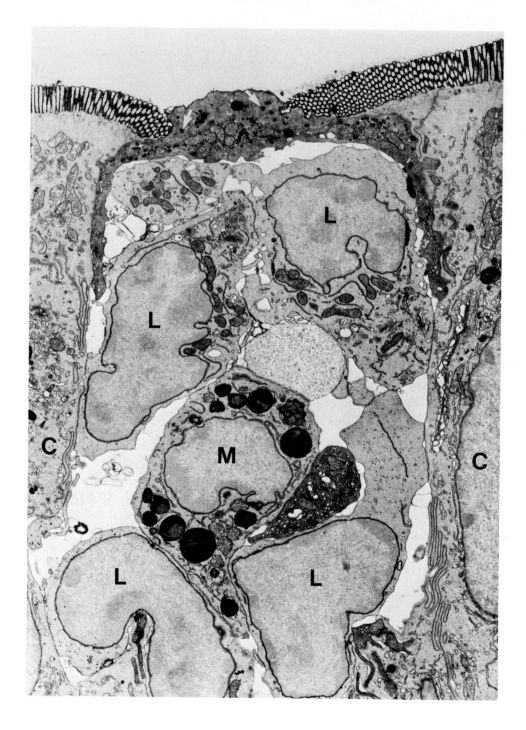

Fig. 10-20. An electron micrograph of the follicular epithelium associated with the nodules of Peyer's patches (mouse ileum). Two columnar cells (C) with microvilli surround a nest of lymphocytes (L) and a macrophage (M). A unique, attenuated cell with a darker cytoplasm joins the two columnar cells, providing a very thin barrier between the lumen and the lymphoid cells. Vesicles (*white arrows*) are seen transporting exogenously administered horseradish peroxidase from the lumen to the lymphoid cells below. A macrophage has also ingested some of this material, which is not localized in its secondary lysosomes. (From R. L. Owen and P. Nemanic. Antigen processing structures of intestinal tract. An SEM study of lymphoepithelial organs. *Scan. Electron Microsc.* 2:367, 1978.)

---

phoid tissue, similar histologically to the tonsils and Peyer's patches. The intestinal crypts above the nodules are often absent or poorly developed (see Fig. 14-15).

OVERVIEW OF IMMUNE RESPONSE MECHANISMS

The immune response is mediated by two major lymphocyte populations: T cells, which require the thymus for maturation and are involved in cell-mediated immunity, and B cells, which mature in the "bursa-equivalent" and are involved in humoral immunity (antibody production). Although T and B cells are not distinguishable morphologically, they can be accurately identified by their unique surface molecules or receptors. T cells can be further subclassified into distinct functional subsets in a similar manner.

The cells that mediate the immune response include macrophages, which clear antigen and initiate the cellular/humoral response by presenting antigens to lymphocytes; helper T cells and suppressor T cells, which regulate the level of responsivity; and effector T cells and B cells, which not only destroy antigens but also attract and activate other leukocytes by the production and secretion of lymphokines and antibodies. The interaction between immunocompetent cells

and soluble mediating factors produces both a positive and a negative feedback mechanism, which regulates the immune response.

Upon interaction with antigen, macrophages initiate the immune response by producing **interleukin 1,** which in turn stimulates helper T cells to proliferate and to produce **interleukin 2.** Elevated levels of this growth factor result in the clonal expansion of effector T cells or B cells. Suppressor T cells modulate the immune response by blocking helper T cell activity by the release of suppressor factors.

NATIONAL BOARD TYPE QUESTIONS

Select the response most closely associated with each numbered item. (The headings may be used once, more than once, or not at all.)

    A. Bone marrow
    B. Thymus
    C. Lymph nodes
    D. Spleen
    E. Peyer's patches

1. Origin of lymphoid stem cells in the adult
2. Produces a hormonelike substance which promotes lymphocyte maturation
3. Site for production of secretory IgA
4. Traps antigens that originate from connective tissue

For the following, select
    A. if only *1, 2, and 3* are correct.
    B. if only *1 and 3* are correct.
    C. if only *2 and 4* are correct.
    D. if only *4* is correct.
    E. if *all* are correct.

5. Which of the following are products of effector T lymphocytes?
    1. Migration-inhibitory factor
    2. Chemotactic factor
    3. Blastogenic factor
    4. Thymopoietin

6. Which of the following is (are) characteristic of mature T lymphocytes?
   1. They are *not* capable of dividing.
   2. They are capable of enhancing as well as suppressing the immune response.
   3. They are involved in allergic reactions.
   4. They are found in lymph nodes.
7. Which of the following is (are) characteristic of epithelial-reticular cells of the thymus?
   1. They are derived from mesoderm.
   2. They provide the structural basis for the blood-thymus barrier.
   3. They are highly phagocytic.
   4. They induce the maturation of T cells.

Select the response most closely associated with each numbered item.
   A. Lymph node
   B. Spleen
   C. Both
   D. Neither

8. Contains "nodular" lymphoid tissue
9. Traps and degrades aged blood cells
10. Contains elaborate lymphatic channels

Select the single best response for each of the following.

11. Which immunoglobulin is produced early in the primary immune response?
    A. IgG
    B. IgM
    C. IgA
    D. IgE
    E. IgD
12. In the spleen, lymphocytes are primarily associated around which structure(s)?
    A. Trabeculae
    B. Red pulp cords
    C. Central arteries
    D. Hilus
    E. Capsule

ANNOTATED ANSWERS

1. A. The bone marrow provides lymphoid stem cells in the adult. The other organs listed are involved in cell maturation or responses to antigens.
2. B. The epithelial-reticular cells of the thymus provide the stimulus for T cell maturation.
3. E. Secretory IgA is a dimeric molecule joined together by a secretory piece provided by epithelial cells. The gut-associated lymphoid tissues provide this kind of arrangement.
4. C. Connective tissues are drained by lymphatic capillaries which carry antigens via afferent lymphatics to the lymph nodes.
5. A. All are lymphokines except thymopoietin, which is a hormonelike product produced by epithelial-reticular cells.
6. C. T cells are found in all secondary lymphoid organs. One of their functions is to regulate the immune response. They can divide after undergoing blastogenesis. Allergic reactions involve plasma cells and mast cells.
7. D. Epithelial-reticular cells produce hormonelike products which induce the maturation of T cells. They are derived from endoderm and are not phagocytic. The blood-thymus barrier is provided by capillaries with tight junctions in the thymic cortex.
8. C. All secondary lymphoid organs contain both nodular (B cells) and diffuse (T cells) lymphoid tissue.
9. B. In addition to trapping bloodborne antigens, the spleen also traps old blood cells which lose their flexibility and therefore cannot pass through the meshwork of the red pulp.
10. A. The lymph nodes are "inserted" into the lymphatic drainage. Lymph passes through the nodes via a system of lymphatic sinuses.
11. B. In a primary immune response, the pentameric antibody, IgM, is produced first. It is later superseded by IgG. The other immunoglobulin classes are more highly specialized in terms of function or location.

12. C. Lymphocytes, which compose the splenic white pulp, are associated with the central arteries. The capsule and trabeculae provide the framework for the organ. The hilus contains the blood supply. Red pulp cords contain a mixture of blood cells, reticular cells, and some lymphoid cells.

BIBLIOGRAPHY

Anderson, A. O., and N. D. Anderson. Studies on the structure and permeability of the microvasculature in normal rat lymph nodes. *Am. J. Pathol.* 80:387, 1975.

Bach, J. F., and M. Dardenne. Studies on thymus products. II. Demonstration and characterization of a circulating thymic hormone. *Immunology* 25:353, 1973.

Berzofsky, J. A. Immune Response Genes in the Regulation of Mammalian Immunity. In R. F. Goldberger (ed.), *Biological Regulation and Development.* New York: Plenum, 1980.

Borysenko, M. Phylogeny of immunity. *Immunogenetics* 3:305, 1976.

Borysenko, M., and J. Borysenko. Stress, behavior, and immunity: Animal models and mediating mechanisms. *Gen. Hosp. Psychiatry* 4:59, 1982.

Boyse, E. A., and H. Cantor. Surface characteristics of T lymphocyte subpopulations. *Hosp. Pract.* 12:81, 1977.

Chen, L. T. Microcirculation of the spleen: An open or closed circulation. *Science* 201:157, 1978.

Cooper, M. D., and A. R. Lawton. The development of the immune system. *Sci. Am.* 231:58, 1971.

Cooper, M. D., et al. The function of the thymus system and bursa system in the chicken. *J. Exp. Med.* 123:75, 1966.

Edelman, G. M. Antibody structure and cellular specificity in the immune response. *Harvey Lect.* 68:149, 1974.

Eisen, N. H. *Immunology.* Hagerstown, Md.: Harper & Row, 1980.

Feldmann, M., A. Rosenthal, and P. Erb. Macrophage-lymphocyte interactions in immune induction. *Int. Rev. Cytol.* 60:149, 1979.

Ford, W. L., and J. L. Gowans. The traffic of lymphocytes. *Semin. Hematol.* 6:67, 1969.

Fudenberg, H. M., et al. *Basic and Clinical Immunology.* Los Altos, Calif.: Lange, 1980.

Golub, E. S. (ed.). *The Cellular Basis of the Immune Response.* Sunderland, Mass.: Sinauer Associates, 1981.

Gowans, J. L. Differentiation of cells which synthesize the immunoglobulins. *Ann. Immunol.* (Paris) 125C:201, 1974.

Haar, J. L. Light and electron microscopy of the human fetal thymus. *Anat. Rec.* 179:463, 1974.

Hood, L. E., I. L. Weissman, and W. B. Wood. *Immunology.* Menlo Park, Calif.: Benjamin-Cummings, 1978.

Jerne, N. K. The immune system. *Sci. Am.* 229:52, 1973.

Katz, D. H. Adaptive differentiation of lymphocytes: Theoretical implications for mechanisms of cell-cell recognition and regulation of immune responses. *Adv. Immunol.* 29:138, 1980.

Katz. D. H. *Lymphocyte Differentiation, Recognition and Regulation.* New York: Academic, 1977.

Katz, D. H., and B. Benacerraf. The regulatory influence of activated T cells on B cell responses to antigen. *Adv. Immunol.* 15:1, 1972.

Lerner, R. A., and F. J. Dixon. The human lymphocyte as an experimental animal. *Sci. Am.* 228:82, 1973.

Mandel. T. Ultrastructure of epithelial cells in the cortex of guinea pig thymus. *Z. Zellforsch. Mikrosk. Anat.* 92:159, 1968.

Miller, J. F. A. P., A. H. E. Marshall, and R. G. White. The immunological significance of the thymus. *Adv. Immunol.* 2:111, 1962.

Moe, R. Electron microscopic appearance of the parenchyma of lymph nodes. *Am. J. Anat.* 114:341, 1964.

Murphy, M. J., et al. Ultrastructural analysis of antibody synthesis in cells from lymph and lymph nodes. *Am. J. Pathol.* 66:25, 1972.

Nossal, G. J. V. The cellular basis of immunity. *Harvey Lect.* 63:179, 1968.

Owen, R. L., and P. Nemanic. Antigen processing structures of the mammalian intestinal tract: An SEM study of lymphoepithelial organs. *Scan. Electron Microsc.* 2:367, 1978.

Paul, W. E., and B. Benacerraf. Functional specificity of thymus-dependent lymphocytes. *Science* 195:1293, 1977.

Raff, M. C. T and B lymphocytes and immune responses. *Nature* 242:19, 1973.

Raviola, E., and M. J. Karnovsky. Evidence for a blood-thymus barrier using electron-opaque tracers. *J. Exp. Med.* 136:466, 1972.

Roitt, I. *Essential Immunology.* Oxford: Blackwell, 1977.

Sell, S. *Immunology, Immunopathology, and Immunity.* Hagerstown, Md.: Harper & Row, 1980.

Trainen, N., and M. Small. Thymic humoral factors. *Contemp. Top. Immunobiol.* 2:321, 1973.

Waksman, B. H. Tolerance, the thymus and suppressor T cells. *Clin. Exp. Immunol.* 28:363, 1977.

Weiss, L. *The Cells and Tissues of the Immune System.* Englewood Cliffs, N.J.: Prentice-Hall, 1972.

Weiss, L. A scanning electron microscopic study of the spleen. *Blood* 43:665, 1974.

Weiss, L., and L. T. Chen. The differentiation of white pulp and red pulp in the spleen of human fetuses. *Am. J. Anat.* 141:393, 1974.

11 Cardiovascular System

The cardiovascular system consists of a muscular pulsatile heart and a system of blood vessels through which blood is pumped to the body. The arteries distribute blood and its dissolved constituents, including oxygen and nutrients, to the capillaries. The veins return the blood to the heart together with carbon dioxide and other metabolites received by the capillary beds and postcapillary venules. Closely associated with the cardiovascular system is the lymphatic system of vessels. The lymphatic fluid (lymph) carried by the lymphatic vessels consists of interstitial fluid drained from the connective tissue and a few circulating lymphocytes. The interstitial fluid is a clear ultrafiltrate of the plasma that escapes from the vascular capillary beds. Since the largest lymphatic vessels drain into the large veins in the neck, the plasma with its circulating lymphocytes is returned to the bloodstream, and solutes originating from the interstitial fluid of the connective tissue are introduced to the bloodstream. It should be appreciated that connective tissue, usually areolar connective tissue, separates arterial capillary beds from blind-ending lymphatic capillaries. Since the venules do not completely drain these connective tissue areas of the fluid that escapes from the arterial capillaries, the lymphatic capillaries absorb the remainder, thereby preventing edema or swelling of the connective tissue space.

This chapter describes the histologic and functional aspects of the heart, blood vessels, and lymphatic vessels.

THE HEART

The human heart consists of four pumping chambers: the right atrium and ventricle, and

247

the left atrium and ventricle. The right atrium pumps blood returning from the superior and inferior vena cava into the right ventricle, which pumps it through the pulmonary artery to the lungs for oxygenation. The left atrium pumps returning oxygenated blood from the pulmonary veins into the left ventricle, which pumps it into the aorta for distribution through the systemic circulation.

The wall of the heart consists of three layers: **endocardium, myocardium,** and **epicardium.** The endocardium is the internal lining of the atrial and ventricular chambers. It consists of an endothelium that is continuous with the endothelium of the incoming veins and outgoing arteries: It covers the surfaces of the atrioventricular, pulmonary, and aortic valves, the chordae tendinae, and papillary muscles. Deep to the endothelium is a dense connective tissue layer consisting of elastic and collagen fibers that also extends into the core of the cardiac valves. Supporting this connective tissue layer is a layer of adipose and irregularly arranged collagen fibers through which blood vessels travel. The deeper portions of the endocardium (**subendocardium**) may also contain smooth muscle bundles in places as well as elements of the cardiac conduction system (see Chap. 7, Fig. 7-17). It is conspicuously thicker in the atrium than in the ventricles.

The myocardium consists of the regular cardiac muscle fibers, each anchored by an endomysium that inserts into the subendocardium. The endomysium within the atria contains significant amounts of elastic fibers that are not common in the ventricular endomysium. Most of the cardiac muscle fibers are anchored to one another by their intercalated disks; others insert into the connective tissue skeleton of the heart.

The connective tissue skeleton of the heart consists of dense collagenous fibers which form rings around the atrioventricular valves (**annuli fibrosi**), reinforce the origins of the aorta and pulmonary artery, and form the fibrous (membranous) part of the interventricular septum. The dense connective tissue of the endocardium,

which extends into the core of the atrioventricular valves, is also part of the connective tissue framework of the heart. The narrow cords of collagen that constitute the chordae tendinae extend from the papillary muscles and insert into the connective tissue core of these valves (Fig. 11-1). The chordae tendinae prevent these valves (tricuspid and mitral) from prolapsing into the atrial chamber during ventricular contraction. The semilunar valves of the pulmonary artery and aorta have significant amounts of elastic fibers on their ventricular surfaces that assist valve closure between ventricular contractions.

The epicardium is a fibroblastic covering that invests the entire outer surface of the heart. The mesothelium of the visceral pericardium is tenaciously attached to the outer surface of the fibrous epicardium. Located just subjacent to the fibrous portion of the epicardium is a looser variety of connective tissue housing the coronary blood vessels, nerves, lymphatic capillaries, and variable amounts of adipose tissue. Connective tissue fibers of the epicardium are continuous with the underlying endomysium of the myocardium.

BLOOD VESSELS

The vascular wall is divided into three compartments or tunics: the **tunica intima,** which includes the endothelium lining the lumen and small amounts of subendothelial connective tissue; the **tunica media,** a middle layer usually consisting of smooth muscle with variable amounts of connective tissue depending on the specific segment of the vascular tree; and the **tunica adventitia,** an outer layer usually consisting of connective tissue, which anchors the vessel to its surrounding tissue. However, there are variations in histologic composition and organization of these three tunics that are characteristic of specific segments of the vascular system and the physiologic functions performed there.

Profiles of venules and arterioles usually occur together in histologic section because they frequently follow a common distribution through-

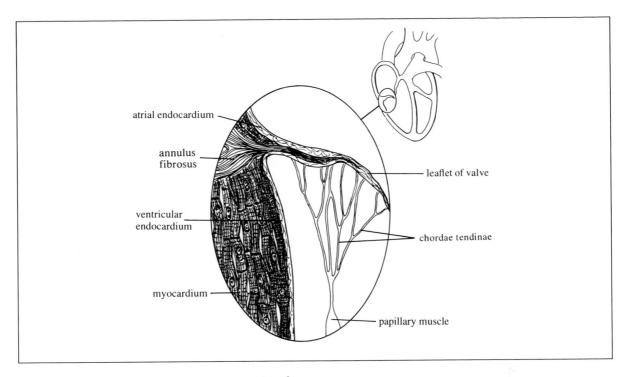

Fig. 11-1. Part of the atrium, ventricle, and valve of the heart, showing the composition of the basic layers.

out the body. In similar fashion, medium-sized arteries and veins travel together. This facilitates comparison of their overall structural appearance and histologic composition. Even at low magnification veins are distinguishable from arteries. Veins have a larger overall diameter, a larger lumen, and a narrower wall than corresponding arteries. Furthermore, the thin venous wall is usually collapsed upon its lumen unless fixed by perfusion, whereas the arterial lumina are often retained in an open, circular profile by their thicker walls. The arterial wall is generally thicker than the venous wall in order to withstand the higher blood pressures that prevail within arteries compared with veins at equal distances from the heart. Consequently, arteries usually display a greater wall-to-lumen ratio than veins. Generally, the thickness of the arterial wall gradually diminishes as blood pressure declines with increasing distance from the heart. Hence the arterial wall becomes thinner with increasing proximity to the capillaries, but the wall-to-lumen ratio becomes greater, which results in increased vascular resistance to flow and therefore decreased blood flow.

Furthermore the histologic composition of the three tunics varies in characteristic ways for specific segments of the arterial and venous circuits, which serve to identify them. The following section is a description of those histologic features.

Arteries

For convenience, arteries are usually divided into three major categories. In sequential order from the heart they are: **elastic arteries** (large or conducting arteries), **muscular arteries** (medium or distributing arteries), and **arterioles** (small arteries). Although each is distinguished by various histologic criteria, it should be appreciated that these categories are inadequate to the extent that the histologic changes occur progressively rather than abruptly along the transition from one type to another.

The **elastic arteries** include the aorta and its largest primary branches (e.g., common carotid and common iliac arteries). Their intima includes the endothelium, which is supported by a thin layer of connective tissue that thickens with advancing age. The tunica media is conspicuous as the largest tunic and for its abundant **elastic laminae.** These elastic membranes alternate with layers of smooth muscle cells and lesser

amounts of collagen. The tunica adventitia is considerably thinner than the media and contains mostly longitudinally arranged collagen fibers (Figs. 11-2, 11-3).

Since diffusion of oxygen from the lumen to the outer layers of the media is inadequate in these largest vessels, the outer layer of the adventitia is supplied by **vasa vasorum,** small arterioles that course through the adventitia and send capillary twigs into the tunica media. The elastic components of the aorta allow it to expand during contraction of the ventricles (systole), thereby storing some of the force of the heartbeat. Between heartbeats (diastole), elastic recoil of the vascular wall continues to propel blood through the vascular system, thereby dampening severe fluctuations in blood pressure and blood flow along the downstream vasculature during the cardiac cycle. The greatest blood pressure occurs in large arteries.

Fig. 11-2. A cross section through the wall of the aorta stained with an elastic stain. The deeply stained, wavy lines are the elastic laminae, which are especially abundant in the tunica media of all large arteries. *TI* = tunica intima; *TM* = tunica media; and *TA* = tunica adventitia.

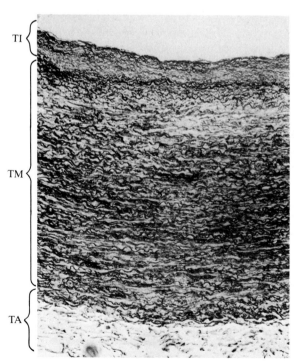

Fig. 11-3. A portion of the tunica media of the aorta viewed with Nomarski optics to provide a more three-dimensional appreciation of the elastic laminae that are abundant there (*arrows*). The darkly stained nuclei belong to smooth muscle cells; the material filling in the intervening spaces between laminae is mostly collagen.

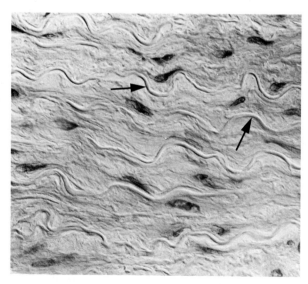

Muscular arteries are branches of elastic arteries (e.g., mesenteric and splenic arteries). They are frequently referred to as medium-sized arteries because they are smaller than elastic arteries but larger than their arteriolar branches. Muscular arteries have a tunica media composed predominantly of circularly or spirally arranged smooth muscle. It is a discrete and easily identified muscular compartment (Figs. 11-4, 11-5).

Fig. 11-4. Cross section through the wall of a muscular artery that has been stained to demonstrate elastic fibers. The wavy internal elastic lamina is conspicuous (*left arrow*). Small dense endothelial nuclei are visible against its surface. In the adventitia there are several elastic lamina (*right arrow*) bordering the outer portion of the media. The muscular media which contains elongate nuclei of smooth muscle cells is between the internal and external elastic laminae. Also within the media are a few scant wavy elastic laminae.

All muscular arteries contain a well-developed **internal elastic lamina** (situated between the intima and media) and a series of thinner **external elastic laminae,** which occupy the adventitia, especially near the media-adventitia border. The internal elastic lamina is commonly considered to be part of the tunica intima. However, since it is probably synthesized by smooth muscle cells of the inner media, it is more appropriately included as part of the media. In this regard, it should be appreciated that smooth muscle cells are capable of producing elastic fibers. In fact, the media of the largest muscular arteries contain a few scattered elastic laminae throughout. In addition, smooth muscle cells produce a few reticular fibers and the proteoglycans present in the tunica media. The adventitia is dominated by abundant longitudinally arranged collagen fibers; however, occasional bundles of longitudinally oriented smooth muscle occur within

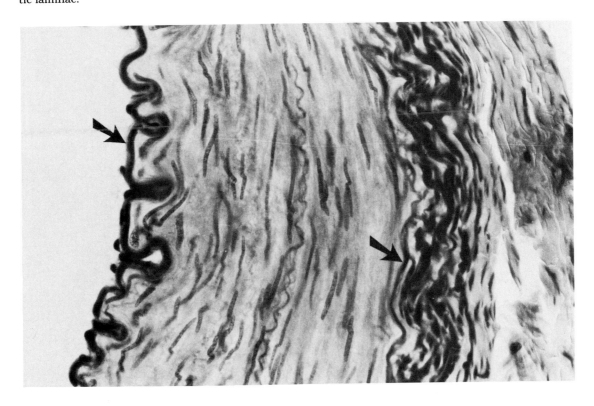

Fig. 11-5. Cross section through the renal artery of the rat, an example of a medium-sized artery or muscular artery. The lumen is on the far left. The artery was fixed by perfusion to keep the lumen open. As a result, the internal elastic lamina (*IEL*) and external elastic lamina (*EEL*) are seen stretched taut, instead of with the wavy appearance they give when there is no intraluminal pressure, as during diastole. There are many smooth muscle cells (*SM*) in the media. The adventitia (*ADV*) is composed mostly of collagen fibers but also contains an autonomic ganglion cell body (*G*) with some attending unmyelinated nerves. *E* = endothelium.

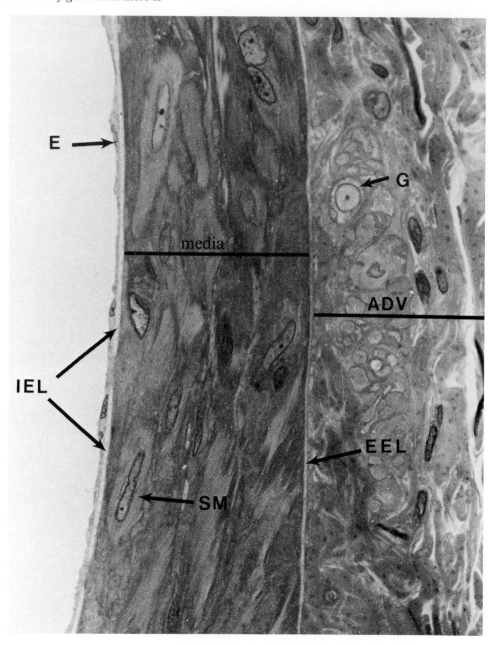

inner adventitia. The adventitia is usually as thick as the media in muscular arteries. Vasomotor nerve fibers, which regulate vascular smooth muscle contraction, travel within the adventitia where their autonomic ganglia are located. From the adventitia, vasomotor nerves penetrate the media for short distances, where they innervate only the outermost layers of smooth muscle. The smooth muscle cells are coupled by gap junctions, which permit depolarizing nerve impulses to spread throughout the deeper, uninnervated medial smooth muscle. Blood flow and blood pressure are regulated by contraction (vasoconstriction) and relaxation (vasodilation) of this muscular media layer, which regulates lumen size. The tough, collage-

nous adventitia reinforces the vascular wall against the stress exerted by the upper levels of intraluminal blood pressure.

Arterioles are the smallest branches of the arteries. They are generally between 20 and 100 μm in diameter. Arterioles regulate blood flow into capillary beds. A well-developed internal elastic membrane separates the intima from a media composed of circular smooth muscle (Figs. 11-6, 11-7). The adventitia is usually poorly developed with little or no external elastic laminae. The medial smooth muscle of arterioles is capable of making dramatic adjustments in lumen diameter that significantly influence blood flow distribution among the capillary beds. With electron microscopy, a few small, unmyelinated vasomotor nerves can be found along the outer circumference of the tunica media (Fig. 11-8).

Fig. 11-6. A small artery with its three tunics identified.

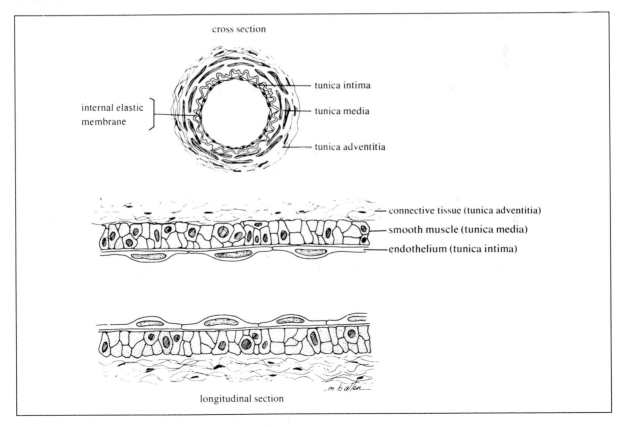

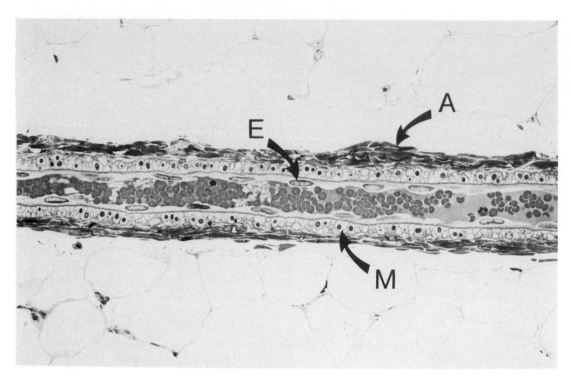

Fig. 11-7. An arteriole coursing through a field of adipose tissue. Erythrocytes can be seen occupying the lumen which is lined by endothelial cells (*E*) oriented with the long axis of the vessel. The smooth muscle cells (*M*) forming the tunica media are cut in cross section since they are circularly arranged around the vessel's long axis. Bundles of collagen constitute the tunica adventitia (*A*). The cells above and below the vessel are fat cells.

Terminal arterioles that give rise to capillaries have a cuff of smooth muscle near the capillary origin. These are **precapillary sphincters,** which regulate blood flow into the capillary bed by vasoconstriction or vasodilation.

Another branch of the terminal arteriole is the **metarteriole.** The metarteriole begins from the arteriole near the origin of the capillary network but drains directly into a venule. Capillaries originate from the metarteriole and anastomose with the capillary network originating from the terminal arteriole. There are precapillary sphinc-

ters at the origin of capillaries from metarterioles also. The metarteriole has single smooth muscle cells scattered along its length except near its confluence with the venule. Nearer the venule its wall contains no smooth muscle and closely resembles a capillary.

Arteriovenous anastomoses are unbranched arteriolar shunts between arterioles and venules that can divert blood flow away from certain capillary networks. They are particularly numerous in the skin, where their constriction can conserve core body heat by diverting blood flow away from cutaneous capillaries.

Capillaries

Most capillaries are 8 to 10 μm wide with a lumen just large enough to permit passage of erythrocytes in single file. The capillary wall is very thin

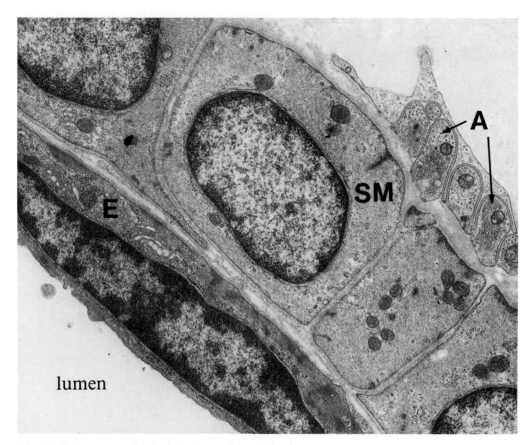

Fig. 11-8. Low-magnification electron micrograph of the wall of an arteriole. *E* = endothelial cell; *SM* = smooth muscle cell; *A* = unmyelinated axons innervating the vascular smooth muscle.

and consists of a single endothelial cell layer supported by a basal lamina and a scant amount of reticular fibers. The endothelial cells have elongate nuclei that are aligned in the longitudinal axis of the capillary. Occasionally associated with the outer circumference of capillaries are a scattered population of **perivascular cells** or **pericytes,** cells with several cytoplasmic processes surrrounding the capillary wall. Pericytes are multipotential mesenchymal stem cells capable of differentiating into vascular smooth muscle cells as well as fibroblasts and other connective

tissue cells. These cells may be responsible for increased muscle cell mass of arteriole walls and for the granulation tissue that is produced when growing capillaries infiltrate an area of tissue undergoing repair.

The endothelial cells that form capillary walls are extremely thin so as to enhance diffusion of oxygen out to surrounding tissues. In addition, several structural modifications occur to facilitate fluid escape from the capillary lumen to the surrounding interstitial space. These specializations identify three categories of capillary: **continuous, fenestrated,** and **sinusoidal** (discontinuous) capillaries.

The **continuous capillary** is the most common type of capillary. Its endothelium is also the type that lines the lumen of all arteries and veins. The endothelial cells of the continuous capillary are joined to one another by incomplete junctions (**fascia occludens**), which permit the escape of limited amounts of plasma from the lumen. These are found abundantly in skin and muscle. Plasmalemmal vesicles invaginate both the luminal surface and the external perivascular surfaces of the endothelium. Although it is believed that these vesicles are involved in transendothelial transport of substances across the vascular wall, the precise mechanism is not established. The prevailing view has been that vesicles participate in transendothelial transport by detaching from one endothelial surface and carrying their contents with them as they migrate across the endothelium to the plasmalemma on the opposite side to liberate their contents by exocytosis. There is some evidence now that the vesicles may not always migrate but rather fuse with one another to form transient or patent transendothelial channels that convey substances across the vascular endothelium. The existence of transendothelial channels is well established. In any case vesicles and transendothelial channels have been associated with transport of macromolecules too large to diffuse across fenestrations. In certain continuous capillaries, such as those forming the blood-brain barrier and the blood-thymus barrier, the intercellular junctions between endothelial cells are of the zonula occludens type, which completely seal the contiguous borders of adjacent endothelial cells. In this type of continuous capillary, pinocytotic vesicles are also scarce so that the escape of plasma into the interstitial space is virtually eliminated.

Fig. 11-9. A composite comparing continuous and fenestrated capillaries.

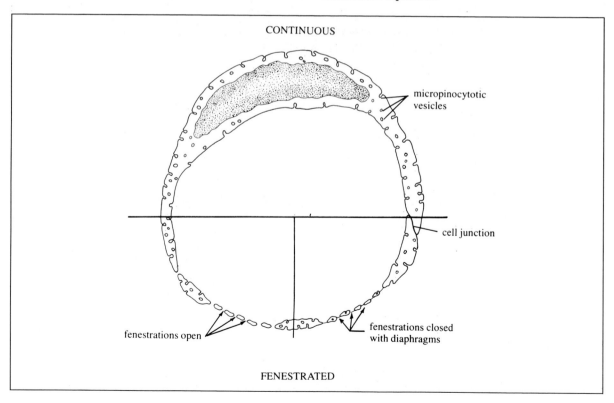

The endothelium of **fenestrated capillaries** has pores (fenestrations) where the cytoplasm is excluded from circular attenuations in the endothelium (Fig. 11-9). The **fenestration** is spanned by a diaphragm consisting of the fused outer leaflets of plasmalemma (Figs. 11-9, 11-10, and 11-11). The weight of evidence suggests that fenestrations increase the permeability of these capillaries to water and dissolved solutes whose molecular weight is less than about 40,000. The presence of fenestrations dramatically accelerates capillary fluid transport compared with continuous capillaries. Fenestrated capillaries are abundant within intestinal villi and especially within endocrine organs, where hormones are secreted in close proximity to capillaries for entry into the bloodstream. Fenestrations devoid of diaphragms are even more permeable. These oc-

cur in the glomerular capillaries of the kidney where rapid filtration of blood plasma is required (see Figs. 11-9, 11-11).

Sinusoids or **discontinuous capillaries** are usually irregularly shaped and depart from the strict tubular geometry of other capillaries. There are large intercellular gaps between endothelial cells that not only permit the escape of plasma, but can also facilitate passage of the formed elements of blood. These gaps are frequently occupied by macrophages. The endothelium has a variable number of fenestrations present. In addition, the basal lamina is either incomplete or entirely absent. Sinusoids are abundant in the liver, spleen, and bone marrow.

The luminal surface of the endothelium has a glycocalyx consisting of sialic acid and heparan sulfate which impart a net negative charge to the

Fig. 11-10. Electron micrograph of a portion of fenestrated capillary. Shown is a cross-section through the endothelium revealing two fenestrations with diaphragms (*arrows*).

Fig. 11-11. Freeze-fractured replica of fenestrated endothelial cell viewed with the electron microscope. The circular perforations in the endothelium are the fenestrations (*arrows*).

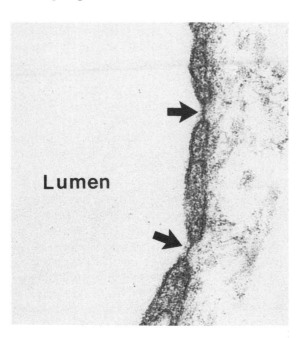

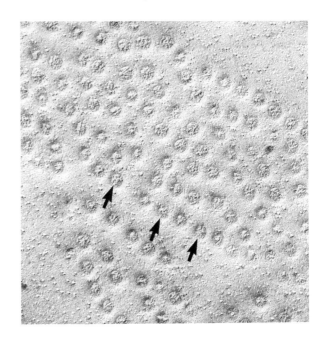

endothelial surface. Since circulating blood cells are also negatively charged, their electrostatic repulsion contributes to the nonthrombogenic character of the endothelium along the healthy vascular wall. However, the glycocalyx avidly binds several plasma proteins such as albumin which constitute an additional filtration barrier to the passage of plasma solutes across the endothelial lining. This has been demonstrated by the leakiness of capillaries where the glycocalyx has been stripped of bound albumin.

Plasma transport across the capillary wall is extensive. The driving force is the net difference between hydrostatic, osmotic, and oncotic pressures across the capillary wall. The hydrostatic pressure is established by the blood pressure within the vascular lumen and is higher than the hydrostatic pressure in the surrounding connective tissue outside the vessel wall nearer the arteriole end of the capillary bed. Thus plasma is lost from the arterial end of the capillaries. Nearer the venule end of the capillary bed, hydrostatic pressure within the lumen diminishes as branching and fluid loss diminish blood pressure. Therefore, at the venule end of a capillary bed, the higher osmotic and oncotic pressures within the vascular lumen tend to pull tissue fluid back into the lumen. The osmotic and oncotic pressures are established by dissolved salts and nondiffusable molecules like albumin.

Veins

Blood returning to the heart from capillary beds flows initially into the **postcapillary venules** and then sequentially through **collecting venules** and **small, medium,** and **large veins.**

The postcapillary venule performs two important functions. First, because blood pressure is lower here than in the capillary bed as well as being lower than the tissue pressure in the surrounding interstitial space, some of the fluid that has escaped from capillaries will return to the circulation by flowing into the postcapillary venules from the surrounding connective tissue areas. The balance of excess interstitial fluid will be drained away by lymphatic capillaries. Sec-

ond, leukocytes migrate into sites of infection by squeezing through the interendothelial spaces in the wall of the postcapillary venule. Histamine released from tissue mast cells renders these venules even more permeable and accelerates the outflow of plasma, which causes the swelling at the sites of inflammation. The wall of the venule consists of an endothelial cell lining surrounded by a basal lamina and a very small amount of collagen. Pericytes are frequently associated with venules.

The larger collecting venules acquire a thicker coat of collagen than postcapillary venules. Somewhat larger venules called **muscular venules** have a single layer of smooth muscle cells in their wall, which is otherwise constructed predominantly of collagenous adventitia.

Small and medium-sized veins are more muscular than venules due to a gradual acquisition of circularly arranged bundles of smooth muscle in the media (Fig. 11-12). However, venous smooth muscle is often interspersed with collagen bundles. Therefore, the media of small and medium-sized veins is never so uniformly muscular or consolidated as the media of arterioles and muscular arteries. The adventitia of small and medium-sized veins, which consists of longitudinally arranged collagen fibers and lesser amounts of elastic fibers, is distinctly thicker than the media. Small and medium-sized veins, particularly those in the arms and legs, exhibit valves that retard the backflow of blood. These valves are semilunar folds of the intima that lie flush against the wall during normal venous blood flow to the heart but resemble cuplike structures projecting into the lumen during backflow of blood.

Large veins, such as the vena cava, have a somewhat thicker subendothelial layer of connective tissue but a poorly developed media. The adventitia is the thickest tunic. Its innermost aspect is distinguished by the presence of longitudinally organized smooth muscle bundles, and its outermost aspect contains longitudinally arranged collagen and elastic fibers (Fig. 11-13). Vasa vasorum travel through the adventitia and penetrate the wall almost to its intima.

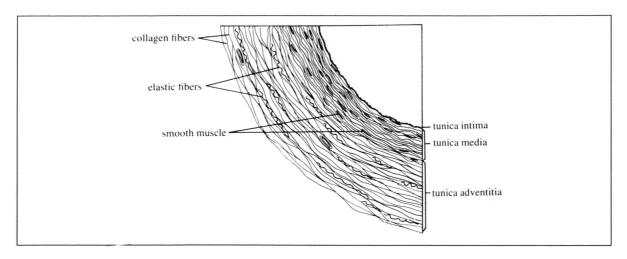

Fig. 11-12. The wall of a medium vein.

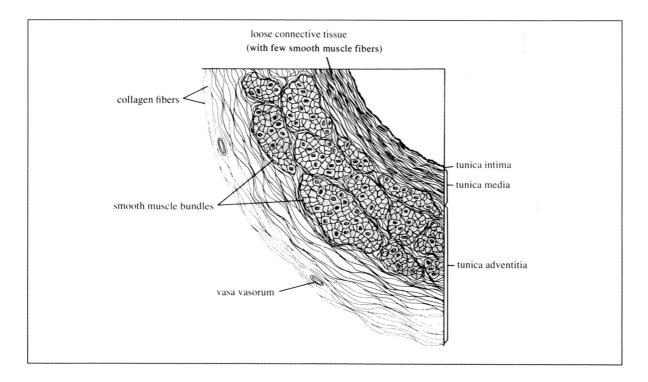

Fig. 11-13. The wall of a large vein.

Regulation of Blood Flow

Blood pressure declines from its highest level in the aorta to its lowest level in the postcapillary venules. The decline in blood pressure is proportional to increasing vascular resistance, which is a function of vascular length and radius (Poiseuille's law). Almost half of the total resistance to blood flow occurs along the small arteries and arterioles, where repeated branching of the vasculature produces an increase in the total surface area of the endothelium relative to the total lumen area. Blood flow is highest in the center of the lumen and lowest near the endothelial lining where frictional resistance is greatest. As a consequence of branching, the same total volume of blood is carried by these smaller vessels as in the larger, less branched vessels, but there is a decrease in blood flow velocity.

Vasoconstriction produced by contraction of vascular smooth muscle is another source of resistance since it reduces lumen size further. Vasodilation or passive distention of the vascular wall increases lumen area and reduces vascular resistance. The distensibility of any specific site along the vascular tree is determined not only by the influence of smooth muscle but also by relative amounts of collagen and elastin present in that vascular segment. The predominance of elastic fibers within the aorta allows its walls to expand with each heartbeat and recoil between beats. The abundance of collagen within the adventitia of muscular arteries places a limit on vasodilation, which may occur there because collagen is much less distensible than either elastic fibers or smooth muscle. Therefore, blood pressure and blood flow are governed by changes in geometry of the vascular wall induced by the degree of vasodilation or vasoconstriction permitted by its various histologic components.

Other factors that regulate blood flow include not only vasomotor innervation of vascular smooth muscle, hemodynamic influences of cardiac performance, and vasoactive hormones, but also local factors such as pH, metabolites, and oxygen availability. Metabolites such as lactic acid produced by surrounding tissue may alter

pH. A relatively small decline in pH toward acidity causes vasodilation, which improves blood flow to that area. Throughout the systemic circulation, local hypoxia (inadequate oxygen) also causes vasodilation (reactive hyperemia). Both of these mechanisms for improving blood flow to metabolically active or oxygen-deficient areas are particularly evident in the coronary circulation. In the special case of the pulmonary circulation, localized hypoxia causes vasoconstriction in order to redirect unoxygenated blood away from lobules that are not properly ventilated by inspired air toward well-ventilated lobules. This ensures that blood returning to the heart is well oxygenated before being pumped throughout the systemic circulation.

SENSORY RECEPTORS REGULATING BLOOD FLOW

Several sites along the cardiovascular system are specialized for detection of changes in blood pressure or oxygen—carbon dioxide tension and participate in reflex responses regulating blood flow. They are the **carotid sinus, carotid body,** and **aortic body.**

The **carotid sinus** is a modification in the vascular wall near the bifurcation of each common carotid artery. At the site of the carotid sinus, the mass of the tunica media is significantly diminished. Consequently, the adventitia bears the stress of intraluminal blood pressure at this site and is distended by increases in blood pressure. Expansion of the sinus due to high blood pressure stimulates branches of the glossopharyn-

Fig. 11-14. Rabbit carotid body. Glomus cell (*arrows*) are clustered near capillaries (*Ca*). Nerve fibers occur in small bundles (*Bnf*) or singly (*Nf*). Collagen (*Col*) is abundant. Inset: Higher magnification comparing differences in nuclear shape of type I cells (*NI*) versus type II cells (*NII*). (From A. Verna, Ultrastructure of the carotid body in the mammals. *Int. Rev. Cytol.* 60:271, 1979.)

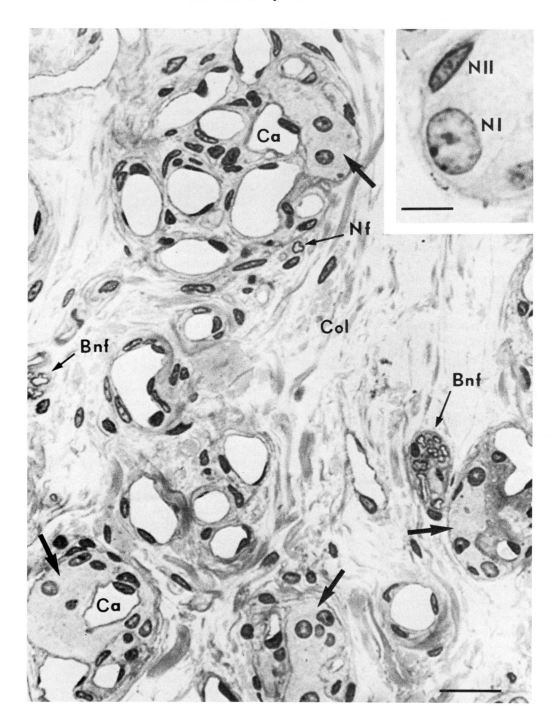

geal nerve (ninth cranial nerve), which innervates the adventitia at this site. Its sensory
impulses are conveyed back to central nervous
system centers that regulate vascular tone. This
provokes a reflex vasodilation of the splanchnic
vasculature and a slowing of the heartbeat, both
of which reduce systemic blood pressure.

The **carotid body** is located on the dorsal aspect of the common carotid bifurcation. It is an
arterial chemoreceptor capable of sensing aci-
demia and reduced oxygen–carbon dioxide tension and making appropriate respiratory and
cardiovascular responses to adjust circulatory
pH and oxygen and carbon dioxide levels. The
carotid body is vascularized by capillaries derived
from the glomic artery, a small branch of the
carotid artery bifurcation, the common carotid
artery, or the external carotid artery. Two types of
cells are clustered together near one side of these
capillaries: **type I cells (glomus cells)** and the
less numerous **type II cells (sustentacular or
sheath cells).** Both cells have a small nuclear-to-
cytoplasmic ratio (Fig. 11-14).

Type I cells are derived from the neural crest,
have a round or spherical nucleus, and contain
cytoplasmic granules that stain with basic dyes.
In electron micrographs, the most conspicuous
feature of type I cells is the abundance of dense-
cored vesicles, which probably contain dopamine. Type II cells have a flattened or reniform
nucleus but no other conspicuous cytologic features. They often envelop type I cells. The carotid
body is innervated by sensory nerves carried
within the **sinus nerve,** a branch of the glos-
sopharyngeal nerve. Most of the axons in the sinus nerve are unmyelinated. The sinus nerve
also innervates the carotid sinus. In addition,
the carotid body has neural connections (gan-
glioglomerular nerves) with the superior cervical
ganglion. These sensory nerves innervate the
type I cells. The transducing mechanism by
which chemical changes in the blood provoke a
response from the carotid body is still controversial. Researchers have proposed two opposing
theories. In one theory the type I cell is the
chemoreceptor; in the other theory the sensory
nerve is the chemoreceptor. However, if dop-

amine is released into the circulation by type I
cells in response to reduced oxygen–carbon dioxide tension or reduced pH in the blood, it may
help to alleviate this condition by reducing vascular resistance and increasing cardiac output
and systolic blood pressure.

The **aortic bodies** are also sensitive to oxygen–
carbon dioxide tension in the blood. They are
histologically similar to the carotid body and are
commonly located in the roof of the aortic arch as
well as in the angle of the subclavian and common carotid arteries on the right.

LYMPHATIC VESSELS

While the blood vessels represent a closed circulation, the lymphatic vessels are simply a **drainage
system.** Lymphatic capillaries end blindly in connective tissue spaces and conduct an ultrafiltrate
of blood plasma, called **lymph,** back to the blood.
Interposed in the lymphatics are a series of
lymph nodes where lymphoid cells proliferate. As
lymph passes through the nodes, the lymph flow
is joined by lymphoid cells and their products
(antibodies). The lymph passes through the
larger lymphatic vessels and the lymphatic ducts,
which join the great veins of the neck. Thus, the
lymphatic system is essential in returning to the
blood water, electrolytes, and proteins, which
have seeped out during metabolic exchanges. In
addition, it supplies the blood with lymphoid
cells and antibodies, which are produced by (or
circulate through) the lymph nodes. Insufficient
drainage by lymphatic vessels results in fluid accumulation in connective tissue; this swelling is
known as **edema.**

Lymphatic capillaries are more variable in size
and shape than blood capillaries, and they are
usually larger in caliber. Unlike blood capillaries,
they branch and anastomose extensively and do
not have perivascular cells associated with them.
Extracellular filaments called **lymphatic anchoring filaments** terminate in the external membrane of the endothelial cells, giving the thin
lymphatics some structural support. Larger
lymphatics resemble veins, except that their lumen diameter is even larger in relation to their

very thin walls, which are composed of endo-thelium (tunica intima), a few smooth muscle cells (tunica media), and a few bundles of collage-nous and elastic fibers (tunica adventitia). Like veins, the lymphatics rely on a system of valves and external musculature to aid in the flow of lymph. The **lymphatic valves** are more closely spaced than venous valves. The **lymphatic ducts** (the thoracic duct and the right lymphatic duct) possess significantly more smooth muscle and elastic fibers in the tunica media. The tunica ad-ventitia, like that of the large veins, contains a longitudinal array of smooth muscle bundles.

ATHEROSCLEROSIS

The pathogenesis of atherosclerosis remains to be fully clarified. It is a lesion of the vascular wall that begins with the deposition of low-density-derived cholesterol esters in the intima. The di-etary intake of these lipids is sufficient to over-load portions of the vascular wall due to factors that are not yet appreciated. As a result the lipids are deposited within the extracellular matrix. Monocytes are believed to migrate into the site, differentiate into macrophages, and phagocytize the lipids. The accumulated lipids are visible with the microscope as profuse vacuoles in the cytoplasm of these macrophages and become known as **foam cells** because of their vacuolated appearance. Smooth muscle cells also accumu-late a smaller portion of the lipids. In addition, it is speculated that a number of multipotential mesenchymal cells called **myointimal cells** also become engorged with lipids. It still remains to identify with certainty all the cells involved at the developing atherosclerotic site (**atheroma**). Nevertheless, the accumulated lipids along the intima produce a yellow fatty streak that is vis-ible with the unaided eye when inspecting the vascular lumen. At this time the atheroma be-comes raised by the accumulated lipids and the cellular infiltration of macrophages. This causes a protrusion of the intima into the bloodstream where sheer forces produced by blood flow may be too high for the endothelium to survive. Damage to the endothelium exposes subendo-thelial basement lamina which is known to have a high affinity for platelets. The attached platelets release platelet-derived growth factor (PDGF) which causes proliferation of nearby vas-cular smooth muscle. This further raises the le-sion and the newly proliferated smooth muscle cells may have unusual constrictive responses to normal vasoactive hormones. Although this last event has not been demonstrated it may be re-sponsible for the vasospasms that occur near dis-eased vessel segments. The fibrocollagenous cap built up over the lesion may be due to the synthe-sis and deposition by the myointimal cells. In various types of atherosclerosis, calcification of the media occurs, a feature of many necrotic tis-sue reactions.

The clot initiated at the site of the atheroma (**mural thrombus**) may become detached from the vascular wall, flow downstream, and occlude the lumen of a smaller vessel. The resulting isch-emic necrosis of tissue where the blood supply has been interrupted is known as an infarct. It is what occurs during a heart attack if the event occurs within the coronary blood vessels, or a stroke if the event occurs within a blood vessel to the brain.

NATIONAL BOARD TYPE QUESTIONS

Select the single best response for each of the following.

1. The basal lamina surrounding the endothe-lium is incomplete or missing around
   A. fenestrated capillaries.
   B. sinusoids.
   C. continuous capillaries.
   D. arterioles.
2. Which of the following vessels contain sig-nificant amounts of longitudinally oriented smooth muscle in the adventitia?
   A. Medium-sized arteries
   B. Small veins
   C. Large arteries
   D. Large veins

3. The tunica media occupied predominantly by elastic lamina with scattered smooth muscle cells throughout is characteristic of:
   A. Arterioles
   B. Medium-sized veins
   C. Large, conducting arteries
   D. Small veins

4. Autonomic ganglia occur in what layer of the muscular arteries?
   A. Intima
   B. Media
   C. Adventitia
   D. Lumen

For the following, select
   A. if only *1, 2, and 3* are correct.
   B. if only *1 and 3* are correct.
   C. if only *2 and 4* are correct.
   D. if only *4* is correct.
   E. if *all* are correct.

5. The glycocalyx associated with the endothelial surface of capillaries
   1. is negatively charged.
   2. consists of glycosaminoglycans.
   3. binds several plasma proteins.
   4. causes the endothelium to become leaky.

6. Which of the following endothelial specializations occur(s) along continuous capillaries of the blood-brain barrier?
   1. Interendothelial gaps
   2. Numerous fenestrations with diaphragms
   3. Numerous fenestrations without diaphragms
   4. Zonula occludens–type junctions

7. Which of the following are features of the carotid sinus?
   1. Its adventitia is innervated by sensory fibers from the ninth cranial nerve.
   2. Attenuation of the tunica media at the location of the sinus near the bifurcation of each common carotid artery.
   3. Its sensory nerves are stimulated during distention of the arterial wall caused by excessive blood pressure.
   4. It is primarily sensitive to oxygen and carbon dioxide levels in arterial blood.

8. Which of the following sites contain(s) smooth muscle?
   1. Precapillary sphincters
   2. Capillaries
   3. Adventitia of large veins
   4. Lymphatic capillaries

9. Arteriovenous shunts
   1. are histologically similar to arterioles.
   2. carry blood which bypasses a capillary bed.
   3. do not have capillary branches.
   4. interconnect an arteriole with a venule.

10. Valves are
   1. semilunar flaps with their free edge directed toward the heart.
   2. never found along lymphatic vessels.
   3. specializations of the tunica intima.
   4. seldom found along veins in the legs.

11. Medium-sized arteries are characterized by
   1. abundant circular smooth muscle in the media.
   2. external elastic lamina.
   3. abundant longitudinally arranged collagen in the adventitia.
   4. an internal elastic lamina.

ANNOTATED ANSWERS

1. B. For further discussion, refer to Capillaries, page 254.
2. D. The adventitia of the other choices is composed of varying amounts of longitudinally oriented connective tissue.
3. C. In other arterial segments elastic fibers are found mostly in the internal and external elastic laminae.
4. C. The vasomotor nerve plexuses also travel within the adventitia.
5. A. For further discussion, refer to page 257.
6. D. The other options are obviously interruptions in the endothelial wall.
7. A. Sensitivity to oxygen and carbon dioxide levels is a feature of chemoreceptors such as the carotid body.

8. B. Only the larger lymphatic vessels contain smooth muscle.
9. E.
10. B. Valves are particularly abundant in veins of the legs except in people with varicose veins.
11. E.

BIBLIOGRAPHY

Aviado, D. M., Jr., and C. F. Schmidt. Reflexes from stretch receptors in blood vessels, heart and lungs. *Physiol. Rev.* 35:247, 1955.

Baez, S. Microcirculation. *Ann. Rev. Physiol.* 39:391, 1977.

Benditt, E. P., and J. M. Benditt. Evidence for a monoclonal origin of human arthrosclerotic plaques. *Proc. Natl. Acad. Sci. U.S.A.* 70:1753, 1973.

Biscoe, T. J. Carotid body: Structure and function. *Physiol. Rev.* 51:437, 1971.

Boss, J., and J. H. Green. The histology of the common carotid baroreceptor areas of the cat. *Circ. Res.* 4:12, 1956.

Boyd, J. D. Observations on the human carotid sinus and the nerve supply. *Anat. Anz.* 84:386, 1937.

Dobrin, P. Mechanical properties of arteries. *Physiol. Rev.* 58:397, 1978.

Dobrin, P. B., and J. M. Doyle. Vascular smooth muscle and the anisotrophy of dog carotid artery. *Circ. Res.* 27:105, 1970.

Keith, A., and M. Flack. The auriculoventricular bundle of the human heart. *Lancet* 2:359, 1906.

Kent, S. Researches on the structure and function of the mammalian heart. *J. Physiol.* 14:233, 1893.

Landis, E. M. Heteroporosity of the capillary wall as indicated by cinematographic analysis of the passage of dye. *Ann. N.Y. Acad. Sci.* 116:765, 1964.

Leak, L. V. Electron microscopic observations on lymphatic capillaries and the structural components of the connective tissue–lymph interface. *Microvasc. Res.* 2:316, 1970.

Majno, G., and G. E. Palade. Studies on inflammation. II. The site of action of histamine and serotonin along the vascular tree: A topographic study. *J. Biophys. Biochem. Cytol.* 11:607, 1961.

Pease, D. C., and W. J. Paule. Electron microscopy of elastic arteries: The thoracic aorta of the rat. *J. Ultrastruct. Res.* 3:469, 1960.

Pritchard, M. M. L., and P. M. Daniel. Arterio-venous anastomoses in the human external ear. *J. Anat.* 90:309, 1956.

Rhodin, J. A. G. The ultrastructure of mammalian arterioles and precapillary sphincters. *J. Ultrastruct. Res.* 18:181, 1967.

Rhodin, J. A. G. Ultrastructure of mammalian venous capillaries, venules, and small collecting veins. *J. Ultrastruct. Res.* 25:452, 1968.

Rhodin, J. A. G., P. Delmissier, and L. C. Reid. The structure of the specialized conducting system of the steer heart. *Circulation* 24:349, 1961.

Roach, M. R. Biophysical analyses of blood vessel walls and blood flow. *Ann. Rev. Physiol.* 39:51, 1977.

Robertson, A. L., Jr., and P. A. Khairallah. Arterial endothelial permeability and vascular disease. *Exp. Mol. Pathol.* 18:241, 1973.

Ross, R., and J. A. Glomset. The pathogenesis of atherosclerosis. *N. Engl. J. Med.* 295:369(Pt. I), 420(Pt. II), 1976.

Simionescu, M., N. Simionescu, and G. E. Palade. Morphometric data on the endothelium of blood capillaries. *J. Cell Biol.* 60:128, 1974.

Simionescu, M., N. Simionescu, and G. E. Palade. Segmental differentiations of cell junctions in the vascular endothelium. The microvasculature. *J. Cell Biol.* 67:863, 1975.

Simionescu, N., M. Simionescu, and G. E. Palade. Structural-functional correlates in the transendothelial exchange of water-soluble macromolecules. *Thromb. Res.* 8 (Suppl. 2):257, 1976.

Simionescu, N., M. Simionescu, and G. E. Palade. Differentiated microdomains on the luminal surface of the capillary endothelium. I. Preferential distribution of anionic sites. *J. Cell Biol.* 90:605, 1981.

Takada, M. Electron microscopic observations on the passage of electrolyte solutions and trypan blue fluid through the walls of venules and capillaries of the venous side. *Nagoya Med.* 9:113, 1963.

Verna, A. Ultrastructure of the carotid body in the mammals. *Int. Rev. Cytol.* 60:271, 1979.

Wollard, H. H., and G. Weddell. The composition and distribution of vascular nerves in the extremities. *J. Anat.* 69:165, 1935.

12 Respiratory System

Objectives

You will learn the following in this chapter:

How to identify, in sequence, the various components of the conducting and respiratory portions of the respiratory system

The composition of the respiratory mucosa and how it provides the mucociliary clearance mechanism

The composition of the olfactory mucosa (compared to respiratory mucosa) and the cells responsible for olfaction

How to identify the distinguishing features of the pharynx and larynx

The layers and contents of the three major layers of the trachea

The various cell types found in the respiratory epithelium and a function for each

The pulmonary vasculature as to the pathway it follows to and from the areas of gas exchange

How to recognize the various segments of the bronchial passages based on key distinguishing features

How to illustrate the composition of an alveolar septum with special reference to the blood-air barrier

The specific functional features of the alveolar epithelium and pulmonary endothelium

Some specific features of the local defense mechanisms of the lung

---

The body depends on the respiratory system to provide oxygen for cellular metabolism and to eliminate carbon dioxide, the primary waste product of metabolism, from the cellular environment. The blood vascular system provides the transport system for gases between the body tissues and the lungs, where the actual exchange of gases takes place; thus respiratory and circulatory functions are closely interdependent.

The respiratory system proper is divided into conducting and respiratory portions. The **conducting portion** consists of the nasal cavity, the pharynx, the larynx, the trachea, and a system of

bronchi, which conduct air from the environment to the respiratory portion of the lungs. The conducting bronchi branch extensively within the lungs (intrapulmonary conducting passages), much as the arterial system branches. The smallest of these branches, the bronchioles, give rise to the **respiratory portion,** which arborizes further and contains the alveoli. Alveoli have ultrathin walls containing extensive capillary beds through which diffusion of gases can readily occur.

In addition, respiration is dependent on a ventilating mechanism, composed of the thoracic cage and the diaphragm, which functions as a bellows, moving air throughout the respiratory system proper.

The components of the respiratory system are illustrated in Figure 12-1.

THE CONDUCTING PORTION

The extrapulmonary conducting portion of the respiratory system, from the nasal cavity to the bronchi, is characterized by a ciliated pseudo-stratified columnar epithelium that is rich in goblet cells. The underlying loose connective tissue contains large numbers of mixed seromucous glands. As the intrapulmonary conducting passages branch and diminish in caliber, the seromucous glands gradually disappear, and the height of the epithelium decreases to a ciliated

simple columnar or cuboidal epithelium. The respiratory membrane of the conducting passages is well suited for entrapment, inactivation, and expulsion of inhaled contaminants that become trapped in the seromucous secretions bathing the epithelium. The seromucous secretion is of a suitable consistency to be moved easily by ciliary action. The cilia move in a wavelike motion, propelling the secretory product in an outward direction (toward the nasal cavity). This mechanical action eliminates inhaled particles and other environmental debris and is termed the **mucociliary clearance mechanism.**

Individuals who suffer from an **immobile cilia syndrome** have a genetic defect resulting in incomplete ciliary composition. They lack either the dynein arms or radial spokes which connect the central pair of microtubules to those of the periphery. Such individuals are prone to chronic lung infections.

The seromucous secretions humidify the air, absorb and detoxify soluble gases, and provide

Fig. 12-1. The components of the respiratory system and their anatomic relationships.

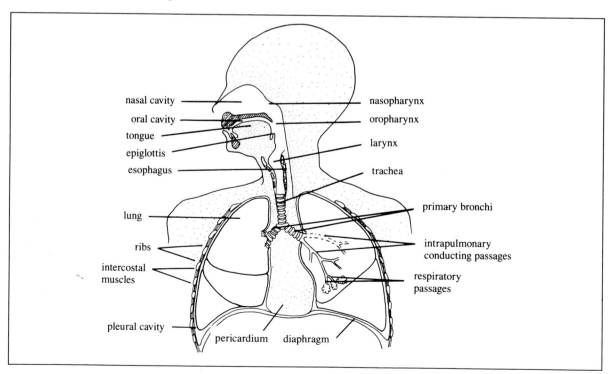

the first line of defense against invasive pathogens. The connective tissue beneath the epithelium (the lamina propria) is rich in lymphoid cells, which form diffuse aggregates and often permeate the epithelium above. Many of these cells produce a secretory immunoglobulin (secretory IgA), which is transported across the epithelium and is effective in killing bacteria and viruses, preventing them from penetrating the epithelium.

Changes in air pressure occur within the conducting passages during inhalation and exhalation. Bone in the walls of the nasal cavities and cartilage in the walls of the larynx, trachea, and bronchi impart a degree of rigidity sufficient to withstand such changes in pressure, preventing collapse or overexpansion. Elastic fibers provide a degree of deformability, permitting elongation of conducting tubes during inhalation, and recoil during passive exhalation. Regulation of aeration volume in response to physiologic demand for oxygen is provided by smooth muscle in the walls of the intrapulmonary conducting passages (secondary bronchi and bronchioles), which is controlled by the autonomic nervous system. Parasympathetic neurons induce muscle contraction, resulting in decrease in luminal diameter and consequently a decrease in aeration volume. Sympathetic neurons induce relaxation of the smooth muscle, resulting in an increase in luminal diameter and thus an increase in aeration volume.

Nasal Cavity

The nasal cavity is a bilaterally symmetric structure separated by the nasal septum. The nasal cavity is separated from the oral cavity by the hard palate. In addition to the **respiratory mucosa** characteristic of this system, the nasal cavity houses the **olfactory mucosa,** which is specialized to receive and transmit stimuli of smell.

THE RESPIRATORY MUCOSA

The respiratory mucosa is composed of a ciliated pseudostratified columnar epithelium and a well-developed underlying connective tissue layer, the lamina propria (Fig. 12-2). Goblet cells are abundant, but unevenly distributed throughout the epithelium. Numerous branched tubuloalveolar glands, resembling small seromucous salivary glands, extend into the underlying connective tissue. The glandular acini are supplied by both sensory and secretomotor nerve endings. A similar arrangement occurs throughout most of the other conducting passages.

Small blood vessels are abundant in the lamina propria. This rich blood supply warms the incoming air. The main respiratory arteries give rise to superficial arcading branches, which in turn give off arterioles that supply a network of capillaries just beneath the epithelium and around the seromucous glands. These capillaries are of the fenestrated variety, allowing rapid diffusion of materials such as gases and nutrients. A similar fenestrated capillary arrangement is found throughout the remaining conducting

Fig. 12-2. The respiratory mucosa. The mucosa of the upper respiratory passages consists of pseudostratified columnar epithelium (*Ep*) with cilia and goblet cells. The underlying lamina propria (*LP*) consists of loose connective tissue and frequently contains large numbers of lymphoid cells, as it does in this instance.

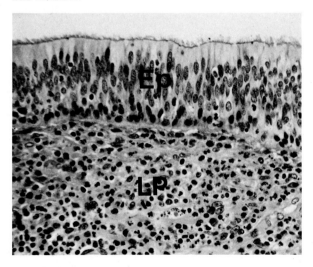

passages. Veins are in close association with the arteries and arteriovenous anastomoses are common in this region. The lymphatic drainage is also well developed.

In some regions the veins resemble erectile tissue and are referred to as **swell bodies.** These specialized veins engorge periodically and alternately occlude one side of the nasal cavity, thereby allowing the nasal mucosa time to recover from desiccation. This cyclic process is under autonomic nervous system control.

THE OLFACTORY MUCOSA

The olfactory mucosa of humans is limited to the roof of the nasal cavity and the upper part of the nasal septum. It is much more extensive in keen-scented animals. The pseudostratified columnar epithelium in this region is thicker than that of the respiratory mucosa. The glands beneath the olfactory epithelium are purely serous, providing a fluid solvent for odoriferous substances. The serous secretions are rapidly washed away, clearing the receptors for new sensory stimuli.

The smell receptors themselves are found at the apical end of certain modified cells of the olfactory epithelium called **olfactory cells.** The other cells are supporting cells. The **supporting cells** are tall with apically located nuclei and often resemble secretory cells. The **basal cells** are short, round cells located at the basal lamina of the epithelium. Basal cells are undifferentiated cells that can divide and differentiate into either of the other two types. Together, the three cell types compose a pseudostratified epithelium that is somewhat thicker than that of the respiratory region (Fig. 12-3).

The olfactory cells are bipolar neurons. The apical portion, a modified dendrite, ends at the

Fig. 12-3. The olfactory epithelium.

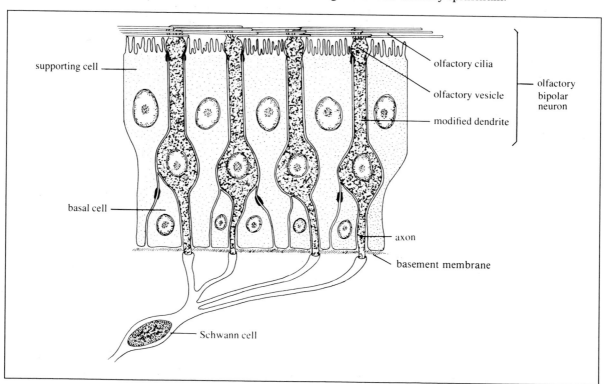

surface of the epithelium in a bulb (the **olfactory knob**) that gives rise to several extremely long cilia. These cilia are nonmotile and usually lie flat against the epithelial surface, rendering them inconspicuous in light microscopic observation. The cilia possess the receptors for smell; olfactory stimulation induces the depolarization of the plasma membrane of the cilia; the impulse is transmitted down the axon of the olfactory cell on the basal side. The axon extends through the basement membrane to join those of other olfactory cells, forming small nerve fascicles. These fascicles join to form about 20 bundles of the olfactory nerve, termed **fila olfactoria,** which pass through the cribriform plate of the ethmoid bone to enter the brain.

The histophysiology of olfaction has not been well elucidated since it is not known precisely how olfactory cells become stimulated or how they are able to discriminate among the extremely wide range of odors. Stimulation of the olfactory cell apparently results from depolarization of the plasmalemma covering the cilia. Scented substances added to the surface of the olfactory mucosa result in a change in electrical potential along the olfactory nerves. There is suggestive evidence that olfactory discrimination is based on the shape of the stimulating molecules. This is the basis of the **stereochemical theory of olfaction,** which suggests that there may be specific receptor proteins along the olfactory cell surface.

The Pharynx

The pharynx is divided into two portions. The first portion, the **nasopharynx,** is continuous with the nasal cavity and is separated from the oral cavity by the soft palate. The lower portion, the **oropharynx,** is both a respiratory and a digestive passage. The mucosa of the nasopharynx, therefore, is similar to the respiratory mucosa of the nasal cavity, a ciliated pseudostratified epithelium with goblet cells and associated seromucous glands. The mucosa of the oropharynx, on the other hand, is characteristic of the digestive tube, particularly the esophagus; thus, the epithelium in the oropharynx is of the stratified squamous variety and the associated glands are of the purely mucous type. Of immunologic import is the **pharyngeal tonsil** located at the roof of the nasopharynx. This tonsil, together with smaller lymphoid aggregates near the openings of the eustachian tubes (**tubal tonsils**), are known as the **adenoids.** Detailed descriptions of the tonsils and other gut-associated lymphoid tissue can be found in Chapter 10.

The Larynx

Below the oropharynx the respiratory and digestive passages separate once again. The larynx (Fig. 12-4) is located anterior to the esophagus and includes a valvelike structure, the **epiglottis,** which prevents food from entering the respiratory passage. The epiglottis contains a core of elastic cartilage attached to the hyoid bone. During swallowing, it closes the opening to the larynx. The larynx also contains the **vocal cords** and is the organ of phonation.

The larynx is a hollow, bilaterally symmetric structure framed by plates of hyaline cartilage and muscle. The **thyroid cartilage** (Adam's apple) protects the anterior aspect, while a smaller, ringlike cartilage, the **cricoid cartilage,** joins the base of the larynx to the trachea. There are several small, paired cartilages as well. These cartilages are held together by skeletal muscle, the **intrinsic muscles,** and dense connective tissue, while the **extrinsic muscles** attach the larynx to the adjacent structures of the throat. The intrinsic muscles alter the shape of the laryngeal cavity and, together with the vocalis muscle, affect the size of the opening between the vocal cords. The mucosa within the larynx forms three pairs of lateral folds reinforced by dense connective tissue cores that project into the laryngeal cavity: superior **aryepiglottic folds,** middle **ventricular folds** (false vocal cords), and the **true vocal cords.** Between the ventricular folds and the vocal cords the walls recess to form the laryngeal ventricles (see Fig. 12-4). The interaction of both vocal cord tension and the shape of the larynx determines the pitch of the sound

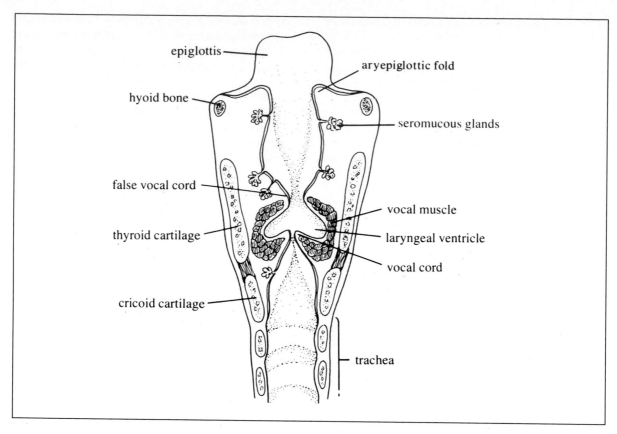

Fig. 12-4. A frontal section of the larynx.

made as the passage of air vibrates the vocal cords.

The mucosa of the larynx is composed primarily of ciliated pseudostratified epithelium, with associated seromucous glands dispersed throughout the lamina propria. However, the stratified squamous epithelium of the pharynx extends into portions of the larynx, where it covers the aryepiglottic folds and part of the epiglottis. The balance of the laryngeal surface is covered by the ciliated pseudostratified variety characteristic of the laryngobronchial mucosa (discussed in more detail later).

The Trachea and Primary Bronchi

The trachea (windpipe) is a rigid tube composed of 16 to 20 segments, each containing a U-shaped piece of hyaline cartilage joined at the free ends and to one another by bands of smooth muscle, the **trachealis muscle,** which runs in a transverse and oblique longitudinal direction (Figs. 12-5, 12-6). The cartilage-free "soft" portion rests against the esophagus posteriorly. The cartilaginous rings are joined together by intersegmental dense connective tissue composed of collagen and elastic fibers that are continuous with the perichondrium of each cartilage ring.

The trachea branches into two primary bronchi, one to each lung. Histologically, the trachea and primary bronchi are very similar, although

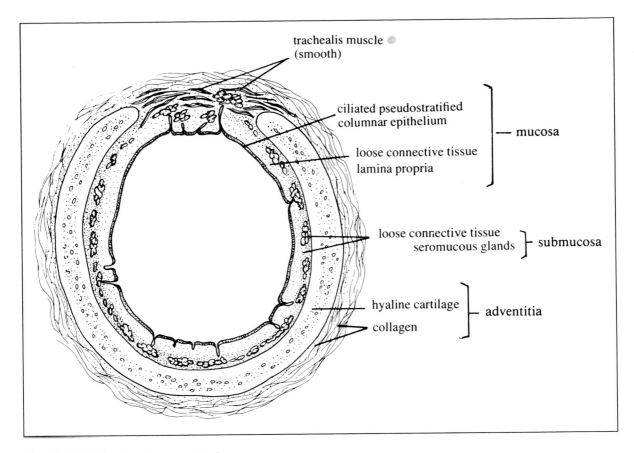

Fig. 12-5. The trachea (cross section).

the cartilage becomes less regular in the distal ends of the primary bronchi. In cross section, they exhibit a well-defined layer pattern that is characteristic of most hollow organs (see Figs. 12-5, 12-6). Each can be subdivided into three layers as follows:

1. Mucosa. The epithelium is the ciliated pseudostratified type, with abundant goblet cells, resting on a thick basement membrane. The lamina propria is composed of loose connective tissue with a significant amount of elastic and reticular fibers and lymphoid cells.

An elastic membrane separates the mucosa from the submucosa. At the distal ends of the primary bronchi the elastic membrane is replaced by a complete ring of smooth muscle, the muscularis mucosa.

2. Submucosa. The submucosa is a loose connective tissue layer containing numerous seromucous glands. Their long ducts project through the mucosa to the lumen. Stellate-shaped myoepithelial cells surround the acini and extend onto part of the ducts.

3. Adventitia. The outer layer contains the U-shaped cartilage and some dense connective tissue. In the "open" region, the submucosal glands tend to be interspersed with the smooth muscle fibers of the trachealis muscle.

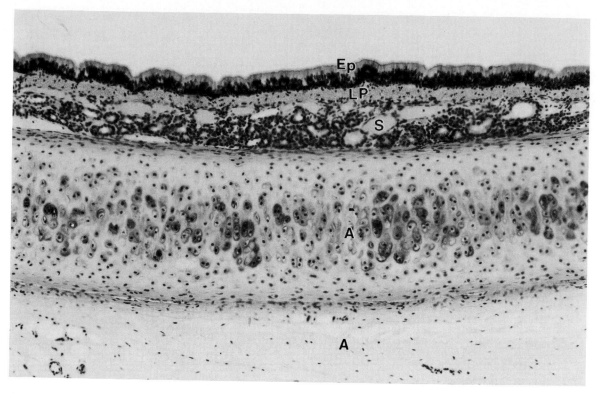

Fig. 12-6. Light micrograph through cartilagenous portion of the trachea. Note the respiratory epithelium (*Ep*) and the underlying lamina propria (*LP*). The submucosa (*S*) contains many seromucous glands, while the adventitia (*A*) contains the cartilage and surrounding connective tissue.

Viewed with the light microscope, the tracheal epithelium appears as a typical pseudostratified epithelium, consisting of ciliated columnar cells, goblet cells, and basal cells with mitotic potential. Two additional cell types can be identified by electron microscopy, **brush cells** and **small granule cells.** Brush cells possess microvilli rather than cilia and are thought to be either immature columnar cells or degranulated goblet cells. A small number of brush cells possess epitheliodendritic synapses with the underlying nerves and therefore are considered to be some

kind of sensory receptors. Small granule cells are located in the basal portion of the epithelium and are filled with small, dense-core granules. Histochemical techniques reveal two general classes of small granule cells. Those that produce catecholamines (epinephrine and norepinephrine) occur in small clusters and appear to be innervated by cholinergic fibers. This class of cells is referred to as **neurosecretory cells.** The second class of cells is known as **protein hormone–secreting cells,** which resemble the enteroendocrine (argentaffin) cells of the alimentary tract. However, the specific cell products and the distribution of cell types in the respiratory tract have not been clearly elucidated. Both classes of secretory cells take up amine precursors and are part of the diffuse neuroendocrine system (see last section, Chap. 17). These cells are also found throughout the epithelia and associated glands of the other bronchial conducting passages. The epithelia of the larynx, trachea, and the bronchi are often referred to collectively as the **laryngo-bronchial epithelium.**

The primary bronchi give rise to several orders of intrapulmonary conducting passages, which in turn give rise to several successive orders of respiratory tubes. The distinguishing features of these passages are summarized in Table 12-1. As the diameter of the passages diminishes, certain histologic structures are modified, corresponding to the lung's functional role at that level. Before we discuss the intrapulmonary bronchial passages, let us first consider the lungs as complete organs.

The Lungs

The lungs are paired organs that are suspended in the pleural cavities of the thorax and covered by a thick, elastic serous membrane known as the **visceral pleura.** The connective tissue within the lungs is rich in elastic fibers and smooth muscle, which permits the lungs to expand when the negative intrathoracic pressure is increased during inspiration. **Elastic recoil** plays a major role in contraction of the lung during expiration.

A primary bronchus and the pulmonary vessels enter each lung at the **hilus.** The right lung has three **lobes** and the left lung two, each lobe receiving a branch of a primary bronchus. Each lobe is subdivided into bronchopulmonary segments, subsegments, and finally into **lobules** of pyramidal shape, arranged pointing superiorly toward the hilus. The base of each lobule faces the surface of the lung. Each subunit is separated by connective tissue septa (Fig. 12-7). The bronchopulmonary segments are not only separated by connective tissue septa but carry their own blood supply. Since the few anomalies that occur in the segments are predictable, the surgeon is able to remove a small diseased segment of the lung while leaving the rest of the organ intact.

The internal structure of the lungs consists of a branching system of conducting passages referred to as the **bronchial tree.**

Table 12-1. Distinguishing Features of the Conducting and Respiratory Passages

	Trachea / primary bronchi	Secondary bronchi	Bronchiole	Respiratory bronchiole	Alveolar duct	Alveolar sac
Position in reference to lung	EXTRAPULMONARY	INTRAPULMONARY				
Mucosa — epithelium	ciliated pseudostratified columnar epithelium	→ ciliated simple columnar	→	ciliated simple cuboidal / simple squamous lining alveoli	→ diffuse	
Mucosa — muscularis mucosa	none	→ diffuse	→ relatively thick	→ thinner		
Submucosa — seromucous glands	numerous	→ sparse	→ none			
Adventitia — cartilage	U-shaped	plates and islands	none			
Presence of alveoli	none			few →	many	
	CONDUCTING PORTION			RESPIRATORY PORTION		

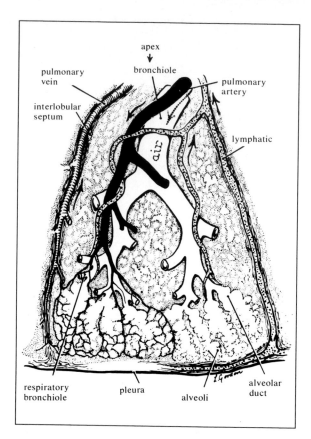

Fig. 12-7. A lobule of the lung, with its base abutting the pleura. The size of the bronchioles and the air passages, as well as that of the blood and lymphatic vessels, is out of proportion. To make it easier to follow the course of the blood vessels and the lymphatics, the former have been omitted from the right side and the latter from the left side. (From A. W. Ham and D. H. Cormack, *Histology* [8th ed.]. Philadelphia: Lippincott, 1979. Reproduced with permission.)

THE PULMONARY VESSELS

The **pulmonary artery** enters the hilus with the primary bronchi and follows the precise branching pattern of these intrapulmonary conducting passages. Thus in cross section, the two structures are always in close alignment and usually share part of their adventitia (see Fig. 12-11). The pulmonary artery and its branches are rather thin-walled, as compared with arteries of similar caliber in the systemic circulation; this is primarily because the pulmonary blood pressure is much lower than that of the systemic circulation.

At the level of the respiratory passages, the branches of the pulmonary artery break up into the alveolar capillaries (Fig. 12-8). The **venous return** follows a separate course from the artery, however. The alveolar capillaries coalesce into small veins in the interlobular septa and join other branches in the intersegmental, interlobular, and bronchopulmonary septa. The bronchopulmonary veins coalesce to form the pulmonary vein. The pulmonary vein finally associates with the artery at the hilus.

The conducting tubes are themselves vascularized by branches of the descending aorta, the **bronchial arteries,** whose small branches are found in their adventitia, much like the vasa vasorum of large blood vessels. Branches of the bronchial arteries terminate at the level of the respiratory bronchioles where they anastomose with branches of the pulmonary arteries. Bronchial veins are present only at the hilus on the dorsal surface of the extrapulmonary bronchi where they drain the bronchial arteries and the visceral pleura. Arteriovenous anastomoses between the bronchial and pulmonary arteries are also present.

Precapillary arterioles are subject to vasoconstriction due to hypoxia. This may be a mechanism for redirecting blood flow away from lobules that are poorly ventilated to those that are sufficiently ventilated. The vasoconstriction is a direct physiologic response to low partial pressure of oxygen. Although definitive chemoreceptors in the pulmonary vasculature for governing

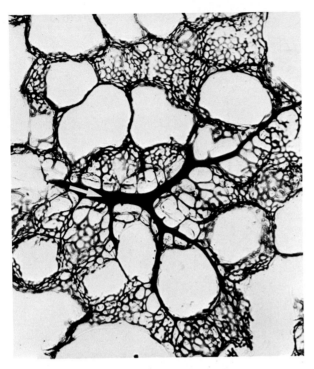

Fig. 12-8. In this preparation, the pulmonary artery was perfused with a latex material. The micrograph shows a terminal branch of the pulmonary artery (*white arrow in direction of blood flow*) giving off a capillary plexus around each of the alveoli in the area. Some alveoli are cut through their walls, advantageously demonstrating the capillary beds.

this response have not been found, the search continues. However, there is a glomuslike structure associated with the pulmonary trunk that histologically resembles the carotid and aortic bodies, which are chemoreceptor organs (see Chap. 11). Its epithelioid cells are innervated by vagal and sympathetic fibers from the deep cardiac plexus. However, its physiologic function is not fully understood.

The lungs possess both a **superficial** and a **deep lymphatic drainage.** The superficial vessels follow the veins in the connective tissue septa, while the deep vessels are associated with the bronchial tree.

The Bronchial Passages

The primary bronchi give rise to several orders of secondary bronchi. The first branches supply each of the pulmonary lobes, three to the right and two to the left. The smaller subdivisions of the secondary bronchi are distributed to the 18 bronchopulmonary segments. Within the bronchopulmonary segments, the branching of the bronchial tree continues for 9 to 12 generations before reaching the respiratory portion.

The tubes of the bronchial tree are classified by three criteria: (1) the diameter of the tube, (2) the number of generations away from the primary bronchus, and (3) the histologic characteristics of the tube wall. We shall concentrate primarily on the third criterion in discussing the features of the bronchial tree.

SECONDARY BRONCHI

Several orders of secondary bronchi represent the first **intrapulmonary** conducting passages. Histologically, the secondary bronchi resemble the primary bronchi and trachea. However, instead of having a continuous piece of cartilage, they possess several smaller discontinuous **cartilaginous plates** in their adventitia. Thus, the rigidity of the conducting tubes is somewhat diminished. The seromucous glands of the submucosa tend to pouch out wherever there is no cartilage, with the result that the two outer layers become less distinct (Figs. 12-9, 12-10).

At this level, the mucosa is composed of ciliated pseudostratified epithelium. After several generations of branching, it diminishes in height. The lamina propria is rich in all connective tissue fiber types and lymphoid cells. Separating the lamina propria from the submucosa is a prominent smooth muscle band interlaced with elastic fibers, the **muscularis mucosa,** which courses in a spiral fashion. The mucosa exhibits marked longitudinal folding when the muscularis mucosa contracts. With successive branching of the secondary bronchi, the cartilaginous component of the adventitia diminishes, while the muscularis mucosa thickens.

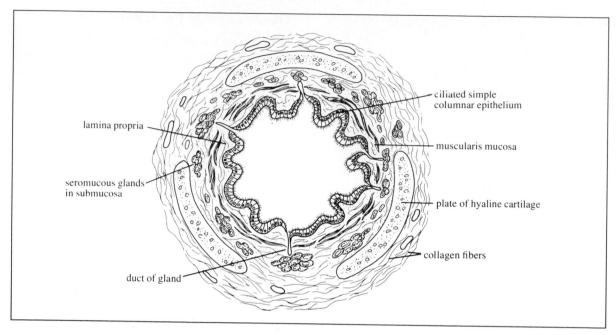

Fig. 12-9. A secondary bronchus (diagram of cross section). This diagram represents a much higher magnification than does Figure 12-5.

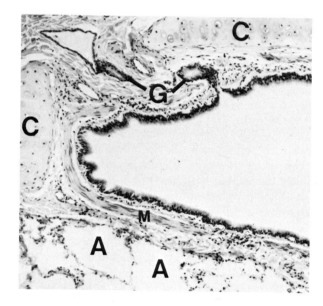

Fig. 12-10. A light micrograph of a secondary bronchus. The muscularis mucosa (*M*) is fairly well developed. Cartilaginous plates (*C*) and seromucous glands (*G*) are present in the outer layers. Alveoli (*A*) are seen adjacently.

It is important to note that there is a gradual transition from one type of passage to another, and thus histologic identification is arbitrary. For example, the last generation of secondary bronchi may possess a few small cartilage plates that may not appear in section, and these secondary bronchi may therefore appear to be bronchioles.

BRONCHIOLES

The last order of secondary bronchi gives rise to several orders of bronchioles (Figs. 12-11, 12-12, 12-13). The tube diameters gradually decrease, and the structure of the walls is simplified. Un-

like the bronchi, bronchioles possess no cartilage plates and very few submucosal seromucous glands. What is left is essentially the mucosa, surrounded by a bit of loose connective tissue (adventitia).

The epithelium is simple columnar. Cilia are still present, but goblet cells gradually disappear distally and are replaced by dome-shaped secretory cells, known as **Clara cells** or simply **bronchiolar secretory cells.** Although their precise function is largely unknown, they possess numerous electron-dense granules that are secreted by exocytosis and contain a proteinaceous substance. Since bronchiolar closure occurs in late expiration, it is thought that reopening may require a lining that is not sticky and has a low surface tension, which the Clara cells provide. The muscularis mucosa is relatively thick in the bronchioles. Elastic fibers increase in number in the lamina propria and among the smooth muscle cells of the muscularis mucosa. These modifications reflect the capacity of bronchioles to alter their luminal diameters. These features are particularly prominent in the last generation of

Fig. 12-11. A low-magnification light micrograph of the lung showing two secondary bronchi (*SB*). Arrows point to the cartilage plates. The associated pulmonary artery (*PA*) branches with the bronchial passages. A bronchiole (*B*) is seen originating from one of the secondary bronchi. It, too, begins to branch before leaving the plane of section. Surrounding these structures are numerous alveoli.

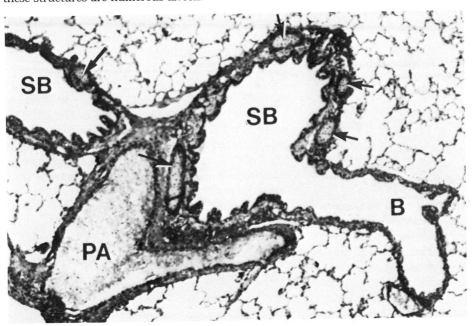

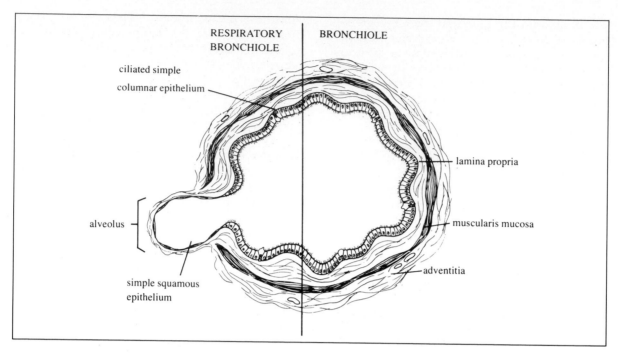

RESPIRATORY
BRONCHIOLE

BRONCHIOLE

ciliated simple

columnar epithelium

lamina propria

alveolus

muscularis mucosa

simple squamous
epithelium

adventitia

Fig. 12-12. A composite of a bronchiole and a respiratory bronchiole (cross section). This diagram represents a much higher magnification than does Figure 12-9.

bronchioles, the **terminal bronchioles,** which give rise to the respiratory portion of the bronchial tree.

The distinguishing features of the conducting and respiratory passages are summarized in Table 12-1.

THE RESPIRATORY PORTION

The terminal bronchioles give rise to two orders of **respiratory bronchioles.** Histologically, they resemble conducting bronchioles, except that they bear thin-walled outpouchings, the **alveoli,** in the part of their walls that is not in contact with the pulmonary artery. Ciliated cuboidal epithelium is still present between alveoli. The muscularis mucosa, heavily laced with elastic

fibers, spirals beneath the epithelium. The number of alveoli increases with each branching. The respiratory bronchioles give rise to the **alveolar ducts** (Fig. 12-14). Here the walls are filled with alveolar outpouchings, without intervening patches of cuboidal epithelium. The tubular shape of the passage still remains, however. What is left of the muscularis mucosa forms a dispersed, anastomosing pattern in the alveolar walls. Smooth muscle cells are somewhat more concentrated at the alveolar openings. The alveolar ducts terminate in a number of **alveolar sacs.** The alveolar sacs are thin-walled structures that contain reticular and elastic fibers but no smooth muscle. Each sac is composed of several alveoli opening into a common chamber, the **atrium** (Fig. 12-15).

The Alveoli

Alveoli are delicate, cup-shaped structures that are lined by an extremely attenuated simple

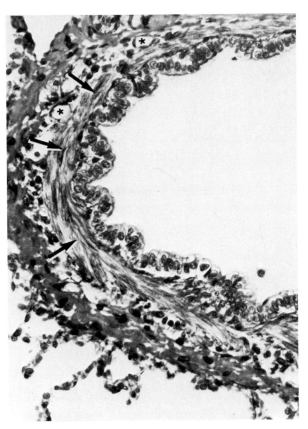

Fig. 12-10. A light micrograph of a bronchiole showing a relatively simple conducting passage wall consisting of a simple columnar ciliated epithelium, a thin lamina propria, and a well-developed muscularis mucosa (*arrows*). The adjacent adventitia contains a number of blood and lymphatic vessels (*asterisks*).

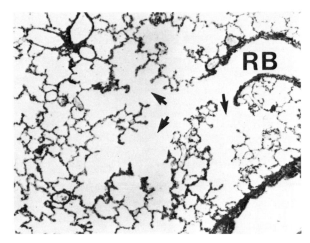

Fig. 12-14. A low-magnification light micrograph of the beginning respiratory portion of the lung, where a respiratory bronchiole (*RB*) is seen giving rise to several alveolar ducts (*arrows*).

squamous epithelium. A single wall, the **interalveolar septum,** is formed between adjacent alveoli. The septum is composed of living cells of adjacent alveoli and the connective tissue between them, which contains numerous reticular and elastic fibers; a few leukocytes, mast cells, and fibroblasts; and an anastomosing network of capillaries. Another cell type, known as the **septal cell,** is also present in the alveolar interstitium, although it superficially resembles the

fibroblast and is thought to have functions related to maintenance of pulmonary connective tissue. Septal cells contain bundles of actin and myosin filaments and contract in response to hypoxia. Whether the septal cells play some physiologic role in the ventilation-perfusion mechanism is unknown.

The alveoli intercommunicate through **alveolar pores,** which equilibrate the air pressure within a lobule and through which infections may spread. Following severe pulmonary infection, the thin connective tissue spaces enlarge and become infiltrated with a variety of inflammatory cells, which immigrate from the blood. Mast cells contribute to the response by releasing histamine, which enhances vascular permeability.

The alveoli are lined by two cell types that are continuous with each other: squamous **alveolar epithelial cells (type I)** and somewhat rounded, cuboidal **secretory cells (type II).** The type I cell is extremely attenuated. At the point where the thin-walled (but continuous) capillaries come in close contact with the epithelium, the endothe-

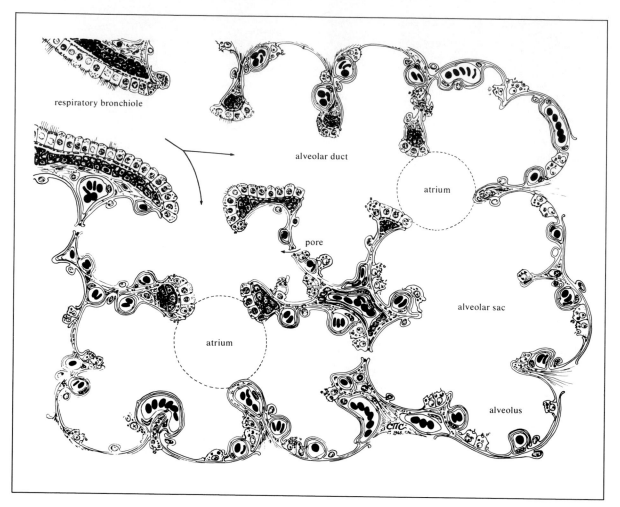

Fig. 12-15. The respiratory unit of the lung: respiratory bronchiole, alveolar ducts, alveolar sacs, and alveoli. The atria indicated by the circles are spaces bounded on one side by the termination of the alveolar duct and on the other by the openings of the alveolar sacs. (After S. Sorokin. In R. O. Greep and L. Weiss [eds.]. *Histology* [4th ed.]. New York: McGraw-Hill, 1977. Reproduced with permission.)

lial cells and type I epithelial cells share a common basement membrane. These form the **alveolar membrane,** the barrier through which gases must pass in the exchange between blood and air (Fig. 12-16). The type II cell contains an organelle complement characteristic of a secretory cell. Especially prominent in type II cells are the **multilamellar bodies** or **cytosomes** (Fig. 12-17). Multilamellar bodies are similar to lysosomes in appearance and in fact possess some lysosomal enzymes. In this regard, they may be considered homologues of residual bodies found in other

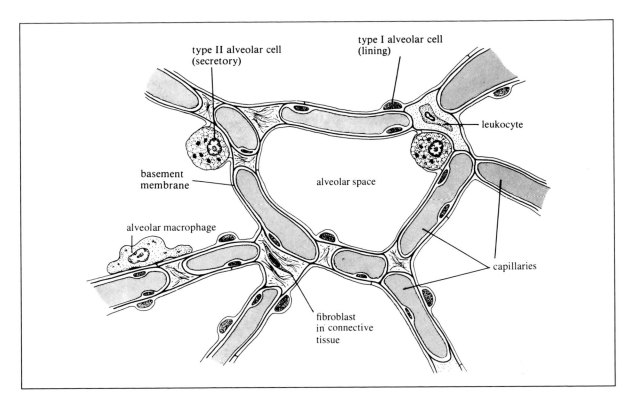

type II alveolar cell (secretory)

type I alveolar cell (lining)

leukocyte

basement membrane

alveolar space

alveolar macrophage

capillaries

fibroblast in connective tissue

Fig. 12-16. An electron microscopic representation of the walls of several alveoli, showing the alveolar membrane, capillaries, and associated cells.

cells. However, multilamellar bodies contain other proteins, as well as some glycosaminoglycans and large amounts of phospholipids. This phospholipid-rich secretion is known as **surfactant.** About 75 to 85 percent of the phospholipids is phosphatidyl choline, which is a surface-active component of surfactant. Surfactant spreads along the epithelial surface, where it forms latticelike complexes with the protein, tubular myelin. It then spreads into a thin film that reduces surface tension at the air-fluid interface. This action stabilizes alveolar diameters, thus preventing their collapse during expiration. As alveolar diameters decrease, the surface concentration is increased and surface tension is reduced. Prema-

ture infants often succumb to **respiratory distress syndrome,** which results from inadequate surfactant production by an immature secretory system.

The Pulmonary Endothelium

The pulmonary endothelium is continuous and nonfenestrated. In addition to its passive role in gas exchange, the capillary endothelium of the lung plays a prominent role in a variety of metabolic functions. The endothelium of small arterioles and venules is also involved in some of these processes. Because the lung receives the entire cardiac output, it is well situated to interact with, alter, and add to the various blood components in a selective manner. The pulmonary endothelium plays an active part in the metabolic transformation of adenine nucleotides, li-

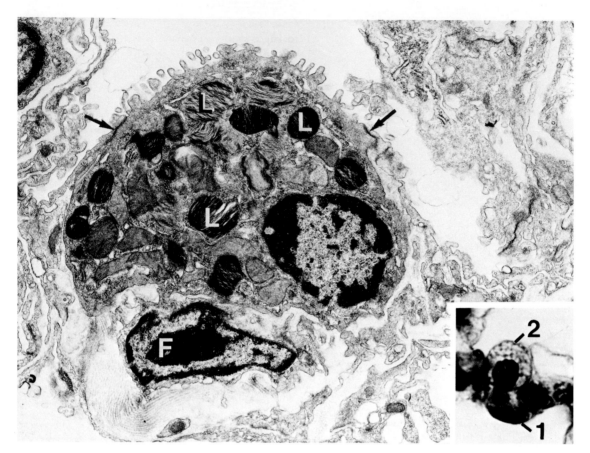

Fig. 12-17. An electron micrograph of a type II alveolar cell from the lung of a mouse. This spherical cell has short microvilli on its free surface and forms junctional complexes (*arrows*) with the adjacent thin type I alveolar epithelial cells that partially cover its surface. The cell contains numerous cisternae of granular endoplasmic reticulum and lamellar bodies (three of which are labeled *L*) in various stages of formation. These contain surfactant, which is secreted on the epithelial surface. In the interstitium below is a fibroblast (*F*). (Courtesy of K. Hitchcock.) Inset: Type I alveolar cell (*1*) and type II alveolar cell (*2*).

poproteins, and prostaglandins as well as the peptides, bradykinin and angiotensin I, and the biogenic amines, serotonin, norepinephrine, and acetylcholine. Many of these substances are metabolized almost completely in a single passage through the lung, suggesting that the metabolism occurs at or near the endothelial plasma membrane. The enzyme dipeptidyl carboxypeptidase, which converts angiotensin I to angiotensin II and inactivates bradykinin, is produced by the endothelial cells. The vasoactive effects of angiotensin II and the homeostatic mechanism of the renin-angiotensin system are discussed in Chapter 16.

LOCAL DEFENSE MECHANISM

Alveolar macrophages are commonly found in the interalveolar septa and on the alveoli themselves (Fig. 12-18, see also Fig. 12-16). In the respiratory passages, the macrophages play an important role in phagocytosis and disposal of particulate matter that reaches the alveoli. Bacteria and viruses are rapidly phagocytized and degraded by alveolar macrophages. Indigestible, inert particles, such as carbon, remain in macrophages for long periods, but they are eventually deposited in islands of collagen (scar tissue). Heavy exposure to asbestos, coal, and other industrial particles can result in pathologic accumulation of particles in such sites. In addition, such particles can also act as carriers for toxic gases, exposing the respiratory membranes to high concentrations of harmful substances. The alveolar fluids are also effective in neutralizing bacteria and viruses by carrying secretory IgA, interferon, and so forth, and by detoxifying harmful gases and organic vapors.

Alveolar macrophages also play a vital role in augmenting specific immune responses of local lymphoid cell populations and those of regional lymph nodes. Lymph nodes are particularly common around the hilus of each lung (hilar lymph nodes). Cigarette smoke and other noxious environmental agents interfere with the normal macrophage and immune functions of the lungs and may increase susceptibility to respiratory infections and other respiratory diseases (see Fig. 12-18).

Both humoral and cell-mediated immunity play a prominent role in the lung's defense against infection. B cells, T cells, macrophages, mast cells, and leukocytes produce various anti-

Fig. 12-18. Electron micrographs of alveolar macrophages obtained by bronchial lavage from the lungs of young adult human subjects. A. Alveolar macrophage of a nonsmoker. B. Alveolar macrophage of a smoker. Note secondary lysosomes filled with tar. (Courtesy of A. J. Ladman and J. B. DeLongo.)

A

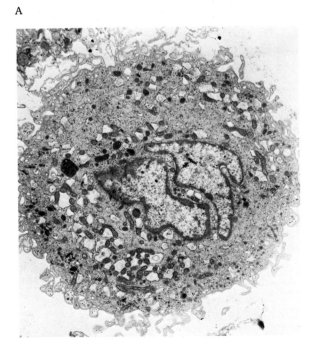

B

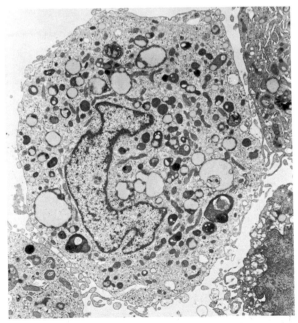

bodies, lymphokines, and other mediators that promote and regulate inflammation and immunity. Apparently, many of these immunologic responses can be expressed autonomously, without extending into systemic immunity. In part, this may be attributed to the close association of the lungs with the regional lymph nodes.

NATIONAL BOARD TYPE QUESTIONS

For the following, select
    A. if only *1, 2, and 3* are correct.
    B. if only *1 and 3* are correct.
    C. if only *2 and 4* are correct.
    D. if only *4* is correct.
    E. if *all* are correct.

1. The olfactory mucosa contains
    1. goblet cells.
    2. serous glands.
    3. cells with motile cilia.
    4. bipolar nerve cells.
2. Which of the following is (are) characteristic of bronchioles?
    1. A ciliated columnar epithelium
    2. A prominent muscularis mucosa
    3. Goblet cells
    4. Cartilage
3. The pulmonary defense system includes which of the following?
    1. Macrophages
    2. Plasma cells
    3. Mast cells
    4. Type II alveolar cells
4. Which of the following is (are) characteristic of pulmonary arteries?
    1. Thick tunica media
    2. Accompany the conducting passages
    3. Carry oxygenated blood
    4. Low pressure, low resistance

5. Which are responsible for converting angiotensin I to angiotensin II?
    1. Clara cells
    2. Type I alveolar cells
    3. Alveolar macrophages
    4. Pulmonary endothelium enzymes

Select the response most closely associated with each numbered item. (The headings may be used once, more than once, or not at all.)
    A. Primary bronchus
    B. Secondary bronchus
    C. Bronchiole
    D. Respiratory bronchiole
    E. Alveolar duct

6. Contains Clara cells
7. Contains numerous alveoli
8. Is extrapulmonary

Select the response most closely associated with each numbered item.
    A. Nasopharynx
    B. Larynx
    C. Both
    D. Neither

9. Contains stratified squamous epithelium
10. Associated with tonsils

Select the single best response for each of the following.
11. How many plasma membranes must a molecule of oxygen cross in order to reach the hemoglobin?
    A. 1
    B. 2
    C. 3
    D. 4
    E. 5
12. Which of the following is characteristic of surfactant?
    A. Produced by alveolar macrophages
    B. Is an immunoglobulin

C. Is composed primarily of phospholipid

D. Increases surface tension

E. None of the above

ANNOTATED ANSWERS

1. C. The olfactory mucosa is of a specialized epithelium containing bipolar nerves. Receptors for odors are located on long non-motile cilia. Serous secretions provide the solvent and mechanisms for clearing the receptors.

2. A. Bronchioles are lined with ciliated columnar epithelium interspersed with goblet cells. A well-developed muscularis mucosa and absence of cartilage allow constriction or dilation of the bronchioles.

3. A. Alveolar macrophages, mast cells, and lymphoid cells serve important functions in immunity and inflammation. The alveolar epithelium provides respiratory functions.

4. C. Pulmonary arteries carry deoxygenated blood from the heart following a course parallel to the bronchial passages. The tunica media is relatively thin since the pulmonary blood pressure is much lower than the systemic.

5. D. A unique function of the pulmonary endothelium is that it provides the specific enzyme necessary to convert angiotensin to a more potent vasoactive form.

6. C. Clara cells secrete proteins thought to promote reopening of bronchioles following expiration.

7. E. Alveolar ducts contain many alveoli; respiratory bronchioles have only a few. The others are conducting passages.

8. A. The primary bronchi are outside the lungs and carry air from the trachea to the lungs.

9. B. Areas of the larynx subject to wear, such as the epiglottis and vocal cords, are covered with stratified squamous epithelium. Other upper conducting passages possess the characteristic pseudostratified ciliated columnar epithelium with goblet cells.

10. A. The pharyngeal tonsil and the smaller tubal tonsils are referred to as adenoids and are located in the nasopharynx, above the soft palate.

11. E. A molecule of oxygen in the alveolar space must pass through five plasma membranes to reach hemoglobin: two of the type I epithelium, two of the capillary endothelium, and one of the erythrocyte.

12. C. Surfactant is a phospholipid-rich substance produced by type II alveolar epithelial cells which decreases surface tension.

BIBLIOGRAPHY

Avery, M. E., N.-S. Wang, and H. W. Taeusch. The lung of the newborn infant. *Sci. Am.* 228:74, 1973.

Belton, J. C., et al. Freeze-etch observations of rat lung. *Anat. Rec.* 170:471, 1971.

Boyden, E. A. Development of the Human Lung. In V. C. Kelly (ed.), *Brennemann's Practice of Pediatrics.* New York: Harper & Row, 1971. Vol. 4.

Brain, J. D., D. F. Proctor, and L. Reid (eds.). *Respiratory Defense Mechanisms.* New York: Marcel Dekker, 1977.

Breeze, R. G., and E. B. Wheeldon. The cells of the pulmonary airways. *Am. Rev. Respir. Dis.* 116:705, 1977.

Clements, J. A. Pulmonary surfactant. *Am. Rev. Respir. Dis.* 101:984, 1970.

Collet, A. J., and G. DesBiens. Fine structure of myogenesis and elastogenesis in the developing rat lung. *Anat. Rec.* 179:343, 1974.

Delahunty, T. S., and J. M. Johnston. The effect of colchicine and vinblastine on the release of pulmonary surface active material. *J. Lipid Res.* 17:112, 1976.

El-Bermani, A.-W., and M. Grant. Acetylcholinesterase-positive nerves of the rhesus monkey bronchial tree. *Thorax* 30:162, 1975.

El-Bermani, A.-W., J. A. Montvilo, and E. I. Bloomquist. Intranuclear rodlets in a pulmonary neuroepithelial body of a rabbit. *Cell Tissue Res.* 220:439, 1981.

Fink, B. R. *The Human Larynx, A Functional Study.* New York: Raven, 1975.

Graziadei, P. P. Cell dynamics in the olfactory mucosa. *Tissue Cell* 5:113, 1973.

Greenwood, M., and P. Holland. The mammalian respiratory tract surface: A scanning electron microscope study. *Lab. Invest.* 27:296, 1972.

Heinemann, H. O. The lung as a metabolic organ: An overview. *Fed. Proc.* 32:1955, 1973.

Hocking, W. G., and D. W. Golde. The pulmonary-alveolar macrophage. *N. Engl. J. Med.* 301:580, 1979.

Hodson, W. (ed.). Development of the Lung. In C. Lenfant (ed.), *Lung Biology in Health and Disease.* New York: Marcel Dekker, 1977. Vol. 6.

Kikkawa, Y. Morphology of the alveolar lining layer. *Anat. Rec.* 167:389, 1970.

Kuhn, C. The Cells of the Lung and Their Organelles. In R. G. Crystal (ed.), *The Biochemical Basis of Pulmonary Function.* New York: Marcel Dekker, 1976. P. 3.

Lauweryns, J. The Blood and Lymphatic Microcirculation of the Lung. In S. C. Sommers (ed.), *Pathology Annual.* New York: Appleton-Century-Crofts, 1971. Vol. 6, p. 365.

Lauweryns, J. M., M. Cokelaere, and P. Theunynck. Serotonin producing neuroepithelial bodies in rabbit respiratory mucosa. *Science* 180:410, 1973.

Macklem, P. T. Airway obstruction and collateral ventilation. *Physiol. Rev.* 51:368, 1971.

Mann, P. E. G., et al. Alveolar macrophages. Structural and functional differences between nonsmokers and smokers of marijuana and tobacco. *Lab. Invest.* 25:111, 1971.

Mathe, A. A., et al. Aspects of prostaglandin function in the lung. *N. Engl. J. Med.* 296:850, 1977.

Matulionis, D. H., and H. F. Parks. Ultrastructural morphology of the normal nasal respiratory epithelium in the mouse. *Anat. Rec.* 176:65, 1973.

Mavis, R. D., J. N. Finkelstein, and B. P. Hall. Pulmonary surfactant synthesis. A highly active microsomal phosphatidate phosphohydralase in the lung. *J. Lipid Res.* 19:467, 1978.

Polyzonis, B. M., et al. An electron microscopic study of human olfactory mucosa. *J. Anat.* 128:77, 1979.

Ryan, J. W., R. S. Niemeyer, and D. W. Goodwin. Metabolic fates of bradykinin, angiotensin I, adenine nucleotidase and prostaglandins E1 and F1 alpha in the pulmonary circulation. *Adv. Exp. Med. Biol.* 21:259, 1972.

Ryan, U. S., et al. Localization of angiotensin converting enzyme (kinase II): II. Immunocytochemistry and immunofluorescence. *Tissue Cell* 8:125, 1976.

Said, S. The lung in relation to vasoactive hormones. *Fed. Proc.* 32:1972, 1973.

Smith, M. N., S. D. Greenberg, and H. J. Spjut. The Clara cell: A comparative study in mammals. *Am. J. Anat.* 155:15, 1979.

Smith, U., and J. Ryan. Electron microscopy of endothelial and epithelial components of the lungs: Correlations of structure and function, *Fed. Proc.* 32:1957, 1973.

Sorokin, S., and J. D. Brain. Pathways of clearance in mouse lungs exposed to iron oxide aerosols. *Anat. Rec.* 181:581, 1975.

Stratton, J. C. The ultrastructure of multilamellar bodies and surfactant in the human lung. *Cell Tissue Res.* 193:219, 1978.

Takaro, T., H. P. Price, and S. C. Parra. Ultrastructure studies of apertures in the interalveolar septum of the adult human lung. *Am. Rev. Respir. Dis.* 119:425, 1979.

Van Golde, L. M. G. Metabolism of phospholipids in the lung. *Am. Rev. Respir. Dis.* 114:977, 1976.

Weibel, E. R. Morphological basis of alveolar-capillary gas exchange. *Physiol. Rev.* 53:419, 1973.

Williams, M. C. Conversion of lamellar body membranes into tubular myelin in alveoli of fetal rat lungs. *J. Cell Biol.* 72:260, 1977.

13 Integument

Objectives

You will learn the following in this chapter:

The three major components (layers) of integument

Some general features of the skin with particular emphasis on physiologic functions

How to identify the five epidermal layers of thick skin and describe their appearance as it relates to cell turnover and keratinization

The basis of skin pigmentation with particular emphasis on formation and distribution of melanin

A function or putative function for the Langerhans cell and Merkel cell

The composition of the dermis and hypodermis, including the cutaneous appendages

How to recognize two different types of glands (sweat and sebaceous) and hair follicles (active and resting) in a histologic section

The integumentary system consists of the organ of body investment—the skin—and a series of suborgans or skin derivatives, which in humans includes glands, hairs, and nails. In other mammals these cutaneous appendages include scales, quills, spines, claws, hooves, and horns.

GENERAL FEATURES AND FUNCTIONS OF THE INTEGUMENT

The skin consists of a superficial epithelial component, the **epidermis,** and underlying connective tissue components, the **dermis** and **hypodermis,** which together virtually invest the entire external body surface. The skin appendages are developmentally derived from the epidermis and are therefore morphologically and functionally related to this epithelium. In the adult, however, some of these structures may be found deep within the dermis.

Some of the features and functions of the skin and its derivatives are summarized in the following outline:

1. The skin is the heaviest and most versatile organ of the body; it accounts for approximately 16 percent of body weight, and as the interface between the body and its environment, it assumes a myriad of functions.
2. The integument is an effective protective shield against a wide range of chemical, physical, and biologic insults. It maintains

body integrity by keeping out foreign substances and microorganisms and keeping body fluids in. The cornified layers of the epidermis render the skin nearly waterproof, which allows the relatively fluid body to exist in dry air without becoming desiccated, to be immersed in fresh water without becoming swollen, and to be immersed in salt water without becoming shrunken. Most substances are poorly absorbed through intact skin; some that gain access include metallic nickel and the resins of poison ivy.

3. The skin is an effective screen against ultraviolet radiation; with the aid of the pigment melanin, it shields the body from potentially harmful doses.

4. The skin has a remarkable regenerative capacity, which allows this organ to heal itself. In addition to reforming itself, the skin carries on other synthetic activities (e.g., vitamin D is produced in the epidermis when the skin is exposed to sunlight).

5. The skin shows great topographic diversity, ranging from thick to thin, rough to smooth, hairy to seemingly hairless.

6. The skin is the organ of personal recognition and sexual attraction; not only do human beings recognize one another by certain surface configurations of face and body, but also the personal "signature" made by ridge patterns on the palmar and plantar surfaces (**dermatoglyphics**) creates a unique means of individual identification.

7. The skin is a remarkably plastic, resilient, and mobile organ; it conforms to all of the varied body contours and readily adapts to constant body movement. Only with age does its elasticity give way to flaccidity.

8. The skin is an important thermoregulatory organ. When the body is warm, cooling is enhanced by evaporation of sweat from its surface and relaxation of the extensive dermal vasculature, which allows maximum cutaneous blood flow; when the body is cold, heat loss is retarded by rapid constriction of blood vessels to reduce cutaneous blood flow.

9. The skin is an incredibly vascular organ that is capable of storing as much as 4.5 percent of the total blood volume. Its vasculature aids in the regulation of blood pressure; through the process of constricting cutaneous capillaries and shunting blood from arteries to veins directly, blood pressure is reduced.

10. The skin is the largest sense organ of the body and maintains an uninterrupted communication between the external and internal environments; sensory functions are carried out by an extensive variety of nerve endings that bring into consciousness the sensations of touch, pain, heat, and cold. Sensory endings are especially prominent in the most naked of body areas (e.g., lips, palmar and plantar surfaces, cornea, and genitalia). In addition, the skin communicates with the external environment by producing odors that attract or repel.

11. The skin is continuous with internal mucous membranes at the eyelids, nares, lips, prepuce, vulva, and anus. These transitional zones are termed **mucocutaneous junctions.**

12. The skin is part of the protective immune system in that its Langerhans cells monitor both the external and internal integumentary environment and are involved in sensitizing lymphocytes against antigens.

THE EPIDERMIS

The epidermal component of the skin consists of a stratified squamous keratinizing epithelium composed of a heterogeneous population of four different cell lines: **keratinocytes, melanocytes, Langerhans cells,** and **Merkel cells.** For pedagogic as well as functional purposes these four groups of cells can be considered to make up a series of epidermal minisystems, as follows: the **keratinizing** or **malpighian system,** the **pigmentary** or **melanocyte system,** the **reticuloepithelial** or **Langerhans system,** and the **Merkel system.**

As seen in vertical section with the light microscope, the stratified epithelium of the epidermis (Figs. 13-1, 13-2) is divided into layers based on the various evolutionary stages of the keratinocyte life cycle. These stages progress from the deepest or most basal layers to the surface. Traditionally, the deeper living layers are termed the **stratum malpighii** and the superficial dead and cornified layers are called the **stratum corneum.** A further subdivision separates the viable layers into the **stratum basale** (also called the **stratum germinativum,** reflecting its functional significance), the **stratum spinosum,** and the **stratum granulosum.** Likewise, the dead keratinized layers can be subdivided into the **stratum lucidum** and the **stratum corneum** proper where they occur (see Figs. 13-1, 13-2). A definitive stratum lucidum is normally found only in the epidermis of "friction surfaces," namely, palms of the hands and soles of the feet. Elsewhere, the keratinized layers are uniformly referred to as simply the **stratum corneum.** This classification scheme and the basic histologic features of the keratinocytes in these layers are summarized in Table 13-1.

Since the epidermis is an epithelium, it contains no blood vessels or lymphatics; it receives all oxygen and nutrients by diffusion from der-

Fig. 13-1. The epidermis of "thick skin" in vertical histologic section, with its various layers.

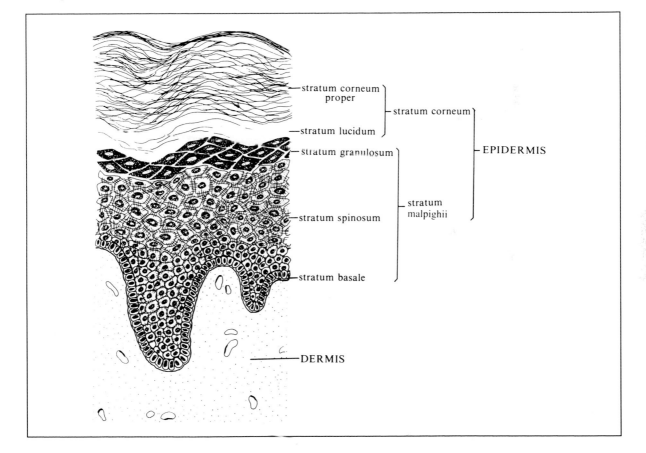

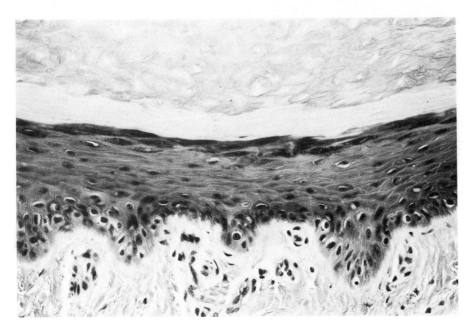

Fig. 13-2. A light micrograph of human thick skin. The five epidermal layers and the underlying dermis can be distinguished. See Figure 13-1 for orientation.

mal vessels. Although the major innervation to the skin is located in the dermis, the epidermis does contain sensory nerve endings, especially in the eyelids and around the genitalia.

Keratinocytes

The first and by far the most abundant population of cells in the epidermis consists of those members that undergo keratinization (Fig. 13-3; see also Fig. 13-2). The morphology of the various stages of these keratinocytes is, of course, the basis for naming the stratified squamous epithelium of the epidermis. The primary function of these cells is to produce a fibrous protein, **keratin,** so that the skin is covered with a protective armor. To perform this task they must constantly participate in a brief life cycle that ulti-

mately leads to cell death. The phases in the cytomorphosis of every keratinocyte are proliferation (mitosis), differentiation, and exfoliation.

The basal or stem cell layer of the epidermis (stratum basale) is an inexhaustible source of new keratinocytes that arise by mitosis. The epidermis, then, is one of the unique body tissues that is continually renewing itself to compensate for cellular loss. In the normal epidermis the proliferation of basal cells is balanced by the exfoliation of surface cells. Using radiolabeled tracers, it has been estimated that the minimum transit time for cells to move from the stratum basale to the stratum corneum is about 14 days in the forearm. In the cheek and oral mucosa, the transit time is substantially shorter, 3 to 4 days. However, the mean turnover (replacement) time for the entire epidermis has been calculated to be approximately 45 days.

Differentiation of the keratinocytes is simply the process of keratinization and the changes that these cells undergo to achieve this end. As the epithelial cells migrate upward and lose their mitotic potential, they begin to synthesize amor-

Table 13-1. Summary of the Layers and Histologic Features of the Epidermis
(Based on the maximum number of layers in thick skin listed in order of deepest to most superficial layers*)

General Layer	Specific Layer	Histologic Features
Stratum malpighii (viable cells)	Stratum basale (stratum germinativum)	Single basal layer of cuboidal or columnar-shaped cells; rests on basement membrane and is in contact with underlying dermis
		Cell axes approximately perpendicular to basement membrane
		Mitosis occurs mainly in this layer, although not restricted to it; serves as a source of stem cells for all new keratinocytes
		Cytoplasmic basophilia
	Stratum spinosum ("prickle cell" layer)	Several layers of polyhedral cells; cells somewhat larger than in basal layer
		Perimeters of cells possess spines ("prickles") that are resolved with the electron microscope as undulations of the plasma membrane that interdigitate with those of adjacent cells and are firmly attached to one another by desmosomes
		Cytoplasmic basophilia
	Stratum granulosum (granular cell layer)	Several layers of flattened cells
		Cell axes approximately parallel to basement membrane
		Cells contain conspicuous basophilic keratohyalin granules
Stratum corneum (horny cells)	Stratum lucidum (clear cell layer)	Several layers of flattened, anucleate cells
		Has hyalin appearance; generally weak cytoplasmic eosinophilia
	Stratum corneum proper	Many layers of very large, flattened, cornified, and anucleate cells; mean horizontal diameter of 45 μm
		Cells in close apposition except in regions of desquamation
		Cytoplasmic eosinophilia

*"Thick skin" occurs on friction (palmar and plantar) surfaces. In "thin skin" (general body surface), the stratum lucidum is usually absent and other strata are thinner, especially the stratum corneum. In both types of skin, keratinocytes contain an abundance of tonofibrils.

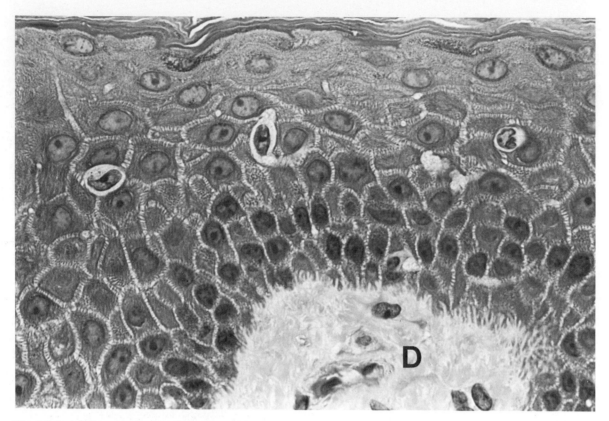

Fig. 13-3. A light micrograph of human epidermis, with the dermis (*D*) below. The keratinocytes are joined together by numerous desmosomes. Due to slight shrinkage, these junctions give the striated appearance around the cells. The three lightly stained cells among the keratinocytes are Langerhans cells.

phous proteins and increasing amounts of fibrillar proteins to form the fibril-matrix complex or "keratin pattern" that fills the cornified cells. In the stratum granulosum, **keratohyalin granules** appear; these structures, which are not membrane-limited, are thought to become part of the interfibrillar matrix of the cornified cells. Some smaller membrane-bound granules also appear in the granulosum; the products of these **membrane-coating granules** or **keratinosomes,** which are discharged extracellularly, are thought to act as binding substances to cement together the cells of the stratum corneum. Finally, dramatic changes in the basic morphology of the keratinocytes occur during the differentiation phase: plasma membranes thicken and toughen, and nuclei or organelles disintegrate. The once-living synthetic cells are now dead cornified plates protecting the body surface.

Exfoliation, the final stage in the keratinocyte life cycle, is the continuous process by which the outermost surface layers of the skin are shed and replaced by the newly differentiated ones below. The shedding mechanism is not fully understood; it is thought that as the cells reach the surface their cementing material becomes less effective, thereby allowing the cornified plates to separate off.

In addition to their function in forming the superficial cornified cells of the epidermis, the basal keratinocytes are the developmental source of the cutaneous appendages.

Melanocytes

The second epidermal cell population is composed of melanocytes (Fig. 13-4). These cells, which are found scattered among the keratino-

cytes throughout the basal layers as well as in hair follicles and dermal connective tissue, are responsible for the production of the pigment **melanin.**

Developmentally, these cells are derived from neural crest ectoderm. Morphologically, they are dendrite-bearing cells with a prominent perinuclear cytoplasm and few to many cytoplasmic processes that extend between adjacent keratinocytes. In routine histologic preparations, melanocytes are difficult to identify. However, in whole mount preparations of the epidermis they can be demonstrated by a histochemical technique known as the **dopa reaction,** which blackens the melanocytes. With the electron microscope they are easily distinguished from surrounding keratinocytes by their paler cytoplasm, lack of tonofilaments, absence of des-

Fig. 13-4. An electron micrograph of a human melanocyte. Note the small electron-dense granules within the cytoplasm. These are pigment-forming organelles or melanosomes. Some have been transferred to an adjacent keratinocyte (*lower right*). (Courtesy of G. Szabo.)

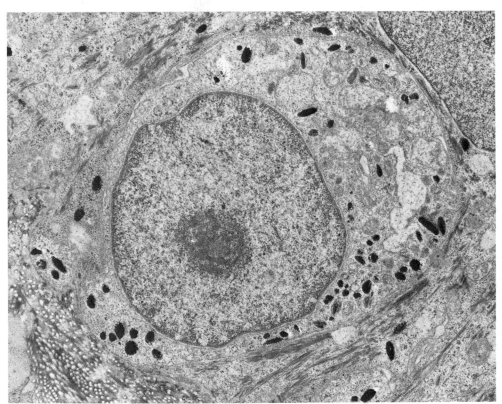

mosomes, and presence of membrane-bound, pigment-forming organelles called the **melanosomes** (see Fig. 13-4).

Melanin is produced by the oxidation of the amino acid tyrosine, and its formation, **melanogenesis,** occurs solely in the melanocytes. Synthesis of melanin occurs in melanosomes that contain the enzyme tyrosinase. When oxidation of precursors and subsequent polymerization of reaction products occur, melanin accumulates in these melanosomes until they are filled with pigment. Once formed, melanosomes and contained melanin are transferred to the keratinocytes, where they function as a screen against ultraviolet radiation. The mechanism of transfer is not known with certainty; either melanocytes inject their pigment into keratinocytes, as is suggested by in vitro studies using time-lapse microphotography, or keratinocytes phagocytize the melanin-containing processes of the melanocytes. In any case, epidermal melanin pigmentation is entirely dependent on the interaction of melanocytes and keratinocytes. For example, when the skin is subjected to prolonged exposure to sunlight, there is an increased synthesis of melanosomes, which are subsequently transferred to keratinocytes to protect the body from future doses of ultraviolet radiation; this process is the mechanism of suntanning. Likewise, if melanocytes are unable to melanize melanosomes, keratinocytes receive colorless granules and **albinism** results; if melanocytes lose their ability to produce melanin or are themselves lost, pigmentation in the epidermis disappears as keratinocytes are sloughed and the cutaneous depigmenting disease **vitiligo** results. Finally, it has been shown that there are no sex or race differences in the approximate number of melanocytes; racial differences in skin color are due to the number and size of the melanosomes and their distribution in keratinocytes.

Langerhans Cells

A third independent epidermal cell population is composed of the Langerhans cells (Fig. 13-5; see also Fig. 13-3). These dendritic cells are found scattered throughout the stratum malpighii, especially among the "prickle cells." Although originally described in the normal human epidermis by Langerhans in 1868, they are identified with certainty only by means of the electron microscope. Their fine structural characteristics include an indented nucleus; a clear cytoplasm; a modest amount of endoplasmic reticulum, mitochondria, and Golgi apparatus; an absence of tonofilaments and melanosomes; and the presence of specific granules. These characteristic intracytoplasmic granules, the so-called Langerhans granules, provide an important means of cell identification; they are rod- or racket-shaped, membrane-limited structures with a central linear density. Often these granules are closely associated or continuous with the cell membrane. The function of Langerhans granules is not known at present. There are no desmosomal contacts between Langerhans cells and adjacent keratinocytes.

Until recently the function of Langerhans cells has been a matter of conjecture. Present evidence favors a bone marrow origin and a function that is related to the primary immune response. Briefly, the Langerhans cells are thought to form a system of reticuloepithelial cells that are involved in clearing antigen from the integument. Recent work suggests that Langerhans cells are traps for externally applied allergens and therefore function in contact allergic hypersensitivity reactions. Essentially, these cells bind and process exogenous antigens and then migrate to lymph nodes, where they stimulate production of specifically sensitized lymphocytes, which in turn migrate to the epidermis and "home in" on the Langerhans traps.

Originally, Langerhans cells were thought to be restricted to the epidermis. However, they have subsequently been found in other stratified squamous epithelia, including the oral mucosa, esophagus, vagina, and cervix, as well as in hair follicles, sebaceous glands and ducts, apocrine ducts, the dermis, the thymus, lymph nodes, and dermal lymphatic vessels. These observations suggest that Langerhans cells are a circulating population, and considerable evidence is now ac-

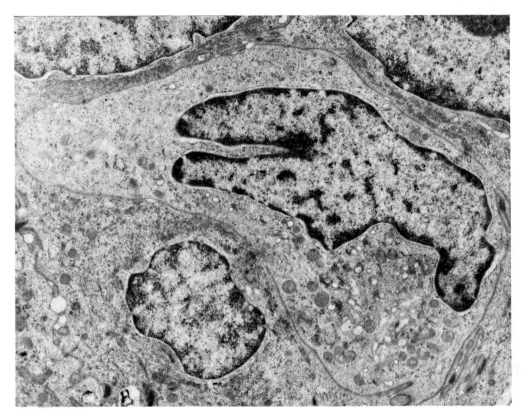

Fig. 13-5. An electron micrograph of a human Langerhans cell. Note the indented nucleus and variety of cytoplasmic organelles. Specific granules are not visible here. (Courtesy of G. Szabo.)

cumulating to suggest that they possess heretofore unrecognized immunologic importance.

Merkel Cells

The fourth cellular population located in the epidermis is composed of distinctive, clear cells called **Merkel cells** (Fig. 13-6). These elements are thought to represent a unique line of neural crest–derived cells that migrate into the epidermis from the dermis during fetal life. They are commonly found in or near the stratum basale and are scattered among the keratinocytes. Although isolated Merkel cells have been described in the epidermis, they occur most often in association with intraepithelial nerve endings. Topographically, Merkel cells have a wide epidermal distribution, occurring in glabrous and haired skin alike. They have also been observed in the dermis and the oral mucosa. However, their presence in the dermis is apparently rare except in embryonic skin.

The structure of the Merkel cells as seen with the electron microscope consists of a cytoplasm that is less electron-dense than adjacent keratinocytes, an irregularly shaped nucleus, small bundles of cytoplasmic filaments, and numerous electron-dense osmiophilic granules. Compared with the abundance of tonofilaments in the keratinocyte cytoplasm, the sparse amount of cyto-

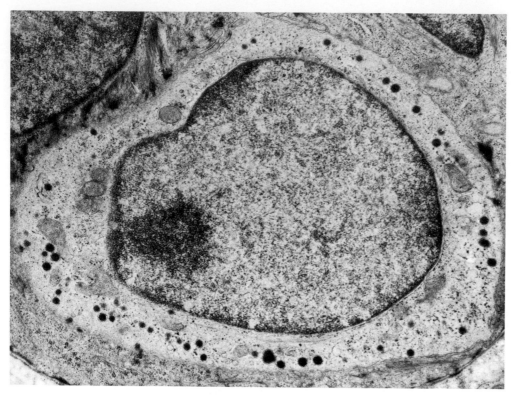

Fig. 13-6. An electron micrograph of a human Merkel cell at the base of the epidermis. Note the characteristic pale cytoplasm and small dense granules. (Courtesy of G. Szabo.)

plasmic filaments in the Merkel cell gives it a "clear" appearance. The Merkel granules are unique among epidermal cells. These membrane-bound particles are concentrated at the side of the Merkel cell facing the underlying dermis. It is the dermal face that is closely associated with a nerve terminus. Unlike the Langerhans cells, Merkel cells are attached to adjacent epithelial cells by desmosomes.

The function of the Merkel cells is not yet known with certainty. Because of their granules and certain histochemical properties, these cells have been compared with polypeptide hormone-producing cells as well as the catecholamine-producing cells of the adrenal medulla and paraganglia. However, their membership in the diffuse neuroendocrine system has not been established. Due to their intimate association with dermal and epidermal nerve fibers that are presumably sensory in function, these cells are thought to be involved in touch reception; such may be the case in many mammals. However, the true significance of Merkel cells in the human epidermis remains to be elucidated.

THE DERMIS

Generally, all epithelia rest on a basement membrane and on underlying connective tissue called the **lamina propria.** Specifically, the connective tissue beneath the stratified squamous epithelium of the epidermis is called the **dermis** (see

Figs. 13-1, 13-2). The interface between these two strata, the **dermoepidermal junction,** varies over the body from relatively smooth in thin skin to highly corrugated in thick skin.

Like the other connective tissue, the dermis is composed of various morphologic and functional frameworks, including collagen, elastic, and reticular fibers (embedded in an amorphous ground substance), nerves, blood vessels, and lymphatics. Also located in the dermis are various cutaneous appendages: sweat glands, sebaceous glands, and hair follicles. Smooth muscle in the dermis is generally associated with hair follicles (arrector pili muscles) and blood vessels, but in some areas (e.g., the scrotum) discrete meshworks of smooth muscle are found. The cellular elements of the dermis are relatively sparse: the most abundant elements are fibroblasts; others include melanocytes, macrophages, mast cells, migratory leukocytes, and adipocytes.

Based on the organization of the various connective tissue fibers, especially collagen, the dermis can be divided into two layers: an outer or superficial **papillary layer** and an inner or deep **reticular layer.** The former is characterized by a loose arrangement of relatively thin fibers embedded in a considerable amount of ground substance; the latter exhibits a dense pattern of thick fibers embedded in a lesser amount of ground substance and fewer cellular elements. The papillary layer derives its name from the fact that it forms the **dermal papillae** that project into the epithelial undulations at the dermoepidermal junction. The reticular layer is considered to be a prototype of dense irregular connective tissue.

Most of the nerve supply and all of the vascular supply of the skin is found in the dermis or the hypodermis. Rich plexuses of capillaries in the dermis not only supply the connective tissue but also are the only source of oxygen and nutrients for the overlying epidermis and its derivatives, whose nourishment is accomplished by diffusion. The dermis also contains many direct anastomoses of arterial and venous vessels that bypass capillary beds; these connections are called **arteriovenous shunts.**

Functionally, the dermis protects and cushions the body, provides resistance to mechanical stress and strain, is a barrier to infections, participates actively in wound healing and inflammation, and has an important inductive effect on the overlying epidermis and its appendages. Its blood supply, including the arteriovenous shunts, plays a major role in the thermoregulatory function of the skin. It should be emphasized that the abundance of blood vessels in the dermis functions primarily for thermoregulation and secondarily for nutrition of the cutaneous tissues.

THE HYPODERMIS

Beneath the dermis is a loose connective tissue layer of variable thickness and composition. Its boundary with the overlying dermis is often indistinct. This subcutaneous layer, which corresponds to the superficial fascia of gross anatomy, is called the **hypodermis.** Depending on several factors, it may be massively infiltrated with adipose tissue where it forms the **panniculus adiposus;** this layer on the ventral abdomen is well-known. It may also contain sheets of skeletal muscle where it forms the **panniculus carnosus.** Although well developed in most mammals, the panniculus carnosus is a vestige in man: all that remains is essentially the platysma of the face and neck. The hypodermis is connected below with underlying deep fascia, aponeurosis, or periosteum.

Functionally, the hypodermis provides support for the overlying skin and attachment to deeper tissues, serves as a storage depot for fat, and contains the large blood vessels that supply the skin.

Large sensory encapsulated receptors, termed **pacinian corpuscles,** are found in the subcutaneous tissues and are especially numerous beneath the dermis of the fingers. They are also prominent in the deep musculoskeletal tissues. Genital corpuscles in the skin of the external genitalia are similar in appearance. A group of smaller sensory receptors, termed **Meissner's corpuscles,** are found in the dermal papillae of hairless skin, particularly in the tips of the fingers and toes. Other morphologic variations of encapsulated endings also occur in integument. Most of these variations are smaller and simpler in construction. See Chapter 8 for further details on these and other sensory receptors.

CUTANEOUS APPENDAGES

At various places on the body, the epidermis forms highly specialized derivatives. In humans, these cutaneous appendages include the sweat glands, sebaceous glands, hairs, and nails. Although developmentally derived from basal ker-

atinocytes, certain of these appendages (e.g., glands and hairs) penetrate deeply into the dermis or the hypodermis (Fig. 13-7).

Sweat Glands

Based on their structure and mode of secretion, two types of sweat glands are distinguished: **eccrine glands** and **apocrine glands.**

ECCRINE GLANDS

The eccrine glands have a wide body distribution and are found throughout the integument except at the lips, beneath the nails, and on the glans penis, glans clitoris, and labia minora; they are most numerous on the palms and soles. However, their distribution in mammals is concen-

Fig. 13-7. Some cutaneous appendages.

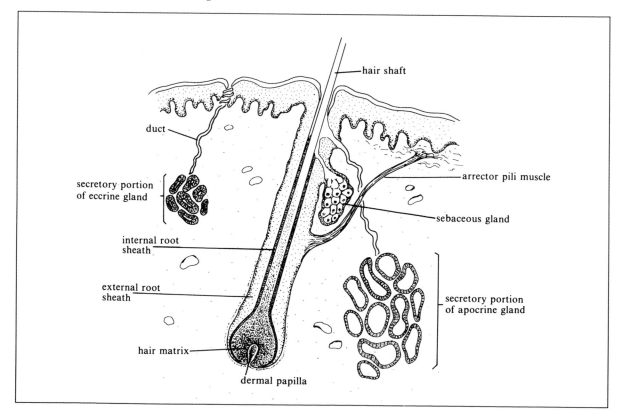

trated in the primates, with the greatest abundance occurring in humans; in nonprimates they are limited to the snout or the digital pads of various species.

Structurally, eccrine glands are simple coiled tubular glands (Fig. 13-8; see also Fig. 13-7). The tightly coiled secretory unit may be located in the dermis or the hypodermis; thus both shallow and deep varieties exist. The corkscrew-shaped duct reaches the surface and opens through an unlined pore on the epidermal surface; it is generally simple, although branching by fusion of the ducts of adjacent glands also occurs. On friction surfaces, eccrine ducts usually open at the apex of epidermal ridges. The diameter of the duct is smaller than the diameter of the secretory coil.

Histologically, the duct is composed of a stratified cuboidal epithelium with two cell layers. The secretory portion consists of a single layer of pyramid-shaped cells; between these cells and the basement membrane is a layer of myoepithelial cells. With the light microscope, two types of secretory cells are visible: "clear" cells and "dark" cells. Fine structural studies show that the clear cells have a broad base that rests on the myoepithelial cells and the basement membrane. They exhibit elaborate intercellular canaliculi, a highly folded basal membrane, and numerous mitochondria. They are presumed to secrete a solute-containing, watery fluid. The dark cells have an inverted pyramidal shape with a broad apex. They exhibit a well-developed rough endoplasmic reticulum, a large Golgi apparatus, and numerous membrane-bound secretory droplets. They are presumed to be mucin-producing cells. Eccrine sweat glands are innervated entirely by sympathetic cholinergic fibers.

Functionally, by responding to thermal stimulation, eccrine glands play a vital role in thermoregulation through the evaporative cooling effects of their secretion. They may also discharge under nervous stress, especially in the palmar and plantar regions. The function of the myoepithelial cells in sweat glands is not known with certainty. Some authors believe that they aid in the expression of secretory material. However,

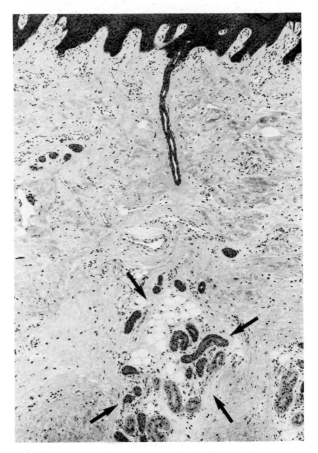

Fig. 13-8. A light micrograph of human integument showing an eccrine sweat gland (*arrows*) deep in the dermis. Part of its duct is visible as it penetrates the epidermis.

others suggest that they are supportive in nature, serving to resist local changes in osmotic pressure that might affect the structural integrity of the intercellular canaliculi. Both properties may be significant. The mode of secretion in eccrine glands is probably by a merocrine process (dark cells) and an active transport-diffusion mechanism (clear cells). Eccrine glands function throughout the life of an individual.

APOCRINE GLANDS

The apocrine sweat glands of humans are far less abundant than the eccrine variety; they are most numerous in the axillary and perianal regions. Unlike eccrine glands, apocrine glands are generally associated with hair follicles.

Structurally, the apocrine gland is also a simple coiled tubular gland (see Fig. 13-7). However, the secretory portions are so large and compact, with diverticula that fuse, that they have been likened to a sponge rather than a coiled tubule. They may be located in the dermis or the hypodermis. The generally straight duct runs approximately parallel to a hair follicle and opens into its upper portion, usually above the entrance of the sebaceous gland. Others, however, open directly onto the surface of the epidermis. As with the eccrine glands, the diameter of the duct is smaller than that of the secretory portion.

Histologically, the duct is similar to those of the eccrine glands. The secretory portion is composed of a single layer of cuboidal or columnar cells resting on myoepithelial cells and a basement membrane. Nuclei are basally placed. Ultrastructurally, the secretory cells are characterized by numerous mitochondria, a well-defined Golgi apparatus, numerous granules, and a highly folded basal plasmalemma. Little is known about the viscous apocrine secretion and its function. All modes of secretion—apocrine, merocrine, and holocrine—are apparently present in apocrine glands. Unlike the glands of the eccrine variety, they only begin to function at puberty.

Some specific apocrine-type glands require special mention: namely, the **ceruminous glands** of the external auditory canals. Together with the sebum from sebaceous glands in this region, their secretions form the earwax (**cerumen**).

Sebaceous Glands

Sebaceous glands are holocrine glands that are found throughout the integument except on the palmar and plantar surfaces and sides. They are located in the dermis and usually discharge their contents by way of a duct into the upper portions of hair follicles (Figs. 13-9, 13-10; see also Fig. 13-7). Some exceptions that are connected directly with the epidermal surface are the sebaceous glands of the lips, the oral and buccal mucosa, the glans penis, the prepuce, the nipples and areolae, the labia minora, and the meibomian or palpebral glands of the eyelids. Of all mammals examined, humans have the largest distribution of sebaceous glands; they are most numerous over the head region and anogenital area.

Structurally, sebaceous glands are simple branched alveolar glands. Histologically, the duct is composed of a stratified squamous keratinizing epithelium that is continuous with the epithelium of the hair canal or the epidermal surface. The secretory portions consist of acinar cells in various stages of differentiation. In the acinar periphery, the cells are small and resemble basal keratinocytes; they rest on a basement membrane. Toward the center of the acini, differentiating cells are enlarged with accumulated lipid; as more and more lipid gathers, the cells eventually die and fragment, and the detritus is secreted. Sebaceous glands are under hormonal control and enlarge at puberty.

Functionally, sebaceous glands are thought to lubricate and to soften hairs and the cornified layers of the skin and to prevent them from drying out. The objection to this notion is that infants and children, whose sebaceous glands are extremely small, have soft and flawless skin. It is probable, rather, that sebaceous glands function in the production of **pheromones.** The scent glands of many mammals are of the sebaceous variety; in humans the source of the different and distinctively pleasant odors of clean bodies is sebum.

Hairs

Hairs (see Figs. 13-7, 13-9) are filamentous projections of fused keratinized cells from the surface of the epidermis. They are produced and located in **follicles,** which are clublike epidermal pockets or invaginations into the dermis or hy-

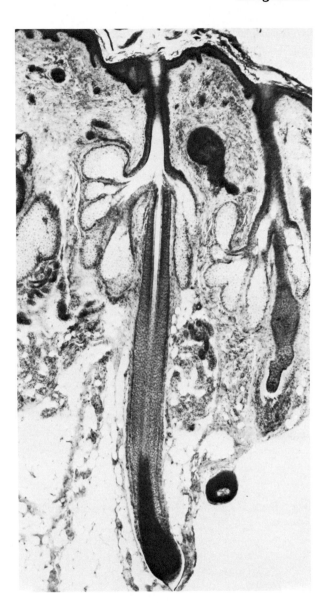

Fig. 13-9. A light micrograph of human thick skin. Two hair follicles extend deep into the dermis. Attached to their upper portions are a number of sebaceous glands, which use the hair follicles as ducts to the surface. The follicle on the right is in its resting phase. See Figure 13-7 for orientation.

Fig. 13-10. A light micrograph of several sebaceous glands attached to a hair follicle (cut in cross section). The cells closest to the follicle have degenerated, reflecting the holocrine mode of secretion.

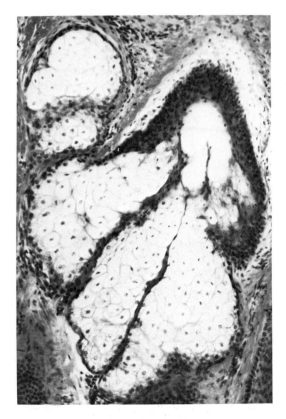

podermis. Hairs are found over most of the body with only a few exceptions. The follicles and associated sebaceous glands are known as **pilosebaceous units.** In general, hairs grow to a certain length, enter into a resting phase, undergo periodic shedding, and subsequently become replaced by new hair; this sequence of events is known as the **hair growth cycle.** Hairs do not form perpendicularly to the epidermal surface but rather occur at a slight angle to it; this explains why it is so difficult to find the "ideal" longitudinal section in histologic preparations. The distribution of hair as well as its texture varies greatly over the body surface.

Projecting into the base of the follicles is a nipplelike indentation that is occupied by a highly vascularized connective tissue. This **dermal papilla** (see Fig. 13-7) has an inductive influence on hair formation, and if it is destroyed no hair will be formed. Located in the base of the follicle (the **hair bulb**) and surrounding the papilla are mitotically active, pluripotential elements derived from the basal epidermal cells. These **matrix cells** (see Figs. 13-7, 13-9) form the **root** of the hair, which in turn gives rise to the keratinized shaft of the hair. Matrix cells also give rise to a "sleeve" of cells that invests the developing hair shaft; this cuff, which is called the **internal root sheath,** extends to about the level of the sebaceous gland duct and aids in the movement of the growing hair. The shaft of the hair consists of

an outer **cuticle,** an inner **medulla,** and an intermediate **cortex;** the medulla may be lacking in thinner hairs. The bulb, root, shaft, and associated internal root sheath are contained in the hair follicle, whose wall, the **external root sheath,** is simply an extension of the basal layers of the epidermis. Melanocytes are located in the bulb and transfer their pigment to the cortex or medulla of the hair, which accounts for its pigmentation.

Extending from the connective tissue surrounding the follicle to the papillary layer of the dermis is a small bundle of smooth muscle fibers. This **arrector pili** muscle forms the third side of a triangle made in conjunction with the follicle and the surface of the skin. A sebaceous gland is usually located within this triangle (see Fig. 13-7). Contraction of the arrector pili muscles in response to cold or fear pulls the follicles inward and the epidermis downward; these muscles make the hairs "stand on end" and elevate the epidermis surrounding the exposed hair shafts, respectively, resulting in the appearance of "goose-flesh."

Functionally, hair plays important roles in protection, thermal insulation, and tactile perception in most mammals; in man its function has

Fig. 13-11. A nail. A. Surface view. B. Longitudinal section.

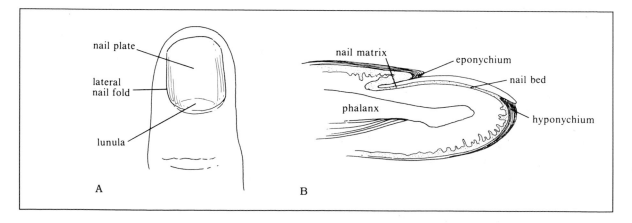

generally been reduced to an aesthetic consideration. However, scalp hair is probably of considerable thermal value when present.

Nails

Nails (Fig. 13-11) are plates of tightly packed keratinized cells that cover the dorsal surfaces of the digits at their distal ends; they occur only in primates. Like the hairs, they have a **matrix** that is located in the dermis, is mitotically active and gives rise to the **nail plate,** and is derived from an invagination of the epidermis. The distal end of the matrix can be seen projecting under the proximal end of the nail as a whitish, crescentic area, the **lunula.** The nail is embedded in a depression in the epidermis and therefore is bounded on all sides, except for its free distal end, by the stratum corneum, which turns under to form the **nail fold.** Where the proximal nail fold turns under, a horny cuticle or **eponychium** is found; where the stratum corneum passes under the distal free margin, the horny **hyponychium** is found. Beneath the plate is the **nail bed,** which has the structure of the stratum basale and stratum spinosum. Melanocytes often occur in the matrix, especially in darker races. Unlike hairs, nails grow continuously. Functionally, nails aid in grasping and manipulating small objects.

NATIONAL BOARD TYPE QUESTIONS

For the following, select
  A. if only *1, 2, and 3* are correct.
  B. if only *1 and 3* are correct.
  C. if only *2 and 4* are correct.
  D. if only *4* is correct.
  E. if *all* are correct.

1. Exposure to ultraviolet light results in an increase in the following:
   1. Tyrosinase activity
   2. Number of melanocytes
   3. Amount of melanin produced
   4. Number of keratinocytes
2. Which of the following is (are) characteristic of Langerhans cells?
   1. Antibody production
   2. Attachment to adjacent cells of desmosomes
   3. Production of hormones or hormonelike substances
   4. Origin from bone marrow
3. Which of the following are functions of integument?
   1. Vitamin D production
   2. Protection
   3. Thermoregulation
   4. Secretion
4. Sebaceous glands are characterized by which of the following features?
   1. Apocrine mode of secretion
   2. Use of hair follicles as secretory ducts
   3. Uniform distribution throughout the body
   4. Secretions high in lipid content
5. Which of the following processes is (are) characteristic of the epidermis?
   1. Proliferation
   2. Differentiation
   3. Exfoliation
   4. Protein synthesis

Select the response most closely associated with each numbered item.
   A. Epidermis
   B. Dermis
   C. Both
   D. Neither

6. Gives rise to the cutaneous appendages
7. Contains large amounts of adipose tissue
8. Contains blood vessels and lymphatics

Select the single best response for each of the following.

9. Which of the following structures do *not* contain keratin?
   A. Stratum corneum
   B. Stratum lucidum
   C. Hair
   D. Dermis
   E. Nails

10. Racial differences in skin color are attributed to which of the following?
    A. Number and size of melanosomes
    B. Number of melanocytes
    C. Thickness of dermis
    D. Thickness of epidermis
    E. None of the above

ANNOTATED ANSWERS

1. B. Exposure of skin to ultraviolet light stimulates melanin production in melanocytes. Increased activity of the enzyme tyrosinase promotes the conversion of the amino acid tyrosine to melanin. The number of melanocytes and keratinocytes (which receive melanosomes) remains unchanged.

2. D. Langerhans cells resemble the monocyte/macrophage in origin, appearance, and function. They are involved in antigen trapping in the epidermis, then migrate to the lymph nodes for further immunologic involvement.

3. E. The skin performs all of the listed functions: (1) vitamin D production—keratinocytes. (2) protection—keratin. (3) thermoregulation—distribution of blood; water (sweat) evaporation. (4) secretion—sweat; lipid.

4. C. Sebaceous glands are usually attached to hair follicles which they use as ducts. They are particularly numerous in the scalp and the anogenital region where they secrete a product rich in lipid (as in greasy hair).

5. E. In the cytomorphosis of keratinocytes, cells go through a brief life cycle in which they divide (stratum basale), differentiate (stratum spinosum and stratum granulosum), and produce the protein keratin (stratum granulosum), which they leave behind when they die. As they reach the cornified surface, they slough off.

6. A. The cutaneous appendages (hair follicles and glands) are located in the dermis and hypodermis, but are epithelial derivatives in their development.

7. D. The hypothermis is a loose connective tissue rich in adipose cells providing support for the dense dermis and attachment to underlying tissues.

8. C. Only the epidermis, like all epithelia, is avascular.

9. D. The dermis is composed primarily of collagen. All others listed are cornified structures.

10. A. Darkly pigmented skin possesses melanocytes, and keratinocytes will contain larger and more numerous melanosomes. The number of melanocytes is approximately the same as in lightly pigmented skin. Thickness of skin makes no difference.

BIBLIOGRAPHY

Allen, T. D., and C. S. Potter. Desmosome form, fate and function in mammalian epidermis. *J. Ultrastruct. Res.* 51:94, 1975.

Braverman, I. N., and A. Yen. Ultrastructure of the human dermal microcirculation. II. The capillary loops of the dermal papillae. *Invest. Dermatol.* 68:53, 1977.

Breathnach, A. S. *An Atlas of the Ultrastructure of Human Skin.* London: Churchill, 1971.

Brody, I. Ultrastructure of the stratum corneum. *Dermatology* 16:245, 1977.

Cairnie, A. B., P. K. Lala, and D. G. Osmond (eds.). *Stem Cells of Renewing Cell Populations.* New York: Academic, 1976.

Elias, M. E., and D. S. Friend. The permeability barrier in mammalian epidermis. *J. Cell Biol.* 65:180, 1975.

Elias, P. M., J. Goerke, and D. S. Friend. Mammalian epidermal barrier layer lipids: Composition and influence on structure. *J. Invest. Dermatol.* 69:535, 1977.

Ellis, R. A. Eccrine Sweat Glands: Electron Microscopy, Cytochemistry and Anatomy. In O. Gans and G. K. Steigleder (eds.), *Normale und Pathologische Anatomie der Haut I.* Berlin: Springer-Verlag, 1969.

Fukuyama, K., K. A. Wier, and W. L. Epstein. Dense homogeneous deposits of keratohyalin granules in newborn rat epidermis. *J. Ultrastruct. Res.* 38:16, 1972.

Guevedo, W. C. Epidermal melanin units: Melanocyte-keratinocyte interactions. *Am. Zool.* 12:35, 1972.

Hashimoto, K. The ultrastructure of the skin of human embryos. VIII. Melanoblast and intrafollicular melanocyte. *J. Anat.* 108:99, 1971.

Hashimoto, K. Fine structure of the Merkel cell in human oral mucosa. *J. Invest. Dermatol.* 58:381, 1972.

Jimbow, K., et al. Some aspects of melanin biology: 1950–1975. *J. Invest. Dermatol.* 67:72, 1976.

Matoltsy, A. G. Desmosomes, filaments and keratohyalin granules: Their role in the stabilization and keratinization of the epidermis. *J. Invest. Dermatol.* 65:127, 1975.

Matoltsy, A. G., and M. N. Matoltsy. The chemical nature of keratohyalin granules of the epidermis. *J. Cell Biol.* 47:593, 1970.

Montagna, W., and F. Hu (eds.). *The Pigmentary System.* Oxford: Pergamon, 1967.

Montagna, W., and P. F. Parakkal. *The Structure and Function of Skin.* New York: Academic, 1974.

Parakkal, P. F. The Fine Structure of Anagen Hair Follicle of the Mouse. In W. Montagna and R. L. Dobson (eds.), *Advances in Biology of Skin.* Oxford: Pergamon, 1969. Vol. 9.

Rowden, G. Immuno-electron microscopic studies of surface receptors and antigens of human Langerhans cells. *Br. J. Dermatol.* 97:593, 1977.

Rowden, G., M. G. Lewis, and A. K. Sullivan. Ia expression of human epidermal Langerhans cells. *Nature* 268:247, 1977.

Seiji, M., and I. A. Bernstein. *Biochemistry of Cutaneous Epidermal Differentiation.* Baltimore: University Park Press, 1977.

Silberberg, I., R. L. Baer, and S. A. Rosenthal. The role of Langerhans cells in allergic contact hypersensitivity. A review of findings in man and guinea pigs. *J. Invest. Dermatol.* 66:210, 1976.

Snell, R. S. An electron microscopic study of melanin in the hair and hair follicles. *J. Invest. Dermatol.* 58:218, 1972.

Spearman, R. I. C. *The Integument.* London: Cambridge University, 1973.

Szabo, G. The Biology of the Pigment Cell. In E. B. Bitlar and B. Bitlar (eds.), *The Biological Basis of Medicine,* New York: Academic, 1969. Vol. 6.

Tarin, D., and C. B. Croft. Ultrastructural studies of wound healing in mouse skin: II. Dermo-epidermal interrelationships. *J. Anat.* 106:79, 1970.

Winkelmann, R. K. The Merkel cell system and a comparison between it and the neurosecretory APUD cell system. *J. Invest. Dermatol.* 69:41, 1977.

Winkelmann, R. K., and A. S. Breathnach. The Merkel cell. *J. Invest. Dermatol.* 60:2, 1973.

Wolff, K., and K. Konrad. Melanin pigmentation: An in vivo model for studies of melanosome kinetics within keratinocytes. *Science* 174:1034, 1971.

Zelickson, A. H. (ed.). *Ultrastructure of Normal and Abnormal Skin.* Philadelphia: Lea & Febiger, 1967.

14 Oral Cavity and Alimentary Tract

Objectives

You will learn the following in this chapter:

How to identify and describe the major components of the tongue, salivary glands, teeth, and tooth-associated structures

The general organizational features of the gastrointestinal tract

The distinguishing features of each segment of the gastrointestinal tract with particular emphasis on the type of epithelium and associated glands found there

How the above distinguishing features reflect the various digestive functions of each segment

The four cell types that compose gastric glands and a function for each

How to identify four specializations of the small intestines which increase the surface area for absorption

The central features of the enteroendocrine system and examples of how their products contribute to the process of digestion

The steps involved in the digestion of carbohydrates, proteins, and fats, and how to identify the cellular source of the enzymes involved

How the above classes of nutrients are absorbed by the epithelium of the duodenum and brought into the circulatory system

---

The digestive system is involved with the intake, mechanical disruption, digestion (chemical breakdown), and absorption of food, and elimination of the nondigestible residue. The end products of digestion are carried through the bloodstream and lymphatics to all the tissues of the body. At their final destination these products are incorporated into individual cells, which may use them for simple turnover of constituents, in various synthetic reactions, or for mitosis.

DIGESTIVE TRACT

The entrance to the digestive tract is the **oral cavity,** where food is masticated, mixed with saliva, and formed into a **bolus,** which passes back into the **pharynx.** The pharynx leads to a slender muscular tube, the **esophagus,** which conveys the bolus to the **stomach.** Muscular contractions of the stomach then mix the food with digestive enzymes and hydrochloric acid and reduce it to a semifluid mass called **chyme.** The chyme is delivered by peristaltic contractions to the proximal part of the small intestine, the **duodenum,** which contains a variety of digestive enzymes made in part by the exocrine pancreas. The products of digestion are ultimately absorbed through the wall of the small intestine and travel through the portal system to the **liver,** where they may be stored, modified, or detoxified before entry into the systemic circulation. The residue passes through to the large intestine, where it is partially dehydrated into **feces** for elimination at the **anus.**

THE ORAL CAVITY
Oral Mucous Membrane

The oral cavity is lined by a stratified squamous epithelium that ranges from **nonkeratinized** to partially or **parakeratinized** depending on location, in terms of wear and tear of the particular region. The epithelium is supported by a relatively cellular connective tissue layer, the **lamina propria.** The epithelium and lamina propria are collectively called the **mucous membrane.** The mucous membrane usually rests on a second loose connective tissue layer, the **submucosa.** In the region of the hard palate, however, against which food is crushed, the submucosa is absent and the lamina propria attaches directly to the periosteum of the bone. The submucosa contains nests of **minor salivary glands,** which may be serous, mucous, or mixed. The ducts of these glands penetrate the oral mucous membrane, where they discharge their secretions. The combined activity of the minor glands and the three major pairs of salivary glands, to be described in the following sections, keeps the oral mucous membrane moist and lubricated.

The Tongue

The tongue (Fig. 14-1) consists of a core of crisscrossing skeletal muscle bundles covered by a mucous membrane. The anterior two-thirds of the tongue is separated from the posterior third by the **terminal sulcus.** The dorsal surface of the anterior portion is characterized by a coating of small protuberances, or **papillae,** of three types:

1. **Filiform papillae** are slender projections that are 2 to 3 mm long. They consist of a connective tissue core covered with stratified squamous epithelium. The surface epithelial cells are parakeratinized; that is, they are filled with keratin as in a true keratinized condition, yet they still retain a shrunken nucleus.

These papillae, which appear whitish due to the parakeratosis of the epithelium, are the most numerous.

2. **Fungiform papillae** are shaped like mushrooms. Because their connective tissue core is highly vascularized, and the surface epithelium is nonkeratinized, they appear as small red dots on the surface of the tongue. These papillae often bear taste buds on their surfaces.

3. **Circumvallate papillae** are the largest, most complex, and least numerous papillae. There are 10 to 12 of them along the terminal sulcus, forming a V that separates the anterior papillate region of the tongue from the smooth posterior portion where the lingual tonsils reside. Each circumvallate papilla is sunk into the surface of the mucous membrane and is surrounded by a deep circular trench. The lateral surfaces of the papillae contain abundant taste buds. The ducts of special **serous glands** (von Ebner's glands) open into the bottom of the trenches, providing a fluid medium in which molecules dissolve to trigger the taste impulse and which constantly washes the trench to ensure continuity of the sense of taste.

TASTE BUDS

Each taste bud is a pale oval body located within the darker-staining epithelium. The taste buds begin at the basement membrane and extend to the free surface, where they open through a small **taste pore** (see Figs. 14-1, 14-2). At the light microscopic level two cell types are commonly described within the taste bud, arranged like the segments of an orange with their long axis parallel to the oval: (1) **neuroepithelial cells,** which are light staining with euchromatic nuclei; and (2) **supporting (sustentacular) cells,** which are dark and thin with heterochromatic nuclei. Both cell types have long **microvilli** that extend into the taste pore. Recent electron microscopic observations have not been able to assign different functions to the two cell types. Nerve endings

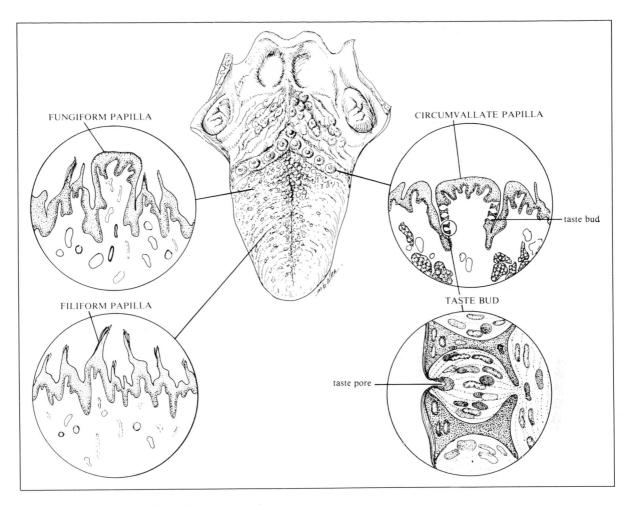

Fig. 14-1. The dorsal surface of the tongue, showing the three different types of papillae.

penetrate and surround the taste buds, carrying the sensation to the olfactory region of the brain. The four primary taste sensations—sweet, salty, bitter, and acid—are not sensed by all taste buds; instead, the perception of these tastes varies regionally over the tongue. Taste buds not only are associated with fungiform and circumvallate papillae but also occur on the soft palate, glossopalatine arch, epiglottis, and posterior wall of the pharynx.

Salivary Glands

In addition to the many continuously secreting **minor glands** located in the submucosa throughout the oral cavity, there are three pairs of large or **major salivary glands** (Fig. 14-3) that secrete only in response to chemical, mechanical, olfactory, or psychologically conditioned stimulation. They are compound glands, consisting of several **lobes** that are further subdivided by connective tissue septa into **lobules.** The secretory portion of the glands may be either acinar (alveolar) or

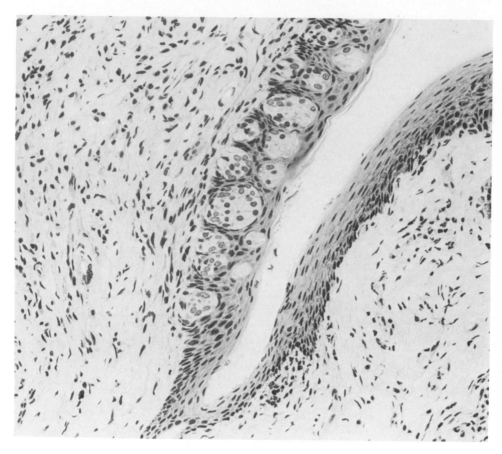

Fig. 14-2. Light micrograph of the lateral aspect of the circumvallate papilla showing numerous taste buds.

tubuloacinar. These glands are located at some distance from the oral cavity, with which they communicate by long excretory ducts. The duct system of the salivary glands is best developed in the parotid glands and least developed in the sublingual glands. The secretion is moved from the glandular acini or tubules into the duct system by the contraction of myoepithelial (basket) cells, which surround the acini or tubules like the tentacles of an octopus. The following outline traces the duct system from the glandular elements to the oral cavity.

1. **Intralobular ducts** are the smallest branches which drain the acini or tubules. Intralobular ducts are defined microscopically as being within a lobule of the gland, surrounded by alveoli. There are two types:
   a. **Intercalated ducts** leave the glandular elements as narrow channels lined with a simple squamous to low cuboidal epithelium. The cells lining the ducts get progressively taller, leading into the second type of intralobular duct.
   b. **Striated ducts** are lined by a simple columnar epithelium that shows basal striations. The striae are caused by mitochondria lined up in infoldings of the plasma

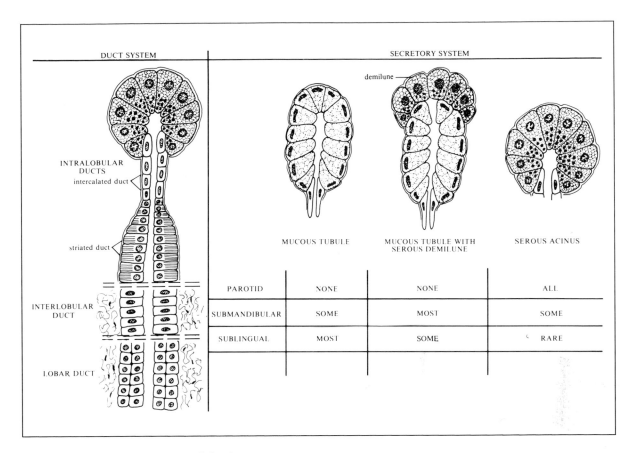

| DUCT SYSTEM | SECRETORY SYSTEM | | |

INTRALOBULAR DUCTS
intercalated duct
striated duct
INTERLOBULAR DUCT
LOBAR DUCT

demilune

	MUCOUS TUBULE	MUCOUS TUBULE WITH SEROUS DEMILUNE	SEROUS ACINUS
PAROTID	NONE	NONE	ALL
SUBMANDIBULAR	SOME	MOST	SOME
SUBLINGUAL	MOST	SOME	RARE

Fig. 14-3. The secretory units and the duct systems of the three major salivary glands. The table lists the relative proportions of the three types of secretory units in each gland.

membrane which yield energy for the ion pumps that actively modify the saliva as it passes through the duct.

2. **Interlobular ducts** arise from the union of intralobular ducts and, as their name implies, run between lobules. They are also lined by a high columnar epithelium but are surrounded by the connective tissue septum defining the lobule. Several interlobular ducts unite to form a **lobar duct,** where the epithelium ranges from high columnar to stratified cuboidal; the lobar duct drains an entire lobe. The lobar ducts join to form the

major excretory duct, which is lined by a stratified epithelium that finally joins with the stratified squamous epithelium of the oral mucosa.

The **parotid glands** are the largest pair of salivary glands; they are located in front of the external ear. The secretory portion is composed entirely of serous acini in the adult, which secrete salts, protein, and the enzyme **ptyalin,** which cleaves starch into smaller carbohydrates.

The **submandibular glands** are compound tubuloacinar in form and mixed seromucous in terms of secretion. Some of the terminal portions of the gland consist of serous acini, others are mucous tubules, while a third arrangement consists of a mucous tubule capped by a hemisphere (**demilune**) of serous cells. The duct system is similar to that of the parotid glands (see Fig. 14-3, and Fig. 3-8 in Chap. 3).

The **sublingual glands,** located in the floor of the mouth, are compound tubuloacinar glands. The secretion is mixed seromucous, but in contrast with the submandibular gland, mucous tubules predominate. Most of the mucous tubules are independent elements, only a minority being capped by serous demilunes. Pure serous acini are quite rare. The duct system is greatly abbreviated in these glands, and the intralobular ducts are very difficult to locate.

The Teeth

The human dentition consists of two sets of teeth; the twenty **deciduous** or **baby teeth** are replaced by the thirty-two **secondary** or **successional teeth.** The two sets are similar microscopically, consisting of a **crown** projecting above the gum (**gingiva**), and one to three roots that fit into a socket or **alveolus** in the bone of the mandible or maxilla. The root of the tooth is attached to the alveolus by a system of collagen bundles called the **periodontal ligament.** The hard tissues of the crown surround a core of loose connective tissue, housed in the **pulp chamber,** which continues into the **root canal** where it communicates with the connective tissue of the peridontal ligament through a small opening, the **apical foramen** (Fig. 14-4).

THE HARD TISSUES

There are three calcified tissues that form the hard substance of the tooth. These tissues vary markedly in structure and embryologic development, as discussed in the following paragraphs.

Dentin

Dentin is similar in composition (but not in structure) to bone tissue, consisting of 20 percent organic and 80 percent inorganic material in the form of calcium salts (hydroxyapatite crystals). The inorganic material is the same as that of bone, except that it is denser and more insoluble. Dentin is present in both the crown and the root of the tooth, surrounding the pulp. During **odontogenesis** (tooth development), dentin is the first hard tissue to form. Although odontogenesis is beyond the scope of this text, it is pertinent to note that the cells forming the dentin (**odontoblasts**) line the pulp cavity (Fig. 14-5). Dentin formation continues throughout life, with the result that the dentin layer becomes thicker at the expense of the pulp. In the case of dental caries (decay), the odontoblasts react by laying down a plug of **reparative dentin,** keeping maximum distance between the decay process and the pulp.

Histologically, the dentin is composed of long **dentinal tubules** running at right angles to the pulp (see Fig. 14-5). Each tubule houses a thin **odontoblastic process,** which is an outgrowth of an odontoblast located at the periphery of the pulp. Between the dentinal tubules are bundles of collagen fibers embedded in a ground substance composed of glycosaminoglycans and protein. The walls of the dentinal tubules (tubular dentin) and the collagenous matrix between tubules (intertubular dentin) are heavily calcified (see Fig. 14-4, inset). Calcification occurs in the form of spherical globules that enlarge and fuse as an advancing front toward the pulp. Calcification is sometimes incomplete, giving rise to hypocalcified areas called **interglobular dentin.** The dentin closest to the pulp is the most recently formed; it is called **predentin** prior to its calcification.

Enamel

Enamel is the hardest substance in the body, being composed of 99.5 percent inorganic matrix. Mature enamel can be seen only in ground sections, since it is completely dissolved away in decalcified sections. (This feature is in contrast to other calcified tissues, which contain enough organic matrix to appear in decalcified sections

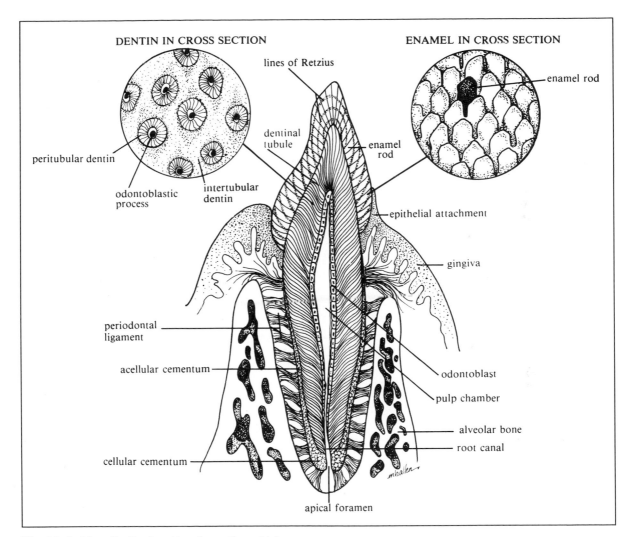

DENTIN IN CROSS SECTION

lines of Retzius

ENAMEL IN CROSS SECTION

enamel rod

peritubular dentin

dentinal tubule

enamel rod

odontoblastic process

intertubular dentin

epithelial attachment

gingiva

periodontal ligament

acellular cementum

odontoblast

pulp chamber

alveolar bone

root canal

cellular cementum

apical foramen

Fig. 14-4. A longitudinal section through an incisor tooth.

as well as in ground sections.) Enamel overlays the dentin, forming the **anatomic crown** of the tooth. Since the crown is most subject to wear and tear, it is functionally appropriate for it to be crafted of the hardest material. The enamel is formed by cells called **ameloblasts,** which are epithelial cells of ectodermal origin. The ameloblasts secrete long, thin enamel **rods** or **prisms** that then become calcified. Unlike odontoblasts, ameloblasts do not persist after the crown is completed; they disappear when the tooth erupts into the oral cavity. The enamel, therefore, has no capacity for regeneration in the case of caries, and damage can be repaired only by the use of foreign filling materials.

Histologically, longitudinal ground sections of enamel reveal long rods extending from the dentinoenamel junction to the free surface. Cut in cross section (see Fig. 14-4, inset), the rods are seen to have a keyhole appearance and look very much like fish scales. Another striking feature of

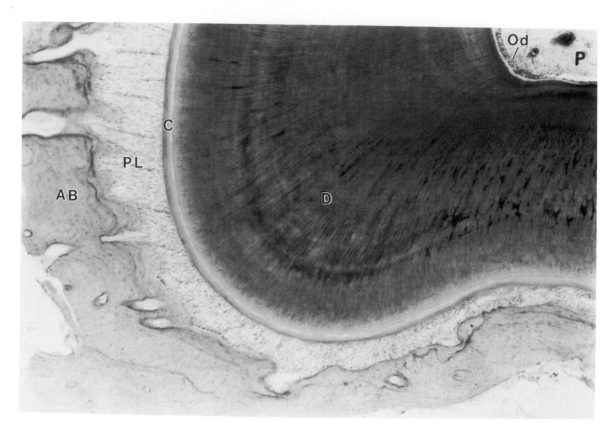

Fig. 14-5. Light micrograph of partial cross-section of a tooth and its associated structures. In the upper right corner is the pulp (*P*). Odontoblasts (*Od*) line the pulp cavity in close contact with the dentin (*D*). Note the dentinal tubules which radiate through the dentin. Since the tooth is cut across the root, one can also see periodontal ligament (*PL*) attaching the cementum (*C*) of the tooth to the surrounding alveolar bone (*AB*).

enamel are the concentric dark bands that run at right angles to the rods in either plane of section. These dark bands, the **lines of Retzius,** are areas of hypocalcification that are thought to reflect minor disturbances in the flow of nutrients to the ameloblasts during development. In those teeth in which the crown starts to develop in utero and finishes after birth, the nutritional disturbance accompanying the first few days following birth is reflected in a pronounced **neonatal line.**

Cementum

Cementum is similar in composition, formation, and structure to bone tissue. The cementum covering the upper portion of the root, near the crown, is thin and acellular (see Fig. 14-5), whereas the cementum surrounding the bottom or **apex** of the tooth is thick and cellular. Cementum is formed by **cementoblasts** that, in the case of cellular cementum, become entrapped by the matrix that they secrete. The trapped cells are then called **cementocytes** and occupy lacunae similar to the osteocytes of bone tissue. Cementum, like dentin, continues to be laid down at the apex of the tooth throughout life. This accounts for the ability of teeth to "drift" slightly, changing their positions relative to one another during the life of the individual.

TOOTH-ASSOCIATED STRUCTURES

The structures associated with the teeth serve to attach and maintain them within the bone of the jaw. These structures consist of the periodontal ligament, gingiva, and alveolar bone.

The **periodontal ligament** is composed of dense collagenous connective tissue whose fibers penetrate into the cementum of the tooth and attach it to the bony wall of the socket (see Fig. 14-5). This arrangement allows limited movement of the tooth and avoids direct transmission of pressure to the alveolar bone, thus preventing its resorption. The relative plasticity of the periodontal ligament allows orthodontic procedures to move teeth in a gradual manner.

The **gingiva** (gums) is a mucous membrane firmly bound to the periosteum of the alveolar bone. It is composed of stratified squamous epithelium that is bound to the tooth enamel. This epithelial attachment resembles a thick basal lamina. Epithelial cells are bound to this attachment by hemidesmosomes. Beneath the epithelium is a fairly dense connective tissue layer. The gingiva comprises what is referred to clinically as **periodontal tissue.**

The portion of bone to which the periodontal ligament attaches is referred to as **alveolar bone.** It is considered to be woven bone since it is not arranged in lamellae. The portion closest to the root of the tooth forms the socket. Blood vessels, lymphatics, and nerves course through the alveolar bone, enter the apical foramen, and pass into the pulp chamber of the tooth, thus providing for its metabolic needs.

ESOPHAGUS AND STOMACH
General Plan of the Digestive Tube

From esophagus to rectum, the digestive tube is a hollow structure following a similar histologic plan, with regional variations based on functional differences. The wall of the tube is composed of four basic, concentrically arranged layers enclosing a lumen (Fig. 14-6).

The **mucosa** is the layer that abuts the lumen. It consists of three parts: (1) a lining **epithelium** that may be specialized for protective purposes (esophagus), or for absorption or secretion (intestines); (2) a **lamina propria** of reticular, lymphoid connective tissue, which both supports the epithelium and functions immunologically; and (3) a **muscularis mucosae,** composed of smooth muscle, which marks the boundary of the mucosa.

The **submucosa** is a relatively thick layer of loose connective tissue. It contains blood vessels, nerve plexuses, and lymphoid nodules.

The **muscularis externa** usually consists of two layers of smooth muscle, an inner circular and an outer longitudinal layer. The two layers are separated by sparse connective tissue containing myenteric nerve plexuses that initiate peristaltic contractions. In the upper portion of the esophagus, skeletal muscle replaces smooth muscle (see The Esophagus, below). In the stomach an extra muscle layer is added, and in the colon the outer layer of the muscularis externa is gathered into three longitudinal bands, the **teniae coli.**

The **adventitia** or **serosa** is the outermost layer of connective tissue, which is either attached directly to surrounding structures (adventitia) in the esophagus and rectum, or bounded by a mesothelium (serosa) if the organ lies within the abdominal cavity.

The Esophagus

The esophagus (Fig. 14-7; see also Fig. 9-3 in Chap. 9), which is approximately 25 cm long, conveys swallowed material from the pharynx to the stomach by rapid peristaltic activity. Specializations of the four layers are described in the following sections.

MUCOSA

The epithelium of the human esophagus is nonkeratinized stratified squamous epithelium, a type found lining moist surfaces that are subject to abrasion. It is supported by a lamina propria

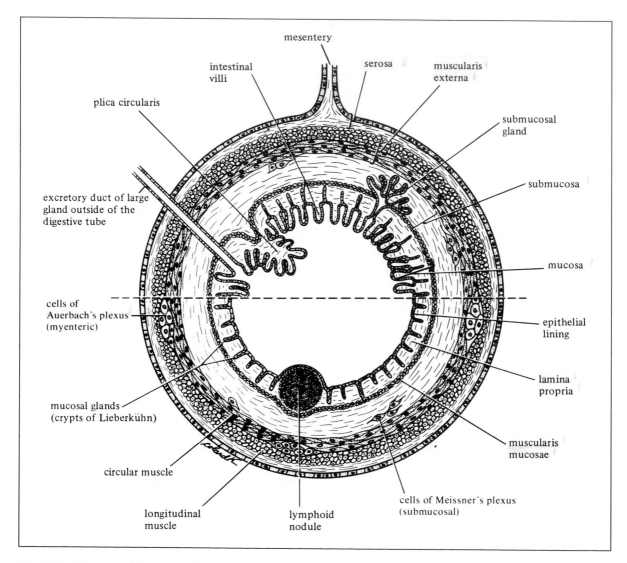

Fig. 14-6. The general features of organization in the gastrointestinal tract. The concentric layers of serosa, muscularis, and mucosa are common to virtually all regions of the tract. In the upper half, the mucosa is depicted with glands and villi as in the small intestine; in the lower half, it is shown with glands only, as in the colon. (From W. Bloom and D. W. Fawcett, *A Textbook of Histology* [10th ed.]. Philadelphia: Saunders, 1975. Reproduced with permission.)

rich in lymphocytes and occasional lymphoid nodules. Since the digestive tract is an open portal of access for microorganisms, the lamina propria of the entire tube is a lymphoid connective tissue. Further information concerning the immunologic and antibacterial functions of this layer is given in Chapter 10.

At the lower margins of the esophagus, **esophageal cardiac glands** may be present in the lam-

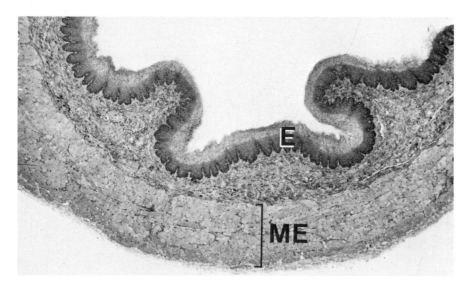

Fig. 14-7. Low-power light micrograph of monkey esophagus, cross section. Note the stratified squamous epithelium (*E*), the well-developed muscularis externa (*ME*), and the intervening connective tissue layers. The muscularis mucosa is not easily distinguishable at this magnification. See Figure 14-4 for orientation.

ina propria; these are compound tubular glands that sometimes react for mucin. Their major ducts are lined by a mucus-secreting columnar epithelium similar to that lining the gastric pits in the stomach. The presence of these glands is subject to individual variation, and they range from well developed to entirely absent.

The **muscularis mucosae** is formed from longitudinally oriented smooth muscle cells supported by delicate elastic fibers.

SUBMUCOSA

The submucosa consists of a dense collagenous and elastic fiber framework that is extremely plastic and resilient. Small mucus-secreting glands, the **esophageal glands proper** (or deep esophageal glands), are located in the submucosa. These are branched tubuloalveolar glands whose ducts penetrate the muscularis mucosae,

discharging mucus onto the epithelial surface to lubricate the esophageal lumen.

The submucosa and mucosa are involved in longitudinal folds that smooth out, opening the lumen during swallowing. Nerve plexuses involved in peristalsis are found throughout the tube in both submucosa and muscularis externa.

MUSCULARIS EXTERNA

The muscularis externa is best understood when viewed in the context of swallowing, an activity that is initiated voluntarily but maintained autonomically. The muscularis externa of the esophagus is unique because it comprises skeletal and smooth muscle, both of which are innervated by autonomic nerves. In the proximal (upper) third of the esophagus, both the inner circular and outer longitudinal muscle layers are skeletal. In the middle third, bundles of smooth muscle begin to replace the skeletal muscle, and the distal (lower) third is composed only of smooth muscle. Innervation of the musculature comes from the vagus nerve and from the cervical and thoracic sympathetic trunks. These nerves form plexuses consisting of fibers and cell bodies, both between muscle layers of the muscularis externa and in the submucosa.

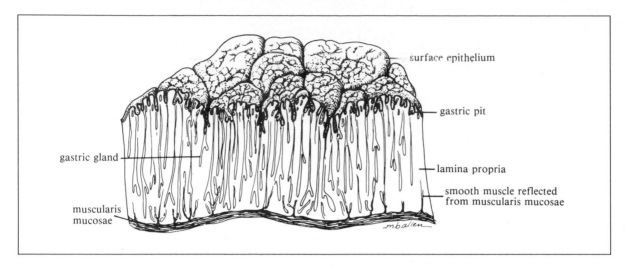

surface epithelium

gastric pit

gastric gland

lamina propria

smooth muscle reflected
from muscularis mucosae

muscularis
mucosae

m.ballen

Fig. 14-8. The surface topography of the stomach and the appearance of mucosa when viewed in cross section at very low magnification.

ADVENTITIA

An adventitia of loose connective tissue covers the proximal portion of the esophagus, connecting it to surrounding structures. The distal portion of the esophagus, below the level of the diaphragm, is suspended within the peritoneal cavity and is covered by a serosa.

The Stomach

The stomach is engaged in both storage and digestion of food. In the upper region of the stomach the food is solid, whereas it is reduced to a partially digested fluid mass, **chyme,** in the distal portion of the organ. Submucosal and myenteric nerve plexuses regulate peristaltic activity, which churns the food, mixes it with digestive enzymes, and delivers small portions of chyme (15–20 ml) from the pyloric region of the stomach to the duodenum. Following a meal about 1,000 ml of gastric fluid, consisting of a salt solution containing mucus, the enzyme **pepsin,** and a glycoprotein called **gastric intrinsic factor,** is secreted. The function of the various components of gastric fluid is discussed later in this section.

When empty, the stomach is contracted and the mucosa is folded into longitudinal ridges (**rugae**), which smooth out when the organ is distended. A finer pattern of shallow furrows, however, divides the mucosa into small, slightly elevated areas 1 to 6 mm in diameter, which are riddled by small **gastric pits (foveolae)** into which the **gastric glands** open (Fig. 14-8).

The mucosa of the stomach is composed of a tall columnar surface epithelium that also dips down to line the gastric pits. The epithelial cells are characterized by an apical **mucous cap** that can be stained with the periodic acid–Schiff (PAS) reaction. The mucus is secreted onto the epithelial surface and forms a barrier against the acidic contents of the stomach. This barrier can be damaged by ingestion of both alcohol and aspirin, increasing the possibility of ulceration of the gastric epithelium. Secretion of acid itself is modulated by the autonomic nervous system and may be increased by stress and anxiety to levels that also cause ulceration of the mucous, or even of deeper layers. Autoradiographic studies have shown that cells of the surface epithelium normally have a very high turnover rate, being renewed approximately every 3 days.

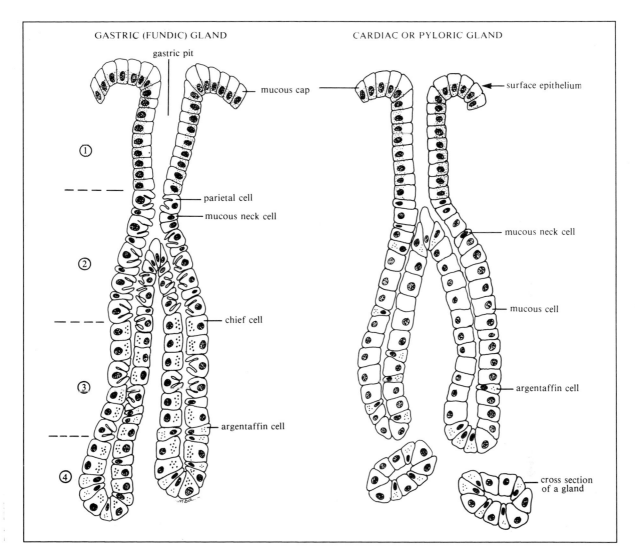

Fig. 14-9. Longitudinal sections of a gastric (fundic) gland and a stylized cardiac or pyloric gland. The four zones on the left correspond to: (1) the gastric pit into which the gland opens, lined by a mucus-secreting surface epithelium; (2) the upper third of the gland, lined by mucous neck cells and parietal cells; (3) the midregion of the gland, lined predominantly by parietal and chief cells; and (4) the bottom of the gland, lined by chief and argentaffin cells. On the right side the cardiac and pyloric glands show only three cell types, as indicated.

The lamina propria is typically lymphoid and supports both the surface epithelium and the numerous gastric glands that open into the gastric pits. These glands are simple or branched tubular glands, and they vary in cellular composition and function depending on their location within the stomach. Three types of glands can be characterized: gastric (fundic) glands, cardiac glands, and pyloric glands (Fig. 14-9).

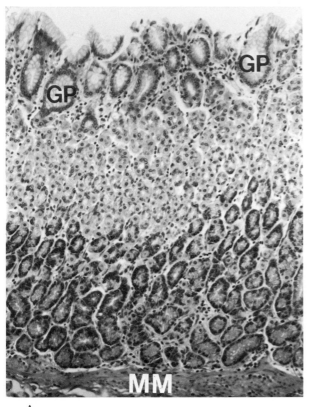

A

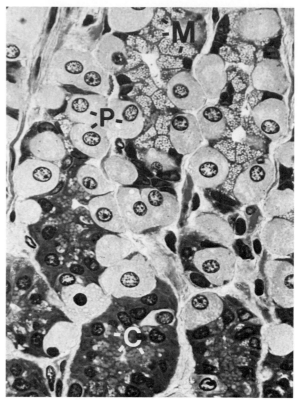

B

GASTRIC (FUNDIC) GLANDS

Gastric glands (Fig. 14-10) are located over the corpus of the stomach and are the most important secretors of gastric juice. Several glands may open into the bottom of one gastric pit. In addition, the terminal ends may divide into two or three branches. Four cell types are located within the gland: chief cells, parietal cells, mucous neck cells, and enteroendocrine cells.

Chief (Zymogenic) Cells

These simple cuboidal or low columnar cells line the lower half or third of the gland. Chief cells elaborate **pepsinogen,** the inactive precursor of **pepsin,** and are basophilic due to the large amount of rough endoplasmic reticulum that is necessary to synthesize this protein. The pep-

Fig. 14-10. The mucosa of the fundic stomach of a monkey. A. Low-power view of the surface epithelium with gastric pits (*GP*). Gastric glands extend down from the pits to the muscularis mucosa (*MM*). The upper portions of the glands stain acidophilically due to the predominance of parietal and mucous neck cells. The basophilic chief cells are seen primarily in the basal region. B. Higher magnification of the mid-region of the gastric glands. Parietal cells (*P*) and mucous neck cells (*M*) predominate in the upper region. In the lower region, chief cells (*C*) are the major cell type.

sinogen is released in response to cholinergic stimulation, and in the low pH of the stomach lumen (pH approximately 2) it is cleaved into the active enzyme pepsin, a proteinase. These cells have the typical structure of any cell involved in the export of protein.

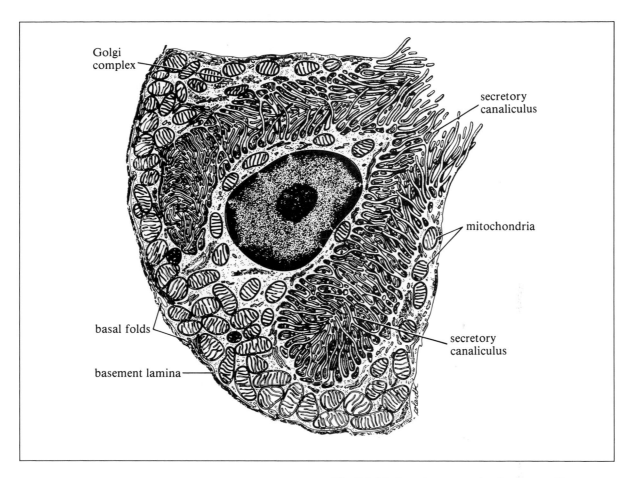

Golgi
complex

secretory
canaliculus

mitochondria

basal folds

basement lamina

secretory
canaliculus

Fig. 14-11. A gastric parietal cell as it would appear under the electron microscope. The numerous large mitochondria and striking intracellular canaliculi are involved in the elaboration of hydrochloric acid. (From W. Bloom and D. W. Fawcett, *A Textbook of Histology* [10th ed.], Philadelphia: Saunders, 1975. Reproduced with permission.)

Parietal (Oxyntic) Cells

These large, pyramidal cells are found lining the upper half of the glands and also wedged between the chief cells. They are easily recognized in hematoxylin and eosin preparations as deeply eosinophilic cells. In the electron microscope they are characterized by a **secretory canaliculus** (Fig. 14-11), which consists of an extensive invagination of the apical cell membrane into the underlying cytoplasm. The canaliculus is lined with long microvilli that greatly amplify the membrane surface area. The secretory canaliculus and abundant large mitochondria found in these cells are involved in the produc-

tion of hydrochloric acid. The pH of gastric juice can range from 0.9 to 2.0. The parietal cells also produce a glycoprotein, gastric intrinsic factor, which binds to dietary vitamin B_{12} and facilitates its absorption in the intestine. Failure to absorb vitamin B_{12} affects maturation of red cells in the bone marrow, leading to pernicious anemia.

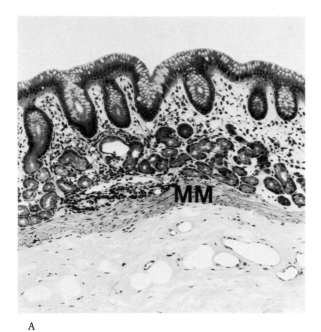

A

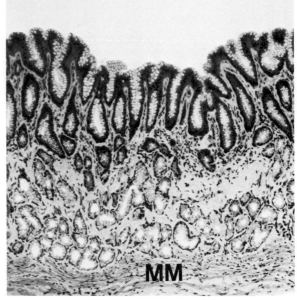

B

Fig. 14-12. The mucosa of the cardiac and the pyloric stomach. A. Cardiac region. Note the simple columnar epithelium composed of mucous cap cells, the gastric pits, and the short mucous glands (cut in cross section) extending to the muscularis mucosae (*MM*). B. Pyloric region. The mucosa is similar to that of the cardiac region, except that the gastric pits are deeper and the mucous glands are longer and more coiled. The muscularis mucosae (*MM*) is seen below.

Mucous Neck Cells

These cells, which are difficult to identify, are lodged between parietal cells in the necks of the glands where they open into the gastric pits. They stain with the PAS reaction, although their mucus differs slightly from that produced by the surface mucous cells (see Fig. 14-10B).

Argentaffin Cells (Enteroendocrine Cells)

See Argentaffin Cells: Cells of the Enteroendocrine System, below.

CARDIAC AND PYLORIC GLANDS

While differing in location, as their names indicate, these glands at the proximal and distal ends of the stomach contain predominantly mucous cells. The gastric pits in the cardiac region are relatively short. Likewise, the glands that extend down from them are primarily short, simple tubular glands. In contrast, the gastric pits of the pyloric stomach are quite deep. The glands are also longer, as well as more branched and coiled (Fig. 14-12). Argentaffin (enteroendocrine) cells are also present. They are particularly prominent in the pyloric region. However, no chief or parietal cells are present in either the cardiac or pyloric stomach.

OTHER LAYERS OF THE STOMACH

The mucosa is bounded by a muscularis mucosae. The submucosa of the stomach is similar to that in the esophagus. The muscularis externa consists of three layers of smooth muscle:

(1) outer longitudinal, (2) middle circular (the most organized layer), and (3) inner oblique. These layers work together to adapt to change in volume within the stomach without changing intragastric pressure and to empty the contents of the stomach into the duodenum. The stomach is covered by a serosa.

THE INTESTINES

Chyme arriving in the small intestine is subjected to an environment very different from that of the stomach. As described in the following chapter on the accessory digestive organs, all of the digestive juices secreted into the small intestine are alkaline and contain a large variety of hydrolytic enzymes that are absent in gastric juice. **Digestion** and **absorption** occur simultaneously in the small intestine. Digestion prepares the food for absorption and consists of two basic steps:

1. Completion of the hydrolysis of large molecules to smaller ones that can be absorbed.
2. Bringing the end products of hydrolysis into an aqueous solution or emulsion. The process of absorption consists of transferring the end products of digestion to the blood or lymph through the intestinal mucosa.

Secretion in the large intestine is limited to a viscid fluid with a high mucin content that acts as a lubricant for the passage of feces.

The Small Intestine

The small intestine is a tube about 4 m long located between the stomach and the large intestine. It is divisible into three segments: the **duodenum,** the **jejunum,** and the **ileum.** Four major layers, as already described, make up the wall of the small intestine. Functionally, the mucosa is the most important layer.

The morphology of the mucosa closely reflects its absorptive function in a number of specializations designed to increase the surface area that is exposed to the intestinal lumen. These specializations are as follows (Figs. 14-13, 14-14):

1. **Plicae circulares.** The mucosa and submucosa together form permanent crescentic folds that extend half to two-thirds of the way around the lumen, effectively increasing the surface area of the mucosa.
2. **Villi.** Fingerlike projections known as villi, 0.5 to 1.5 mm long, cover the mucosal surface in a dense mat numbering 10 to 40 per square millimeter. They give the small intestine a characteristic velvety appearance when seen as a whole specimen.
3. **Intestinal crypts (Lieberkühn's crypts).** The amount of surface epithelium is increased not only by raised villi but also by invagination to form tubular glands, or crypts, extending almost to the muscularis mucosae (see Fig. 14-14).
4. **Microvilli.** The apical surfaces of the simple columnar cells that form the mucosal epithelium are covered by a dense mat of microvilli known as the **striated border** (see Fig. 3-10). These microvilli amplify the surface area about 30-fold and constitute the major specialization that facilitates absorption.

MUCOSA

Epithelium of Villi

Three cell types form the covering of the villi:

1. **Columnar absorptive cells** have a well-developed striated border of microvilli whose plasma membranes are covered by a network of branching glycoprotein filaments, or a **surface coat.** This coat functions not only to protect the underlying cells from proteolytic and mucolytic agents but also to provide binding sites for specific substances that are to be absorbed. Enzymes catalyzing the final breakdown of proteins and carbohydrates (peptidases and disaccharidases) are actually located in the membrane of the microvilli. The products of digestion pass from the intestinal lu-

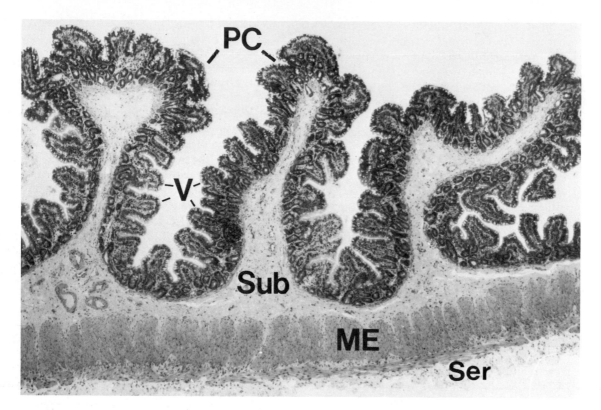

Fig. 14-13. Low-power light micrograph of longitudinal section of monkey small intestine (jejunum). Note the large folds, the plicae circulares (*PC*), covered by numerous smaller projections, the villi (*V*). The underlying tissue layers include the submucosa (*Sub*), muscularis externa (*ME*), and the serosa (*Ser*).

men through the epithelium and gain access to either blood or lymphatic channels in the underlying lamina propria. Additional details concerning the digestion and absorption of carbohydrates, protein, and fats, as well as the role of epithelial cells in those processes, are given in the summary of digestive processes at the end of this chapter.

2. **Goblet cells** are unicellular mucous glands scattered among the absorptive cells. These flask-shaped cells secrete mucus that lubricates and protects the epithelium.

3. **Argentaffin cells (enteroendocrine cells).** See below.

Epithelium Lining Crypts

The epithelium covering the villi continues down to line the crypts along their upper halves (see Fig. 14-14). The bottoms of the crypts, however, contain two additional cell types (Fig. 14-15):

1. **Undifferentiated stem cells** at the base of the crypts undergo mitosis to replace those cells that are shed from the tips of the villi. Mitotic cells that differentiate in the crypts make their way up to the surface of the villi, where they are shed in about 5 days.

2. **Paneth cells** occur in groups at the base of the crypts. They are large, striking cells containing an abundance of large secretory granules that stain deep red with eosin (see Fig. 14-15). These cells are long-lived and thus are not replaced so often as the other cell types. At present, the function of these secretory cells and

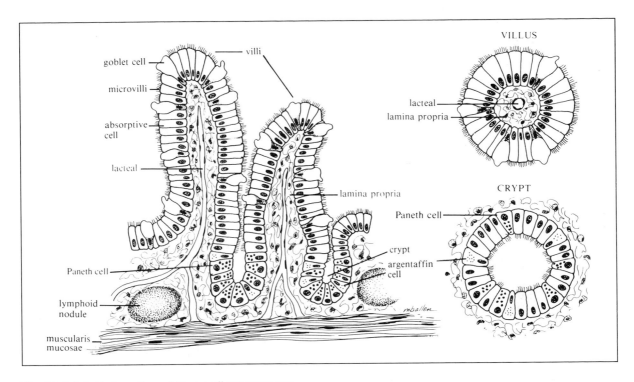

Fig. 14-14. Left: A section of the small intestine mucosa showing two villi and two crypts. Right: Cross sections through a villus and a crypt.

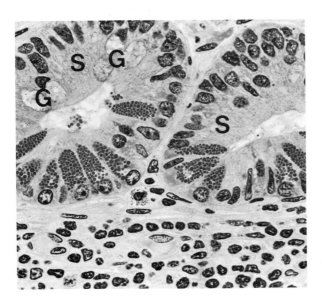

Fig. 14-15. A light micrograph of the basal regions of two intestinal crypts (monkey). Note the Paneth cells with large serous granules, the undifferentiated stem cells (S), and a few goblet cells (G). The lamina propria below contains numerous lymphoid cells.

the identity of their product are unknown, although some studies have suggested that these cells make **lysozyme,** which is an agent that is capable of lysing bacteria.

The **lamina propria** fills the spaces between the crypts and forms the cores of the villi. It resembles the reticular connective tissue of lymphoid organs in fiber content and in its large cellular component. Large numbers of **lymphocytes, macrophages, plasma cells,** and **eosinophils** are located in the fiber framework. In addition, many lymphocytes penetrate the epithelium itself. Many of the plasma cells in the lamina propria have been shown to produce IgA, an immunoglobulin that is then passed toward the lumen, attached to a protein synthesized by the epithelial cells (secretory piece). This complex may then have a protective function in preventing viral and bacterial infection. Isolated **lymphatic nodules** also occur throughout the small intestine, although they reach their greatest numbers in the ileum. Large nodules may even penetrate the muscularis mucosae and extend into the submucosa. In the ileum, groups of nodules called **Peyer's patches** aggregate together. There are 30 to 40 nodules per patch, and the patches always occur on the side of the ileum opposite the mesenteric attachment. Therefore, they may or may not be present in a microscopic section, depending on what side of the ileum the preparation was excised from.

The smooth muscle of the **muscularis mucosae** is reflected in thin strands back up into the lamina propria situated in the cores of the villi. Here the smooth muscle surrounds the central **lacteal,** a lymphatic vessel, which is the terminal branch of the lymph plexus that provides the pathway for assimilation of absorbed lipid. Contraction of the muscle cells facilitates emptying of the lacteals.

SUBMUCOSA

The submucosa is composed of dense connective tissue that contains nerve plexuses (Meissner's plexus). In the duodenum, large mucous glands (**Brunner's glands**) are located in the submucosa (Fig. 14-16). They secrete an alkaline fluid, rich in bicarbonate, which is thought to buffer and protect the duodenal mucosa from the acid gastric juice. It also provides a favorable pH for digestion to continue, since enzymes contributed by the pancreas to the duodenum have a higher pH optimum than those of the stomach.

MUSCULARIS EXTERNA

The inner circular and outer longitudinal layers of smooth muscle are separated by connective tissue containing the **myenteric nerve plexus** (Auerbach's plexus). The muscularis externa is covered by a layer of loose connective tissue bounded by a mesothelium that is continuous with the mesentery at its point of attachment.

MICROSCOPIC IDENTIFICATION OF SPECIFIC AREAS

Clues to microscopic identification of specific areas of the small intestine are as follows:

1. Duodenum: Brunner's glands in the submucosa
2. Ileum: Peyer's patches

If you see either of the above, you know exactly where the section is from. If you see neither of the above, all you can say is that the specimen is **not** duodenum. (Peyer's patches are located only on the side of the ileum opposite the mesenteric attachment, so if you do not see them you cannot **rule out** ileum.)

The Appendix

The appendix (Fig. 14-17) is a fingerlike blind pouch, an evagination of the cecum, so that it is histologically similar to the colon. It follows the four-layered pattern of the digestive tube and is characterized chiefly by its small lumen and by an extensively developed lymphoid tissue in the lamina propria and submucosa. The mucosa of the appendix, like that of the colon itself, differs

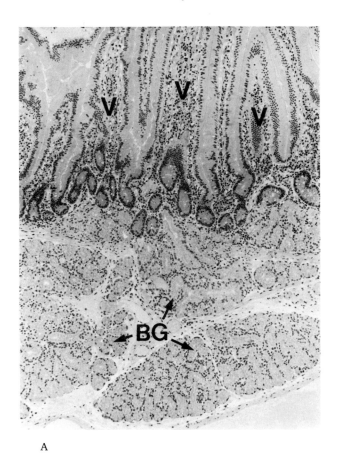

A

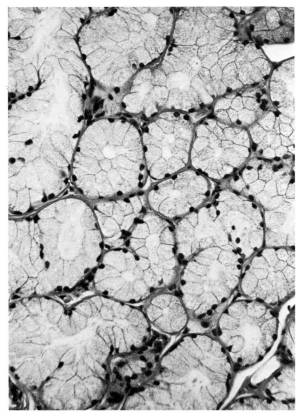

B

Fig. 14-16. The human duodenum. A. A light micrograph of the mucosa and submucosa. Note the villi (*V*), and the large mucous-producing Brunner's glands (*BG*) in the submucosa. B. Higher magnification of a Brunner's gland. It is a branched tubular gland composed almost entirely of mucous cells.

from that of the small intestine in that it does have crypts, but no villi. The epithelium contains a cell population similar to that of the small intestine: columnar cells with microvilli, goblet cells, Paneth cells, enteroendocrine (argentaffin) cells, and undifferentiated (basal) cells. The appendix by itself is considered to be a lymphoid organ of minor immunologic significance, but it is part of a larger and important defense system, which includes the tonsils and Peyer's patches, known as the gut-associated lymphoid tissues (see Chap. 10).

The Large Intestine (Colon)

The main function of the colon (Figs. 14-18, 14-19) is the absorption of water and minerals, converting the residual chyme that enters into semisolid feces. Certain vitamins are also absorbed, some of which are synthesized by the large numbers of endogenous bacteria.

Although amino acids can be absorbed by the colon, nearly all absorption of digestive products occurs in the small intestine. Many of the specializations of the mucosa that amplify surface area in the small intestine, therefore, disappear at the level of the colon. There are no plicae circulares or villi in the colon, and the striated

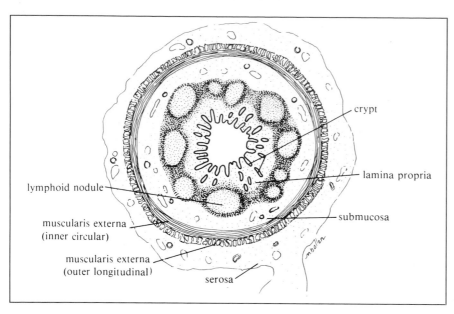

Fig. 14-17. Cross section of the appendix.

Fig. 14-18. Cross section of the colon (low magnification).

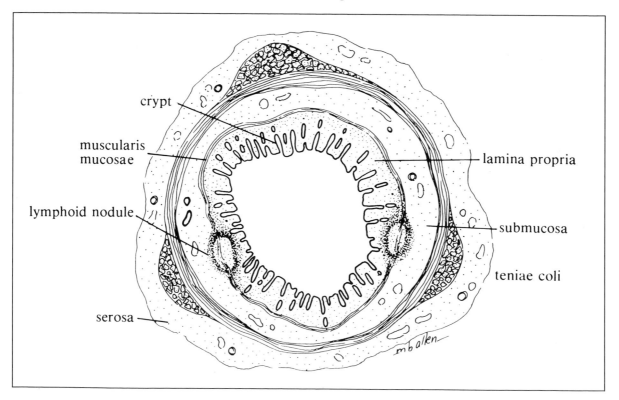

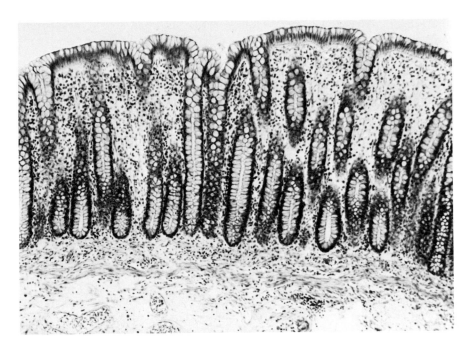

Fig. 14-19. A light micrograph of the human colon mucosa. Note the absence of villi. Long crypts extend down to the muscularis mucosa. The surface cells and those lining the crypts are primarily goblet cells.

borders of the epithelial cells are shorter than in the small intestine. The intestinal crypts, on the other hand, persist and are quite deep. They differ from those of the small intestine in their greater number of goblet cells and lack of Paneth cells. Since goblet cells produce a lubricant mucus, more goblet cells appear in the distal portions of the gastrointestinal tract as the feces become more solid.

The structure of the lamina propria in the colon is similar to that of the small intestine. Lymphoid nodules continue to occur, often extending into the typical submucosa through the well-developed muscularis mucosae.

The outer longitudinal layer of the muscularis externa is characteristically reorganized into three thick longitudinal bands, the **teniae coli,** which persist to the level of the rectum where the muscularis assumes its typical arrangement.

The colon is covered by a serosa. At the distal end of the colon, the tract is modified into a straight canal, called the **rectum.** Here there are no plicae circulares and the crypts are fewer and deeper. The rectum joins the anal canal.

In the anus, the mucosa assumes longitudinal folds known as the **rectal columns of Morgagni.** The crypts shorten, and the epithelium suddenly becomes a stratified squamous type as the transition to skin is made. A large plexus of veins in the lamina propria of this region may become distended and varicose, presenting as hemorrhoids.

Argentaffin Cells: Cells of the Enteroendocrine System

Small granulated cells occur in the epithelia of the stomach and the small and large intestine as well as in the ducts of the pancreas and liver. They are particularly prominent in the pyloric stomach and in the duodenum of the small intestine. **Argentaffin** is an archaic but popular term referring to the silver-staining properties of these cells. These cells are now more properly referred to as **enteroendocrine** cells and are known to be hormone producing cells belonging to the **APUD system** (having **a**mine **p**recursor **u**ptake and **d**e-carboxylation properties). Because such endocrine cells are scattered throughout several organ systems, they are included in a larger category of cells known collectively as the **diffuse neuroendocrine system** (see Chap. 17). In the digestive system alone, over a dozen different hormone-producing cells have been described.

Argentaffin or enteroendocrine cells are difficult to distinguish light microscopically without silver staining. But when appropriately stained, it can be seen that most of the enteroendocrine cell cytoplasm, which is full of minute granules, is basally oriented, adjacent to the lamina propria into which the cell discharges its products. At the ultrastructural level, enteroendocrine cells as a group resemble peptide hormone-producing cells, with well-developed rough endoplasmic reticulum and Golgi membranes. The secretory vesicles are small and membrane-bound. Several distinct cell types have been described, based on secretory granule characteristics. This suggests that each may have a different endocrine function. Although such a direct correlation has not yet been established, immunocytochemical techniques have been used specifically to localize the various hormone-producing cells. Figure 14-20 shows an electron microscopic view of a "typical" human enteroendocrine cell.

In the stomach, cells of the enteroendocrine system are located at the base of the glands, scattered singly among the other cell types (see Fig. 14-9). Here they produce a number of peptide hormones and vasoactive amines. One of the peptides, **gastrin,** increases gastric motility as well as secretion of both hydrogen chloride and pepsinogen. Another peptide, **somatostatin,** inhibits the function of gastrin and several other hormones. The stomach also contains **insulin**-producing cells and **glucagon**-producing cells (often termed **enteroglucagon**), which resemble A cells of the endocrine pancreas and are directly involved in insulin regulation. **Histamine** stimulates gastric secretion and increases vascular permeability, while another amine, **serotonin,** inhibits gastric secretion and is a potent vasoconstrictor.

Enteroendocrine cells are also located basally between absorptive cells of the small and large intestines. Like those of the gastric mucosa, these cells produce a variety of peptide hormones and amines. In addition to enteroglucagon and serotonin, the enteroendocrine cells of the intestines also produce **secretin** and **pancreozymin** (or **cholecystokinin**), which control the secretions of the accessory digestive organs (as discussed in the next chapter); **motilin,** which increases contractility of the smooth musculature; and **neurotensin,** which decreases smooth muscle contractility and modulates glucoregulatory systems, leading to rapid hyperglycemia. There are many other hormones produced by intestinal cells, but their functional roles in digestive physiology have not been elucidated as yet.

It is of interest to note that several of the peptide hormones present in the gut are also found in the central nervous system and in peripheral nerves. This probably represents an intricate neuroendocrine linkage, in which products of the enteroendocrine system provide both local hormonal regulation of digestive processes by affecting neighboring cells (**paracine** function) and control of distant functions by discharging these products into the bloodstream (**endocrine** function).

Enteroendocrine cells can also be regarded as sensory cells that receive stimuli from the gut lumen through tuftlike long microvilli projecting into the gut lumen (see Fig. 14-20, **inset**). Physical as well as chemical agents may serve as stimuli. However, enteroendocrine cells are not

Fig. 14-20. An electron micrograph of an enteroendocrine (argentaffin) cell from the human colon. Note that the cell is polarized toward the basal lamina. The electron-dense secretory granules are released into the lamina propria below. (Courtesy of P. Colony.) Inset: an enteroendocrine cell from the small intestine of a guinea pig stained with silver, showing a cytoplasmic extension to the lumen of the intestinal crypt.

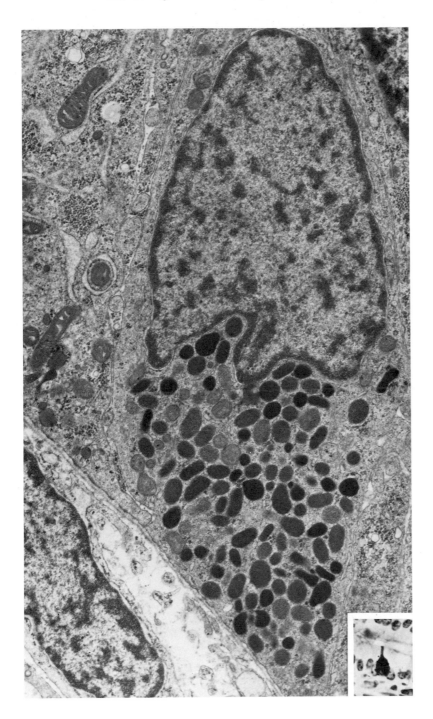

intimately connected to either the underlying nerves or capillaries; hence, they are significantly different from classic endocrine cells not only with respect to mode of stimulation but also with respect to mode of action. The morphologic and functional similarities among sensory, neuroendocrine, and enteroendocrine cells are numerous. Thus, the hormones of enteroendocrine cells can also be considered neurotransmitters. This view is supported by the fact that some polypeptide hormones are common to both the gastrointestinal tract and the central and peripheral nervous systems.

SUMMARY OF THE DIGESTIVE PROCESSES

The products of digestion pass from the lumen of the gastrointestinal tract to the circulation. The physiology of these transfer reactions is beyond the scope of this discussion, except to mention that the processes involved include **pinocytosis** and **active transport.** The large concentration of products on the luminal side, of course, yields a large gradient favoring rapid diffusion to the blood. Many substances, however, are actively transported and others are secreted by the mucosal epithelium. The small intestine is richly vascularized to receive absorbed nutrients (Fig. 14-21).

The biochemical process of digestion is now known in some detail. The glycoprotein coat, which covers the microvilli of the duodenal epithelium, acts as a matrix to which digestive enzymes bind in their inactive forms. **Enterokinase,** produced by the absorptive epithelium itself, locally activates trypsinogen to trypsin. In turn, trypsin activates all of the other inactive digestive enzymes. This is referred to as the **cascade activation mechanism.**

Carbohydrates

Starch (a glucose polymer) and its derivatives are the major polysaccharides digested by the human. The disaccharides **sucrose, lactose,** and **maltose** and the monosaccharides **glucose** and

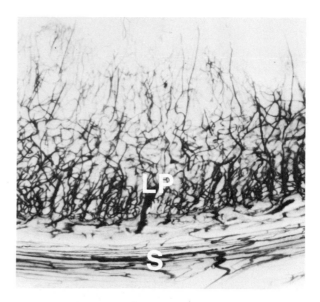

Fig. 14-21. A light micrograph of an unstained guinea pig small intestine. The vasculature was perfused with a latex material to allow visualization of the blood supply. Note the blood vessels in the submucosa (*S*) and the lamina propria (*LP*). Capillaries extend from the lamina propria into the villi.

fructose are the principal simple sugars. Starch is partially reduced to **dextrins** by the action of **ptyalin** in the saliva. In the small intestine, it is degraded to disaccharides by **pancreatic amylase.** The disaccharides are further split into monosaccharides by enzymes that are located on the striated border of intestinal epithelial cells; they are then absorbed by various mechanisms into the blood.

Proteins

Pepsinogen produced by the chief cells of the gastric glands is converted to the active enzyme pepsin by hydrochloric acid elaborated by the parietal cells. It cleaves proteins to smaller polypeptide fragments. The action of pepsin is terminated by the alkaline pH of pancreatic secretions released into the duodenum. Trypsin, chymotrypsin, and carboxypeptidase, components of pancreatic juice, and intestinal aminopeptidases and dipeptidases split the polypeptides into amino acids.

Infants of many species, including humans, are able to absorb some proteins directly by pinocytosis without first digesting them. The protein antibodies of maternal colostrum, which may confer passive immunity to the infant, are absorbed from the intestine. As the gastrointestinal tract matures, the cells lose their ability to absorb proteins by pinocytosis. For this reason, protein foods such as eggs and wheat should not be given to small infants, who may absorb them and develop allergies against them.

Fats

Pancreatic lipase digests dietary triglycerides into free fatty acids and monoglycerides in the duodenum (Fig. 14-22). These products are emulsified by bile salts to form micelles about 2 nm in diameter that diffuse across the apical border of mucosal absorptive cells and accumulate in the cytoplasm. The micelles are picked up by the smooth endoplasmic reticulum (SER), whose membranes contain enzymes for the resynthesis of triglycerides from fatty acids and monoglycerides. The resynthesized triglyceride accumulates within the SER; it is then transported to the Golgi apparatus where it is further processed

Fig. 14-22. The pathway of lipid absorption by the intestinal epithelium. (*1*) Lipid droplets consisting primarily of triglycerides are hydrolyzed by pancreatic lipase in the lumen of the small intestine, yielding free fatty acids and monoglycerides. (*2*) Free fatty acids and monoglycerides are bound by bile salts into micelles, which diffuse across the microvillous membrane into the apical cell cytoplasm where they gain access to the smooth endoplasmic reticulum (SER). In the lumen of the SER they are again esterified into triglycerides. (*3*) The triglycerides are transported to the Golgi apparatus, where they are modified by the addition of protein and sugar moieties into complex glycolipoprotein granules called chylomicra. (*4*) Chylomicra are released from the lateral borders of the cells by exocytosis. They cross the basement membrane and finally enter lymphatic vessels in the lamina propria.

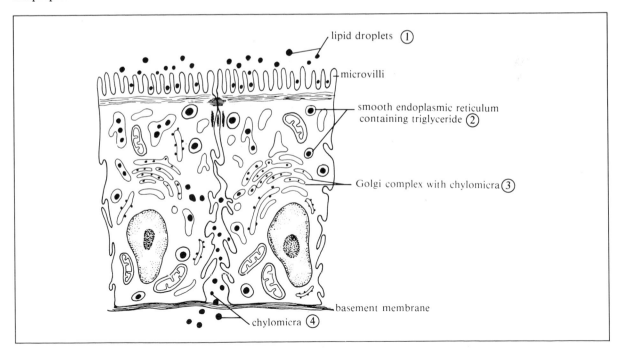

lipid droplets ①

microvilli

smooth endoplasmic reticulum containing triglyceride ②

Golgi complex with chylomicra ③

basement membrane

chylomicra ④

into complex, membrane-bound glycolipoprotein droplets or **chylomicra.** The chylomicra fuse with the lateral plasma membranes of the absorptive cells and are discharged into the extracellular space between neighboring absorptive cells. They then move down, cross the basal lamina, and enter the small lymphatic vessels in the lamina propria of the intestinal villi. These lymphatics drain into the central lacteals, which are periodically emptied by contractions of the villus, occurring about 6 times per minute.

NATIONAL BOARD TYPE QUESTIONS

For the following, select
   A. if only *1, 2, and 3* are correct.
   B. if only *1 and 3* are correct.
   C. if only *2 and 4* are correct.
   D. if only *4* is correct.
   E. if *all* are correct.

1. Regarding circumvallate papillae, which of the following statements is (are) correct?
   1. They contain more taste buds than fungiform papillae.
   2. They are distributed uniformly throughout the dorsal surface of the tongue.
   3. They are associated with serous glands.
   4. They are the most numerous type of papillae.
2. Which of the following statements regarding dentin is (are) correct?
   1. It contains more inorganic material than enamel.
   2. It is derived from ectoderm.
   3. It is attached directly to the alveolar bone.
   4. It can be repaired by increased matrix production of odontoblasts.
3. In the gastrointestinal tract, glands occur in the
   1. epithelium.
   2. lamina propria.

3. submucosa.
4. muscularis mucosae.
4. An individual deficient in parietal cells will exhibit which of the following symptoms directly related to that cell type?
   1. Pernicious anemia
   2. Decrease in the mucous coat lining the stomach
   3. Elevated pH in the lumen of the stomach
   4. Decrease in production of gastrin
5. Which of the following cells are found in gastric glands (in fundic stomach)?
   1. Enteroendocrine cells
   2. Zymogen (chief) cells
   3. Mucous neck cells
   4. Goblet cells

Select the single best response for each of the following.

6. In what order do the complex fats encounter the following components of the lipid processing system: (1) lacteals, (2) lipases/bile salts, (3) microvilli of intestinal absorptive cells, (4) chylomicrons, (5) basolateral surface of intestinal absorptive cells.
   A. 4, 3, 5, 1, 2
   B. 2, 3, 4, 5, 1
   C. 2, 4, 5, 3, 1
   D. 3, 2, 4, 5, 1
   E. 3, 2, 5, 1, 4
7. Which structures are present in the large intestine and not in the small intestine?
   A. Goblet cells
   B. Absorptive cells
   C. Paneth cells
   D. Enteroendocrine cells
   E. Autonomic ganglia
8. In which segment of the gastrointestinal tract does one find the most rapid turnover of epithelium?
   A. Esophagus
   B. Fundic stomach
   C. Pyloric stomach
   D. Small intestine
   E. Colon

9. Enterokinase, produced by intestinal absorptive cells, serves which function?
   A. Elevates the pH in the lumen
   B. Induces secretion of pancreatic enzymes
   C. Converts trypsinogen to trypsin
   D. Facilitates lipid uptake
   E. Regulates water absorption

Select the response most closely associated with each numbered item. (The headings may be used once, more than once, or not at all.)
The following are products of the enteroendocrine system:
   A. Gastrin
   B. Enteroglucagon
   C. Somatostatin
   D. Serotonin
   E. Secretin

10. Induced secretion of accessory digestive organs
11. Vasoconstrictor
12. Increases secretions of hydrogen chloride and pepsinogen

ANNOTATED ANSWERS

1. B. Circumvallate papillae form a well-defined ridge in the midregion of the tongue. They are the least numerous of the papillae, but are the largest and contain the most taste buds.
2. D. Unlike enamel, which is 99.5 percent inorganic, ectodermally derived, and incapable of repair, dentin is less hard, mesodermal in origin, and repairable by odontoblasts which reside in the pulp. The periodontal ligament attaches the cementum of the tooth to the alveolar bone.
3. A. Unicellular glands occur within the epithelium itself, while more complex glands are found in the underlying connective tissue layers.
4. B. Parietal cells produce hydrogen chloride, responsible for the low pH of stomach secretions, and gastric intrinsic factor, responsible for facilitating absorption of vitamin B_{12}. This vitamin is essential for the maturation of erythrocytes.
5. A. Goblet cells are not present in the stomach. Mucus is produced by cells of the surface epithelium and by mucous neck cells.
6. B. Lipases and bile salts digest and emulsify lipids in the lumen. They are absorbed by microvilli, processed into membrane-bound droplets called chylomicrons which are discharged basolaterally and taken up by lymphatic vessels in the connective tissue.
7. C. Paneth cells are not present in the colon. All others listed are found throughout the small and large intestine.
8. D. The most rapid renewal of epithelium occurs in the small intestine. For this reason, the first side effects of chemotherapy are usually malabsorption and diarrhea which occur in 3 to 4 days.
9. C. The function of enterokinase is to convert trypsinogen to trypsin, its active form. Trypsin, in turn, activates all the other inactive digestive enzymes.
10. E. Secretin induces secretion of digestive enzymes by the pancreas and release of bile by the gallbladder.
11. D. Serotonin inhibits gastric secretion and is a potent vasoconstrictor.
12. A. Gastrin has a direct stimulatory effect on cells of the gastric glands.

BIBLIOGRAPHY

Bhaskar, S. N. (ed.). *Orban's Oral Histology* (8th ed.). St. Louis: Mosby, 1976.
Cardell, R. R., S. Badenhausen, and K. R. Porter. Intestinal absorption in the rat. An electron microscopic study. *J. Cell Biol.* 34:123, 1967.

Clementi, S. W., and G. E. Palade. Intestinal capillaries. I. Permeability to peroxidase and ferritin. *J. Cell Biol.* 41:33, 1969.

Craig, S. W., and J. J. Cebra. Peyer's patches: An enriched source of precursors for IgA-producing immunocytes in the rabbit. *J. Exp. Med.* 134:188, 1971.

Davenport, H. W. *Physiology of the Digestive Tract.* Chicago: Year Book, 1971. P. 85.

Eastwood, G. L. Gastrointestinal epithelial renewal. *Gastroenterology* 72:962, 1977.

Edwards, D. A. W. The esophagus. *Gut* 12:948, 1971.

Erlandsen, S. L., J. A. Parsons, and T. D. Taylor. Ultrastructural immunocytochemical localization of lysozyme in the Paneth cells of man. *J. Histochem. Cytochem.* 22:401, 1974.

Fault, W. P. Peyer's patches: Morphologic studies. *Cell. Immunol.* 1:500, 1970.

Friedman, M. H. F. (ed.). *Functions of the Stomach and Intestines.* Baltimore: University Park Press, 1975.

Fujita, T. S., and S. Kobayashi. The structure and function of gut endocrine cells. *Int. Rev. Cytol.* 6(Suppl.):187, 1977.

Garrett, J. R., J. D. Harrison, and P. J. Stoward. *Histochemistry of Secretory Process.* London: Chapman Hall, 1977.

Gray, G. M. Carbohydrate digestion and absorption: Role of small intestine. *N. Engl. J. Med.,* 292:1225, 1975.

Greider, M. H., V. Steinberg, and J. E. McGuigan. Electron microscopic identification of the gastrin cell of the human antral mucosa by means of immunocytochemistry. *Gastroenterology* 63:572, 1972.

Grossman, M. J. Gastrin and its activities. *Nature* 228:1147, 1970.

Grube, D., and W. G. Forssman. Morphology and function of the enteroendocrine cells. *Horm. Metab. Res.* 11:589, 1979.

Hand, A. R. Nerve-acinar cell relationships in the rat parotid gland. *J. Cell Biol.* 47:540, 1970.

Hashimoto, K., R. J. Dibella, and G. Shklar. Electron microscopic studies of the normal human buccal mucosa. *J. Invest. Dermatol.* 47:512, 1966.

Hingson, D. J., and S. Ito. Effect of aspirin and related compounds on the structure of mouse gastric mucosa. *Gastroenterology* 61:156, 1971.

Isselbacher, K. J. The intestinal cell surface: Properties of normal, undifferentiated, and malignant cells. *Harvey Lect.* 69:197, 1973–1974.

Ito, S. Anatomic Structure of the Gastric Mucosa. In C. F. Code and W. Heidel (eds.), *Handbook of Physiology.* Baltimore: Williams & Wilkins, 1967. Vol. 2, p. 705.

Ito, S. The fine structure of the gastric mucosa. In *Gastric Secretion: Mechanisms and Control.* Oxford: Pergamon, 1967. P. 3.

Ito, S., and G. C. Schofield. Studies on the depletion and accumulation of microvilli and changes in the tubulovesicular compartment of the mouse parietal cells in relation to gastric acid secretion. *J. Cell Biol.* 63:364, 1974.

Johnson, L. R. (ed.). *Gastrointestinal Physiology.* St. Louis: Mosby, 1977.

Larsson, L. I. Peptide secretory pathways in GI tract: Cytochemical contributions to regulatory physiology of the gut. *Am. J. Physiol.,* 239:237, 1981.

Leblond, C. P. Life history of cells in renewing systems. *Am. J. Anat.* 160:113, 1981.

Leblond, C. P., and M. Weinstock. A Comparative Study of Dentin and Bone Formation. In G. H. Bourne (ed.), *Biochemistry and Physiology of Bone.* New York: Academic, 1976. Vol. 4, p. 517.

Mattern, C. F. T., W. A. Daniel, and R. I. Henkin. The ultrastructure of the human circumvallate papilla: I. Cilia of the papillary crypt. *Anat. Rec.* 167:175, 1970.

Merzel, J., and C. P. Leblond. Origin and renewal of goblet cells in the epithelium of the mouse small intestine. *Am. J. Anat.* 124:381, 1969.

Mooseker, M. S., and L. G. Tilney. Organization of an actin filament—membrane complex, filament polarity and membrane attachment in the microvilli of intestinal epithelial cells. *J. Cell Biol.* 67:725, 1975.

Moxey, P. C., and J. S. Trier. Endocrine cells in the human fetal small intestine. *Cell Tissue Res.* 183:33, 1977.

Murray, R. G., A. Murray, and S. Fujimoto. Fine structure of gustatory cells. *J. Ultrastruct. Res.* 27:444, 1969.

Ockner, R. K., and K. J. Isselbacher. Recent concepts in intestinal fat absorption. *Rev. Physiol. Biochem. Pharmacol.* 17:107, 1974.

Owen, R. L., and A. L. Jones. Epithelial cell specializations within human Peyer's patches: An ultrastructural study of intestinal lymphoid follicles. *Gastroenterology* 66:189, 1974.

Palay, S. L., and L. J. Karlin. An electron microscopic study of the intestinal villus. I. The fasting animal. II. The pathway of fat absorption. *J. Biophys. Biochem. Cytol.* 5:363, 373, 1959.

Rubin, W., W. D. Gershon, and L. L. Ross. Electron microscope radioautographic identification of serotonin-synthesizing cells in the mouse gastric mucosa. *J. Cell Biol.* 50:399, 1971.

Samloff, I. M. Pepsinogens, pepsins, and pepsin inhibitors. *Gastroenterology* 60:586, 1971.

Schofield, G. C., S. Ito, and R. P. Bolender. Changes in

membrane surface areas in mouse parietal cells in relation to high levels of acid secretion. *J. Anat.* 128:669, 1979.

Slaven, H. C., and L. A. Baretta (eds.). *Developmental Aspects of Oral Biology.* New York: Academic, 1972.

Solcia, E., C. Capella, G. Vassallo, and R. Buffa. Endocrine cells of the gastric mucosa. *Int. Rev. Cytol.* 42:223, 1976.

Thorn, N. A., and O. H. Petersen (eds.). *Secretory Mechanisms of Exocrine Glands.* New York: Academic, 1975.

Trier, J. S. Morphology of the Epithelium of the Small Intestine. In C. F. Code and W. Heidel (eds.), *Handbook of Physiology.* Washington, D.C.: American Physiological Society, 1968. Vol. 3, Chap. 63.

Walker, W. A., and R. Hong. Immunology of the gastrointestinal tract. Part I. *J. Pediatr.* 83:517, 1973.

15 Accessory Digestive Organs

Objectives

You will learn the following in this chapter:

The histologic organization of the exocrine and endocrine portions of the pancreas

Ultrastructural aspects of digestive enzyme secretion from the exocrine acinar cells of the pancreas

The various cell types of the islets of Langerhans and their hormones

The histologic organization of the liver with particular emphasis on blood supply and bile ducts

The ultrastructure of the hepatocyte and its multiple roles in digestion and regulation of plasma constituents

The ultrastructure of the Kupffer cell and its role in the reticuloendothelial system as a phagocytic cell

The histologic organization of the gallbladder and its role in storage and secretion of bile

In addition to the salivary glands, three other organs extrinsic to the alimentary canal are connected to it by ducts: the **pancreas, liver,** and **gallbladder.** In the embryo, these glands form as diverticula from the primitive foregut and remain attached by excretory ducts to the duodenum in the adult. The substances dispensed through these ducts are important participants in the digestive and absorptive processes occurring in the intestines. Since these substances are conveyed through ducts to an external body surface (intestinal canal) and eventually eliminated from the body in the feces, the glands producing them are included in the category of **exocrine glands.**

However, the pancreas is not an exocrine gland exclusively but also consists of endocrine tissue that produces hormones and releases them into the circulation. Nor is the liver exclusively an exocrine gland. Although it excretes bile, it also synthesizes a profusion of substances that it contributes to the bloodstream.

THE PANCREAS

The pancreas performs two important functions: (1) the synthesis and release of digestive enzymes (exocrine function), and (2) the synthesis and release of several hormones that influence carbohydrate metabolism (endocrine function). These separate tasks are performed by histologically distinct areas of the pancreas. The exocrine pancreas accounts for the bulk of the parenchyma, which is punctuated by small, discrete islands of

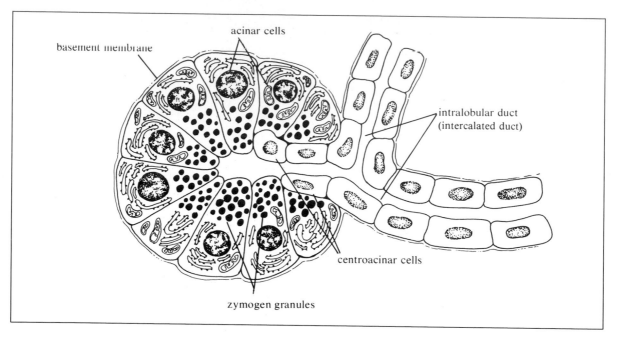

Fig. 15-1. Exocrine acinus of the pancreas.

endocrine tissue (islets of Langerhans). These two functions are discussed separately.

Exocrine Pancreas

HISTOLOGIC ASPECTS

The exocrine part of the pancreas is a compound acinar gland. It is composed of secretory acini deployed at the ends of a branching duct system; the ducts eventually coalesce to form the **main pancreatic duct** (duct of Wirsung) and an accessory duct (Santorini), which drain into the duodenal lumen.

Although the pancreas is retroperitoneal, there is peritoneal mesothelium associated with part of its surface. It has an incomplete connective tissue capsule that when present is thin enough to reveal convolutions of the underlying lobulation. Septa extend from this connective tissue capsule, subdividing it into incomplete lobules with considerable variation in size.

The **secretory acinus** is composed of pyramidal epithelial cells arranged around the terminus of an **intralobular duct** (intercalated duct).

Epithelial cells of the acinus are joined together on their lateral surfaces by junctional complexes, rest on a basal lamina, and are supported by reticular fibers (Fig. 15-1).

When properly fixed and stained, the apical and basal portions of the acinar cells display opposite affinities for acid and basic dyes. The apical portion contains acidophilic granules and the basal portion contains an amorphous basophilic material (Figs. 15-2, 15-3). Electron microscopy indicates that the granular eosinophilia in the apical part of the cell is due to membrane-bound secretory granules containing digestive enzymes that are localized there, and that the basophilia near the base of the cell is attributable to the abundance of rough endoplasmic reticulum (RER) localized there (see Figs. 15-1, 15-2). In addition, filamentous mitochondria frequently give the basal part of the cell a striated appearance. The nucleus occupies a position somewhat basal in the cell; it has a prominent nucleolus and peripherally placed chromatin. The Golgi apparatus is supranuclear. Microtubules are present in the apical region of the cell.

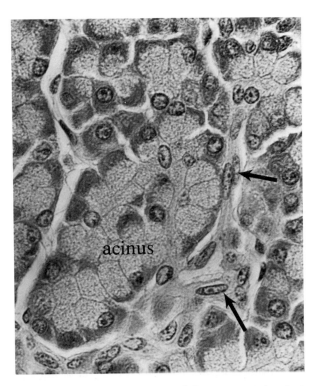

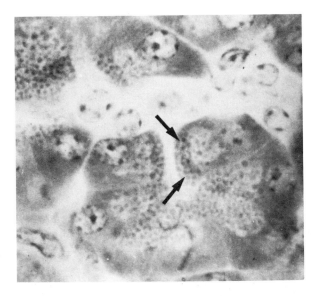

Fig. 15-3. Exocrine acinus within the pancreas. A half a dozen or more cells make up this particular acinus. Notice the zymogen granules located within the apical cytoplasm (*arrows*).

Fig. 15-2. Exocrine portion of the pancreas showing a large acinus. Basal portion of the exocrine cells are basophilic, while the apical portion is acidophilic or lighter staining in this micrograph. An intralobular duct is present with relatively flat epithelial cells (*arrows*).

The intralobular ducts are composed of a low cuboidal to cuboidal epithelium that stains poorly relative to the acinar cells, making them easily identified even at low magnification (see Fig. 15-2). The larger **interlobular ducts** display tall columnar epithelium. They course through the interlobular connective tissue, increasing in size as more and more ducts join to them. These larger ducts have occasional goblet cells and argentaffin cells. The main duct of Wirsung, surrounded by dense collagenous connective tissue, traverses the length of the pancreas and opens into a recess of the duodenal lumen (the **ampulla of Vater**), either alone or together with the common bile duct. The wall of this terminal part of the duct is composed of longitudinal and circularly arranged smooth muscle (the **sphincter of Oddi**), which regulates the flow of digestive enzymes from the pancreas as well as bile flow from the gallbladder.

INNERVATION

The human pancreas receives neural contributions from the **vagal** (parasympathetic) and **splanchnic** (sympathetic) nerves, which penetrate the periphery of its superior and inferior borders to travel within the interlobular connective tissue. The nerves terminate within parasympathetic and sympathetic ganglia, which are also located in the interlobular septa. Postganglionic axons penetrate the parenchyma and distribute to the acini, islets, and blood vessels.

Axons have been observed by electron microscopy to penetrate the basal lamina around acini and establish contact with the basal surfaces of the acinar cells. Since vagal stimulation and cholinergic agonists provoke secretion of pancreatic enzymes, it is probable that these axons innervating the acinar epithelium are vagal in origin. However, accumulating evidence indicates that our understanding of pancreatic innervation is incomplete and that a peptidergic pathway exists in addition to cholinergic and adrenergic ones. Immunocytochemistry has revealed the presence of peptidergic nerves containing **vasoactive intestinal polypeptide** (VIP). VIP nerves have been observed in association with both exocrine and endocrine portions of the pancreas. It is a potent vasodilator of splanchnic vasculature and, therefore, causes systemic hypotension.

VASCULATURE

Arterial blood is supplied by the pancreaticoduodenal arteries (plus branches of the splenic and hepatic arteries), which form arcades around the pancreas. Smaller branches from these arcades travel within the interlobular connective tissue and then penetrate the lobules, where they distribute to the acini and islets. Branching arterioles supply the islets and acini separately. However, the outflow from the islets drains through several capillaries into the exocrine capillary network, producing an **insular-acinar portal system.** This portal system is the morphologic basis for a possible endocrine influence by islets on the exocrine portion of the pancreas. The venous drainage follows the arterial course in reverse fashion, ultimately emptying into the portal and splenic veins.

FUNCTIONAL CONSIDERATIONS

The pancreas synthesizes a complete range of digestive enzymes required to break down proteins, fats, and starches into smaller molecules that can be absorbed by the intestine. These enzymes include trypsinogen, chymotrypsinogen, procarboxypeptidases, proelastase, amylase, various lipases, deoxyribonuclease, and ribonuclease. The enzymes are stored in the secretory vesicles (zymogen granules) that accumulate in the apical cytoplasm (see Fig. 15-3).

Digestive enzymes are synthesized on the rough endoplasmic reticulum and released into its lumen. **Transport vesicles** containing the newly synthesized proteins pinch off from the smooth portion of the endoplasmic reticulum and migrate to the Golgi apparatus, where they coalesce with the forming face of the Golgi. **Condensing vacuoles** containing the dilute enzyme products pinch off from the concave secretory face of the Golgi and concentrate them into dense membrane-bound granules (zymogen granules). The zymogen granules are in the secretory vesicles that are stored in the apical portion of the cell before being discharged into the acinar lumen. The membrane of a few vesicles will fuse with the apical plasmalemma. The part of the plasmalemma to which the secretory vesicle fuses ruptures and the contents of the vesicles are discharged into the lumen of the acinus, which is continuous with the lumen of the intralobular duct. This vesicle-mediated release of substances from a cell is called **exocytosis** (emiocytosis). Exocytosis of a digestive enzyme normally occurs at a liminal pace but is dramatically accelerated by vagal and hormonal stimuli that depolarize the acinar cell (stimulus-secretion coupling).

Since microtubule-disrupting drugs interfere with the secretion of digestive enzymes, there is some evidence that microtubules may participate in cell secretion by ferrying secretory vesicles from the Golgi region to the apical cell membrane prior to exocytosis.

Secretion of pancreatic fluid is provoked by vagal and hormonal stimulation although it is not clear which stimulus is more important in the human pancreas. The hormonal stimulation is provided by two hormones: the oligopeptide **pancreozymin** (also known as **cholecystokinin**) and **secretin.** Both are produced by the duodenal mucosa and released in response to the entry of acidified stomach contents into the duodenum. These hormones must enter the circulation to reach the pancreas. Because vagotomy increases the latency of pancreatic response to intraduodenal stimulation, the early phase of pancreatic enzyme release is probably vagally mediated.

Pancreozymin and secretin act upon two different cellular targets. Pancreozymin initiates release of digestive enzymes from the acinar cells. Secretin causes the duct cells to release an aqueous bicarbonate solution that becomes the fluid vehicle carrying pancreatic enzymes to the duodenum. The alkaline pH of the ductal solution maintains the released enzymes in an inactive state until they reach the duodenum, thus preventing autodigestion of the pancreas. The mixing of this alkaline pancreatic juice with the acidic contents of the stomach creates a neutral pH within the duodenum. The neutral pH allows **enterokinase,** an enzyme associated with the intestinal mucosa, to convert the inactive trypsinogen to the active trypsin. Trypsin in turn activates the other precursor proteolytic enzymes. The lipases and amylase are apparently released in the active form.

Endocrine Pancreas

HISTOLOGIC ASPECTS

The endocrine cells of the pancreas are aggregated into small spherical clusters known as **islets of Langerhans,** which are scattered among the exocrine acini and ducts. The cells of the islets are arranged into compact anastomosing cords that are extensively vascularized by fenestrated capillaries, as would be expected of endocrine tissue (Figs. 15-4, 15-5). In contrast with the exocrine pancreas, there are no ducts associated with the islets. Each islet cell is closely apposed to a capillary so that hormones are released directly into the pericapillary space.

Several cell types have been identified in the islets of the human pancreas but routine histologic stains such as hematoxylin and eosin do not distinguish them from one another. However, certain stains distinguish cells based on differential staining of their cytoplasmic granules. After chrome alum hematoxylin, the

Fig. 15-4. Islet of Langerhans.

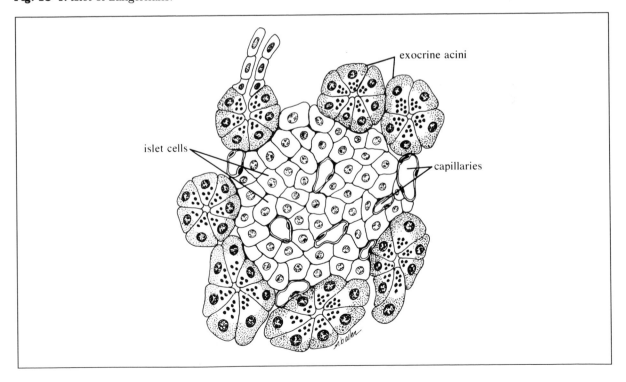

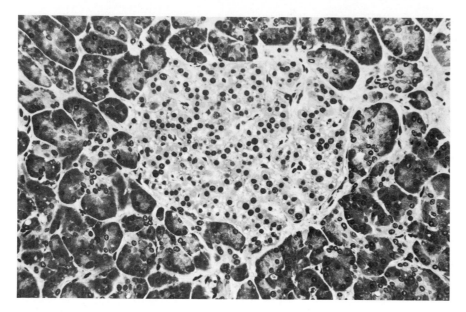

Fig. 15-5. A light micrograph of a pancreatic islet surrounded by acinar cells of the exocrine pancreas.

glucagon-producing alpha cells (A cells) stain red, and the **insulin-producing beta cells** (B cells) stain blue. Alpha and beta cells represent 20 and 75 percent of the islet cell population, respectively. With more complex staining mixtures two other cells are identified: the **delta cells,** which account for 5 percent of the islet cell population, and a clear cell (C cell) type without stainable granules. **Somatostatin** has been located in granules of the delta cell by immunocytochemistry and is known to inhibit the release of insulin and glucagon. Somatostatin is apparently involved in nutrient homeostasis. Delta cells appear to be identical with somatostatin cells of the duodenal mucosa. Somatostatin is also secreted from the hypothalamus and blocks release of growth hormone from the pituitary.

More recently another human islet cell has been identified by immunocytochemistry. It secretes **pancreatic polypeptide** (PP). Cells secreting PP are located preferentially in the ventral portion of the head of the pancreas. They are mostly deployed within the islet periphery, but single cells are also scattered through the exo-crine tissue in this area. PP is released in response to ingestion of food. It stimulates secretion of gastric enzymes, and inhibits bile secretion and intestinal peristalsis. However, excessive amounts of PP have been implicated in the pathophysiology of diabetes mellitus. Secretion is apparently under control of adrenergic nerves.

FUNCTIONAL ASPECTS

Glucagon and insulin are hormones that exert powerful effects on carbohydrate metabolism, most notably in adipose tissue, muscle, and the liver. These two hormones exert an antagonistic influence on blood glucose levels.

Glucagon is a **hyperglycemic-glycogenolytic hormone** that is released in response to low blood glucose levels. Its primary action is in the liver, where it causes glycogenolysis (breakdown of glycogen to glucose). The mobilized glucose is released into the bloodstream causing a transient hyperglycemia. It acts by stimulating adenyl cyclase, thereby increasing the intracellular concentration of cyclic AMP, which activates glycogen phosphorylase.

Insulin, on the other hand, is released in response to elevated blood glucose levels. Insulin reduces blood glucose levels by facilitating the transport of glucose across cell membranes of liver, muscle, and fat cells in particular, leading to glycogen deposition in these tissues by activating glycogen synthetase. It also inhibits lipolysis. During insulin deficiency, as in diabetes mellitus, blood glucose becomes elevated to the point where it cannot be completely reabsorbed by the kidney and escapes into the urine. Diabetes mellitus results most commonly from an insufficient population of B cells or from inadequate production of insulin by B cells.

THE LIVER

The primary cellular constituent of the liver is the hepatocyte, which accounts for about 80 percent of the cellular population. Since the hepatocyte is both an exocrine cell and a secretory cell, it is intimately associated with a duct system for the excretion of bile and a sinusoid system for secretion of substances into the bloodstream. Its intimate association with sinusoids also allows recovery of nutrients arriving from the intestines through the portal circulation. Hepatocytes store these nutrients and dispense them back into the sinusoids for distribution to the body as required. Glucose is stored in the form of glycogen and fats are stored as triglycerides.

Additionally, the hepatocyte synthesizes most of the circulating plasma proteins, including albumin, blood clotting factors such as prothrombin and fibrinogen, globulins (except the immunoglobulins), angiotensinogen, and most lipoproteins (except for the chylomicrons produced by the intestinal epithelium). Hepatocytes also detoxify many lipid-soluble drugs and remove certain waste products from the blood.

Certain sinusoidal lining cells, the **Kupffer cells,** phagocytose foreign particulate matter from the circulation, assist the excretion of bilirubin, and assist in the conservation of iron from deteriorating erythrocytes.

Histologic Aspects

The liver has four incompletely separated lobes that are invested with an extremely thin connective tissue capsule (Glisson's capsule). The peritoneal mesothelium is reflected onto most of its surface. Its hilus (**porta hepatis**) is an entryway for blood vessels as well as an exit for the common hepatic duct. It receives a dual blood supply, the larger volume composed of venous drainage from the intestines, stomach, and spleen arriving through the **portal vein,** and a lesser volume of arterial blood arriving through the **hepatic artery.**

The parenchyma of the human liver is not circumscribed by connective tissue into discrete

Fig. 15-6. A light micrograph of part of a classical liver lobule (monkey) showing cords of hepatocytes separated by anastomosing sinuses. Blood flows (*arrows*) from vessels in the peripheral connective tissue (*arrowheads*) toward the central vein (*C*).

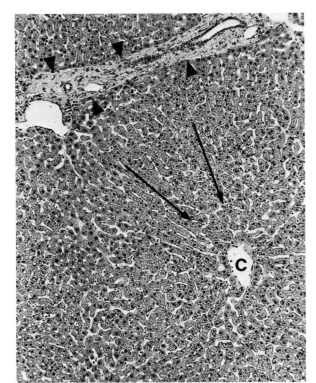

compartments or lobules. The hepatocytes are organized into anastomosing **plates** or **laminae,** deployed around two axes that serve as histologic landmarks for our concept of a classic liver lobule (Fig. 15-6). These two axes are the **portal triad** and the **central venule.** The portal triad consists of three structures (a branch of the **portal vein,** a branch of the **hepatic artery,** and a branch of the **bile duct**) that invariably accompany one another in their distribution throughout the liver. These three structures are bound together by a sheath of collagen referred to as the **portal canal,** which also contains small lymphatics and nerves (Figs. 15-7, 15-8). In histologic section, an imaginary line can be drawn connecting these triads and subdividing the liver parenchyma into contiguous hexagonal areas, each with a central axis occupied by a central venule. These areas represent sections through a liver lobule. The hepatic plates, separated by sinusoids, extend from the periphery of the lobule and converge at the central axis where the sinusoids drain into the central venule (Fig. 15-9; see also Figs. 15-6, 15-7, 15-8).

The direction of blood flow proceeds from the periphery of the lobule where branches of the portal vein terminate in its sinusoids. Branches of the hepatic artery empty either into the portal veins or directly into the sinusoids. The sinusoids form an anastomosing network that allows blood from a few terminal portal veins and hepatic arterioles to perfuse a large network of sinusoids within the lobule. The sinusoids traverse the lobule and drain into a **central venule** that runs along the long axis of the

Fig. 15-8. Portion of a classic liver lobule. Plates of hepatocytes occupy the space between the central venule (*CV*) and elements of the portal triad. *BD* = bile duct; *HA* = hepatic arteriole; *PV* = portal venule. The plates of hepatocytes are separated by sinusoids.

Fig. 15-9. Low-magnification electron micrograph showing hepatocytes (*H*) organized into hepatic plates, which are separated by sinusoids (*S*). Also conspicuous are several profiles of bile canaliculi (*arrows*). *KC* = Kupffer cell. (Courtesy of E. Wisse.)

Fig. 15-7. Portion of a classic liver lobule.

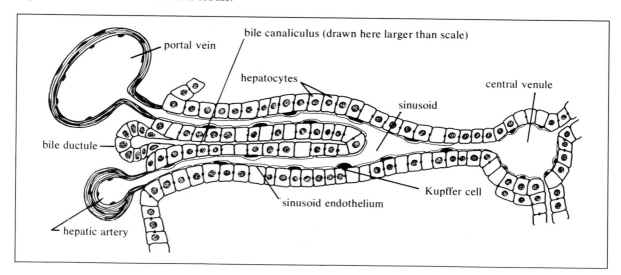

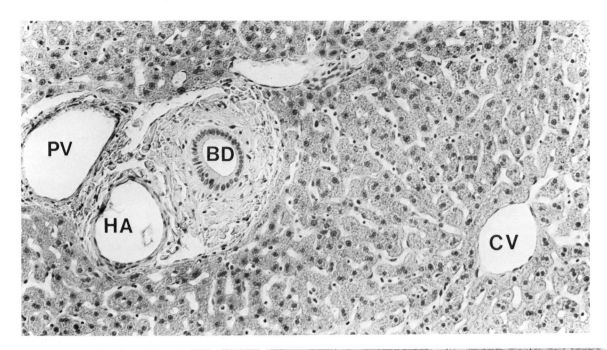

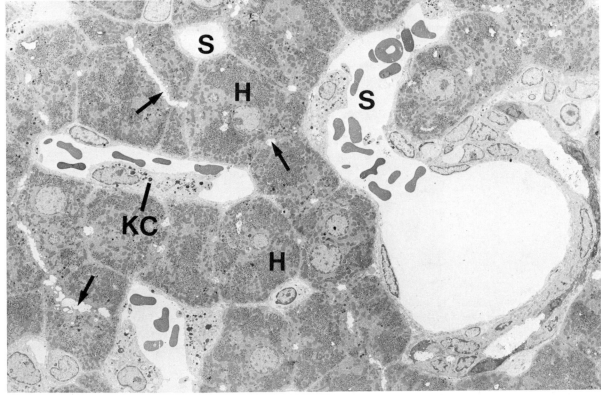

lobule. The central venules emerging from neighboring lobules join to form **intercalated veins (sublobular veins)**, which enter other lobules and eventually form the hepatic vein that drains the liver.

Routine paraffin sections of the liver reveal that the hepatocyte is a polyhedral cell with a central nucleus that is often polyploid. Of the total hepatocyte population, 65 percent are mononucleated and 35 percent are binucleated. The cytoplasm is often poorly stained because glycogen is dissolved out during preparation of the tissue, leaving behind irregular translucent spaces. Rough endoplasmic reticulum is responsible for most of the cytoplasmic basophilia. Abundant smooth endoplasmic reticulum is visible with electron microscopy.

The intralobular passageways that carry bile from its site of formation within the lobule to the bile ducts at the periphery of the lobule are the **bile canaliculi.** Electron microscopy reveals that their walls are formed by the indented plasmalemmas of contiguous hepatocytes (Figs. 15-10, 15-11, 15-12). Tight junctions involving the plasmalemmas of apposing hepatocytes form impermeable seals along the length of the canaliculi. This structural arrangement segregates bile flow from blood flow within the lobule. Numerous desmosomes and gap junctions are also present along apposing hepatocyte plasmalemmas. The canaliculus is difficult to resolve with the light microscope because its lumen, which is small in diameter, may be collapsed. However, the canaliculi are well displayed by staining with gold chloride or by staining for the presence of al-

Fig. 15-10. Hepatocyte.

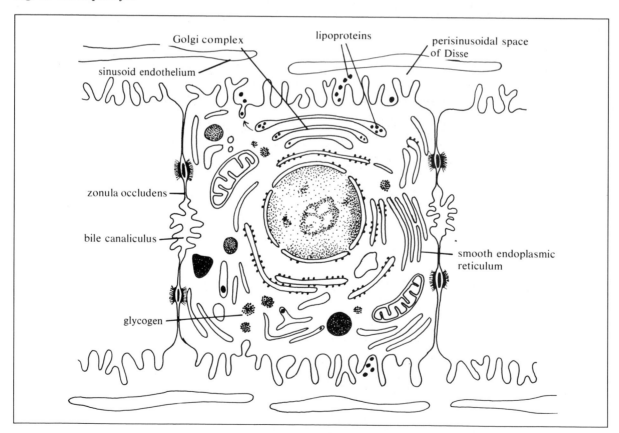

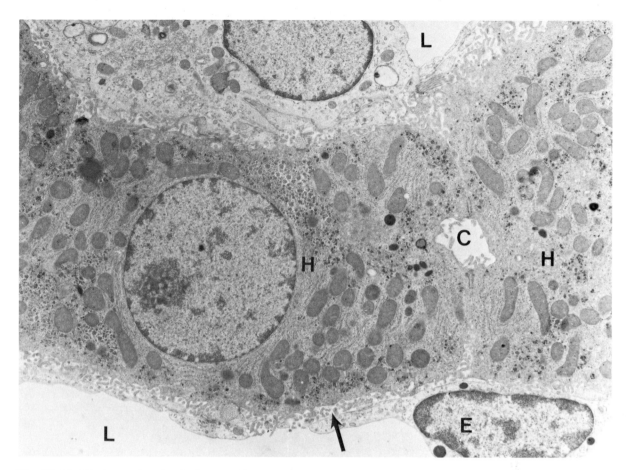

Fig. 15-11. Electron micrograph showing the spatial relationship of the bile canaliculus (*C*) with adjacent hepatocytes (*H*) and the sinusoid lumen (*L*). *E* = endothelial nucleus; arrow indicates space of Disse. (Courtesy of E. Wisse.)

kaline phosphatase. These techniques provide the best appreciation of the anastomosing, three-dimensional character of the canaliculi as they interpose between adjacent hepatocytes. The canaliculus is more visible in the instance of biliary obstruction that causes damming of bile flow and dilation of the canaliculus.

At the periphery of the lobule the bile canaliculus joins the small terminal bile ductules (cholangioles). The cholangioles have a low cuboidal epithelium and empty into larger inter-lobular bile ducts with cuboidal to columnar epithelium in the portal canals. The ductules often have short extensions (**canals of Hering**) composed of simple squamous epithelium that enter a short distance into the lobule, where their lumina become continuous with the lumen of the canaliculus. Because of their small diameter, canals of Hering are relatively difficult to see with the light microscope.

The ultrastructural relationship between the liver cell and the sinusoidal endothelium appears to be designed for the easy exchange of substances between the hepatocyte and the bloodstream. The sinusoid endothelium is discontinu-

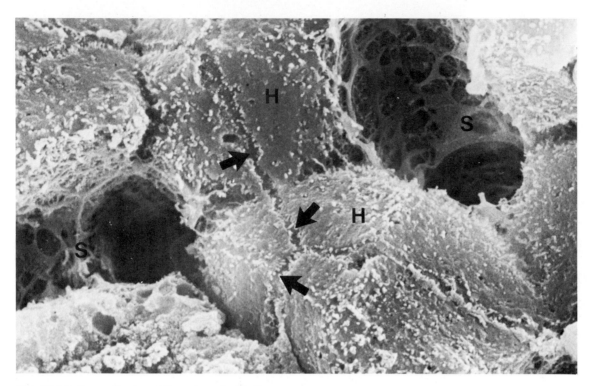

Fig. 15-12. Freeze-fractured liver viewed with the scanning electron microscope. Contiguous hepatocytes (*H*) have been fractured apart to reveal the pathway of a bile canaliculus (*arrows*). *S* = sinusoids. (From P. M. Motta, The three-dimensional fine structure of the liver as revealed by scanning electron microscopy. *Int. Rev. Cytol.* [Suppl. 6]:347, 1977.)

ous with open fenestrations (0.1–1 μm in diameter), allowing plasma to percolate freely through the **perisinusoidal space** (space of Disse). The perisinusoidal space separates the endothelium from the liver cell and contains only a few reticular fibers, an incomplete or absent basal lamina, and short microvilli that project from the liver cell into the space of Disse (see Figs. 15-10, 15-11, 15-12). Only the formed elements of the blood are excluded from the space of Disse; this allows plasma to flow against the liver cells, which may then receive nutrients from the portal circulation or dispense substances into the circulation. For instance, chylomicrons (1,500–4,000 Å in diameter), which are com-

posed of dietary triglycerides reesterified by the intestinal epithelium and transported to the liver, are small enough to cross the sinusoidal endothelium into the space of Disse where they are phagocytized by the hepatocyte. Lipoproteins formed from these triglycerides are first released into the space of Disse and then gain access to the sinusoids.

The lining of the hepatic sinusoids consists of two cell types: (1) flat **endothelial cells** with dense nuclei, and (2) larger, stellate **Kupffer cells** with vesicular nuclei. It has already been stated that the endothelium of the liver is discontinuous with open fenestrations. The unique feature of the hepatic sinusoids is the presence of the Kupffer cell, which is a fixed macrophage that is part of the reticuloendothelial system. Kupffer cells are derivatives of monocytes that emigrated from the bloodstream and insinuated themselves between endothelial cells of the sinusoidal lining (Fig. 15-13; see also Fig. 15-9). A cytoplasmic process projecting into gaps between endothelial cells secures the Kupffer cells in place. They tend to bulge slightly into the sinusoidal lumen, which distinguishes them from the flatter endothelial cells. The Kupffer cells clear the blood

perfusing the liver by actively phagocytizing foreign particulate matter. They are easily identified in electron micrographs by the presence of numerous lysosomes in the cytoplasm for processing the phagocytized material (see Fig. 15-13). Like cells of the monophagocyte system elsewhere (spleen, bone marrow, lymph nodes), the Kupffer cells recognize and phagocytize remnants of disintegrating red blood cells. In this respect they are actively engaged in the metabolism of hemoglobin, producing iron (which is stored in the cytoplasm as **hemosiderin**) and **bilirubin,** a noniron-containing breakdown product of hemoglobin. The bilirubin is released into

Fig. 15-13. Electron micrograph of Kupffer's cell (*KC*) projecting into the sinusoidal lumen (*L*). Its cytoplasm contains many secondary lysosomes. *H* = hepatocytes; perisinusoidal space of Disse (*arrows*). (From K. Wake, Perisinusoidal stellate cells (fat-storing cells, interstitial cells, lipocytes), their related structure in and around the liver sinusoids, and vitamin A–storing cells in extrahepatic organs. *Int. Rev. Cytol.* 66:303, 1980.)

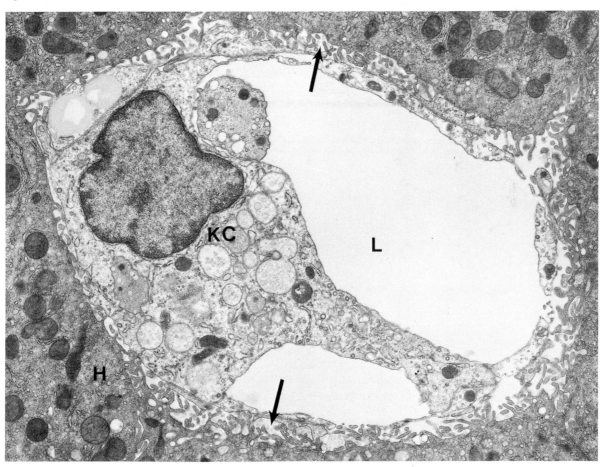

the circulation and retrieved by hepatocytes, which conjugate it and excrete it into the bile. Kupffer cells are capable of mitosis and increase in number significantly after stimulation of the reticuloendothelial system.

Another cell associated with the sinusoids is the **lipocyte,** a fat-storing cell that contains fat droplets and stores vitamin A (Fig. 15-14). Lipocytes are found in small numbers in the perisinusoidal spaces.

Fig. 15-14. Electron micrograph of hepatic lipocyte within the perisinusoidal space. Its cytoplasm is replete with lipid droplets surrounding the nucleus. L = sinusoid lumen; H = hepatocyte. (From K. Wake, Perisinusoidal stellate cells (fat-storing cells, interstitial cells, lipocytes), their related structure in and around the liver sinusoids, and vitamin A–storing cells in extrahepatic organs. *Int. Rev. Cytol.* 66:303, 1980.)

Innervation of the Liver

Most of the nerves in the human liver are unmyelinated, cholinergic vasomotor fibers. They enter the liver at its hilus and become associated with the adventitia of the hepatic artery. Some of these nerves are associated with hilar ganglia. Microscopic evidence of nerve fibers coursing through the portal canal in association with the vessels and bile ducts is substantial, but nerve fibers have not been found innervating the hepatic parenchyma in the human. More detailed information concerning the innervation of the liver is needed.

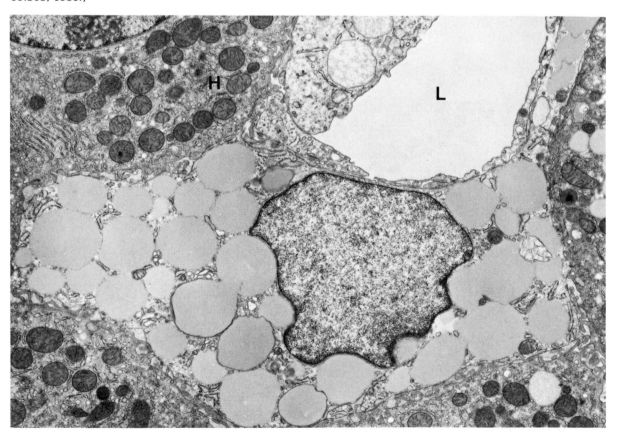

Ultrastructural Correlates of Liver Function

Because hepatocytes produce most of the plasma proteins, their high rate of protein synthesis is reflected by the abundance of rough endoplasmic reticulum (RER) and free ribosomes in the cytoplasm. Proteins destined to be secreted into the circulation are assembled on membrane-bound polysomes (RER), while proteins for the internal use of the hepatocyte are assembled on free ribosomes. During synthesis of the various classes of lipoproteins, such as the very low-density lipoproteins (VLDL), the apoprotein is assembled on the RER, joined to lipid in the smooth endoplasmic reticulum (SER), and packaged into secretory vesicles by the Golgi apparatus. Secretory vesicles that bud off from the mature face of the Golgi apparatus release the lipoprotein particles by exocytosis into the perisinusoidal space. From there they flow through the fenestrated sinusoidal endothelium and are incorporated into the circulation.

SER is also abundant and enzymes associated with it perform some of the most important functions of the hepatocyte: (1) glycogenolysis, (2) synthesis of lipids and cholesterol compounds, (3) reesterification of free fatty acids into triglycerides for storage, (4) the degradation of lipid-soluble drugs and toxic substances, and (5) glucuronide conjugation of bilirubin. In the last instance, lipid-soluble substances that are toxic at elevated concentrations are rendered harmless by enzymes of the SER, which modify them by oxidation, hydroxylation, or conjugation before they are excreted in the bile. For instance, bilirubin is conjugated with glycuronide by glucuronyl transferase, an enzyme of the SER, prior to being excreted as a bile pigment. Without this protective mechanism, bilirubin would accumulate to toxic levels in the blood (**hyperbilirubinemia**).

Normally, drugs, steroids, and lipid-soluble toxins that are metabolized by enzymes of the SER also cause dramatic proliferation of the SER and its associated enzymes so that the liver can increase its capacity to metabolize that substance. This phenomenon is the basis of induced drug tolerance, which requires that dosages of therapeutic drugs may have to be progressively increased in certain instances to counteract the liver's increasing capacity to metabolize them and to reduce effective blood levels of the drug. In other instances the metabolizing capacity of the liver may be increased intentionally by the administration of drugs, such as barbiturates, which stimulate proliferation of the SER and its enzymes (e.g., glucuronyl transferase). This procedure augments the liver's capacity to detoxify and may be appropriate in conditions such as severe hyperbilirubinemia where blood levels of bilirubin must be reduced rapidly. However, increasing levels of barbiturate addiction can eventually exceed the capacity of the SER to detoxify them. Furthermore, overdoses of such drugs can be insidiously dangerous, especially when an abrupt interruption in habitual use allows the SER to decline to the extent where it is incapable of metabolizing the drug when the habit is suddenly resumed at its peak level.

Fasting is another instance where proliferation of SER occurs. During fasting, the circulating insulin-glucagon ratio declines. The increased pancreatic glucagon arriving in the portal blood stimulates proliferation of SER rich in glucose 6-phosphatase activity, glycogenolysis, and the release of free glucose into the sinusoids.

The Functional Lobule in Health and Disease

As already described, the structural and functional unit of the human liver (and most mammalian livers) is not easily defined because the parenchyma is not subdivided into independent functional lobules by connective tissue. In the pig, connective tissue delineates the hexagonal shape that is recognized as the **classic liver lobule,** in which elements of the portal triads are situated at the periphery, usually at the trigonal points of the hexagon. A central venule occupies its central axis. However, this structural concept fails to account for the fact that terminal branches of portal vessels and biliary ducts distribute to adjacent portions of neighboring hexagonal liver lobules, not exclusively to the parenchyma within a single hexagonal lobule. The structural concept of the classic liver lobule has been useful because it is perhaps the best scheme to describe the two-dimensional image obtained from histologic sections of liver. However, a more accurate appreciation of liver function is provided by the concept of the **liver acinus** or **microcirculatory unit,** which is based on the three-dimensional path followed by substances injected into the portal or hepatic vessels and bile ducts. These studies corroborate that the portal vessels contribute blood to portions of three adjacent hexagonal liver lobules simultaneously. The liver acinus consists of the parenchymal mass between two central venules and is arranged around a central axis consisting of terminal branches of the portal vein, hepatic artery, and

bile duct. The **complex acinus** consists of three liver acini each occupying portions of three contiguous hexagonal fields and having axes that are terminal branches of the same preterminal portal vein, hepatic artery, and bile duct (Fig. 15-15).

The concept of the liver acinus is consistent with observations of normal and pathologic liver function. Hence, hepatocytes closest to the axis are the first to receive blood and are therefore less susceptible to hypoxic damage and the first to regenerate after many types of liver trauma. Three concentric zones have been identified around the axis of the acinus; these zones display different levels of resistance to various pathologic conditions. The zone located farthest from the terminal hepatic artery is usually the most vulnerable. The changing histologic patterns seen in developing pathologic lesions are more easily understood together with an adequate understanding of the simple and complex liver acinus. Since the distribution of necrosis throughout the liver follows either the vascular

Fig. 15-15. A complex liver acinus superimposed on the hexagonal shape of classic lobules. The shaded areas are the three zones of the simple liver acinus supplied by terminal branches of the hepatic artery and portal vein. *CV* = central vein; *PC* = portal canal.

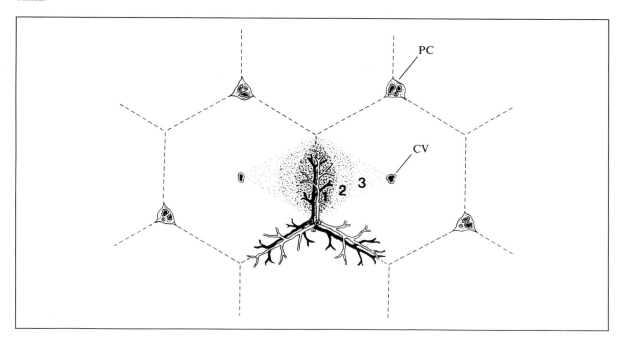

branches (hypoxia, nutrient deficiency, toxicity), biliary branches (infection), or lymphatic branches (infection), which together constitute the axis of the liver acinus, the geometry of the acinus provides a more accurate appreciation of the lobule's response to pathologic influences. For a detailed description of these pathologic changes and their associated effects on the liver acinus, consult Rappaport (see Bibliography for this chapter).

One concept of liver construction emphasizing its exocrine nature is the **portal lobule.** Its peripheral limits are defined by imaginary lines connecting three central venules; its central axis is the interlobular bile duct. The portal lobule is sometimes invoked to explain certain biliary tract pathologies.

Regeneration of the Liver

If only a portion of the liver is damaged or surgically excised, unaffected hepatocytes are capable of replenishing the parenchymal cell mass by both hypertrophy and hyperplasia. However, parenchymal areas that are badly damaged or necrotic allow the connective tissue to collapse. In this instance, regeneration of hepatocytes begins but overproduction of collagen by fibroblasts produces excessive connective tissue that becomes a barrier to reestablishing adequate vascular and biliary connections. This process, known as **cirrhosis,** interferes with regeneration and restoration of liver function.

Jaundice

Jaundice describes the yellow appearance of the skin produced by abnormally high levels of bile pigments in the blood. Excess circulating bilirubin has three major causes: (1) excessive hemolysis of erythrocytes, with production of bilirubin by macrophages exceeding the normal retrieval capacity of hepatocytes (hemolytic jaundice); (2) inadequate ability of hepatocytes to retrieve, process, or excrete bilirubin; and (3) obstruction of the biliary tract.

THE GALLBLADDER

Since bile is continually being produced by the liver (but is needed only after ingestion of food), a distensible and contractile organ like the gallbladder is required to store and dispense bile. The gallbladder rests against the inferior surface of the liver, where excretory ducts from both organs join to form the common bile duct.

Histologic Aspects

The mucosa consists of a simple columnar epithelium with central elongate nuclei. Short microvilli extend from their apical surfaces. Adjacent epithelial cells are attached to one another by tight junctions on their adjacent membranes near their apical surfaces. The mucosa forms anastomosing folds, which generate the appearance of epithelially lined pockets in section (Figs. 15-16, 15-17). This gives the false impression that glands are frequently found in the lamina propria underlying the epithelium. However, these intricate mucosal folds disappear to some extent as the organ becomes distended with bile. True glands, however, are not observed except in the neck region of the gallbladder near the cystic duct, where simple tubuloalveolar glands connecting with the bile duct are present in the lamina propria and the perimuscular layer.

There is no true muscularis mucosa, only a **muscular lamina** consisting of irregular, anastomosing bundles of smooth muscle running in longitudinal, circular, and oblique directions. These smooth muscle bundles are separated from one another by intervening collagenous, elastic, and reticular connective tissue. External to this layer is a relatively thick **perimuscular layer** consisting mostly of collagenous and some elastic fibers. Fibroblasts and a variable number of fat cells are also present in this layer. Lymphatics and blood vessels traverse the perimuscular layer before reaching the mucosa. Covering most of the perimuscular layer is the serosa, which is continuous with that covering the liver (see Fig. 15-16).

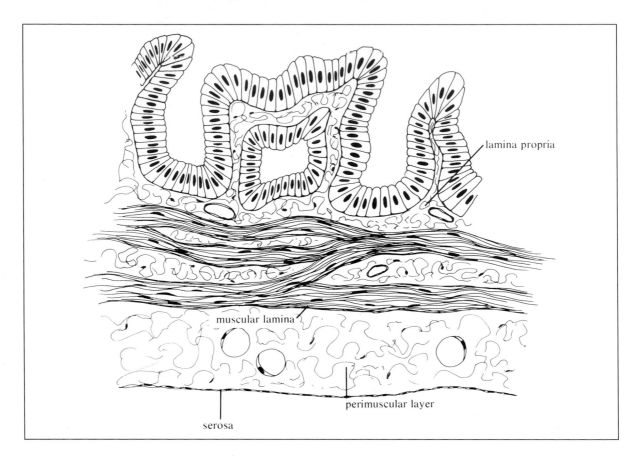

Fig. 15-16. The wall of the human gallbladder.

The neck of the gallbladder is joined to the **cystic duct,** its excretory duct. The cystic and common hepatic ducts join to form the **common bile duct** (ductus choledochus), which transmits bile to the ampulla of Vater in the duodenum. The common bile duct consists of tall columnar epithelium and occasional scattered smooth muscle bundles, which are not prominent until the terminus of the duct in the duodenum. Here the smooth muscle component is well developed into the **sphincter of Oddi.** This sphincter is a variable composite of smooth muscle around the terminus of the common bile duct within the duodenal wall (the choledochoduodenal junction), and usually also around the terminus of the associated main pancreatic duct. The sphincter of Oddi is composed of circular and longitudinal smooth muscle within the wall of the duodenum. It generally consists of four parts, which vary within individuals:

1. **Sphincter choledochus:** annular sheath around the bile duct; contraction prevents the flow of bile
2. **Sphincter pancreaticus:** annular sheath around the terminal segment of the main pancreatic duct; contraction stops the flow of pancreatic enzymes
3. **Fasciculi longitudinales:** longitudinally arranged muscle that facilitates the flow of bile when contracted by shortening and widening the lumen of the duct
4. **Sphincter ampullae:** smooth muscle surrounding the ampulla of Vater

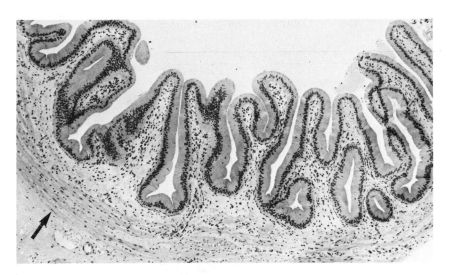

Fig. 15-17. Monkey gallbladder. The mucosa is composed of anastomosing folds. The epithelium is simple columnar. Part of the muscularis (*arrow*) is seen below.

Functional Aspects

Bile is an aqueous solution composed of pigments (principally bilirubin), salts, lecithin, and cholesterol. The bile salts emulsify fatty substances, making them more soluble and facilitating their absorption by the small intestine. Bile salts released by the gallbladder are usually reabsorbed by the intestine and used again (**enterohepatic circulation**).

Bile is stored in a concentrated form due to the ability of the epithelium to withdraw water and inorganic ions from the bile. It is believed that these salts are transported across the apical epithelium and released into the lateral intercellular spaces basal to the tight junctions. Water passively follows, resulting in dilation of the intercellular spaces. Water is then picked up and carried away by subepithelial capillaries, which often appear dilated in section.

The release of **secretin** and **cholecystokinin** from the duodenal mucosa is stimulated by the presence of fatty substances in the bolus entering from the stomach. Cholecystokinin activates contraction of the gallbladder, causing it to dispense bile into the duodenum via the common bile duct. These same hormones also induce relaxation of the sphincter of Oddi. Secretin acts on the bile ducts, causing them to release a watery bicarbonate solution that mixes with and dilutes the bile. Secretin release is stimulated by the entry of the acidic chyme into the duodenum.

NATIONAL BOARD TYPE QUESTIONS

For the following, select
- A. if only *1, 2, and 3* are correct.
- B. if only *1 and 3* are correct.
- C. if only *2 and 4* are correct.
- D. if only *4* is correct.
- E. if *all* are correct.

1. The apical cytoplasm of the pancreatic acinar cell is
   1. basophilic due to the presence of rough endoplasmic reticulum.
   2. acidophilic due exclusively to the presence of numerous mitochondria.
   3. basophilic due to the presence of the nucleus.
   4. acidophilic due to the presence of secretory (zymogen) granules.

2. Which of the following biologic actions is (are) caused by cholecystokinin?
   1. Contraction of the gallbladder
   2. Contraction of the sphincter of Oddi
   3. Secretion of digestive enzymes for pancreatic acinar cells
   4. Secretion of an aqueous, alkaline bicarbonate solution from cells forming intralobular pancreatic ducts

3. The intercalated ducts of the pancreas
   1. consist of columnar epithelium.
   2. drain the secretory acinus.
   3. contain goblet cells.
   4. consist of low cuboidal epithelium.

4. The smooth endoplasmic reticulum of the liver
   1. esterifies free fatty acids into triglycerides.
   2. degrades lipid-soluble drugs.
   3. proliferates in response to barbiturates.
   4. participates in glucuronide conjugation of bilirubin.

5. Kupffer cells
   1. are lodged within the discontinuities of hepatic sinusoids.
   2. recognize and phagocytize remnants of disintegrating erythrocytes.
   3. are derivatives of monocytes.
   4. metabolize phagocytized hemoglobin but do not store the iron in any form.

6. The plasmalemma of a hepatocyte is bounded by
   1. a bile canaliculus.
   2. a contiguous hepatocyte.
   3. the space of Disse (perisinusoidal space).
   4. the hepatic artery.

7. Which of the following statements regarding the liver is (are) true?
   1. The perisinusoidal space is located between sinusoidal endothelium and hepatocyte plasmalemma.
   2. The sinusoids consist of a discontinuous endothelium with open fenestrations.
   3. The sinusoids carry blood from branches of the portal vein and hepatic artery to central venules.
   4. The perisinusoidal space contains a well-developed basement membrane.

8. The bile canaliculus
   1. becomes enlarged as a result of biliary tract obstruction.
   2. is formed by the plasmalemmas of adjacent hepatocytes.
   3. does not normally leak bile because it is sealed by the zonula occludens.
   4. is lined by simple squamous epithelium throughout its entire length.

9. Which of the following is (are) located in the portal canal?
   1. Branches of the hepatic artery
   2. The central venule
   3. Branches of the portal vein
   4. Hepatic sinusoids

10. Regarding the islets of Langerhans:
    1. Alpha cells are the most abundant cell type.
    2. Beta cells represent approximately 70 to 75 percent of islet cells and release insulin.
    3. Islet cells release their hormones into intercalated ducts.
    4. Delta cells secrete somatostatin.

11. The gallbladder
    1. has a lumen lined by simple columnar epithelium.
    2. lacks a serosa.
    3. has a muscular lamina but no muscularis mucosa.
    4. contains numerous glands throughout the lamina propria.

ANNOTATED ANSWERS

1. D. The rough endoplasmic reticulum in the base of the pancreatic acinar cell makes that area basophilic; the acidophilic zymogen granules monopolize the apical portion.

2. B. Cholecystokinin and secretin cause relaxation of the sphincter of Oddi. Secretin induces secretion from the pancreatic ducts.

3. C. Columnar cells and goblet cells are present in the interlobular ducts.

4. E.
5. A. Iron is present in Kuppfer cells as hemosiderin.
6. A. Branches of the hepatic artery travel within the portal canals and are separated from hepatocytes by collagen.
7. A. A basement membrane is either poorly developed or entirely absent from the perisinusoidal space.
8. A. The bile canaliculus is formed by contiguous plasmalemmas of adjacent hepatocytes.
9. B. The central venule and sinusoids are present within the classic liver lobule parenchyma.
10. C. As with all mature endocrine tissue, duct systems do not drain endocrine parenchyma.
11. B. True glands are not present except within the neck region where they communicate with the bile duct.

BIBLIOGRAPHY

Alumets, J., F. Sundler, and R. Hakanson. Distribution, ontogeny and ultrastructure of somatostatin immunoreactive cells in the pancreas and gut. *Cell Tissue Res.* 185:465, 1977.

Andersson, S. Secretion of gastrointestinal hormones. *Ann. Rev. Physiol.* 35:431, 1973.

Baum, J. B., et al. Localization of glucagon in the alpha cells in the pancreatic islet by immunofluorescent techniques. *Diabetes* 11:371, 1962.

Bishop, A. E., et al. The location of VIP in the pancreas of man and rat. *Diabetologia* 18:73, 1980.

Bloom, W. A new type of granular cell in the islets of Langerhans of man. *Anat. Rec.* 49:363, 1931.

Brauer, R. W. Liver circulation and function. *Physiol. Rev.* 43:115, 1963.

Cardell, R. R., Jr. Smooth endoplasmic reticulum in rat hepatocytes during glycogen deposition and depletion. *Int. Rev. Cytol.* 48:221, 1977.

Caro, L. G., and G. E. Palack. Protein synthesis, storage and discharge in the pancreatic exocrine cell: An autoradiographic study. *J. Cell Biol.* 20:473, 1964.

Dallner, G., P. Siekevitz, and G. E. Palade. Biogenesis of endoplasmic reticulum membranes. I. Structural and chemical differentiation in developing rat hepatocyte. *J. Cell Biol.* 30:73, 1966.

Floyd, J. C., Jr., et al. A Newly Recognized Pancreatic Polypeptide: Plasma Levels in Health and Disease. In R. O. Greep (ed.), *Recent Progress in Hormone Research.* New York: Academic, 1977. Vol. 33, p. 519.

Fujita, T., and T. Murakami. Microcirculation of the monkey pancreas with special reference to the insulo-acinar portal system. A scanning electron microscope study of vascular casts. *Arch. Histol. Jpn.* 35:255, 1973.

Gepts, N., J. DeMey, M. Marichal-Pipeleers. Hyperplasia of "pancreatic polypeptide" cells in the pancreas of juvenile diabetics. *Diabetologia* 13:27, 1977.

Jamieson, J. D., and G. E. Palade. Intracellular transport of secretory proteins in the pancreatic exocrine cell: I. Role of the peripheral elements of the Golgi complex. *J. Cell Biol.* 34:577, 1967.

Jamieson, J. D., and G. E. Palade. Intracellular transport of secretory proteins in the pancreatic exocrine cell: II. Transport to condensing vacuoles and zymogen granules. *J. Cell Biol.* 34:597, 1967.

Jamieson, J. D., and G. E. Palade. Condensing vacuole conversion and zymogen granule discharge in pancreatic exocrine cells: Metabolic studies. *J. Cell Biol.* 48:503, 1971.

Jamieson, J. D., and G. E. Palade. Synthesis, intracellular transport and discharge of secretory proteins in stimulated pancreatic exocrine cells. *J. Cell Biol.* 50:135, 1971.

Johnson, L. R. Gastrointestinal hormones and their functions. *Ann. Rev. Physiol.* 39:135, 1977.

Lacy, P. E. The pancreatic beta cell: Structure and function. *N. Engl. J. Med.* 276:187, 1967.

Motta, P. M. The three-dimensional fine structure of the liver as revealed by scanning electron microscopy. *Int. Rev. Cytol.* (Suppl. 6):347, 1977.

Novikoff, A. B., et al. Studies of the secretory process in the mammalian exocrine pancreas. I. The condensing vacuoles. *J. Cell Biol.* 75:148, 1977.

Novikoff, P. M., and A. Yam. Sites of lipoprotein particles in normal rat hepatocytes. *J. Cell Biol.* 76:1, 1978.

Orci, L., et al. Somatostatin in the Pancreas and the Gastrointestinal Tract. In T. Fujita (ed.), *Endocrine Gut and Pancreas.* Amsterdam: Elsevier, 1976. P. 73.

Palade, G. Intracellular aspects of the process of protein synthesis. *Science* 189:347, 1975.

Paulin, C., and P. M. Dubois. Immunohistochemical identification and localization of pancreatic polypeptide cells in the pancreas and gastrointestinal tract of the human fetus and adult man. *Cell Tissue Res.* 188:251, 1978.

Rappaport, A. M. The structural and functional unit in the human liver (liver acinus). *Anat. Rec.* 130:673, 1958.

Rappaport, A. M. Acinar Units and the Pathophysiology of the Liver. In C. H. Rouiller (ed.), *The Liver*. New York: Academic, 1963.

Striffler, J. S., E. L. Cardell, and R. R. Cardell, Jr. Effects of glucagon on hepatic glycogen and smooth endoplasmic reticulum. *Am. J. Anat.* 160:363, 1981.

Wake, K. Perisinusoidal stellate cells (fat-storing cells, interstitial cells, lipocytes), their related structure in and around the liver sinusoids, and vitamin A-storing cells in extrahepatic organs. *Int. Rev. Cytol.* 66:303, 1980.

Wisse, E. and D. L. Knook. The Investigation of Sinusoidal Cells: A New Approach to the Study of Liver Function. In H. P. Popper and F. Schaffner (eds.), *Progress in Liver Diseases*. New York: Grune & Stratton, 1979. Vol. VI.

16 Urinary System

Objectives

You will learn the following in this chapter:

The general histologic organization of the kidney, ureter, and urinary bladder

The structure and function of distinct segments of the uriniferous tubule, the structural unit of the kidney

The interrelationship of the vascular system with each segment of the uriniferous tubule

The ultrastructure and function of the renal corpuscle and its filtration barrier

The structure of the proximal and distal tubules and the ultrastructural mechanisms involved in the reabsorption of glomerular filtrate

The cooperative roles of Henle's loop and the collecting duct in the concentration of urine and the conservation of water

---

The urinary system includes the **kidneys** and their excretory ducts, the **ureters,** plus the **urinary bladder** and its excretory duct, the **urethra.** The kidneys regulate the composition and volume of body fluids by constantly adjusting blood plasma volume and constituents that circulate through them. This regulation is accomplished by the retention of important circulating substances, the excretion of certain metabolic waste products, the variable retention of body water, the differential regulation of salt content, and the maintenance of acid-base balance. The formation of urine is essentially the by-product of these continuous renal processes that preserve the internal fluid environment of the body against disruptive external influences. By regulating the volume and composition of the circulating plasma, the kidneys also influence the immediate fluid environment bathing every cell in the body. Therefore, compromised kidney function result-

ing from disease is often signaled by systemic toxemia, edema, or dehydration.

THE KIDNEYS
General Organization and Function

The paired human kidneys are retroperitoneal and occupy a posterior position within the abdominal cavity. They are invested with a thin but tough collagenous capsule.

The functional and structural units of the renal parenchyma are the **uriniferous tubules.** The uriniferous tubules are arranged radially around a cavity called the **renal sinus,** thereby producing a bean-shaped organ. The renal sinus contains an expanded portion of the ureter (the **renal pelvis**), which branches to form several **major** and **minor calyces** for collecting urine. Adipose tissue supports the renal pelvis. The ureter emerges from the kidney through a hilus, the same area

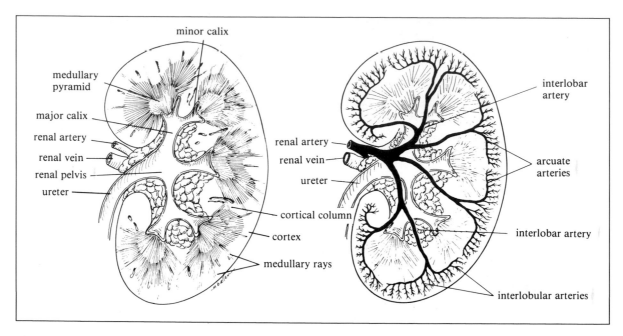

Fig. 16-1. Hemisected kidney. *Left,* parenchyma and excretory passages. *Right,* blood supply.

through which blood vessels and nerves enter the kidney (Figs. 16-1, 16-2).

Uriniferous tubules receive a portion of the circulating plasma that is routinely filtered away from the incoming blood supply to the kidney. The epithelium of these tubules modifies the filtered plasma as it passes through various segments of the tubules. Most of the water and essential constituents are reabsorbed by the tubules and returned to the bloodstream; but the rest, containing mostly toxic metabolytes, is concentrated and excreted as urine into the calices. Consequently, the histologic picture of the renal parenchyma is an intimate morphologic relationship between the renal vasculature and all segments of the uriniferous tubule. Capillary tufts from the incoming vasculature are associated with the end of the uriniferous tubule involved

with filtration. The excretory end of the uriniferous tubules opens into the minor calices.

Because specific regions of the uriniferous tubules tend to occupy specific regions of the parenchyma, they impart a characteristic pattern to the glandular part of the hemisected kidney. This pattern produces a reddish-brown **cortex** lying under the capsule and a lighter **medulla** next to the renal pelvis (see Fig. 16-1). Specific segments of uriniferous tubules are located only within the cortex; other segments are located in the medulla.

The medulla consists of approximately a dozen **renal pyramids,** a name that refers to their pyramidal geometry and triangular shape in histologic section. The base of each pyramid faces the cortex. Numerous medullary rays extend up into the cortex. The apex or papilla of each pyramid projects into the funnel-shaped lumen of a minor calix. The medullary pyramids are sepa-

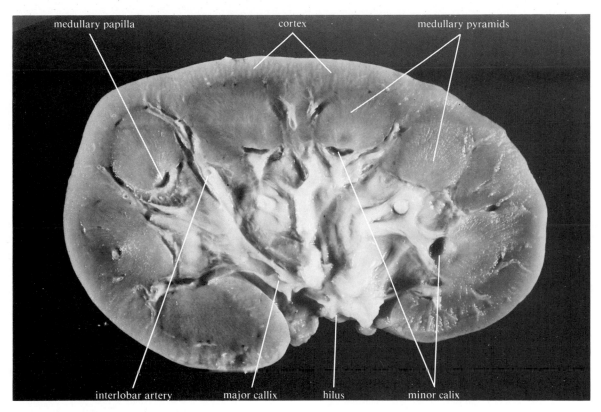

medullary papilla

cortex

medullary pyramids

interlobar artery

major callix

hilus

minor calix

Fig. 16-2. Hemisected human kidney with several macroscopic structures identified.

rated from one another laterally by columns of cortex (**cortical columns**) that extend between them. A **renal lobe** consists of each pyramid and the cortical tissue associated with its sides and base (see Figs. 16-1, 16-2).

The human kidney is multilobed and consists of approximately a dozen lobes (± 6). Each lobe is associated with a minor calix that receives urine from the terminal portions of uriniferous tubules of that lobe. The uriniferous tubules of each lobe terminate on the apex of each medullary pyramid in such a way that their lumina appear as orifices on the surfaces of the papilla (the **area cribrosa,** L. *cribrum,* "sieve"). While renal lobes can be recognized according to structural and functional criteria, they are not delineated by connective tissue boundaries.

Uriniferous Tubules

The uriniferous tubules are composed of two distinct functional regions: the **nephron,** which is involved in the production of urine, and the **collecting tubule,** which is involved in the hypertonic concentration of urine. These two segments arise from separate embryonic primordia. In the mature kidney several nephrons fuse with and empty into a single collecting duct or tubule.

The nephron is a continuous tubule consisting of histologically and functionally distinct regions along its length, which will be briefly described, beginning with the end involved in filtration.

Within the cortex, where filtration occurs, a tuft of capillaries (**glomerular capillaries**) occupies an indented blind-ending portion of the nephron called **Bowman's capsule.** Together, these two elements, glomerular capillaries and capsule, constitute the **renal corpuscles,** which are located exclusively in the cortex (Fig. 16-3). The renal corpuscle is an intimate structural association between the incoming renal arterial supply and the nephron, whose ultrastructural design allows for filtration of plasma from arterial blood. This ultrafiltrate of blood plasma is called **glomerular filtrate.** It is sometimes called **provisional urine** because its composition is modified during its passage through the remainder of the tubule by exchange of substances between various segments of the tubule and its closely associated capillaries.

The glomerular filtrate flows from the lumen of Bowman's capsule through the other tubular segments of the nephron in the following sequence: **proximal convoluted** and **proximal straight tubules, thin segment,** and **distal straight** and **distal convoluted tubules** (see Fig. 16-3). Both proximal and distal convoluted portions are found within the cortex along with renal corpuscles. The proximal and distal straight portions and their connecting thin segments form **Henle's loops,** which extend into the medulla from the cortex.

Within the cortex, several distal convoluted tubules join each collecting duct through short arched collecting tubules. The collecting duct continues into the medulla, extending all the way to the papilla. Within the cortex the collecting ducts and Henle's loops (together with vascular loops to be described later) are clustered together in small parallel groups, called **medullary rays,** before entering the medulla. The medullary rays appear as extensions from the base of the medullary pyramid into the cortex. Each medullary ray and its surrounding cortical tissue constitute a **renal lobule.** A lobule is composed of those portions of a nephron within each medullary ray (i.e., Henle's loops and collecting ducts) and its associated cortical structures (renal corpuscles, proximal and distal convoluted tubules). Specific segments of each uriniferous tubule are therefore contained within the cortex, the medullary rays, or the medullary pyramids (Fig. 16-4).

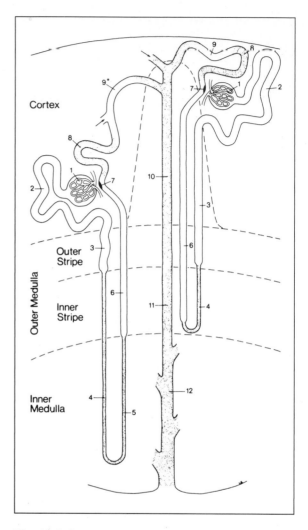

Fig. 16-3. Diagram of a short-looped and long-looped nephron emptying into a collecting duct system. Within the cortex the dashed line indicates the boundary of a medullary ray. *1* = renal corpuscle, *2* = proximal convoluted tubule, *3* = proximal straight tubule, *4* = descending thin limb, *5* = ascending thin limb, *6* = distal straight tubule (thick ascending limb), *7* = macula densa, *8* = distal convoluted tubule, *9* = connecting tubule, *9** = connecting tubule of juxtamedullary nephron that forms an arcade, *10* = cortical collecting duct, *11* = outer medullary collecting duct, *12* = inner medullary collecting duct (papillary duct). (From W. Kriz and L. Bankir, A standard nomenclature for structures of the kidney, *Am. J. Physiol.* 254:F1, 1988)

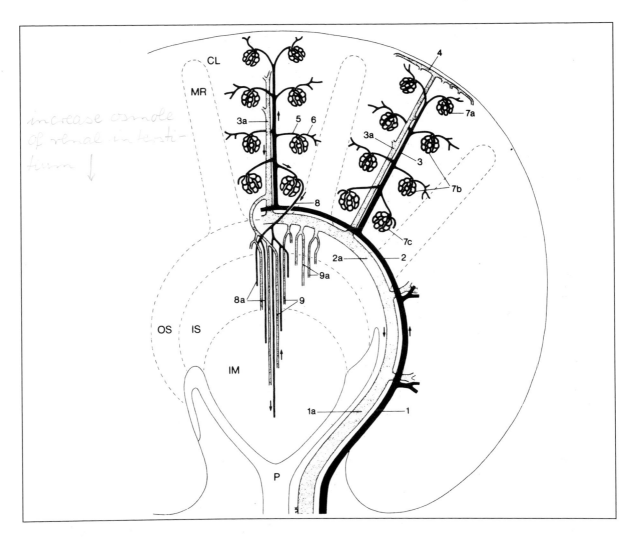

increase osmole of renal intersti- tium ↓

Fig. 16-4. Diagram of intrarenal vasculature (peritubular capillaries derived from the efferent arteriole are not shown). Within the cortex the medullary rays are distinguished from the cortical labyrinth by a dashed line. *OS* = outer stripe, *IS* = inner stripe, *IM* = inner medulla, *P* = renal pelvis. *1 & 1a* = interlobar artery and vein, *2 & 2a* = arcuate artery and vein, *3 & 3a* = interlobular or cortical radial artery and vein, *4* = stellate vein, *5* = afferent arteriole, *6* = efferent arteriole, *7a, 7b, & 7c* = superficial, midcortical and juxtamedullary glomerulus, *8 & 8a* = juxtamedullary efferent arteriole and descending vasa recta, *9 & 9a* = ascending vasa recta. (From W. Kriz and L. Bankir, A standard nomenclature for structures of the kidney. *Am. J. Physiol.* 254:F1, 1988.)

Blood Supply

After entering the hilus of the kidney, the renal artery splits into dorsal and ventral branches. These branches divide into several **interlobar arteries,** which penetrate the cortical columns between pyramids and extend radially toward the corticomedullary junction (see Figs. 16-1, 16-2). At the corticomedullary junction the interlobar arteries bifurcate into **arcuate arteries,** which travel between the cortex and the base of the pyramids. The arcuate arteries give rise to smaller

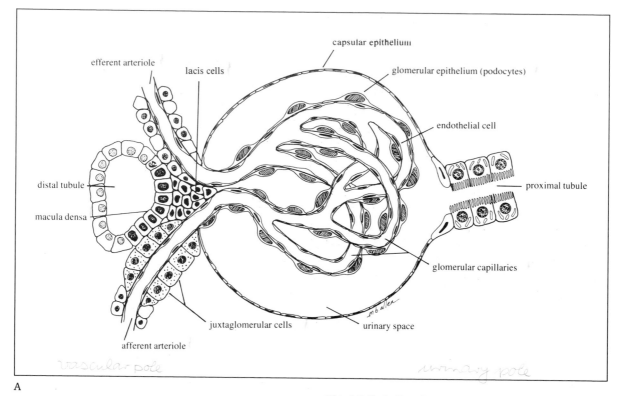

A

vascular pole   urinary pole

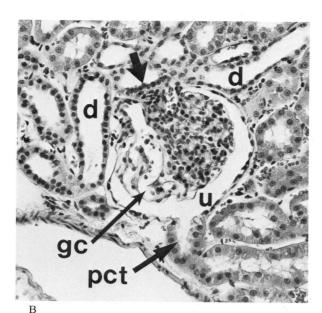

B

Fig. 16-5. A. Renal corpuscle. B. Light micrograph of a renal corpuscle. A tuft of glomerular capillaries (*gc*) forms a glomerulus, which is surrounded by the urinary space (*u*). The urinary space is continuous with the lumen of the proximal convoluted tubule (*pct*) at the urinary pole of the corpuscle. The macula densa (*unlabeled arrow*) is the compact plate of cells forming a portion of the wall of the distal convoluted tubule (*d*), which is weaving in and out of the plane of section. The portion of the distal convoluted tubule formed by the macula densa occupies the space between the afferent and efferent arterioles, both of which are just outside the plane of section.

Fig. 16-6. Corrosion cast of a renal glomerulus from the rat kidney. Renal blood vessels were injected with a plastic resin that hardens to preserve glomerular capillary geometry. The tissue is eroded away in a strong alkali bath to reveal the vascular cast, which is viewed with the scanning electron microscope. *AA* = afferent arteriole; *EA* = efferent arteriole. (From T. Murakami, Vascular arrangement of the rat renal glomerulus. A scanning electron microscope study of corrosion casts. *Arch. Histol. Jpn.* 34:87, 1972.)

interlobar arteries (cortical radial arteries), which traverse the cortex between medullary rays. Along their path toward the renal capsule, the interlobular arteries give rise to the **afferent arterioles,** which then break up into the glomerular capillary tufts of each renal corpuscle (see Fig. 16-3). The glomerular capillaries coalesce to form the efferent arterioles draining each renal corpuscle (Figs. 16-4, 16-5, 16-6). From this point the efferent vessels of outer cortical and **juxtamedullary glomeruli** distribute differently (see Fig. 16-4).

Each efferent arteriole emerging from outer cortical glomeruli forms a **peritubular capillary**

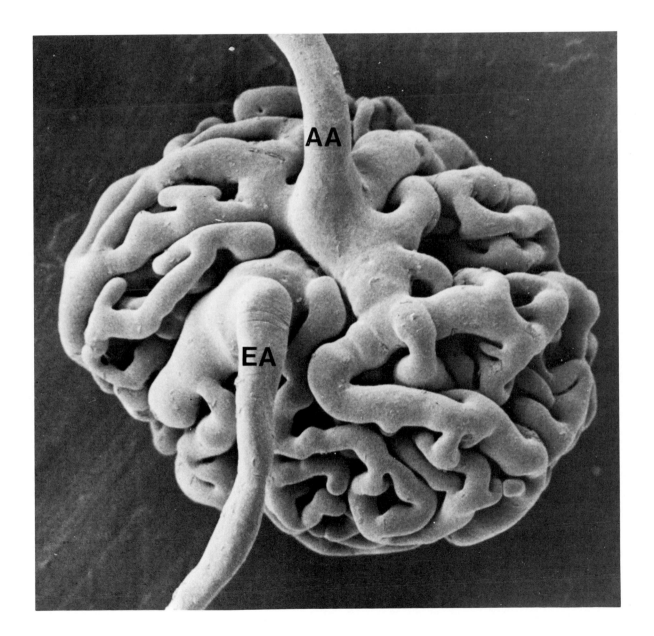

plexus, which travels among the convoluted tubules in the cortex, and a capillary plexus associated with the medullary rays. The peritubular capillaries from the outer cortical glomeruli drain into **stellate veins** near the surface of the kidney, which converge upon and drain into **interlobular veins** (then into arcuate, interlobar, and renal veins). Each efferent arteriole emerging from juxtamedullary glomeruli also forms peritubular capillaries that travel among the convoluted tubules, and in addition gives off long recurrent capillary loops called **vasa recta**, which accompany structures within the medullary rays and extend within medullary rays deep into the medulla. The descending limbs of the loops are the **arteriolae rectae** and the ascending limbs are the **venae rectae.** On ascending to the corticomedullary junction the venae rectae drain into arcuate or interlobular veins. The arterial and venous vasa recta act as countercurrent exchangers and are referred to as the **rete mirabile.** The proximity of these capillary branches of the efferent arterioles to all segments of the nephron and collecting ducts facilitates the exchange of substances among them during modification of the glomerular filtrate.

Histology of the Renal Corpuscle and Ultrastructure of the Filtration Barrier

Beginning with the renal corpuscle, the histology and function of each segment of the uriniferous tubule will be described.

The structures responsible for filtering plasma away from the incoming blood supply, the **renal corpuscles,** are constructed of two histologic elements: (1) **glomerular capillaries** contributed by the afferent arterioles, and (2) **Bowman's capsule,** the indented blind-ending portion of the nephron that encases the glomerular capillaries. Bowman's capsule thus has double walls. The outer wall is the **parietal epithelium (capsular epithelium)**. At the point where the capsule becomes indented to accommodate the entry of a tuft of glomerular capillaries, the capsular epithelium is reflected back onto the surface of

the glomerular capillaries as the **visceral epithelium (glomerular epithelium)** (see Fig. 16-5). Filtration occurs across the glomerular capillaries and glomerular epithelium into the **urinary space,** which separates the glomerular and capsular epithelium. The urinary space that receives the glomerular filtrate is continuous with the lumen of the proximal convoluted tubule, the next segment along the nephron. Consequently, the structure of the renal corpuscle has two poles: a **vascular pole** where the afferent and efferent arterioles are located and a **urinary pole** where the capsule becomes continuous with the proximal convoluted tubule. The urinary space is confluent with the lumen of the proximal convoluted tubule (see Figs. 16-5, 16-7).

Fig. 16-7. Scanning electron micrograph of fractured rat kidney revealing a renal corpuscle (*RC*) encased in its parietal epithelium. Both urinary (*U*) and vascular (*V*) poles are indicated. In the lower left hand corner is another renal corpuscle with its parietal epithelium torn, revealing the underlying glomerulus. A glomerulus is shown at higher magnification in figure 16-7. (From P. Andrews and K. Porter, A scanning electron microscopic study of the nephron. *Am. J. Anat.* 140:81, 1974.)

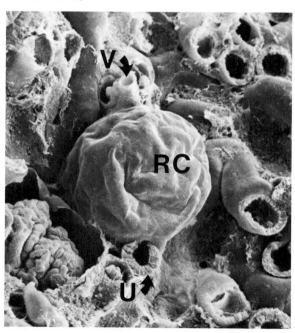

The capsular epithelium is a simple squamous variety. At the urinary pole, it ends abruptly where the epithelium of the proximal convoluted tubule begins; at the vascular pole, it is continuous with elaborately branched cells of the glomerular epithelium (the **podocytes**). In histologic section, the glomerulus appears as an anastomosing capillary network whose flat endothelial cell nuclei are easily distinguished from the larger oval nuclei of the podocytes. Details of the podocytes are not easily observed with light mi-

croscopy, but electron microscopy reveals that podocytes have large **primary processes** that clasp the glomerular capillaries (Figs. 16-8, 16-9). From these processes, smaller **secondary processes (foot processes** or **pedicels)** extend around the capillaries, interdigitating with the secondary processes of the other podocytes (Fig. 16-10). Spaces between the intertwining network of secondary processes are called **slit pores** and are only 25 nm wide. A **slit membrane** spans the distance between pedicels. An unusually thick basal lamina intervenes between the fenestrated capillary endothelium and the podocyte

Fig. 16-8. Three-dimensional relationship between glomerular capillary and podocytes (visceral epithelium). Visceral epithelium is drawn incompletely to expose fenestrations in the underlying glomerular capillary.

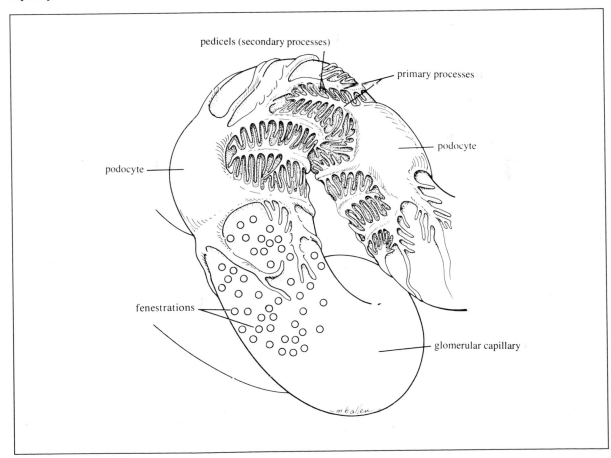

pedicels (secondary processes)

primary processes

podocyte

podocyte

fenestrations

glomerular capillary

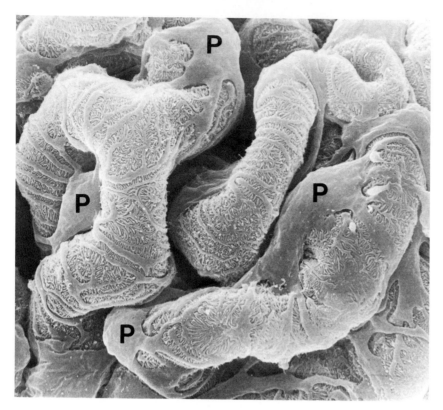

Fig. 16-9. Scanning electron micrograph of glomerular epithelial podocytes (*P*) extending around the circumference of glomerular capillaries. (From P. Andrews, Studies of kidney glomerular epithelial foot process loss in the nephrotic state and experimental situations. *Biomed. Res.* 2 [Suppl.]:293, 1981.)

processes. Together these three structures (fenestrated glomerular endothelium, podocyte slit membranes, and the intervening basal lamina) constitute the filtration barrier within each renal corpuscle (Fig. 16-11).

Mechanisms of Filtration

The fenestrations in the glomerular capillary endothelium have no diaphragms and permit rapid flow of plasma across the capillary wall but prevent the passage of blood cells. The blood plasma next encounters the basal lamina, which ex-

cludes the passage of molecules according to molecular weight and molecular size. The passage of molecules much larger than 10 nm in diameter across the basal lamina is restricted; and molecules near the molecular weight of albumin (68,000) or larger are also restricted. However, smaller molecules—such as simple sugars, metabolites, amino acids, and even small peptides—pass freely across the basal lamina. The next barrier is the filtration slit, which also restricts passage according to molecular size and weight, but its specific filtration properties have been difficult to distinguish from those of the basal lamina. It has been established, however, that molecules are also restricted according to electrostatic charge, since polyanions are signifi-

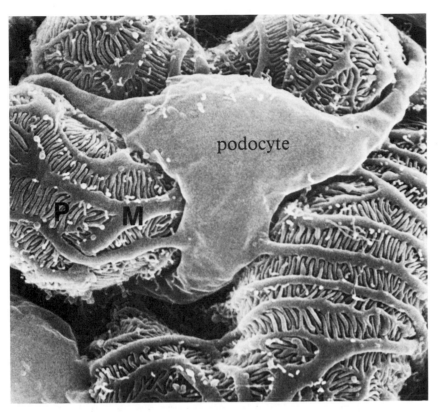

Fig. 16-10. Scanning electron micrograph of glomerular epithelial podocyte with its major processes (*M*) and pedicels (*P*). (From P. Andrews, A scanning and transmission electron microscopic comparison of puromycin aminonucleoside-induced nephrosis to hyperalbuminemia-induced proteinuria with emphasis on kidney podocyte pedicel loss. *Lab. Invest.* 36:183, 1977.)

cantly more retarded than polycations. This is owing to the presence of negatively charged acidic glycoproteins on the podocyte epithelium and its slit membrane as well as on the glomerular endothelium and matrix of the basal lamina, which electrostatically oppose the passage of negatively charged molecules such as albumin. The acidic glycoprotein responsible for the negative charge on the podocyte plasmalemma is podocalyxin, a sialoglycoprotein. The negative charge on the glomerular basement membrane is due to heparin sulfate. Masking this negative charge increases the permeability of the filtration barrier to anions such as albumin.

The driving force for filtration is the net difference in the sum of hydrostatic pressure (blood pressure) and colloid osmotic pressure across the filtration barrier. Of the 1,200 ml of blood flowing through the kidneys per minute, approximately 20 percent of the plasma arriving through the afferent arteriole is routinely filtered away by the renal corpuscles. Therefore, approximately 130 ml of plasma or glomerular filtrate enters the urinary space per minute. This amount is known as the glomerular filtration rate and is an important clinical index of renal function. For a given individual with normal kidneys, glomerular filtration

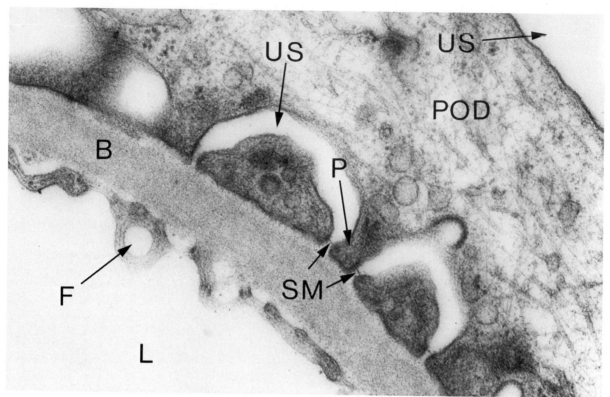

Fig. 16-11. High-magnification electron micrograph of the filtration barrier in a renal glomerulus of the rat. *POD* = podocyte, *B* = basal lamina; *F* = fenestration in endothelium of glomerular capillary; *L* = lumen of glomerular capillary; *P* = pedicel; *SM* = slit membrane, *US* = urinary space.

rate remains constant over a wide range of blood pressure. This is due to the kidney's ability to maintain its intrinsic blood flow constant over a wide range of systemic blood pressure. Hence, glomerular filtration rate and renal blood flow are said to be **autoregulated.** The kidney regulates glomerular filtration rate over a wide range of blood pressures by adjusting the relative degree of vasoconstriction and vasodilation of the afferent and efferent arterioles. Renal failure occurs when blood pressure falls below the lowest level at which autoregulation can occur.

Proximal Tubule

At an average glomerular filtration rate, approximately 180 liters of glomerular filtrate is formed daily and enters the proximal convoluted tubule. During passage through the uriniferous tubules, most of this volume and its dissolved constituents are absorbed by the tubules and returned to the bloodstream; the remainder is concentrated so that only 1 to 2 liters of urine are formed each day. In mammals, about 85 percent of the glomerular filtrate is reabsorbed by the proximal tubule and secreted into the interstitial space where it is retrieved by the peritubular capillaries. The distal tubule handles whatever else is to be reabsorbed.

Compositional modification of provisional urine occurs as a result of the exchange of substances between proximal and distal tubules and their closely associated peritubular capillaries. Two processes operate toward this end; **secretion** and **reabsorption.** Substances are added to the provisional urine after being secreted from peritubular capillaries into the renal interstitium, where they are retrieved by the tubular epithelium and added to the tubular lumen. Substances are removed from the provisional urine after being reabsorbed by the tubular epithelium, pumped into the interstitium, and retrieved by capillaries.

Among the constituents of the glomerular filtrate that are reabsorbed by the proximal tubule are electrolytes such as sodium, potassium, and chloride and bicarbonate ions; glucose, amino acids, and small proteins; and ascorbic acid, all of which diffuse into the peritubular capillaries. Sodium is actively transported into the interstitium against an electrochemical gradient. Since this process requires energy, the cells of the proximal tubule are characteristically packed with mitochondria. Nitrogenous waste products such as urea, uric acid, ammonia, and creatinine are not reabsorbed and consequently are excreted in the urine.

Both the **convoluted** and **straight segments** of the proximal tubule are composed of a simple cuboidal epithelium whose lateral cellular surfaces interdigitate in a complex fashion with adjacent epithelial cells of the tubule. Their apical or luminal surface is characterized by a **brush border,** which is shown by electron microscopy to consist of long microvilli that are required for reabsorption (Figs. 16-12, 16-13). Apical canaliculi originate between and at the base of the microvilli and extend into the cytoplasm, where they are associated with vacuoles. These structures are apparently involved in the absorption and subsequent concentration of protein from the glomerular filtrate. These vacuoles fuse with lysosomes, which degrade the protein to amino acids that can be secreted and retrieved by the peritubular capillaries. In addition, peptidases anchored in the brush border plasmalemma hy-

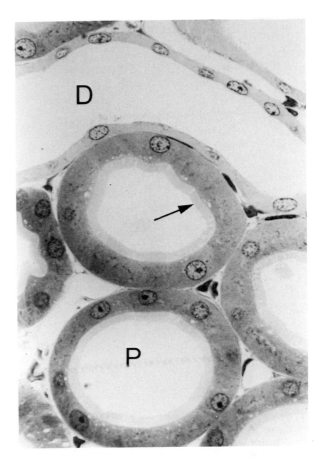

Fig. 16-12. Proximal (*P*) and distal (*D*) convoluted tubules in cortex of rat kidney. Because this kidney was fixed by perfusion, the brush border (*arrow*) has been well preserved on the apical surface of the epithelium of the proximal convoluted tubules. The distal tubules lack a brush border.

drolyze small peptides into amino acids before they are absorbed by the proximal tubule.

Since most of the reabsorption occurs here, the proximal tubule characteristically displays the best-developed brush border of any segment of the uriniferous tubules (see Fig. 16-12). A spherical nucleus usually occupies a central location in the cell. Numerous elongate mitochondria occupy the basal portion of the cell, with their long axes oriented perpendicular to the tubule

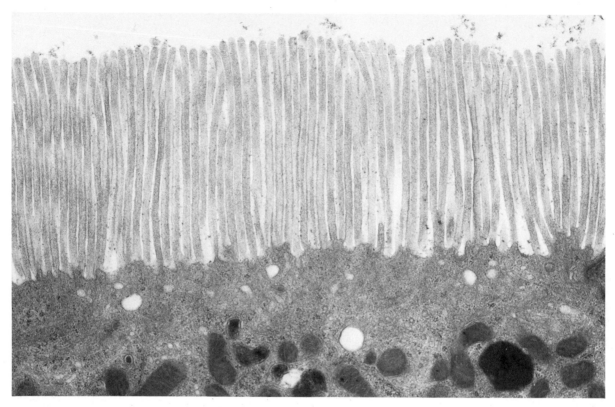

Fig. 16-13. Electron micrograph demonstrating the microvilli projecting from the apical surface of the proximal convoluted tubule.

axis. The cytoplasm stains well with eosin. Unless perfusion fixation is used, the brush border is poorly preserved, and remnants of it tend to obliterate the tubule lumen.

Distal Tubule

The distal tubule consists of three parts: the **distal straight portion,** the **macula densa,** and the **distal convoluted portion.** The straight portion is the ascending thick segment of Henle's loop. This straight segment can be followed from the medulla back into the cortex, where a small specialized region of its wall, the macula densa, establishes a contiguous relationship with the vascular pole of its renal corpuscle (see Figs. 16-3,

16-5). From here the convoluted portion of the tubule begins. It follows a tortuous course within the cortex before joining to a collecting duct in the medullary rays through a short arched collecting duct.

The distal tubule has a larger lumen due to the absence of occluding microvilli and to the low cuboidal shape of its epithelial cells. The significant reduction in number and length of microvilli reflects the diminished reabsorptive role played by the distal tubule as compared with the proximal tubule (see Figs. 16-12, 16-14). Long mitochondria are present in the individual cells, giving a striated appearance to the basal part of the cell. Mitochondrial numbers are significantly reduced in comparison with the proximal tubule, which partly explains the relatively lighter cytoplasmic eosinophilia of distal tubules. The nuclei

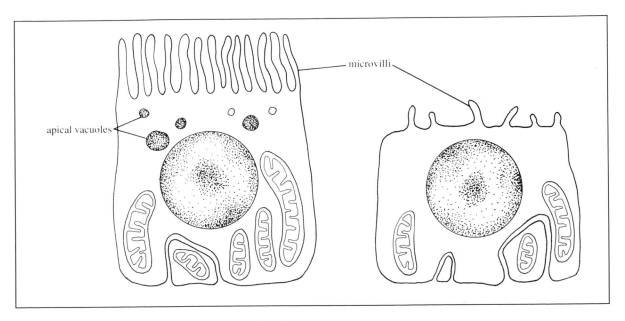

Fig. 16-14. Epithelial cells of the proximal (*left*) and distal (*right*) convoluted tubules.

of the distal tubules are slightly displaced toward the apical surface of the cell.

The **macula densa** (see Figs. 16-3, 16-5) is a short portion of the distal tubule where it is interposed between afferent and efferent arterioles at the vascular pole of each renal corpuscle. The macula densa cells are smaller than the other cells along the distal tubule so they are more densely packed together. This produces a more closely packed array of oval nuclei. These specialized epithelial cells form the relatively flattened wall of this portion of the distal tubule. The macula densa is closely applied to the outer wall of the afferent arteriole and to a lesser extent to the efferent arteriole. Macula densa cells have been implicated as sensors of sodium content in the glomerular filtrate as it passes through this segment of the distal tubule. Their function is discussed below in conjunction with the juxtaglomerular apparatus.

Juxtaglomerular Apparatus and Blood Pressure Regulation

The part of the wall of the afferent arteriole to which the macula densa is applied is composed of specialized smooth muscle cells (myoepithelial cells) called **juxtaglomerular cells** (**JG cells**) (see Fig. 16-5). Immunocytochemistry indicates that these cells contain **renin** within large cytoplasmic granules of variable size. With conventional staining techniques these granules and hence the JG cells themselves are difficult to identify with the light microscope. However, there are appropriate stains devised to display these granules and to identify JG cells with the light microscope. The JG cells occupy the tunica media of the afferent arteriole, replacing the smooth muscle cells that would normally be located there. Since there is usually no basal lamina supporting the macula densa cells, there is virtually nothing to separate JG cells from macula densa cells. The macula densa and JG cells are believed to cooperate in the regulation of blood volume, extracellular fluid volume, and ultimately blood pressure. The intimate histologic relationship of the JG cells and macula densa cells is known as the **juxtaglomerular apparatus.**

Lacis cells (Goormaghtigh cells, polkissen cells) are similar in appearance to JG cells, but with agranular cytoplasm. They are found between the walls of the afferent and efferent arterioles, forming a nest of cells (extraglomerular mesangium) lodged between the macula densa and Bowman's capsule (see Fig. 16-5). They are continuous with a population of **mesangial cells** (intraglomerular mesangium) scattered along the interstices of the glomerular capillary endothelium and the podocytes. The function of both these cells is unclear, but mesangial cells seem to police the filtration barrier by phagocytosis of various kinds of occluding debris. Clinically, mesangial cells are important as a source of potential tumors.

The juxtaglomerular cells are innervated by unmyelinated adrenergic fibers. It is believed that these nerves participate in renin secretion, since beta-adrenergic antagonists, which presumably bind to receptors on the JG cell surface, interfere with renin release. In addition to this neural regulatory component there are two physiologic cues responsible for triggering renin secretion from JG cells: (1) a decline in blood pressure within the afferent arteriole sensed by the JG cells, and (2) a decline in sodium concentration within the distal convoluted tubule sensed by the macula densa. ⌐ increase

Once released into the bloodstream, renin engages in a cascade of reactions that ultimately increase blood pressure. Renin catalyzes the conversion of **angiotensinogen** (**renin substrate**) to **angiotensin I.** Angiotensinogen is a peptide produced by the liver that is present in the circulation. Angiotensin I has little biologic action. However, it is converted to **angiotensin II** by a converting enzyme present in the blood and on the endothelium of some capillary beds, most notably the pulmonary endothelium. Angiotensin II is the most potent vasoconstrictor produced by the body. The vasoconstriction produced by angiotensin II increases blood pressure immediately. However, it also stimulates the release of aldosterone from the zona glomerulosa of the ad-

renal gland. Aldosterone acts on the distal tubule to increase its rate of sodium reabsorption, which permits the retention of water and a commensurate increase in vascular fluid volume (and hence blood pressure) as well as extracellular fluid volume.

Apparently the JG cells act as local baroreceptors, becoming stretched or contracted according to changes in blood pressure within the afferent arteriole. With a decline in blood pressure, the JG cells are allowed to contract, which causes the release of renin. Once the action of renin increases blood pressure, the afferent arteriole is expanded, which stretches the JG cells and thereby curtails renin release. This mechanism can be demonstrated by researchers wanting to induce hypertension. By tying a suture around the renal artery tightly enough to reduce the size of its lumen, the blood pressure within the afferent arteriole is proportionately reduced, which stimulates excess renin secretion (Goldblatt hypertension). Stenosis of the renal artery produces the same effect.

The role played by the macula densa is less well understood. However, the close proximity of the macula densa to the JG cells indicates that the macula densa cells may be able to trigger release of renin from the JG cells when the concentration of sodium within the distal tubule is reduced significantly. Once aldosterone causes more renal retention of sodium, a negative feedback loop curtails renin secretion.

Henle's Loop

Comparative studies have shown that the loop of Henle is a structural feature associated with animals whose kidneys concentrate urine to hypertonicity relative to blood plasma. Animals whose kidneys do not have these loops do not produce concentrated urine. Although the concentration of urine occurs in the distal convoluted tubule and mostly in the collecting ducts under the influence of antidiuretic hormone (ADH), the capacity of these tubules to concentrate urine depends strictly on the existence of a hypertonic interstitial environment within the medulla which is established by the loops of Henle. This will be discussed in more detail after the histology of the loops and of the collecting ducts is described.

The thin segments join the **proximal straight tubule (descending thick segment)** to the **distal straight tubule (ascending thick segment)** (see Fig. 16-3). Together these three structures constitute Henle's loop. Henle's loops are found within the medullary rays and medulla. The length of Henle's loop varies with increasing proximity of its renal corpuscle to the corticomedullary junction. Due mostly to an increase in the thin segment length, the loops of juxtamedullary nephrons are longer compared with those nearer the capsule. The loops of juxtamedullary nephrons extend into the medulla, whereas those nearest the capsule may not reach the medulla at all (see Fig. 16-3).

The juncture of descending thick segments (60 μm in diameter) with the thin segments (15 μm in diameter) is marked by a sudden attenuation of tubule diameter. The transition between the thin segment and the ascending thick segment (35 μm in diameter) is likewise abrupt (see Fig. 16-3). The histologic appearance of the straight descending portion of Henle's loop is similar to the proximal convoluted tubule with which it is continuous. And the histologic appearance of the straight ascending portion of Henle's loop is similar to the distal convoluted tubule with which it is continuous. However, the thickness of the straight segments is somewhat less than their convoluted counterparts.

The thin segment is composed of simple squamous epithelium with a nucleus that bulges slightly into its lumen. There are short, thinly scattered microvilli on its apical surface that are visible only with the electron microscope. The cytoplasm contains only a few visible organelles, mostly mitochondria. In the human each epithelial cell has a single flagellum projecting into the lumen. Under the light microscope, the wall of the thin segment is only slightly thicker than the wall of neighboring vasa recta, which appear as typical capillaries. With practice they can be distinguished rather easily.

The bend in the longest loops of Henle occurs along the thin segment, whereas the bend in the smaller loops usually occurs along the ascending thick segment distal to the thin segment. The longer loops of Henle associated with juxtaglomerular nephrons extend a considerable distance into the medulla, with some thin segments almost reaching the apex of the papilla. The thin segments invariably extend deeper into the medulla than the thick segments. In contrast, the loops of superficial nephrons extend only slightly into the medulla or are confined to the medullary rays.

The ascending thick segment extends further into the medulla than the descending thick segment, producing two macroscopically recognizable zones within the medulla: an **outer** and an **inner zone.** The boundary between these two zones is the juncture between the ascending thick segment and the ascending thin segment. The outer zone contains mostly ascending thick segments with some descending thick segments, plus the descending portion of the thin segments. The inner zone contains only thin segments. In addition, both zones contain numerous vasa recta and collecting ducts (see Figs. 16-3, 16-4).

Collecting Tubules

The collecting duct is the principal site of action of ADH, although the distal convoluted tubule is also influenced. ADH increases the permeability of the collecting duct so that water may be drawn out from its glomerular filtrate by the hypertonic medullary interstitium established by Henle's loop. The result is further concentration of the glomerular filtrate. This function will be discussed more completely after a description of the collecting duct histology.

Within the medullary rays, connecting tubules that are continuous with the distal convoluted tubules join nephrons to their collecting ducts. The collecting ducts run the length of the medullary rays to enter the medulla. Within the inner medulla several collecting ducts coalesce to form the larger **papillary ducts** (inner medullary collecting ducts), which open onto the surface of the papilla and form the **area cribrosa.**

The cells of the smaller collecting ducts are cuboidal with distinct cellular boundaries. However, the epithelium gradually becomes taller along the larger tubules and is columnar in the papillary ducts (Fig. 16-15). The nucleus occupies a basal location, which is especially evident in the taller duct cells of the papillary ducts. With the light microscope, the apical surface of each papillary duct cell is convex, bulging noticeably into the lumen. The columnar epithelium of the papillary ducts often continues onto the surface of the papilla at the area cribrosa. Near the juncture where the papilla joins the minor calix, the epithelium becomes transitional, as it is in the major calices, ureter, and urinary bladder.

Most often with conventional formalin and paraffin embedding procedures, the cells of the collecting ducts appear to be a homogeneous population of cells that are either clear or stain less intensely than the cells of the nephron. This is due to the paucity of stainable organelles within the cells of the collecting duct generally. However, with superior fixative and embedding procedures, two distinct cell types are identified: **principal cells (light cells)** and **intercalated cells (dark cells).** The lightly stained principal cells are the most common cell type of the collecting ducts. The intercalated cells are found in greatest numbers within the outer zone of the medulla (40% intercalated cells vs. 60% principal cells) or in smaller numbers along the terminal part of the distal convoluted tubule, but are entirely absent from the papillary ducts, which are formed exclusively of principal cells. In light micrographs, intercalated cells stain darker than principal cells due to the presence of numerous large mitochondria; this also distinguishes them in electron micrographs. Electron microscopy also reveals that the basal and lateral plasmalemmas of both cell types are folded into interlocking undulations that serve to increase their basal surface areas. The extracellular space between these folds of plasmalemma is known as the **basal** and **lateral labyrinth** (Fig. 16-16).

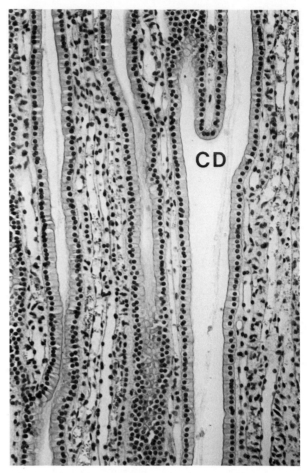

Fig. 16-15. Papillary region of human renal medulla. Several collecting ducts are longitudinally sectioned. Two collecting ducts are converging to form a larger duct. The basal location of nuclei within the columnar epithelium make these ducts conspicuous. Two other collecting ducts are unlabeled. *CD* = collecting duct.

Fig. 16-16. Collecting duct of the rat showing its two cell types, the intercalated cell (*IC*) and the principal cell (*PC*). The large arrow points to the basal labyrinth. The three small arrows point to the occluding junctions between cells that seal the lumen (*L*) of the duct from the intercellular space between cells. Coated vesicles (*cv*) occupy the apical portion of the intercalated cell. Mitochondria are characteristically more abundant in the intercalated cell than in the principal cell.

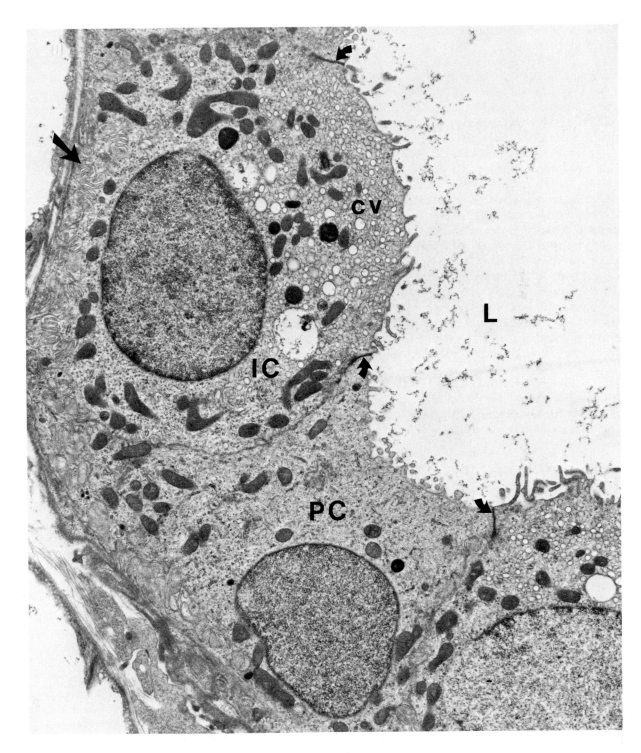

The principal cells are responsible for the ADH-induced permeability of the collecting ducts. Since principal cells are also scattered in small numbers along the distal convoluted tubules, ADH also has an effect on water permeability there, albeit less than in the collecting ducts. ADH increases the permeability of the luminal membrane of the duct cells to water even though it reacts with receptors on the basal membrane. The basal membrane is freely permeable to water even in the absence of ADH. Under the influence of ADH, the passage of water into the cells from the collecting duct lumen causes them visibly to expand. It has been demonstrated by electron microscopy that the lateral labyrinth dilates substantially as water flows out from the principal cells during ADH stimulation. However, the tight junctions joining the lateral membranes of adjacent duct cells near their apical surfaces remain intact. This demonstrates that the ductal epithelium does not allow water to flow between cells but rather through them under the influence of ADH.

It is not known with certainty to what extent intercalated cells respond to ADH, but experimental evidence suggests that they may play a role in potassium reabsorption.

Concentration of Urine

The mechanism that is postulated to be responsible for the concentration of urine is called the **countercurrent hypothesis of urine concentration.** It involves the cooperation of three structural regions of the uriniferous tubules: the loop of Henle, the distal convoluted tubule, and the collecting ducts. The functional capacity of the collecting tubules to concentrate urine depends strictly on the existence of a hypertonic medullary interstitium that is established by the loops of Henle. This hypertonic medullary environment is actually a continuous gradient that increases from isotonic at the corticomedullary junction to very hypertonic at the medullary papilla. Under the influence of ADH, which increases the permeability of the distal tubule and collecting ducts, water is drawn out from these tubules by the hypertonic environment of the medullary intersti-

tial space. The arterial and venous vasa recta located here cooperate in the retrieval of water entering the medullary interstitium from the collecting ducts. Hence, by the action of ADH, urine is concentrated and the body conserves water that would otherwise be lost in the urine.

To understand this process, it helps to know what happens to the glomerular filtrate as it passes through the uriniferous tubule. The isotonic glomerular filtrate entering the loop of Henle becomes increasingly concentrated as it moves down the descending limb. As it moves up the ascending limb, it actually becomes slightly hypotonic with respect to blood plasma. Because the thin ascending limb is impermeable to water but permeable to sodium chloride, salt from the tubular lumen diffuses into the medullary interstitium, the tubular fluid becomes increasingly less hypertonic as it moves up the ascending limb, and a hypertonic gradient is established within the medullary interstitium. To assist this process the thick ascending limb pumps reabsorbed chloride into the medullary interstitium. Because the descending limb is permeable to water, water diffuses passively out of this portion of the loop, thereby increasing the concentration of tubular fluid moving down the descending limb. Sodium is believed to diffuse back into the descending limb of Henle's loop but at a slower rate than it is being pumped out of the ascending limb. As a result, sodium accumulates within the medulla. This recirculation of sodium ions between descending and ascending segments of Henle's loop and the medullary interstitium is referred to as **countercurrent multiplication.** The end result is the establishment of an osmotic gradient in the medullary interstitium that is determined almost entirely by sodium chloride and urea. Reabsorbed urea escapes from the collecting duct to contribute to medullary hypertonicity. Without the osmotic gradient, the fluid flowing through the distal convoluted tubules and collecting tubules could not be concentrated.

The distal convoluted tubules and collecting tubules are essentially impermeable to water except under the influence of ADH. Since the collecting tubule runs through the hypertonic interstitium produced by Henle's loop, an increase in water permeability produced by ADH allows water to diffuse passively down its concentration gradient, moving out of the collecting duct along with urea into the interstitium. The degree to which urine is concentrated depends on the amount of circulating ADH, but the urine can never become more hypertonic than the medullary interstitium. The accompanying ascending vasa recta retrieve the conserved water.

The cue for the release of ADH is an increase in the osmolality of the blood. When the antidiuretic influence of ADH has reduced the osmolality of the blood to normal, ADH release is proportionately reduced or terminated.

Innervation of the Kidney

The kidney has a rich vasomotor innervation consisting mostly of unmyelinated adrenergic nerves of sympathetic splanchnic origin. These nerves are associated with the renal artery and all its branches up to and including the afferent arteriole where the JG cells are also innervated. A small number of myelinated nerves invariably accompany the unmyelinated ones within the adventitia of the larger renal vessels. Stimulation of renal nerves produces a reduction in renal blood flow that involves a redistribution away from the outer cortex toward the juxtamedullary glomeruli and medulla. A similar redistribution of blood flow occurs during hemorrhagic hypotension.

There is also a less well-developed cholinergic nerve supply to these vessels, perhaps of vagal origin. Nerve cell bodies are scattered throughout the adventitia of the renal artery.

URINARY EXCRETORY PASSAGES

The minor and major calyces, renal pelvis, ureter, and bladder are similar in histologic organization. The primary distinction is a progressive thickening of the muscular component in their walls from calices to bladder. The mucosal lining of these structures is composed of transitional epithelium and a thin lamina propria. In the human, no muscularis mucosa is present. Instead, the connective tissue of the lamina propria extends into the external muscular layer, where it becomes enmeshed among bundles of anastomosing smooth muscle. In the upper ureter this muscular layer consists of two distinct layers, an inner longitudinal layer and an outer circular layer (the opposite arrangement occurs in the intestines). In the lower third of the ureter, however, an additional outer layer of longitudinal smooth muscle is present, which becomes especially prominent in the bladder. Slow peristaltic contractions of smooth muscle in the walls of the calyces and ureter move urine from the papilla into the bladder.

Blood vessels penetrate the adventitia and muscle coat of the ureter on their way to supply an abundant capillary network subjacent to the epithelium. Elastic fibers present in the connective tissue of the lamina propria constrict the mucosa of the empty ureter into longitudinal folds. As a result, the mucosa presents a conspicuously corrugated appearance in cross section. An extensive nerve plexus, including ganglia with numerous nerve cell bodies, travels within the adventitia and muscular layer of the ureter. Most of these nerves supply this smooth muscle layer.

A fold of mucous membrane at the oblique entry of the ureter into the bladder performs a valve function; the mucous membrane is forced against the urethral orifice by the urine present in the bladder, thus preventing reflux back into the ureter. The intramural portion of the ureter has only a longitudinal muscle coat, which, when contracted, opens the ureteral orifice to facilitate introduction of urine into the bladder.

Occluding junctions between surface epithelial cells help to establish a permeability barrier between the hypertonic urine present within the bladder lumen and the plasma circulating within the capillaries of the lamina propria.

No glands are present in the excretory passages, with the exception of intraepithelial mucous glands in the bladder, especially near the urethral orifice.

A plexus of sympathetic nerves in the adventitia of the bladder contributes to the motor innervation of the muscular layer and to the sensory innervation of the mucosa.

NATIONAL BOARD TYPE QUESTIONS

For the following, select
    A. if only *1, 2, and 3* are correct.
    B. if only *1 and 3* are correct.
    C. if only *2 and 4* are correct.
    D. if only *4* is correct.
    E. if *all* are correct.

1. Which of the following structures is (are) lined by simple squamous epithelium?
   1. Bowman's capsule
   2. Vasa recta
   3. Thin segment of Henle's loop
   4. Minor calyx

2. Proximal convoluted tubules
   1. are absent from cortical columns.
   2. have a more prominent brush border than distal convoluted tubules.
   3. are located in medullary rays.
   4. have peptidases anchored in their apical plasmalemma.

3. Which of the following statements regarding renal collecting ducts is (are) true?
   1. The collecting duct system is located in both medullary rays and medullary pyramids.
   2. The apical plasmalemma of the principal cell is impermeable to water except under the influence of antidiuretic hormone.
   3. Papillary ducts empty into minor calyces.
   4. Intercalated cells are present throughout the entire length of the collecting duct system.

4. Which of the following statements concerning the loop of Henle is (are) true?
   1. It has a descending thick segment which is continuous with the distal convoluted tubule.
   2. Juxtamedullary nephrons have loops with the shortest thin segments.
   3. Loops from superficial nephrons are longest and penetrate more deeply into the medulla.
   4. It is responsible for establishing the hypertonic environment of the medullary interstitium.

5. Juxtaglomerular cells
   1. are located primarily in the tunica media of the efferent arteriole.
   2. release renin in response to inadequate blood pressure in the afferent arteriole.
   3. lack an innervation.
   4. are in close contact or proximity with macula densa cells.

6. Macula densa cells
   1. are located at the junction of the ascending limb of Henle's loop with the beginning of the distal tubule.
   2. are capable of sensing the sodium concentration in the glomerular filtrate at that site.
   3. trigger the release of renin from juxtaglomerular cells when sodium concentration is too low at that site.
   4. have distinctive cytoplasmic granules.

7. Which of the following statements regarding the filtration barrier in the kidney is (are) true?
   1. The negative charge which retards the passage of polyanions is due to acidic glycoproteins distributed over the surface of the glomerular basement membrane and podocyte plasmalemma.
   2. The basal lamina retards passage of molecules with the molecular weight of albumin and larger.
   3. The slit membrane spans the distance between adjacent pedicels.
   4. Fenestrae of the glomerular endothelium retard the passage of erythrocytes but allow the passage of most plasma solutes.

8. Peritubular capillaries in the kidney
   1. are branches of the efferent arteriole.
   2. are branches of the afferent arteriole.
   3. retrieve solutes reabsorbed from the glomerular filtrate by the proximal convoluted tubules.
   4. have a common distribution with the vasa recta.

9. Which of the following statements concerning the vasa recta is (are) true?
   1. Descending limbs of vasa recta originate

from the efferent arteriole associated with juxtamedullary nephrons.

2. Ascending limbs of vasa recta retrieve water reabsorbed by inner medullary collecting ducts.

3. Ascending limbs of vasa recta drain into arcuate or interlobular veins.

4. Descending limbs of vasa recta originate from the afferent arteriole of superficial nephrons.

10. Peritubular capillaries
1. are branches of vasa recta.
2. are closely associated with proximal convoluted tubules.
3. play no role in retrieval of plasma constituents reabsorbed by the distal convoluted tubule.
4. are branches of the efferent arteriole.

11. Which of the following statements regarding urinary excretory passages is (are) true?
1. The upper segment of the ureter contains an inner longitudinal and an outer circular layer of smooth muscle.
2. Its adventitia lacks autonomic ganglia.
3. Its mucosa is lined by transitional epithelium.
4. It contains a well-developed muscularis mucosa.

12. The urinary bladder
1. has a mucosa lined with transitional epithelium.
2. is devoid of an autonomic nerve supply.
3. has intraepithelial mucous glands.
4. has an epithelium devoid of zonula occludens—type junctions.

ANNOTATED ANSWERS

1. A. The minor calyx is lined by transitional epithelium.
2. C. There are no convoluted tubules in the medulla or medullary rays.
3. A. Intercalated cells are absent from the papillary collecting ducts.

4. D. For a broader discussion see Henle's loop on page 378.
5. C. Juxtaglomerular cells are located primarily in the afferent arteriole and are innervated by unmyelinated adrenergic nerves.
6. A. Juxtaglomerular cells contain the stainable cytoplasmic granules consisting of renin.
7. E.
8. B. Vasa recta are associated with the structures in the medullary rays and medulla but not with the convoluted tubules which are associated with peritubular capillaries in the cortex.
9. A. Review Figure 16-3.
10. C. Peritubular capillaries are intimately associated with the proximal and distal convoluted tubules to facilitate retrieval of substances reabsorbed by those tubules.
11. B. The ureter has a rich autonomic innervation but no muscularis mucosa.
12. B. The musculature of the urinary bladder is well innervated. The leakproof quality of the bladder is ensured by zonula occludens junctions throughout the epithelium.

BIBLIOGRAPHY

Andrews, P. A scanning and transmission electron microscopic comparison of puromycin aminonucleoside-induced nephrosis to hyperalbuminemia-induced proteinuria with emphasis on kidney podocyte pedicel loss. *Lab. Invest.* 36:183, 1977.

Andrews, P. Studies of kidney glomerular epithelial foot process loss in the nephrotic state and experimental studies. *Biomed. Res.* 2 (Suppl.):293, 1981.

Andrews, P. M., and K. R. Porter. A scanning electron microscopic study of the nephron. *Am. J. Anat.* 140:81, 1974.

Aukland, K. Renal blood flow. *Int. Rev. Physiol.* 11:23, 1976.

Barajas, L. Anatomy of the juxtaglomerular apparatus. *Am. J. Physiol.* 237:F333, 1979.

Barajas, L. The ultrastructure of the juxtaglomerular apparatus as disclosed by three-dimensional reconstructions from serial sections. *J. Ultrastruct. Res.* 33:116, 1970.

Barajas, L., and J. Müller. The innervation of the juxtaglomerular apparatus and surrounding tubules: A quantitative analysis by serial section electron microscopy. *J. Ultrastruct. Res.* 43:107, 1973.

Barajas, L., and P. Wang. Localization of tritiated norepinephrine in the renal arteriolar nerves. *Anat. Rec.* 195:525, 1979.

Barger, A. C., and J. A. Herd. Renal Vascular Anatomy and Distribution of Blood Flow. In J. Orloff and R. W. Berliner (eds.), *Handbook of Physiology.* Baltimore: Waverly, 1973. P. 349.

Bialestock, D. The extra-glomerular arterial circulation of the renal tubules. *Anat. Rec.* 129:53, 1957.

Bulger, R. E., R. E. Cronin, and D. C. Dobyan. Survey of the morphology of the dog kidney. *Anat. Rec.* 194:41, 1979.

Daniel, P. M., C. N. Peabody, and M. M. L. Prichard. Cortical ischaemia of the kidney with maintained blood flow through the medulla. *Q. J. Exp. Physiol.* 37:11, 1952.

Davis, J. O., and R. H. Freeman. Mechanisms regulating renin release. *Physiol. Rev.* 56:1, 1976.

Fray, J. C. S. Stretch receptor model for renin release with evidence from perfused rat kidney. *Am. J. Physiol.* 231:936, 1976.

Goldblatt, H. Experimental hypertension induced by renal ischemia. *Harvey Lect.* 33:237, 1937–1938.

Grantham, J. J., et al. Paths of transtubular water flow in isolated renal collecting tubules. *J. Cell Biol.* 41:562, 1969.

Graves, F. T. The anatomy of the intrarenal arteries and its application to segmental resection of the kidney. *Br. J. Surg.* 42:132, 1954.

Handler, J. S., and J. Orloff. The Mechanism of Action of Antidiuretic Hormone. In J. Orloff and R. W. Berliner (eds.), *Handbook of Physiology.* Baltimore: Waverly, 1973.

Hatt, P. Y. The Juxtaglomerular Apparatus. In A. J. Dalton and F. Haguenau (eds.), *Ultrastructure of the Kidney.* New York: Academic, 1967. P. 101.

Hayslett, J. P. Functional adaptation to reduction in renal mass. *Physiol. Rev.* 59:137, 1979.

Jorgensen, F. *The Ultrastructure of the Normal Human Glomerulus.* Copenhagen: Munksgaard, 1966.

Kanwar, Y. S., and M. G. Farquhar. Presence of heparin sulfate in the glomerular basement membrane. *Proc. Natl. Acad. Sci.* 76:1303, 1979.

Kriz, W., and L. Bankir. A standard nomenclature for structures of the kidney. *Am. J. Physiol.* 254:F1–8, 1988.

Kriz, W., J. M. Barrett, and S. Peter. The renal vasculature: Anatomical-functional aspects. *Int. Rev. Physiol.* 11:1, 1976.

McKenna, O. C., and E. T. Angelakos. Adrenergic innervation of the canine kidney. *Circ. Res.* 22:345, 1968.

Maunsbach. A. B. Cellular mechanisms of tubular protein transport. *Int. Rev. Physiol.* 11:145, 1976.

Morel, F., and A. Doucet. Hormonal control of kidney functions at the cell level. *Physiol. Rev.* 66:377, 1986.

Munkácsi, I., and M. Palkovits. Study of the renal pyramid, loops of Henle, and percentage distribution of their thin segments in animals living in desert, semidesert and water-rich environment. *Acta Biol. Acad. Sci. Hung.* 17:89, 1966.

Murakami, T. Vascular arrangement of the rat renal glomerulus. A scanning electron microscope study of corrosion casts. *Arch. Histol. Jpn.* 34:87, 1972.

Myers, C. E., et al. Human renal ultrastructure: IV. Collecting duct of healthy individuals. *Lab. Invest.* 15:1921, 1966.

Orci, L., et al. Membrane ultrastructure in urinary tubules. *Int. Rev. Cytol.* 73:183, 1981.

Ordoñez, N. G., and B. H. Spargo. The morphologic relationship of light and dark cells of the collecting tubule in potassium-depleted rats. *Am. J. Pathol.* 84:317, 1976.

Pitts, R. F. *Physiology of the Kidney and Body Fluids.* Chicago: Year Book, 1963.

Rennke, H. G., and M. A. Venkatachalam. Structural determinants of glomerular permselectivity. *Fed. Proc.* 36:2619, 1977.

Ryan, G. B., S. J. Hein, and M. J. Karnovsky. Glomerular permeability to proteins. *Lab. Invest.* 34:415, 1976.

Spinelli, F. Structure and development of the renal glomerulus as revealed by scanning electron microscopy. *Int. Rev. Cytol.* 39:345, 1974.

Staehelin, A., F. J. Chlapowski, and M. A. Bonneville. Luminal plasma membrane of the urinary bladder: I. Three-dimensional reconstruction from freeze-etch images. *J. Cell Biol.* 53:73, 1972.

Stein, J. H. The Renal Circulation. In B. M. Brenner and F. C. Rector (eds.), *The Kidney.* Philadelphia: Saunders, 1976. Vol. 2, p. 215.

Thoenes, W., and K. H. Langer. Relationship Between Cell Structures of Renal Tubules and Transport Mechanisms. In K. Thurau and H. Kahrmarker (eds.), *Renal Transport and Diuretics.* Berlin: Springer Verlag, 1969, P. 37.

Tisher, C. C. Anatomy of the Kidney, In B. M. Brenner and F. C. Rector (eds.), *The Kidney.* Philadelphia: Saunders, 1976. Vol. 1, p. 3.

Tisher, C. C., R. E. Bulger, and B. F. Trump. Human renal ultrastructure: I. Proximal tubule of healthy individuals. *Lab. Invest.* 15:1356, 1966.

Trump, B. F., and E. P. Benditt. Electron microscope

studies of human renal disease; observations of normal visceral glomerular epithelium and its modification in disease. *Lab. Invest.* 11:753, 1962.

Wågermark, J., V. Ungerstedt, and A. Ljunggvist. Sympathetic innervation of the juxtaglomerular cells of the kidney. *Circ. Res.* 22:149, 1968.

Wilson, W. A new staining method for demonstrating the granules of the juxtaglomerular complex. *Anat. Rec.* 112:497, 1952.

17 Endocrine System

Objectives

You will learn the following in this chapter:

The general histologic organization of the major endocrine glands: thyroid, parathyroid, adrenal, hypophysis, and pineal

The ultrastructural mechanisms utilized by thyroid follicle cells during synthesis, storage, and release of thyroid hormone

The structure of the parafollicular cell in the thyroid and its release of calcitonin to regulate calcium homeostasis

The structure of the principal cells of the parathyroid and its role in calcium homeostasis

The zonation of the adrenal cortex and its role in the synthesis and release of mineralocorticoids and glucocorticoids

The structure and development of the adrenal medulla and its role in amplification of the body's sympathetic nervous system

The vascular and neural basis for the hypothalamic regulation of the pituitary; hypophyseal hormones that influence diverse target areas in the body

The role of the pineal in diurnal and seasonal regulation of endocrine-mediated processes

General description of the diffuse neuroendocrine system

The endocrine organs are responsible for regulating and coordinating important physiologic functions of the body through small-molecular-weight hormones, which they synthesize and release into perivascular spaces. After crossing the vascular wall, circulating hormones can exert influences on target cells remote from their site of release. Many hormones, such as proteins, which are not lipid-soluble and therefore unable to diffuse across the plasmalemma of target cells, influence those cells by first reacting with specific membrane-receptor molecules that activate adenyl cyclase. This latter membrane enzyme increases intracellular concentrations of cyclic adenosine monophosphate (cAMP); cyclic AMP acts as an internal or second "messenger" by phosphorylating enzymes that catalyze particular cellular responses. Other hormones, such as steroids, are lipid-soluble and diffuse across the plasmalemma to exert their influence directly within the target cell. Still other hormones, such as epinephrine, exert their influence on the electrogenic plasmalemmas of muscle and nerve cells, which become depolarized or hyperpolarized depending on the type of receptor present or stimulated. Because of the ability of distinct cell types to respond in different ways to the same hormone through different receptors, a single circulating hormone can evoke either one response from a discrete cell type alone or various responses from several different cell types as it circulates throughout the body. This capability allows the endocrine system to operate with an economy that does not require bulky nerve tracts as does the peripheral nervous system, the other great integrator of bodily functions. Nevertheless, certain neurosecretory cells of the central nervous system are also part of the endocrine system.

In contrast to the exocrine glands, which secrete substances into a system of ducts, endocrine organs lack ducts of any kind. However, endocrine tissue is absolutely dependent on the circulatory system and without exception is highly vascularized by fenestrated capillaries, which apparently facilitate entry of hormones into the circulation. The action of a hormone often results in the adjustment of circulating concentrations of some other biologically active substance, which in turn inhibits hormone release by the endocrine organ. This feedback inhibition is often a vascular-mediated function also.

Although isolated bits of endocrine tissue are found within the parenchyma of larger organs that are not primarily endocrine in nature (e.g., the islets of the pancreas and the interstitial cells of the testis), this chapter addresses itself to organs that are exclusively endocrine: the thyroid, parathyroid, adrenals, pituitary, and pineal, and the diffuse neuroendocrine system.

THE THYROID

The thyroid consists of follicles whose constituent epithelial cells secrete two iodinated amino acids collectively termed **thyroid hormone: tetraiodothyronine** (thyroxine) and **triiodothyronine.** The former is released in considerably larger quantity as the principal circulating hormone, whereas the latter is more potent and is released in a smaller quantity.

Thyroid hormone produces several principal effects:

1. Thyroid hormone stimulates oxidative metabolism in certain tissues, thereby raising the basal metabolic rate (BMR). This effect is substantial on cardiac and skeletal muscle and the liver, whereas the brain, gonads, and smooth muscle are not responsive.
2. Thyroid hormone is involved in thermoregulation of the body. In collaboration with other hormones, it can elevate body temperature by mobilizing energy substrates such as fat for conversion into heat.
3. Thyroid hormone promotes tissue maturation. It exerts tremendous influence on the development of the nervous, musculoskeletal, and reproductive systems. Although this function is often performed in concert with other hormones, the absence of thyroid hormone during neonatal development leaves these systems in an infantile state.

Histologic Organization

The histologic organization (Figs. 17-1, 17-2) of the thyroid is relatively simple. There is a thin, fibrous capsule whose projections invade the gland and partition it into poorly defined lobules. The parenchymal cells, which produce thyroid hormone, are organized into numerous structural units called **follicles.** Follicles consist of a single layer of epithelial cells which completely enclose a central lumen. The follicle is essentially an epithelial sphere whose lumen functions as an extracellular storage site for an inactive polymer of thyroid hormone. The stored hormone occupying the follicle lumen appears histologically as an amorphous, homogeneous colloid (see Fig. 17-1). The follicles are surrounded by a basal lamina and reticular fibers. A network of blood vessels, including fenestrated capillaries, courses through the sparse connective tissue between follicles. Small unmyelinated nerves running within the interfollicular space are primarily vasomotor nerves. However, some sympathetic fibers have been observed that are closely apposed to follicular epithelial cells, with only an intervening basal lamina. This relationship indicates the possibility of a neural stimulus for thyroid secretion in addition to that known to occur in response to thyroid stimulating hormone.

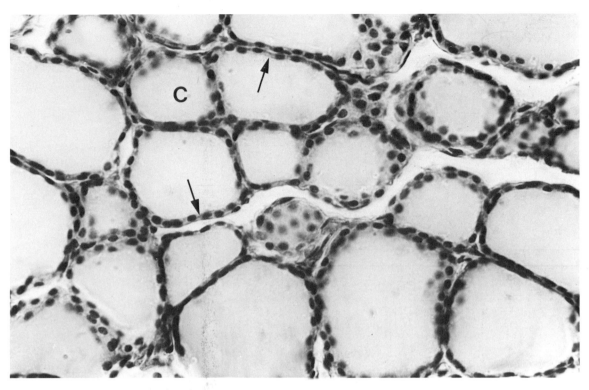

Fig 17 1. Light micrograph of human thyroid gland. Follicles are composed of simple cuboidal epithelial cells (*arrows*) and are filled with colloid (*C*). The colloid is an extracellular storage site for thyroglobulin.

The epithelial cells vary in height from low cuboidal to columnar, but the former appearance is more common. When the follicle is in an active state, the epithelium is tallest and the free apical surface facing the colloid displays scattered but well-developed microvilli. The follicle cells are bound together laterally near their apical surfaces by junctional complexes. Gap junctions involving lateral membranes of adjacent follicle cells have also been observed with freeze-fracturing, indicating the possibility that all epithelial cells within a follicle are coupled in their secretory responses.

Parafollicular cells in the human are a much smaller population of cells enclosed between the basal surface of the follicular epithelium and its basal lamina. Consequently, they have no sur-

face in contact with the follicle lumen and are not involved in production of thyroid hormone. They produce **calcitonin,** an important hormone involved in calcium homeostasis. In some species the parafollicular cell is called a C cell in reference to its clear cytoplasm. In these species a parafollicular cell is easily distinguished at the light microscopic level from follicular epithelial cells, which stain darker. Their identification is further facilitated by their interfollicular location, as in the case of dogs. However, in the human thyroid the parafollicular cell is not easily distinguished from the regular follicular cells unless it is stained by immunohistochemical methods for calcitonin (Fig. 17-3). However, when viewed with the electron microscope, its cytoplasm contains numerous membrane-bound granules that are electron-dense and believed to consist of cal-

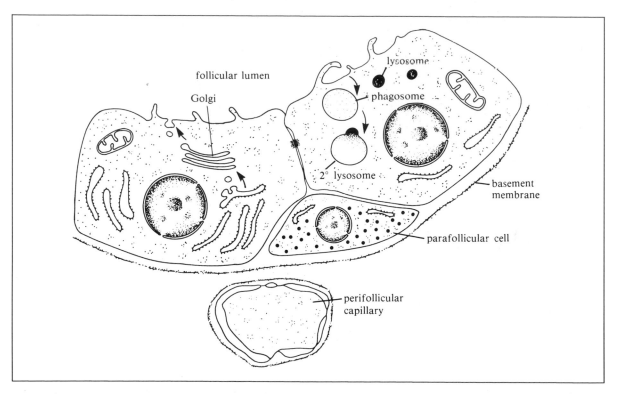

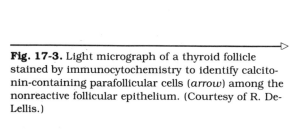

Fig. 17-2. Two follicular epithelial cells from the thyroid. One cell (*left*) shows the organelles involved in the synthesis and transfer of thyroglobulin to the apical plasmalemma, where it is deposited by exocytosis into the follicular lumen. The other cell (*right*) shows the organelles involved in the retrieval of thyroglobulin by endocytosis. Lysosomes fuse to the phagosome, mixing proteases with thyroglobulin and thereby releasing the active tetraiodothyronine and triiodothyronine subunits. A parafollicular cell is also shown enclosed in the same basement membrane that circumscribes the basal aspect of the follicle. The dense granules represent calcitonin.

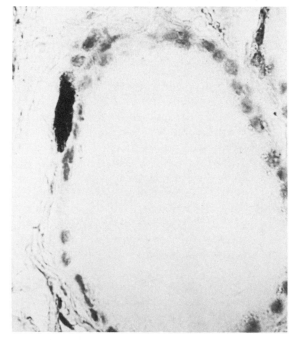

Fig. 17-3. Light micrograph of a thyroid follicle stained by immunocytochemistry to identify calcitonin-containing parafollicular cells (*arrow*) among the nonreactive follicular epithelium. (Courtesy of R. De-Lellis.)

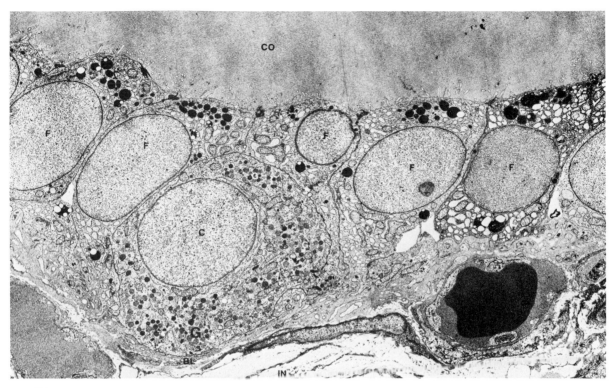

Fig. 17-4. Wall of human thyroid follicle exhibiting both follicular epithelial cells (*F*) and a parafollicular cell (*C*). The parafollicular cell is separated from the luminal colloid (*CO*) by follicular cell cytoplasm and contained within the basal lamina (*BL*) enclosing the follicle. The granules (*G*) within the cytoplasm of the parafollicular cell contain calcitonin. *IN* = interfollicular space. (From R. DeLellis, G. Nunnemacher, and H. Wolfe, C-cell hyperplasia, an ultrastructural analysis. *Lab. Invest.* 36:237, 1977. © 1977. U.S.-Canadian Division of International Academy of Pathology.)

citonin (Fig. 17-4; see also Figs. 17-2, 17-3). It has been shown that parafollicular cells are concentrated in the central region of both lobes of the thyroid but are relatively scarce in the superior and inferior poles.

In most nonmammalian groups parafollicular tissue forms a distinct gland, the **ultimobranchial body,** which serves the same purpose. In mammals, evidence is strong that parafollicular cells are ultimately of neural crest origin, cells of which migrate into the last branchial pouch of the developing pharynx before becoming incorporated into the thyroid and giving rise to C cells.

Synthesis and Secretion of Thyroid Hormone

The follicular epithelial cells synthesize an inactive, polymeric form of thyroid hormone called **thyroglobulin,** which is released and stored extracellularly within the follicle lumen (see Fig. 17-1). The protein part of thyroglobulin is synthesized by the rough endoplasmic reticulum, which is located basally and laterally within the cell. The carbohydrate (mostly galactose) is added within the Golgi complex, which is located in the supranuclear part of the cell where the thyroglobulin precursors are also polymerized. Secretory vesicles (15–20 nm) containing this noniodinated glycoprotein polymer carry it to the apical surface of the cell, where it is released into the follicular lumen for storage. Autoradiographic evidence indicates that thyroglobulin may be iodinated within the follicle lumen near the luminal membrane (see Fig. 17-2).

Nerve fibers to follicular epithelial cells have been observed, indicating the possibility of a neural stimulus for thyroid secretion. However, the best understood mechanism for thyroid secretion is that initiated by **thyroid-stimulating hormone (TSH)**, a hormone released by the pituitary. TSH simultaneously stimulates synthesis and release of thyroid hormone. It increases: (1) the uptake of iodide from the bloodstream by follicular epithelium, (2) the synthesis of thyroglobulin and its deposition into the follicular lumen, (3) iodination of thyroglobulin, (4) phagocytosis or retrieval of thyroglobulin-containing colloid, and (5) secretion of thyroid hormone into the bloodstream. A negative feedback mechanism assures that elevated levels of circulating thyroid hormone curtail TSH release from the pituitary. Histologically, the influence of TSH is reflected by hypertrophy of the follicular epithelium, diminished volume of extracellular colloid, and an increase of intracellular colloid droplets.

Upon stimulus provided by TSH, colloid-containing thyroglobulin is retrieved from the follicle lumen by phagocytosis (see Fig. 17-2). These large thyroglobulin-containing phagosomes (50–400 nm) fuse with smaller electron-dense vesicles, which have been identified as primary lysosomes based on positive staining for acid phosphatase. Lysosomal proteases mixing with thyroglobulin split the inactive macromolecule into its biologically active components, tetraiodothyronine (T_4) and triiodothyronine (T_3). The thyroid hormones are then released at the basal side of the cell, where they gain access to the perifollicular capillaries and become blood-borne. The monoiodinated and diiodinated precursors are not released but are reutilized in the synthesis of more hormone.

The pathologic consequences of iodine deficiency include **goiter,** a chronic enlargement of the thyroid. The increased size of the gland is due initially to hypertrophy and hyperplasia of the follicular epithelium as a result of increased release of TSH (**parenchymal goiter**). The increased release of TSH is caused by the lack of circulating thyroid hormone, which cannot be synthesized in the absence of iodine. When normal dietary iodine intake is resumed, thyroid hormone can again be produced, terminating TSH release. However, the increased storage capacity of the proliferated follicular epithelium in parenchymal goiter permits an excessive accumulation of colloid, increasing the size of the thyroid further (**colloid goiter**). **Adenomas** of the thyroid secrete thyroid hormone but are insensitive to TSH regulation.

Hypothyroidism during infancy or in late pregnancy (which may occur due to congenital absence of the thyroid or maternal iodine deficiency) results in a condition known as **cretinism,** which is characterized by physical and mental retardation. The bony skeleton grows slowly and incompletely, and the reproductive system remains infantile. Thyroid deficiency has its most severe consequences during infancy, especially in the neonate when thyroid hormone is required for proper development of these systems. If thyroid deficiency is recognized early enough, replacement therapy may be instituted and the effects reversed. However, if thyroid hormone is administered after a critical period has passed, during which time target cells are receptive to the influence of thyroxine, defects become irreversibly established. Hypothyroidism in the adult results in less severe consequences (**myxedema**), since the body's systems have already developed fully. Under these circumstances, thyroid deficiency is characterized by lethargy, weakness, fatigability; slowed thinking and speech processes; intolerance to cold; dry, thick yellow skin; and interstitial edema rich in protein and proteoglycans (from which the term **myxedema** is derived).

PARAFOLLICULAR CELLS

The parafollicular cells of the thyroid are involved in hormonal regulation of calcium levels in the bloodstream. These parafollicular cells or C cells produce **calcitonin** (previously known as **thyrocalcitonin**), a hypocalcemic factor that lowers plasma calcium concentration by suppressing resorption of bone by osteoclasts and osteocytes, thereby diminishing the return of calcium to the blood. This process facilitates the kidney's task of eliminating excess calcium from the bloodstream. The antagonistic effects of calcitonin and parathyroid hormone operate alternatively to rigorously maintain blood calcium concentration. Parafollicular cells are stimulated to release calcitonin by hypercalcemic blood; unlike the follicular cells, they are not under the minute-to-minute control of the pituitary. There is evidence, however, that hypophyseal growth hormone stimulates the release of calcitonin, which increases the number of differentiating osteoblasts required for bone growth in the young.

THE PARATHYROID

Histologic Aspects

The parathyroid glands develop from the third and fourth pharyngeal pouches. The four tiny glands are generally found within the capsule of the thyroid, one each at the superior and inferior poles of both lobes. The parathyroids possess a thin capsule of their own whose trabeculae extend into the gland and divide it into incomplete lobules. Most of its blood vessels enter through these trabeculae. The parenchymal cells form irregular anastomosing cords or groups that are supported by reticular fibers. Less frequently, they may form follicles containing colloid. Fat cells may also be present and increase in number with age.

Two parenchymal cells can be distinguished histologically, a major population of **principal** or **chief cells** and a minor population of **oxyphil cells** (Fig. 17-5). Principal cells are uniformly

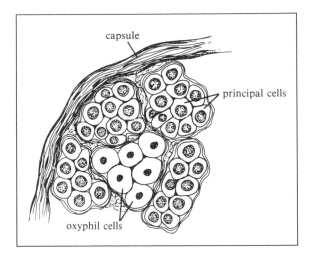

Fig. 17-5. Parathyroid gland. The cells are arranged in cords by loose connective tissue. The principal cells are predominant in number. Oxyphil cells are recognized by their smaller, more condensed nuclei and larger relative cytoplasmic volume.

small (8–10 μm) and polyhedral in shape, with uniformly round nuclei. The cytoplasm is slightly acidophilic. Electronic micrographs reveal the presence of membrane-bound granules that appear to be secretory vesicles containing **parathyroid hormone.** These granules stain with iron-hematoxylin and are also argyrophilic. There are only small numbers of mitochondria, and Golgi body development depends on the synthetic state of the cell.

Two types of principal cells can be distinguished, presumably based on the state of secretory activity. One type has fewer membrane-bound granules and large glycogen deposits, whereas a second type has much less glycogen but a preponderance of membrane-bound granules.

Oxyphil cells do not appear until somewhat before puberty and increase in number with age. They occur singly or in small clusters. These cells have a strongly acidophilic cytoplasm that stains well with eosin due to the presence of numerous mitochondria. The nuclei are slightly smaller

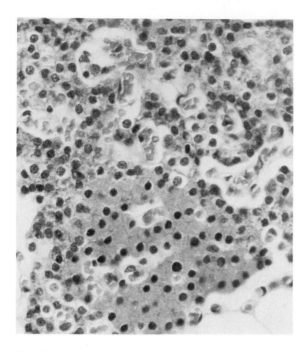

Fig. 17-6. A region of the parathyroid gland showing a nest of oxyphil cells in the lower half of the photo and principal cells in the upper half. The acidophilic cytoplasm of the principal cells causes them to appear darker in this photo. The oxyphil cells are easily recognized by their smaller nucleus-to-cytoplasmic ratio.

than those of the principal cells, and their chromatin may be more condensed. The cytoplasmic volume is also slightly larger, so that the nucleus-to-cytoplasm ratio of oxyphil cells is somewhat smaller than that of principal cells (see Figs. 17-5, 17-6). Hence oxyphil cells are distinguished from the principal cells by their greater affinity for acid dyes and their larger cytoplasmic volume. The functional significance of oxyphil cells is not known.

Histophysiology of Parathyroid Hormone

Parathyroid hormone is released in response to deficient blood calcium levels (hypocalcemia). It maintains calcium levels in the plasma by increasing the normal rate of calcium mobilization from bone, the body's largest pool of calcium. It acts by increasing the rate of osteoclastic resorption and by increasing osteocytic osteolysis. In addition, parathyroid hormone promotes absorption of dietary calcium from the small intestine and reabsorption of calcium by the proximal tubules in the kidney.

Vitamin D is also important in promoting absorption of calcium from the intestine. In vitamin D-deficient rickets, the principal cells hypertrophy in an attempt to recover normal calcium levels (**secondary hyperparathyroidism**). The hypercalcemia owing to **primary hyperparathyroidism** is most commonly caused by a benign tumor (adenoma) of the parathyroid and by hyperplasia of the principal cells. It can be alleviated by surgical excision of the involved parathyroid tissue. The hypercalcemia associated with primary hyperparathyroidism is due to excessive bone resorption carried out by osteoclasts under the influence of abnormally high levels of circulating parathyroid hormone.

The control of blood calcium levels within certain limits is critical. Normal plasma levels are about 4 to 5 mEq/liter. Hypercalcemia may cause disturbances in the cardiac conduction system and calcium deposition in the kidney, resulting in kidney failure. Hypocalcemia can also produce spontaneous neuromuscular excitability and tetanic convulsions leading to death. These effects reflect the important role calcium plays in stabilizing ionic gradients across electrogenic membranes, such as the plasmalemma of muscle and nerve cells. Since calcium is also required for the release of neurotransmitter from neurosecretory vesicles in the axon terminals of motor neurons, there is a quantitative relationship between extracellular calcium and the amount of neurotransmitter release.

It is important to bear in mind that the secretory activity of both parafollicular cells and the parathyroid is a direct response to blood calcium levels and that neither seems to be controlled by the pituitary.

THE ADRENALS

The adrenals are contained within the perirenal adipose tissue on the medial cranial pole of each kidney. They are actually two endocrine glands contained within a common connective tissue capsule: an outer **cortex** and an inner **medulla.** In submammalian species this contiguous association of adrenocortical tissue with medullary chromaffin tissue does not exist; consequently, it should not be surprising that they have separate embryologic origins. The adrenal cortex is derived from coelomic mesodermal epithelium. The chromaffin cells are ectodermal in origin, ultimately derived from neural crest cells that migrate into the developing adrenal anlage from nearby sympathetic ganglia. The cortex is essential for life; the medulla, while important, is not.

Adrenal Cortex

HISTOLOGIC ORGANIZATION

Prior to birth the human adrenal cortex displays two distinct zones: an outer poorly developed permanent zone and inner well-developed fetal zone. Shortly after birth the fetal zone begins to degenerate and soon disappears while the permanent zone (adult zone) begins to differentiate into the three zones characteristic of the mature adrenal.

The mature adrenal cortex consists of three concentric zones: first, an outer **zona glomerulosa,** a thin zone of spherical groups of pyramidal to columnar cells immediately subjacent to the capsule and continuous with the more extensive **zona fasciculata,** consisting of long, radially arranged cords or columns of polyhedral cells; finally, there is the **zona reticularis,** the innermost zone consisting of an anastomosing network of cellular cords that rest on the medulla (Figs. 17-7, 17-8).

The cortical cells are supported by delicate reticular fibers. They have acidophilic cytoplasm with round nuclei that are centrally located. Electron microscopy indicates that an abundance of smooth endoplasmic reticulum is a common feature of these cortical cells, and that the mitochondria have tubular cristae characteristic of steroid-producing cells. Cells from all three zones are vacuolated to some degree, most notably those from the zona fasciculata (Fig. 17-9). These numerous vacuoles contain lipid droplets in situ, which are composed primarily of cholesterol acyl esters used in the synthesis of steroids by the cortex. Vacuolation is an artifact resulting from the dissolution of lipids by the organic solvents used in conventional paraffin-embedding procedures.

The high concentration of lipids in the zona fasciculata imparts a yellow color to the fresh, unfixed adrenal cortex. In hypersecretory diseases of the adrenal cortex, these lipids are depleted because their metabolic turnover is so high. In these instances the adrenal cortex has a brown coloration.

VASCULATURE

The adrenal vasculature is highly variable even among mammals. The blood supply of the human adrenal arises from numerous adrenal arterial branches that ramify over the surface of the adrenal capsule. Branches of these adrenal arterioles penetrate the capsule to form a thin **subcapsular plexus** from which straight **cortical capillaries** originate. Cortical capillaries separate cellular cords of the **zona fasciculata,** and drain into a plexus of capillaries within the zona reticularis. This plexus is drained by a few channels, which empty into the **medullary sinuses** (in effect forming a portal system between cortex and medulla). The medullary sinuses drain into larger venous sinuses, which empty into the **central vein (adrenal vein).**

The walls of the central vein and its major branches are distinctive because they possess bundles of longitudinally oriented smooth muscle, which occupy one side of the venous wall and are significantly reduced in the wall on the opposite side of the lumen. The larger venous sinuses join the central vein between these pillars of smooth muscle. Some of the larger venous sinuses also have eccentric muscular pillars, but

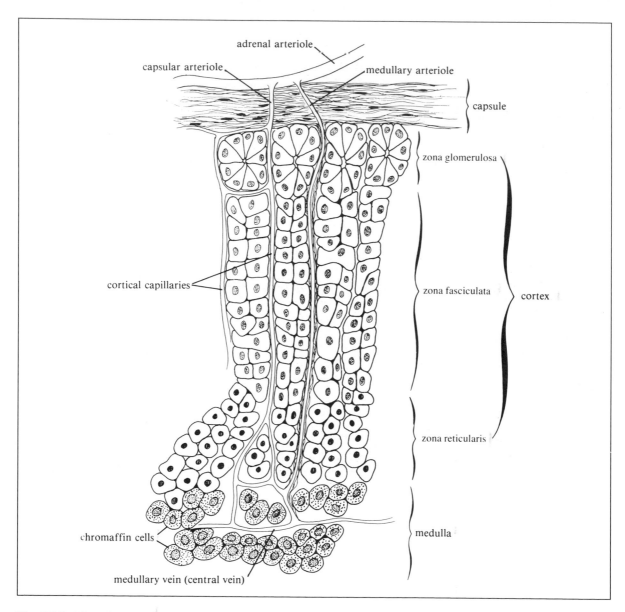

Fig. 17-7. Adrenal gland. The blood supply to the cortex and medulla is shown.

all have elastic fiber reinforcement. The muscular component of the central vein diminishes in thickness along its course from the head of the adrenal, where it is thickest, to the tail of the adrenal, where it disappears entirely. In the tail, the cortex is reflected onto the central vein, forming a cuff of cortical tissue along the length of the vein.

It has been postulated that the muscular pillars associated with the central vein and its major branches regulate medullary blood flow.

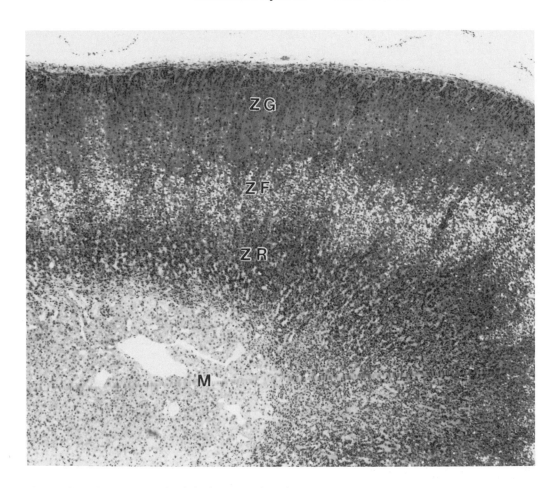

Fig. 17-8. Light micrograph of the human adrenal. The gland is covered by a capsule (*C*). The cortex contains three histologically distinct zones: zona glomerulosa (*ZG*), zona fasciculata (*ZF*), and zona reticularis (*ZR*). Deep to the cortex is the medulla (*M*). Note the distended capillaries in the medulla (*arrows*).

According to this hypothesis, blood can be prevented from draining out through the central vein when the large venous sinuses become compressed between contracting muscular pillars of the central vein. As a consequence, blood is pooled in the medullary sinuses. After relaxation, the elastic fibers of the medullary sinuses propel blood forcefully out through the central vein. The pooling of blood would allow medullary hormones to accumulate in greater concentration before being expelled in the venous effluent. An alternate route of venous flow is provided by **emissary** veins in the tail region that link the venous system with external capsular veins. However, our understanding of adrenal vascular mechanics remains to be clarified.

Other branches of the adrenal arterioles, **medullary arterioles,** penetrate the cortex within trabecular extensions of the capsule and drain directly into the medullary sinuses without

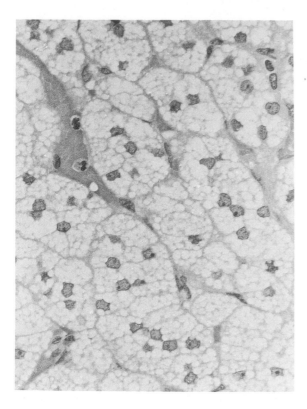

Fig. 17-9. The zona fasciculata of the adrenal at higher magnification to show the highly vacuolated cytoplasm of the cells in this region.

supplying the cortex. Consequently, the medulla has a dual blood supply arriving from cortical capillaries and medullary arterioles. The cortical capillaries and medullary sinuses of the adrenal are all fenestrated.

INNERVATION

Small vasomotor nerves are responsible for regulating blood flow through the adrenal cortex and medulla. Preganglionic sympathetic nerves that are destined to innervate the medullary chromaffin cells enter the adrenal through splanchnic nerves, which traverse the cortex within thin connective tissue trabeculae. Parenchymal cells of the adrenal cortex are not innervated.

HISTOPHYSIOLOGY

The adrenal cortex produces three classes of steroid hormones: The zona glomerulosa produces **mineralocorticoids (aldosterone** and **deoxycorticosterone),** which influence electrolyte balance, and the zona fasciculata and reticularis produce mostly **glucocorticoids,** which influence carbohydrate and protein metabolism, as well as some **androgens** or male hormones. Small amounts of androgens are synthesized by the reticularis but in certain disorders can exert a masculinizing effect on developing genitalia.

The most clearly understood mineralocorticoid produced by the zona glomerulosa is **aldosterone,** a hormone that regulates the body's sodium retention. Aldosterone acts upon the distal tubule of the kidney, causing reabsorption of sodium ions with a proportional loss of potassium. It apparently exerts this effect on most other cells of the body, including also the salivary glands and sweat glands. This indispensable homeostatic mechanism is hormonally regulated by the **renin-angiotensin system.** Renin is released by the juxtaglomerular cells of the kidney in response to a signal from the afferent arteriole indicating a fall in blood pressure or from the macula densa indicating reduced sodium load in the distal tubule. Renin then catalyzes the transformation of serum **angiotensinogen** into **angiotensin I,** a biologically inactive decapeptide. Angiotensin I is then converted into **angiotensin II,** a biologically active octapeptide, by a converting enzyme present in the plasma and in the endothelium of various vascular beds, notably the pulmonary endothelium of the lung.

No other substance produced by the body is a more potent vasoconstrictor than angiotensin II. Consequently, blood pressure is raised immediately by the vasoconstrictive action of angiotensin II on vascular smooth muscle. Secondly, angiotensin II provokes the secretion of aldosterone from the zona glomerulosa, thereby elevating blood pressure on a more long-term basis through renal retention of sodium, which results in increased intravascular fluid volume. The resulting increased blood pressure causes a reduction or shutdown of renin release by the juxtaglomerular cells by a negative feedback mechanism. If this mechanism for maintaining blood pressure is compromised, shock may ensue.

The zona fasciculata (and the zona reticularis to a limited extent) is responsible for production of **glucocorticoids,** the most important of which are cortisol, cortisone, and corticosterone. In the liver, glucocorticoids stimulate the conversion of protein to carbohydrate, the accumulation of glycogen, and the release of excess glucose into the blood. Glucocorticoids also increase the turnover of lipid in fat cells. This catabolic influence on the liver and adipose tissue increases the body's supply of molecular substrates for sufficient energy to combat various types of physical and emotional stress. The secretion of glucocorticoids is a useful and necessary bodily response to stress, but when released in excessive amounts or without respite, its catabolic influence eventually exerts a deleterious effect on the body. Excessive glucocorticoid secretion suppresses the immune response of depleting lymphatic organs of lymphocytes and diminishing antibody synthesis; it inhibits the inflammatory response; and it retards growth.

The release of glucocorticoids by the zona fasciculata and zona reticularis is governed by adrenocorticotropin (ACTH), a hormone produced by the pituitary. ACTH stimulates steroid synthesis and release, as well as hypertrophy of these two zones. ACTH is released from the pituitary during periods of stress caused by fear, pain, anxiety, or other related stimuli. When the blood levels of glucocorticoids become sufficiently elevated as a result of ACTH stimulus, release of ACTH is shut down by a negative feedback mechanism. However, ACTH has *no* direct effect on the zona glomerulosa or on aldosterone release, which is governed by the renin-angiotensin system.

The independent hormonal control mechanisms governing secretory activity of the zona glomerulosa versus the zona fasciculata and zona reticularis are underscored in primary and secondary adrenocortical insufficiency. In **primary adrenocortical insufficiency** (Addison's disease, chronic hypocorticism), all three zones of the adrenal cortex are atrophied as a result of their incomplete development or elimination by severe infection. Histologically, the adrenal cortex appears as an extremely shrunken zone surrounding a normal medulla. **Secondary adrenocortical insufficiency** is a disease caused by insufficient release of ACTH by the pituitary. The primary deficit originates in the pituitary rather than in the adrenal cortex. It can also result from intensive glucocorticoid therapy, which exerts a negative feedback upon ACTH release. As a result, the synthesis and release of glucocorticoids from the zona fasciculata is diminished without directly affecting the secretion of mineralocorticoids from the glomerulosa, which is not regulated by hypophyseal ACTH. This dual control of the zona glomerulosa versus the zona fasciculata and zona reticularis is further illustrated by observations that hypophysectomy causes atrophy of the zona fasciculata and reticularis but has no appreciable effect on the glomerulosa. This atrophy is reversed by administration of ACTH which will cause hyperplasia in the fasciculata but not in the glomerulosa. In the instance of Cushing's syndrome, which is characterized by hypersecretion of ACTH, hyperplasia of the fasciculata and reticularis occurs without appreciable changes in the glomerulosa cells. However, when diffuse adrenocortical hyperplasia is accompanied by hyperaldosteronism, cells similar to those in the glomerulosa are found.

Adrenal Medulla

HISTOLOGIC ASPECTS

The chromaffin cells of the adrenal medulla are irregularly shaped epithelioid cells. The cells are named after a histochemical reaction that utilized potassium bichromate to oxidize catecholamines to a yellow-brown reaction product. Two such cell types are identifiable by more sophisticated histochemical procedures; one producing **epinephrine** and another producing norepinephrine. Cells containing norepinephrine are autofluorescent and stain well with silver and iodine, whereas cells producing epinephrine are not autofluorescent and stain weakly with silver and iodine. It has been shown that membrane-bound granules visible with electron microscopy contain the catecholamines, which are discharged by exocytosis upon stimulation of the sympathetic nerves innervating these cells. These catecholamines are subsequently found in the venous effluent. In electron micrographs of glutaraldehyde-fixed tissue, the norepinephrine granules are more electron-dense due to better preservation, whereas epinephrine granules are less so due to loss by diffusion. In the human adrenals approximately 80 percent of the cells are of the epinephrine type. Glucocorticoids perfusing the medulla from the cortex are believed to cause induction of the enzyme that converts norepinephrine to epinephrine in chromaffin cells.

Chromaffin cells are analogous to postganglionic neurons because of their neural crest origin and their innervation by preganglionic sympathetic fibers.

FUNCTIONAL ASPECTS: PHYSIOLOGIC AND METABOLIC ACTIONS OF CATECHOLAMINES

The release of catecholamines from the adrenals can be elicited not only by stimulation of the splanchnic nerves but also by physical and emotional stress. Most of the physiologic effects are striking enough to be recognized by anyone who has experienced stimuli such as pain, fear, or severe cold leading to epinephrine discharge. Epinephrine causes an abrupt increase in heart rate, cardiac output, and blood pressure as well as stimulating respiration. It facilitates breathing by dilating the bronchi. It also redistributes blood flow by constricting blood vessels to the skin and dilating those to skeletal muscle. The generalized effect is to reinforce and prolong the effects of the sympathetic nervous system. Its metabolic effects include the increase of lipolysis in fat cells and increased glycogenolysis in the liver by the activation of phosphorylase. This general systemic response of the body has been called the "fight or flight" response because it prepares the body for action under threatening conditions of various types.

THE HYPOPHYSIS

The hypophysis (pituitary) is a remarkable endocrine organ because of the broad range of diverse physiologic functions that it subserves. Because it regulates the secretory activity of any other endocrine organs and tissues, it has been called the "master gland." However, this term is misleading because it is now known that the hypophysis itself is under the hormonal regulation of the hypothalamus. The hypothalamus forms that part of the floor of the third ventricle of the brain from which the hypophysis is suspended.

Development and General Organization

The hypophysis is composed of two histologically distinct regions of different developmental origins: (1) the **adenohypophysis,** that part derived from oral ectoderm (as a dorsal outpocket of Rathke's pouch), and (2) the **neurohypophysis,** derived from neural ectoderm (as a downgrowth of the diencephalon).

During embryonic development before the bones of the skull form, the presumptive adenohypophysis evaginates and detaches from the roof of the oral cavity and migrates to a position contiguous with and anterior to the neurohypophysis, which retains its neural connection to the developing brain. Subsequently, the adenohypophysis and neurohypophysis become joined as a single organ within a common collagenous capsule. Occasionally, cells of the adenohypophysis fail to migrate completely and remain at the site of Rathke's pouch to become what is known as a pharyngeal hypophysis.

Since the pituitary is composed of several regions, it is necessary to become familiar with its structural organization before discussing it further. These regions are depicted in Figure 17-10 and listed in the following scheme:

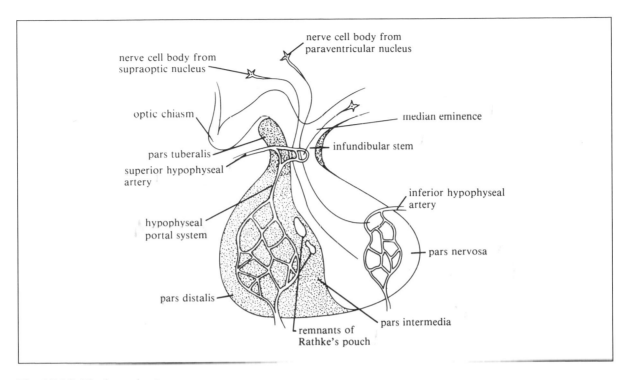

Fig. 17-10. The hypophysis.

Adenohypophysis	Pars tuberalis
	Pars distalis (anterior lobe)
	Pars intermedia
Neurohypophysis	Neural stalk (infundibulum)
	Median eminence
	Infundibular stem
	Pars nervosa

When development is complete in the human, the pars intermedia, which is developmentally part of the adenohypophysis, fuses with the pars nervosa to form a posterior lobe. Usually interposed between the posterior lobe and the anterior lobe are large cystlike remnants of Rathke's pouch with an epithelial lining and usually containing an amorphous colloid. The pars tuberalis is an extension of the anterior lobe, which forms a sleeve around the infundibular stem.

The entire pituitary rests in a small depression in the sphenoid bone, which is covered over by a dural diaphragm. A perforation in this diaphragm is traversed by the infundibulum, which is a continuation of the hypothalamus into the pars nervosa. It will become clear that this structural association of the hypophysis with the hypothalamus is a necessary one on which the function of the hypophysis depends.

The blood supply to the anterior lobe is from the **superior hypophyseal artery,** which forms a capillary network in the **pars tuberalis** and median eminence. A system of portal venules, the **hypophyseal portal system,** traverses the ventral aspect of the neural stalk connecting the capillary bed in the median eminence with a sinusoidal capillary plexus in the pars distalis. This portal system provides the vascular basis for hormonal regulation of the pars distalis by the hypothalamus (see Fig. 17-10). Short axons from nerves of hypothalamic origin terminate around the capillary plexus in the median eminence, where they release hormones called **releasing factors** and **inhibiting factors;** these hormones are carried by the hypophyseal portal system to the pars distalis where they regulate secretion of specific hormones from specific cells within the anterior lobe.

The blood supply to the pars nervosa is provided by the **inferior hypophyseal artery.** The venous drainage is carried to capsular veins, which empty into dural sinuses.

Pars Distalis

HISTOLOGIC ASPECTS

The parenchyma of the anterior lobe consists of cords or small irregular groups of cells supported by a sparse reticular network. Sinusoidal capillaries are distributed among these cellular cords (Fig. 17-11).

At least six hormones of major importance are produced by cells of the anterior lobe. The cells may be identified by immunohistochemical staining, using antibodies prepared against any one of the isolated and purified hypophyseal hormones. This technique has made it possible to identify cell types on the basis of ultrastructural criteria such as granule size, cell shape, and preferential distribution within the anterior lobe. In addition, an array of more traditional histochemical procedures can be used to identify cell types. However, only three cell types are recognized with conventional hematoxylin and eosin staining, based on the affinity of cytoplasmic granules for these dyes: **acidophils, basophils,** and **chromophobes.**

The large granules of acidophils stain brightly with eosin, giving the cytoplasm a distinct, granular appearance. The acidophil population includes two cells types: **somatotropes,** which produce growth hormone, and **mammotropes,** which produce prolactin.

Although basophils stain well with basic dyes, they stain in mediocre fashion with hematoxylin, which is not a true base. Because these cells secrete glycoprotein hormones, they stain well with the periodic acid–Schiff reaction for carbohydrates. The population of basophils includes several cell types: **thyrotropes,** which produce TSH, **corticotropes,** which produce adrenocorticotropin, and **gonadotropes,** the cell that produces

Fig. 17-11. Light micrograph of monkey pituitary showing three regions: the pars distalis (*PD*), the pars intermedia (*PI*), and the pars nervosa (*PN*).

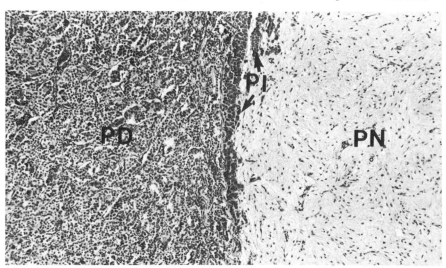

follicle-stimulating hormone and luteinizing hormone.

Chromophobes stain so poorly with hematoxylin and eosin that the cytoplasm appears virtually translucent, making them easily identifiable. Electron microscopy indicates the presence of a few granules, however, leading to the general conclusion that these cells are degranulated as a result of having released most of their hormonal contents. Chromophobes also display some of the ultrastructural features of various chromophils, indicating they may be a heterogeneous population of degranulated acidophils and basophils.

FUNCTIONAL ASPECTS

Release of any one of the anterior lobe hormones is induced by the influence of a corresponding releasing hormone produced in the hypothalamus, which gains access to the anterior lobe through the hypophyseal portal system. The anterior lobe hormones and their principal effects are enumerated in the following list:

1. **Growth hormone** (somatotropin, STH). A simple protein that stimulates body growth by increasing protein synthesis in most cell types. Its most prominent effect is to promote proliferation of cartilage cells in the epiphyses of growing bones. Variations in circulating levels of this hormone are reflected by striking changes in physical stature. During childhood, before the epiphyseal plates have closed, a deficiency of STH results in **dwarfism,** whereas excessive secretion produces **gigantism.** After the epiphyseal plates have closed, excessive STH produces **acromegaly,** a condition characterized by an enlargement of the bones in the hands, feet, and skull, especially the mandible. Excess secretion of STH is often associated with adenoma tumors of somatotropes.

   STH apparently acts through a molecular intermediary, **somatomedin,** which is probably formed in the liver. Somatomedin promotes growth by stimulating mitosis. It participates in a negative feedback loop by reducing STH release from the adenohypophysis and by stimulating release of somatostatin from the hypothalamus.

2. **Prolactin** (lactogenic hormone). A simple protein that initiates secretion by alveoli in the lactating mammary gland and stimulates development of the mammary gland. The cells that secrete prolactin, **mammotropes,** are more numerous in females than in males, and they are most numerous during pregnancy. Prolactin is secreted in greatest amounts in women who breast-feed their babies. During pregnancy and lactation, hyperactive prolactin-secreting cells hypertrophy and become hyperplastic.

3. **Adrenocorticotropin** (ACTH). A polypeptide that stimulates hypertrophy of the zona fasciculata and zona reticularis in the adrenals as well as the release of glucocorticoids produced there. The cells producing ACTH also produce **lipotropin** (LTH), a polypeptide that mobilizes fat in some species but has no confirmed function in the human. A potent opiate similar to morphine, **endorphin,** is also produced by these cells. Within the ACTH cells located in the intermedia, ACTH is broken down to melanocyte-stimulating hormone. Accordingly, all four of these hormones are produced by the same cell.

4. **Thyroid-stimulating hormone** (thyrotropin, TSH). A glycoprotein that stimulates the secretion of thyroid hormone.

Gonadotropins

5. **Follicle-stimulating hormone** (FSH). A glycoprotein initiating growth of primordial follicles in the female and spermatogenesis in the male.

6. **Luteinizing hormone** (LH), **interstitial cell-stimulating hormone** (ICSH). A glycoprotein that acts on the interstitial cells of the gonads. In the human female, it stimulates the theca interna to secrete estrogen, brings about ovulation (in conjunction with FSH), causes luteinization of the granulosa and theca interna following ovulation, and thereafter initiates

and maintains the secretion of progesterone from the corpus luteum. In the male, it stimulates the release of testosterone from the interstitial cells of the testis. Both gonadotropins (FSH and LH) are synthesized by the same cell called a **gonadotrope.**

FEEDBACK INHIBITION OF HORMONES RELEASED BY THE ANTERIOR LOBE

Increased circulating levels of hormones produced by a target organ such as the thyroid serve to inhibit secretion of the corresponding hypophyseal hormones (in this instance, TSH). Inhibition is exerted directly on the pituitary and also apparently by preventing the release of appropriate hypothalamic releasing hormones. It should be recognized that inhibitory factors are also released by the hypothalamus.

One of the histologic indications of hormonal interdependence displayed by cells of the anterior lobe is the hypertrophy that follows surgical removal of their corresponding target organs. This effect is most obvious with the basophils that produce glycoprotein hormones. Castration produces hypertrophic gonadotropes (castration cells, gonadectomy cells), which display significantly dilated Golgi apparatuses, appearing as large negative images with the light microscope. The same result occurs with thyrotropes following removal of the thyroid. This phenomenon is a consequence of the absence of adequate circulating hormones produced by target organs that exert feedback inhibition on the particular cells of the anterior lobe.

Pars Intermedia

In certain fish and amphibians and in the monkey, the pars intermedia is a distinct, well-developed region of the pituitary. Its cells produce **melanocyte-stimulating hormone** (MSH). In amphibians, MSH increases pigmentation of the skin surface by causing dispersion of melanosomes within melanophore cells.

In the human, the pars intermedia is rudimentary and appears as a diffuse region of slightly basophilic cells that also produce MSH (see Fig. 17-11). MSH increases melanin synthesis and increases the number of melanosomes in epidermal melanocytes, resulting in increased skin pigmentation. The cells of the intermedia are dispersed among other cells in the adjacent area of the anterior and posterior lobes. It has recently been established by immunocytochemistry that ACTH and MSH are produced and released by the same cell type in the human pituitary. Also present in these cells are **endorphins,** an endogenous painkiller, and **lipotropin,** a hormone regulating fat metabolism. All these hormones are produced as posttranslational products from a common precursor molecule. The release of MSH and ACTH from the same cell may explain the increased skin pigmentation associated with Addison's disease. An equally likely cause may be due to the identical sequence of amino acids found in portions of both ACTH and MSH, which provides each with some of the other's biologic activity. As a result, high levels of ACTH in Addison's disease may be able to exert a limited amount of MSH-like activity on skin pigmentation.

Small, unmyelinated axons to the cells of the pars intermedia may be involved in release of MSH of amphibians and may also play a role in secretion of the cells in the human rudimentary intermedia.

Neurohypophysis

The pars nervosa is primarily a dense bundle of unmyelinated axon terminals (see Fig. 17-11). These axons originate from cell bodies located in the hypothalamus. This tract of nerves is called the **hypothalamic-hypophyseal tract,** named by convention after the location of its cell bodies and the destination of its axons (see Fig. 17-10).

Two hormones are released in the pars nervosa: **antidiuretic hormone (ADH, vasopressin)** and **oxytocin.** These hormones are octapeptides that are synthesized by cell bodies of the hypothalamic-hypophyseal tract, conveyed down its axons by axoplasmic transport, and released in the pars nervosa. The axons of this tract originate from two separate locations within the hypothalamus and converge as they travel together down the infundibular stem into the pars nervosa. ADH is synthesized primarily, but not exclusively, by nerve cell bodies forming the **supraoptic nucleus;** and oxytocin is synthesized predominantly by nerve cell bodies forming the **paraventricular nucleus.** However, these nuclei are not homogeneous, and each contains some cell bodies producing the other hormone. The two hormones are produced by separate cell bodies and therefore are released from separate axon terminals. Both ADH and oxytocin are covalently bound to different carrier peptides called **neurophysins.**

Within the nervosa, individual axons are separated from one another by **pituicytes,** similar to glial cells of the central nervous system. It is unclear what functions are performed by pituicytes. The histologic picture of the pars nervosa is one similar to that of any unmyelinated nerve, staining relatively poorly with hematoxylin and eosin. The only well-stained structures are the nuclei of pituicytes, since their cytoplasmic processes are also difficult to visualize with the light microscope. With the electron microscope, the nerve terminals are seen to contain membrane-bound granules that contain ADH in one population of axons and oxytocin in another population of axons. Groups of these neurosecretory granules can be demonstrated at the light microscopic level with the chrome alum hematoxylin as blue-black **Herring bodies** in axonal varicosities where they are concentrated. The axon terminals are closely apposed to the capillary plexus fed by the inferior hypophyseal artery. These neurosecretory granules containing ADH and oxytocin are apparently released into the perivascular space by exocytosis in response to the arrival of an action potential (excitation-exocytosis coupling). The only structures interposed between the fenestrated endothelium and the axon terminal are their basal lamina and reticular fibers.

FUNCTIONAL ASPECTS

ADH causes the kidney to produce concentrated urine, thereby conserving water. It accomplishes this by increasing water permeability of the distal convoluted tubules and collecting ducts, segments of the uriniferous tubules that are normally impermeable to water. The resulting effect is the passive movement of water down its concentration gradient into the hypertonic medullary interstitium, to be subsequently reabsorbed by blood vessels. This process diminishes the water content of the urine. Large volumes of water are lost in the urine during the absence of ADH, an uncommon condition known as **diabetes insipidus.** An increase in the osmolality of body fluids, which occurs after water deprivation, is the stimulus for synthesis and release of ADH; a decrease in body fluid osmolality has the reverse effect.

Oxytocin stimulates the contraction of uterine smooth muscle during the final stages of pregnancy. It also causes the contraction of myoepithelial cells surrounding the alveoli in the mammary gland. This mechanical thrust forces milk into the ducts and lactiferous sinuses during suckling. The release of oxytocin from the pars nervosa is initiated by the **suckling reflex.** Stimulation of the nipple as a result of suckling produces afferent or sensory stimuli conducted by nerves to the brain, where they generate a nerve impulse along axons from cell bodies within the paraventricular nucleus. These impulses are propagated along the hypothalamo-hypophyseal tract and cause release of oxytocin from axon terminals within the pars nervosa.

THE PINEAL

During evolution, the epithalamus has been a parietal eye and a sensor of ambient temperature. However, in mammals the epithalamus has become the pineal gland, whose secretory activity is determined by photoperiod information relayed to it by nerve tracts from the eye. The pineal produces a number of substances including the indole derivative **melatonin,** to which some of the physiologic functions of the pineal are attributed. In amphibians, melatonin blanches the skin by causing melanosomes to aggregate; it has no similar effect in mammals. The human pineal is believed to influence the rhythmic secretory activity of certain endocrine organs in a manner that is dependent on the relative length of light and dark periods during a 24-hour day (**circadian rhythms**) or during annual or seasonal fluctuations in light and darkness. For instance, more ACTH is released during morning hours than evening hours. Many of these effects may be exerted indirectly by the action of melatonin on the hypothalamus, which exhibits the highest affinity for melatonin within the central nervous system. This may be the case for birds and mammals, in whom melatonin's distinct inhibitory effect on the gonads is apparently achieved by interference with the release of hypophyseal gonadotropins. Melatonin is rapidly taken up by the nervous system and is known to relieve symptoms of epilepsy and parkinsonism. These anticonvulsant effects of melatonin may result from its influence on the sodium and potassium balance in the brain.

Histologic Organization

The pineal is a dorsal outgrowth of the diencephalon attached by a short stalk to the posterior roof of the third ventricle. Its surface is covered with pia mater from which connective tissue trabeculae extend into the parenchyma, forming irregular lobules. Nerves and blood vessels enter the organ through these trabeculae.

The **pinealocyte** is derived from neuroepithelium of the diencephalic roof. It is the primary parenchymal cell and is arranged into irregular cords and follicles. These cells have large nuclei that are irregularly folded into various configurations. The cytoplasmic processes are slightly basophilic but are difficult to observe with conventional staining procedures for the light microscope. These cytoplasmic processes extend to the connective tissue trabeculae, where they terminate as bulbous expansions near blood vessels.

Areas containing intercellular calcified organic matrix concentrically organized into oval elements are common. These opaque concentrations are often referred to as **brain sand** or **corpora arenacea** (Fig. 17-12). Their functional significance is not known. However, the pineal is of clinical significance because its calcified concretions are easily located in x-rays of the skull. Since the pineal is a midline structure, any nearby space-occupying lesion such as a tumor would apply sufficient pressure to shift the appearance of the calcifications away from the mid-

Fig. 17-12. Light micrograph of the human pineal containing large opaque concretions.

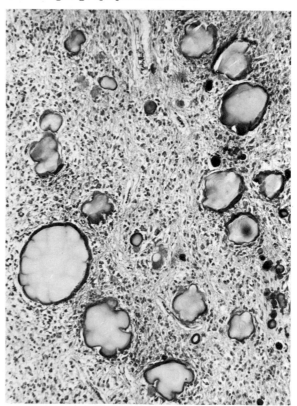

line in x-rays. This is helpful to the radiologist in determining the presence and location of the lesion.

The pineal is well innervated by sympathetic adrenergic fibers from the superior cervical ganglion. Surgical interruption of pineal innervation causes striking changes in its physiologic activity.

A small population of a second cell type, the **interstitial cell,** represents only about 5 percent of the total cell number. These cells are distinguished from pinealocytes by their more elongate nuclei and condensed chromatin.

Functional Aspects

Although other indolamines are known to be produced and released by the pineal, melatonin is the most clearly understood at the present time. Fluctuations in its concentration in the bloodstream appear to regulate various endocrine mediated biologic processes with respect to diurnal and seasonal cycles, most notably perhaps in the reproductive functions of birds and rodents: it synchronizes parturition with that part of the year when the newborn are most likely to survive. Many other important pineal functions remain to be elucidated, especially in the human.

The pineal exhibits an inherent secretory rhythmicity resulting in elevated blood plasma concentrations of melatonin during darkness and minimal concentrations during daylight hours. This alternating secretory activity occurs even in continuous darkness, but the amount and duration of release are dependent on diurnal changes in ambient illumination. Constant light depresses pineal activity by reducing the concentration of enzymes that form melatonin. **Photic stimuli** are carried to the pineal by the sympathetic nervous system, specifically by nerves arriving from the superior cervical ganglion. Consequently, bisection of these sympathetic nerves innervating the pineal would prevent it from responding to diurnal changes in environmental illumination. Normally, nervous influence is exerted on the pineal by diurnal changes in the ac-

tivity of these nerves concurrent with alternating day and night cycles. This influence is recorded within the pineal by coordinated fluctuations in *N*-acetyltransferase activity, the rate-limiting enzyme required for melatonin synthesis. During darkness, norepinephrine is released from nerve endings, which stimulates the production and secretion of **indoles.**

DIFFUSE NEUROENDOCRINE SYSTEM

A **diffuse neuroendocrine system** (DNES) composed of endocrine cells and neuronal cell bodies produces many physiologically active peptides and amines. These cells are part of the **amine precursor uptake and decarboxylation** (APUD) system that decarboxylates amine precursors into dopamine or serotonin. This system consists of a central division that includes the neuroendocrine cells of the hypothalamic-hypophyseal axis (adrenocorticotrophs and melanotrophs) and the pineal gland (pinealocytes); and a peripheral division that includes the chief cells of the parathyroid gland, the parafollicular cells of the thyroid chromaffin cells of the adrenal medulla, ganglion cells of the sympathetic nervous system, type I cells of the carotid body, the melanocyte, and the large population of **gastroenteropancreatic** (GEP) endocrine cells. The 18 widely scattered cells of the GEP system originate from endoderm of the primitive gut wall and produce gastrin, serotonin, secretin cholecystokinin, insulin, enteroglucagon, and many other hormones. Many of these cells are the argentaffin, argyrophilic, and enterochromaffin cells of the gastrointestinal tract (see Chap. 14). Wherever their location, cells of the APUD system are not easily identified by conventional staining techniques unless dense granules can be visualized in their basal cytoplasm. However, they are revealed effectively by fluorescence microscopy after formaldehyde fixation.

Within the category of APUD cells, some are not innervated while others are innervated by visceral efferent axons or visceral afferent dendrites.

NATIONAL BOARD TYPE QUESTIONS

For the following, select
- A. if only *1, 2, and 3* are correct.
- B. if only *1 and 3* are correct.
- C. if only *2 and 4* are correct.
- D. if only *4* is correct.
- E. if *all* are correct.

1. The hypophyseal portal system
   1. consists of long straight venules.
   2. is located in the pars tuberalis.
   3. carries releasing factors to the anterior lobe of the pituitary.
   4. connects a capillary bed in the median eminence to a capillary plexus in the anterior lobe.

2. Which of the following statements about cells in the hypophysis is (are) true?
   1. Follicle-stimulating hormone and luteinizing hormone are both released from gonadotropes.
   2. Chromophobes stain intensely with basic dyes.
   3. ACTH is produced by cells located within the pars intermedia.
   4. The acidophils of the anterior lobe represent a single cell type.

3. The hypothalamic-hypophyseal tract
   1. has its nerve cell bodies in the pars nervosa.
   2. consists of myelinated axons.
   3. releases oxytocin and antidiuretic hormone from the same axon terminals.
   4. releases oxytocin in response to suckling.

4. Which of the following statements about the pineal is (are) true?
   1. It contains intercellular, calcified concretions.
   2. It secretes less melatonin during periods of darkness.
   3. It is innervated by nerves arriving from the superior cervical ganglion.
   4. It secretes more melatonin during periods of constant illumination.

5. Which of the following areas of the pituitary is (are) derived from oral ectoderm?
   1. Pars tuberalis
   2. Pars intermedia
   3. Pars distalis
   4. Pars nervosa

6. The human parafollicular cell
   1. contains cytoplasmic membrane-bound granules.
   2. is located within the basal lamina surrounding thyroid follicles.
   3. releases calcitonin in response to hypercalcemia.
   4. releases calcitonin in response to a hypophyseal hormone in the adult.

7. Which of the following statements about the thyroid is (are) true?
   1. Thyroid-stimulating hormone (TSH) stimulates retrieval of colloid from the follicle lumen.
   2. Prolonged TSH stimulation causes both hypertrophy and hyperplasia of follicle cells.
   3. Lysosomes must fuse with phagosomes before T_3 and T_4 are enzymatically liberated from thyroglobulin.
   4. TSH stimulation causes release of calcitonin from parafollicular cells.

8. The cells of the zona glomerulosa
   1. are innervated by sympathetic axons.
   2. release aldosterone in response to angiotensin II.
   3. undergo hyperplasia in response to ACTH.
   4. atrophy in Addison's disease.

9. Which of the following zones of the adrenal atrophy as a result of long-term cortisone treatment?
   1. Zona glomerulosa
   2. Zona fasciculata
   3. Medulla
   4. Zona reticularis

10. Chromaffin cells of the adrenal medulla
    1. are innervated by sympathetic axons.
    2. have no membrane-bound granules in the cytoplasm.
    3. are derivatives of neural crest tissue.
    4. atrophy during Addison's disease.

11. Which of the following statements about the zona fasciculata is (are) true?

    1. It secretes mineralocorticoids in response to ACTH

    2. It secretes glucocorticoids in response to ACTH

    3. It atrophies during Cushing's syndrome

    4. It shows hyperplasia and hypertrophy during hypersecretion of ACTH

12. The diffuse neuroendocrine system

    1. is part of the amine precursor uptake and decarboxylation system.

    2. includes the argentaffin cells of the gastrointestinal tract.

    3. includes cells with cytoplasmic granules that are visible by fluorescence microscopy after formaldehyde fixation.

    4. includes sympathetic ganglionic neurons.

ANNOTATED ANSWERS

1. E.

2. B. Mammotropes and somatotropes are both acidophils. Chromophobes have no stainable cytoplasmic granules.

3. D. The hypothalamic-hypophyseal tract consists of unmyelinated axons whose cell bodies are located in the hypothalamus.

4. B. Blood plasma concentrations of melatonin are elevated during darkness and minimal during daylight hours.

5. A. The nervosa is derived from neural ectoderm and evaginates from the diencephalon.

6. A. In the adult calcitonin is not controlled by the hypophysis.

7. A. See Question No. 6.

8. C. Cells of the glomerulosa are not innervated.

9. C. Since the zona fasciculata and zona reticularis undergo hypertrophy in response to ACTH, the negative feedback of cortisone on ACTH release would allow these two zones to atrophy.

10. B. Chromaffin cells have abundant cytoplasmic granules containing epinephrine and norepinephrine. Addison's disease is a developmental defect in the cortex which does not involve the medulla.

11. C. Mineralocorticoids are released from the zona glomerulosa. The zona fasciculata hypertrophies during hypersecretion of ACTH (Cushing's syndrome).

12. E.

BIBLIOGRAPHY

Anderson, E. The anatomy of bovine and ovine pineals: Light and electron microscope studies. *J. Ultrastruct. Res.* Suppl. 8, May 1965.

Burgers, A. C. J. Melanophore-stimulating hormones in vertebrates. *Ann. N.Y. Acad. Sci.* 100:669, 1963.

Busch, W. Die arterielle Gefässversorgung der Nebenniere, zugleich ein Beitrag zur Anatomie der Nebenniere. *Z. Microsk. Anat. Forsch.* 6:159, 1955.

Dobbie. J. W., and T. Symington. The human adrenal gland with special reference to the vasculature. *J. Endocrinol.* 34:479, 1966.

Dupouy, J. P. Differentiation of MSH-, ACTH-, endorphin-, and LPH-containing cells in the hypophysis during embryonic and fetal development. *Int. Rev. Cytol.* 68:197, 1980.

Farquhar, M. G. Processing of Secretory Products by Cells of the Anterior Pituitary Gland. In H. Heller and K. Lederis (eds.), *Endocrine Tissues*. London: Cambridge University, 1971.

Gagnon, R. The arterial supply of the human adrenal gland. *Rev. Can. Biol.* 16:421, 1957.

Ham, A. W., et al. Physiological hypertrophy of the parathyroids, its cause and its relation to rickets. *Am. J. Pathol.* 16:277, 1940.

Henderson, E. F. The longitudinal smooth muscle of the central vein of the suprarenal gland. *Anat. Rec.* 36:69, 1927.

Herlant, M. The cells of the adenohypophysis and their functional significance. *Int. Rev. Cytol.* 17:299, 1974.

Hewer, E. E., and M. F. L. Keene. Observations on the development of the human suprarenal gland. *J. Anat.* 61:302, 1927.

Hirsch, P. F., and P. L. Munson. Thyrocalcitonin. *Physiol. Rev.* 49:548, 1968.

Idelman, S. Ultrastructure of the mammalian adrenal cortex. *Int. Rev. Cytol.* 27:181, 1970.

Kutschera-Aichbergen, H. Nebennierenstudien. *Frankf. Z. Pathol.* 28:262, 1922.

von Lawzewitsch, I., et al. Cytological and ultrastructural characterization of the human pituitary. *Acta Anat.* 81:286, 1972.

Li, J. Y., M. P. Dubois, and P. M. Dubois. Ultrastructural localization of immuno-reactive corticotropin, β-lipotropin, α- and β-endorphin in cells of the human fetal anterior pituitary. *Cell Tissue Res.* 204:37, 1979.

Long, J. A., and A. L. Jones. Observations on the fine structure of the adrenal cortex of man. *Lab. Invest.* 17:355, 1967.

McMillan, P. J., W. M. Hooker, and L. J. Deftos. Distribution of calcitonin-containing cells in the human thyroid. *Am. J. Anat.* 140:73, 1974.

Merklin, R. J. The arterial supply of the suprarenal gland. *Anat. Rec.* 44:359, 1962.

Møller, M. The ultrastructure of the human fetal pineal gland. *Cell Tissue Res.* 151:13, 1974.

Møller, M. Presence of a pineal nerve (nervus pinealis) in the human fetus; a light and electron microscopical study of the innervation of the pineal gland. *Brain Res.* 154:1, 1978.

Munger, B. L., and S. I. Roth. The cytology of the normal parathyroid glands of man and Virginia deer: A light and electron microscopic study with morphological evidence of secretory activity. *J. Cell Biol.* 16:379, 1963.

Nadler, N. J., et al. Elaboration of thyroglobulin in the thyroid follicle. *Endocrinology* 74:333, 1964.

Nonidez, J. F. The origin of the "parafollicular" cells, a second epithelial component of the thyroid gland of the dog. *Am. J. Anat.* 49:479, 1932.

Nussdorfer, G. G. Cytophysiology of the adrenal cortex. *Int. Rev. Cytol.* vol. 98, 1986.

Pearse, A. G. E., and A. F. Carvalheira. Cytochemical evidence for an ultimobranchial origin of rodent thyroid C cells. *Nature* 214:929, 1967.

Rasmussen, H., and M. A. Pechet. Calcitonin. *Sci. Am.* 223:42, 1970.

Reiter, R. J. The mammalian pineal gland: Structure and function. *Am. J. Anat.* 162:287, 1981.

Salazar, H., and R. R. Peterson. Morphologic observations concerning the release and transport of secretory products in the adenohypophysis. *Am. J. Anat.* 115:199, 1964.

Symington, T. *Functional Pathology of the Human Adrenal Gland.* Baltimore: Williams & Wilkins, 1969.

Wurtman, R. J., and J. Axelrod. The pineal gland. *Sci. Am.* 213:50, 1965.

Zeckwer, I. T. Possible functional significance of the longitudinal muscle in the adrenal veins in man. *Arch. Pathol.* 20:9, 1935.

18 Male Reproductive System

Objectives

You will learn the following in this chapter:

The histologic organization of the testis and its basic units, the seminiferous tubules

The stages of spermatogenesis that result in haploid spermatozoa: spermatocytogenesis, meiosis, and spermiogenesis

The ultrastructural components of the spermatozoon and their roles in fertilization

The Leydig cells, occupants of the interstitial tissue between seminiferous tubules, and their role in the hormonal regulation of spermatogenesis

The blood-testis barrier

The structure and function of the excurrent ducts of the testis and the accessory glands

The structure and function of the penis

The adult male reproductive system (Fig. 18-1) is composed of **primary sex organs** and **secondary** or **accessory sex organs.** The primary organs are the paired, scrotal **testes,** and the accessory organs consist of a series of **excurrent ducts** punctuated along their length with numerous **glandular modifications** and ultimately terminating in the organ of copulation, the **penis.**

The testes are composed of many small, convoluted tubes called **seminiferous tubules** and abundant intertubular or **interstitial tissue.** Functionally, these glandular organs contain various cells that (1) produce the motile male gametes called **spermatozoa,** (2) isolate, protect, nurture, and support the developing germ cells, (3) produce particular steroid hormones called **androgens** that are responsible for male characteristics, and (4) are phagocytic in nature.

The excurrent duct system includes the bilateral **tubuli recti, rete, ductuli efferentes, ductus epididymidis, ductus deferens, ampulla,** and **ejaculatory duct** and the singular **urethra.** Functionally, these complex tubular structures (1) store spermatozoa, (2) provide an environment for the "maturation" of the spermatozoa, and (3) play both passive and active roles in the transmission of the male gametes to the outside of the body.

The glandular modifications include the **ampullary diverticula,** the **seminal vesicles,** the **prostate,** the **bulbourethral glands** (of Cowper), the **urethral glands** (of Littre), and the **preputial glands** (of Tyson). Functionally, the accessory glands are primarily concerned with (1) producing the majority of the fluid matrix of the final secretory product of the male reproductive system, a suspension of spermatozoa called the **semen,** (2) providing factors that are required for sperm metabolism and energetics, (3) lubricating certain of the excurrent ducts, and (4) se-

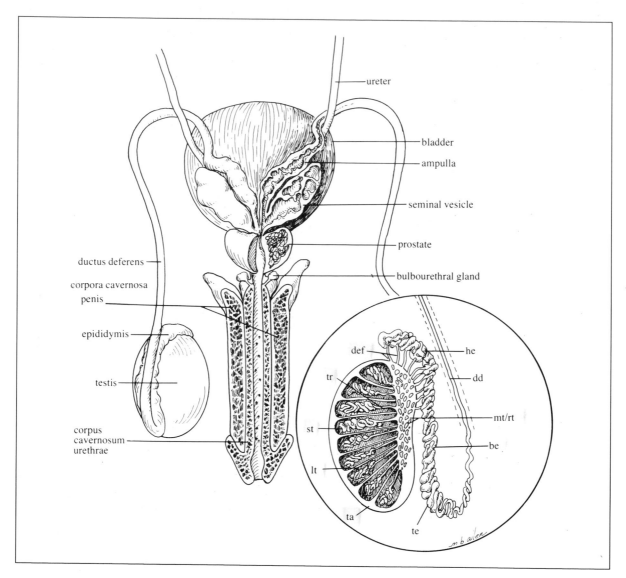

Fig. 18-1. Human male reproduction system; dorsal view. Insets shows cut view of right testis and associated structures. *ta* = tunica albuginea; *It* = septum separating testis into lobules; *st* = seminiferous tubule; *tr* = tubulus rectus; *mt/rt* = mediastinum containing rete testis; *def* = ductuli efferentes; *he* = head of epididymidis; *be* = body of epididymidis; *te* = tail of epididymidis; *dd* = ductus deferens.

creting substances that may increase the effectiveness of the spermatozoa within the female reproductive tract.

The penis is a body of erectile tissue; its function is to ensure that the spermatozoa are delivered directly into the female reproductive tract during semen expulsion, a process called **ejaculation.**

DEVELOPMENT

Developmentally, the male reproductive system has complex origins: it arises from splanchnic mesoderm, mesodermal mesenchyme, endoderm, and ectoderm. The diversity of embryonic origins undoubtedly contributes to the wide variety of epithelial cell types and structures encountered in this system.

If the tubes and tubules of the entire male reproductive tract could be straightened out, an essentially Y-shaped arrangement would be evident. Each upper wing of the Y would consist of the mesodermal derivatives (seminiferous tubules and surrounding intertubular tissue, tubuli recti, rete, ductuli efferentes, ductus epididymidis, ductus deferens, ampulla, seminal vesicle, ejaculatory duct); the base of the Y would consist of the endodermal derivatives (prostate, prostatic urethra, membranous urethra, bulbourethral glands, cavernous urethra) and the ectodermal components (glandular urethra, prepuce, preputial glands, the skin covering the penis). In addition, the mesodermal component of the seminiferous tubules becomes invaded during development with elements that are destined to give rise to the germ cells at sexual maturity. Although these **primordial germ cells** (or **gonocytes** as they are called when they take up residence in the primitive testis) arise in the yolk sac, their origin can be considered as distinct from the three primary germ layers.

STRUCTURE AND FUNCTION OF THE TESTIS

The testis is a "bipartite" glandular organ, with both exocrine and endocrine compartments. Its exocrine function is to produce male germ cells; its endocrine function is mainly to produce male hormones, the major one of which is **testosterone.** Like any other "epithelial" organ, the testis consists of parenchyma (the germinal or seminiferous epithelium) and stroma (the supporting connective tissue). However, in this organ both of these entities can be considered to be special—that is, the parenchyma is composed of seminiferous tubules derived from primordial germ cells (nongerm layer origin?) and supportive or **Sertoli cells** (splanchnic mesodermal origin); the stroma is not only connective and supportive but also secretory, in that it contains the epithelioid endocrine cells called the **interstitial cells of Leydig** (mesenchymal origin). Indeed, the Leydig cells are parenchymal in a functional sense.

Stroma

Each testis is surrounded by a dense, fibrous connective tissue capsule, the **tunica albuginea** (see Fig. 18-1). This layer consists of fibroblasts, collagen fibers, and some smooth muscle cells; the smooth muscle cells are more numerous on the side of the testis next to the epididymis. On the posterior border of the testis, the tunica albuginea thickens and projects inward as the **mediastinum testis** (see Fig. 18-1). This region where the testicular blood vessels enter supports a series of labyrinthine passages called the **rete testis.** Like the tunica albuginea, the mediastinum also consists of fibroblasts, collagenous connective tissue, and some smooth muscle cells. From the mediastinum, thin connective tissue septa radiate into the testis, dividing it into incomplete lobules or compartments. These **lobules** contain one or more seminiferous tubules that empty into the rete (see Fig. 18-1). The innermost portion of the testicular capsule is composed of a thin, delicate layer of loose connective tissue and blood vessels. This layer, called the **tunica vasculosa,** is continuous with the interstitial connective tissue of the intertubular regions.

Seminiferous Tubules

The seminiferous tubules are highly convoluted exocrine tubes lined with a special epithelium called the **germinal** or **seminiferous epithelium.** This epithelium consists of two distinct populations of cells: (1) a renewing, stratified population of **spermatogenic cells** derived from primordial germ cells, and (2) a nondividing,

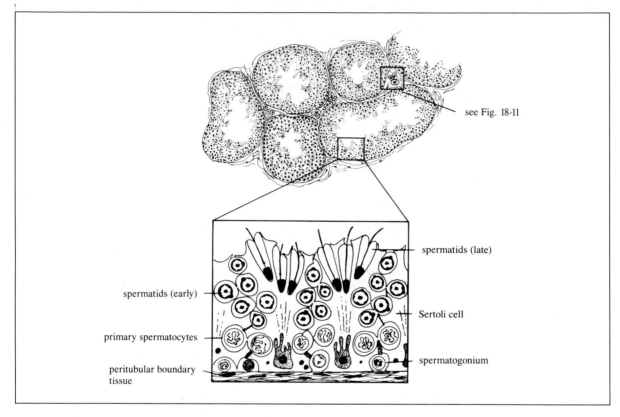

see Fig. 18-11

spermatids (late)

spermatids (early)

Sertoli cell

primary spermatocytes

spermatogonium

peritubular boundary
tissue

Fig. 18-2. A portion of the testis in histologic section. Above, a low-magnification view of the seminiferous tubules and interstitial tissue; below, a high-magnification view of the portion in the seminiferous tubule above, showing the various elements of the germinal epithelium.

unilaminar population of nongerminal, supportive **Sertoli cells** (Figs. 18-2, 18-3, 18-4). There are approximately 500 seminiferous tubules in each human testis.

SPERMATOGENIC CELLS

Like other renewing epithelia, the seminiferous epithelium contains stem cells, proliferating cells, differentiating cells, and exfoliating cells. The most immature elements are located at or near the basement membrane, whereas the more differentiated ones are near the surface (i.e., the luminal surface of the seminiferous tubules). The successive orders of spermatogenic cells arranged from the basement membrane to the lumen include **spermatogonia, spermatocytes,** and **spermatids.** The exfoliated cells become the male gametes or **spermatozoa** (see Figs. 18-2, 18-4).

Spermatogenesis

The process by which spermatogonia are transformed into spermatozoa is called **spermatogenesis.** The cytomorphosis of the spermatogenic cells can be divided into three major phases: spermatocytogenesis, meiosis, and spermiogenesis. The life cycle of the spermatogenic cells is summarized in Table 18-1.

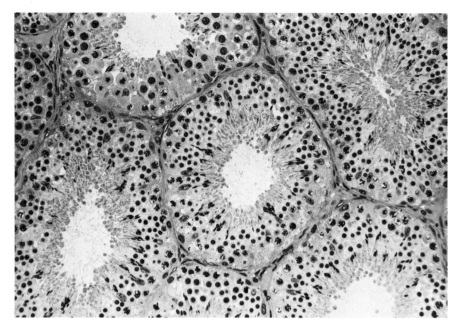

Fig. 18-3. Light micrograph of monkey testis showing several cross-sectional profiles of seminiferous
tubules. The epithelium is composed primarily of
spermatogenic cells in various stages of development.
Each tubule is surrounded by connective tissue (interstitial tissue).

Fig. 18-4. Light micrograph of monkey testis seminiferous epithelium. Sertoli cells (S) are closely associated with several spermatogenic cell stages: spermatogonia (1), primary spermatocytes (2), early
spermatids (3), and late spermatids (4). Discharged
cytoplasmic bodies are present in the lumen (arrows).

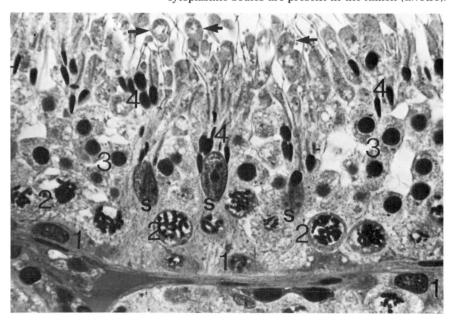

Table 18-1. Life Cycle of Spermatogenic Cells

| Cell Generation | Ploidy | | Comments |
	Chromosomes	DNA	
Primordial germ cells	2n	2n	Arise in yolk sac, migrate to developing testis, and take up residence in primitive seminiferous tubules (cords)
Gonocytes	2n	2n	Primordial germ cells in the testicular cords; they give rise to prospermatogonia that populate the prepubertal testis
Spermatogonia (type A; type B)	2n	2n	Spermatocytogenesis: these cells divide mitotically to renew themselves and ultimately yield primary spermatocytes
Primary spermatocytes	2n	4n ⎤	Meiosis: "reduction divisions" to yield haploid (n) spermatids
Secondary spermatocytes	n	2n ⎦	
Spermatids	n	n	Spermiogenesis: morphologic transformation of these cells to form spermatozoa
Spermatozoa	n	n	Adult male gametes

1. **Spermatocytogenesis** is the phase in which spermatogonial stem cells generate the spermatocytes as well as replace themselves. In humans, three types of spermatogonia are recognized: **type A dark, type A pale,** and **type B** spermatogonia, classified according to the staining properties of their nuclei (Fig. 18-5). Type A dark (Ad) cells have an ovoid nucleus that stains darkly; type A pale (Ap) cells have an ovoid nucleus that stains lightly. Type B spermatogonia have a more spherical nucleus with darkly staining heterochromatin arranged in patches, primarily along the nuclear envelope. The Ad cells probably serve as reserve stem cells, or at least do not divide frequently. Type Ap spermatogonia, however, divide mitotically to form type B as well as other type A cells to ensure that their numbers are not exhausted during a process that continues throughout most of the life of an individual. Type B cells divide mitotically to form preleptotene spermatocytes. In general, spermatogonia rest upon the basement membrane of the seminiferous tubules.

2. **Meiosis** is a special type of nuclear division that takes place *only* in the germ cell lines. It is a process that occurs in anticipation of fertilization. In order to maintain the normal diploid (2n) condition of chromosomes in many organisms, it is necessary that the male and female gametes—which are derived from diploid (2n) precursors—be "reduced" to a haploid (n) condition prior to their union during fertilization in order to form a diploid (2n) zygote. Meiosis is therefore a reduction division, in contrast to mitosis, in which the daughter cells are the same "ploidy" as the parent cell. Furthermore, instead of simply separating chromosome pairs into maternal and paternal members, the meiotic mechanism has evolved a means of achieving genetic variation by a process called "crossing-over," in which segments of complementary chromosomes are exchanged. This exchange ultimately ensures that offspring are significantly different from their parents. However, since the crossing-over step occurs after all of the DNA is duplicated and a tetraploid (4n) cell is formed, *two* nuclear divisions are

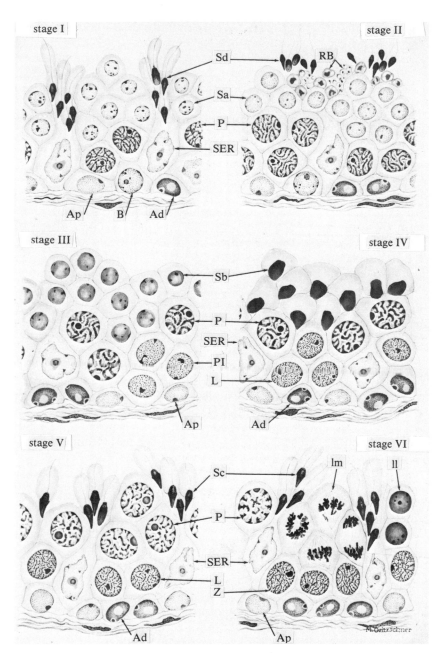

Fig. 18-5. Six typical types of cellular associations found repeatedly in human seminiferous tubules. *Ser* = nucleus of Sertoli cell; *Ap* and *Ad* = pale and dark type A spermatogonia; *B* = type B spermatogonia; *Pl* = preleptotene primary spermatocyte; *L* = leptotene primary spermatocyte; *Z* = zygotene primary spermatocyte; *P* = pachytene primary sper-matocyte; *Im* − primary spermatocyte in division; *II* = secondary spermatocyte in division; *Sa, Sb, Sc, Sd* = spermatids at various stages of spermiogenesis; *RB* = residual bodies. (From Y. Clermont, The cycle of the seminiferous epithelium in man. *Am. J. Anat.* 112:35, 1963.)

needed to reach the haploid (n) requirement for a gamete. Thus meiosis is a process consisting of two divisions of the genetic material: the first to separate analogous, genetically mixed chromosomes, and the second to separate the duplicated DNA (chromatids). An added bonus with two divisions is that twice as many haploid (n) cells result from a single diploid (2n) stem cell.

In spermatogenesis the first and second meiotic divisions occur in the **primary** and **secondary spermatocytes,** respectively. With respect to DNA content in the nucleus, the sequence of events is as follows: a diploid (2n) primary spermatocyte derived from the mitotic division of a diploid (2n) type B spermatogonium duplicates its DNA to become a tetraploid (4n) primary spermatocyte. A prolonged series of events or subphases collectively called **prophase** ensues, in which crossing-over occurs to "mix" the genetic information. Metaphase, anaphase, and telophase of the first meiotic division follow, whereby the tetraploid (4n) primary spermatocyte forms two diploid (2n) secondary spermatocytes. Further genetic variation is achieved by random orientation of the genetic material on the plate in metaphase I and therefore by random selection of the "analogues" during the first meiotic division. Since no DNA replication or crossing-over occurs in secondary spermatocytes, prophase II through telophase II proceed quickly, resulting in the second meiotic division and four haploid (n) spermatids. The meiotic process with its various phases and subphases of prophase I are summarized in Table 18-2.

In retrospect, meiosis has three important functional features: (1) A haploid (n) gamete is formed to ensure the formation of diploid (2n) offspring; (2) genetic variation of the offspring is achieved by the crossing-over process in prophase I and the random selection of genetic material during the first meiotic division; and (3) a greater number of spermatids per spermatogonium is possible with the two meiotic divisions.

Histologically, primary and secondary spermatocytes are distinguished from each other by their overall size and nuclear characteristics. Primary spermatocytes are large cells with distinct "threads" of chromatin in their nuclei; their nuclear appearance during prophase I has no parallel in secondary spermatocytes. Secondary spermatocytes are much smaller cells, with nuclear chromatin occurring in a granular form in prophase II.

3. **Spermiogenesis** is the phase that generates the sperm. It is not a cellular division but essentially a cytologic transformation of the spermatids from roughly spherical, nonmotile cells to the streamlined spermatozoa that will be capable of motility. This phase occurs in the upper layers of the seminiferous epithelium, where it is characterized by the following events: (1) formation of the **acrosome,** a caplike envelope of hydrolytic enzymes important for fertilization that covers the nucleus anteriorly and laterally; (2) condensation and elongation of the nucleus; (3) formation of the flagellum to provide the structure for motility; and (4) discharge of organelles and cytoplasm that are no longer required. The spermatozoa are then released into the lumina of the seminiferous tubules, from which they are carried to the ductus epididymidis for further maturation and storage. The various stages in the development of the spermatozoa occur in typical cellular associations, which appear in the human seminiferous tubules as six different patterns (see Fig. 18-5).

Clonal Nature of the Developing Germ Cells

From electron microscopic studies of the spermatogenic process, it is now known that male germ cells from type A spermatogonia to late-stage spermatids develop syncytially. Thus in all of the subsequent divisions from a single spermatogonium, cytokinesis is incomplete and the daughter cells are connected through delicate cytoplasmic "bridges" (see Fig. 18-2) approximately 2 μm in width. This condition is probably responsible for the close synchrony of spermatogenic development in various areas of the seminiferous tubules.

Table 18-2. Summary of Meiosis

Cell Generation		
Phase	*Subphase*	*Description*
Primary Spermatocyte		Undergoes reductional division: separation of homologous ("maternal" vs. "paternal") chromosomes; centromeres do not divide. Newly formed preleptotene primary spermatocytes resemble type B spermatogonia; DNA synthesis begins
Prophase I		Approximately 22 days in duration; nuclear and cytoplasmic size increases during this "growth" phase
	Leptotene	Early: DNA synthesis completed; this is now tetraploid (4n) cell, although chromosomes appear single
		Late: spiralization of chromosomes to form threadlike structures
	Zygotene	Homologous chromosomes pair (synapsis) and form synaptonemal complexes where crossing-over can occur; "maternal" and "paternal" analogues now genetically different from maternal and paternal chromosomes of previous germ cell generations or somatic cells
	Pachytene	Pairing is complete, which creates appearance that chromosome number is halved when actually it is not; this association of 2 paired chromosomes is called a bivalent. Chromosomes contract and become shorter and thicker; at the end of pachytene each chromosome of bivalent splits longitudinally into 2 chromatids (dyad) attached by a centromere; the bivalent therefore consists of 4 chromatids. Chromatids are structural evidence of DNA replication
	Diplotene	Synaptonemal complexes absent, indicating that crossing over is complete; maternal and paternal centromeres (kinetochores) of bivalent separate slightly (i.e., tetrad begins to separate into 2 dyads); incomplete separation due to areas of chromosome overlap (chiasmata) where crossing-over occurred; chromosomes continue to shorten and thicken; nucleus reaches maximum size
	Diakinesis	Bivalents appear thickest and shortest; chiasmata have moved to ends of chromosomes
Metaphase I		Nuclear membrane absent; tetrads of bivalents are randomly arranged at the equatorial plate
Anaphase I		Centromeres of each analogous pair of chromosomes (bivalent) move to opposite poles of cell, taking dyads (sister chromatids) along with them (i.e., tetrads are completely separated into dyads)
Telophase I		Results in formation of secondary spermatocytes: if chromosome number is considered, this is haploid (n) cell; however, this is really a diploid (2n) cell with respect to DNA content (dyad = 2 × n chromatids)
Secondary Spermatocyte		Undergoes equational division: separation of sister chromatids; centromeres divide
Prophase II		No DNA replication or crossing-over; nucleus contains granular chromatin Dyads arrange themselves at equatorial plate
Metaphase II		Dyads arrange themselves at equatorial plate

Table 18-2. (continued)

Cell Generation		
Phase	Subphase	Description
Anaphase II		Centromeres now divide and each chromatid (monad) moves to opposite poles of cell
Telophase II		Results in formation of spermatids; these are haploid (n) cells with respect to chromosome number *and* DNA content; however, DNA is different from either parental DNA

Fig. 18-6. Spermatozoa in the epididymis of the bat. Note the stereocilia projecting from the apical surface of the epithelium (*E*). *N* = nucleus of sperm within lumen of epididymis; *M* = mitochondrial sheath of middle piece. (Courtesy of A. Gustafson)

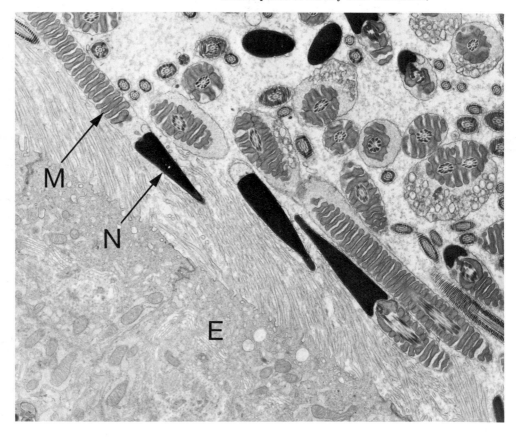

The Mature Spermatozoon

The mature spermatozoa (Figs. 18-6, 18-7) are the male gametes. Their production is the purpose of spermatogenesis, and thus they are the principal exocrine product of the testis. Approximately 95 million spermatozoa are produced by each testis daily. The human spermatozoon is approximately 60 μm in length and consists of head and tail portions (see Fig. 18-7). The **head** (4–5 μm) contains the nucleus with its haploid (n) genetic material and the **acrosome** (Figs. 18-8, 18-9). The **tail** is subdivided from anterior to posterior into four segments: (1) the **neck,** an area of connection between head and tail; the neck contains a pair of centrioles, the distal one degenerating in the mature sperm; (2) the **middle piece** (5–7 μm), a region whose outer circumference contains a sheath of mitochondria that provide the energetics for motility; (3) the **principal piece** (45 μm), a region whose outer circumference contains a fibrous sheath that aids in support of the tail region; and (4) the **end piece** (5 μm), the terminal segment of the tail. Located in the core of the tail portion from the base of the neck through most of the end piece is the microtubular axoneme of the flagellum. It consists of nine doublet microtubules surrounding a central pair of microtubules. The central pair of microtubules extends anteriorly to the transversely oriented proximal centriole within the neck piece. The axoneme is the source of propulsion for the sperm. Closely associated with the outer aspect of the nine microtubules of the axoneme are nine **outer dense fibers.** These outer dense fibers confer rigidity to the tail, helping it to straighten between beats of the axoneme.

CAPACITATION OF SPERM

After mammalian sperm have been deposited within the female reproductive path a series of events must occur in the sperm before they are capable of binding to and penetrating the egg. These series of reactions are collectively referred to as **capacitation.** While not fully understood, capacitation involves the release of an epididymal

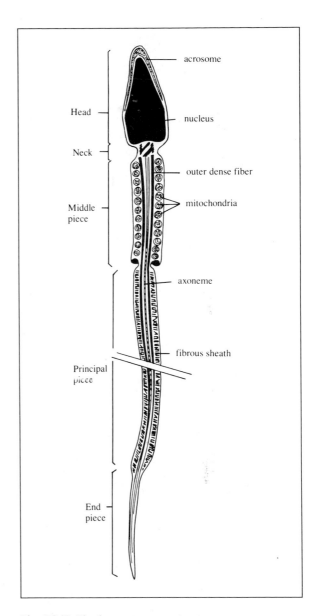

Fig. 18-7. The human spermatozoa.

glycoconjugate from the surface of the sperm which exposes binding sites for the zona pellucida, an extracellular coating of the egg consisting of mucopolysaccharides. After release of the glycoconjugates the sperm also become motile. After binding to the zona pellucida, the acro-

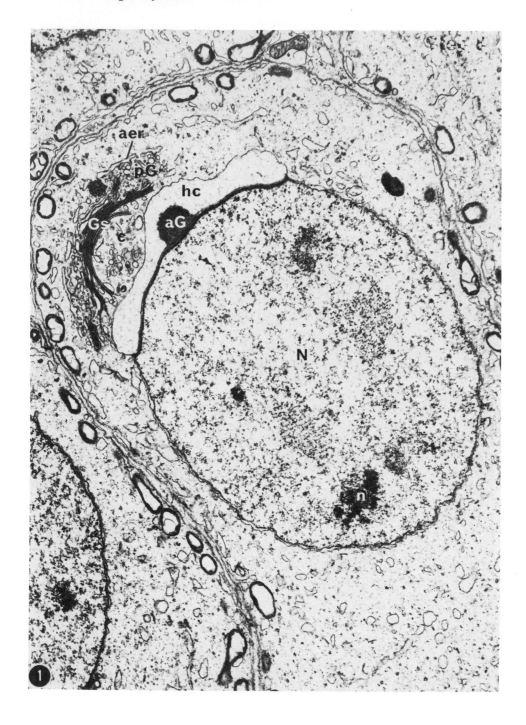

Fig. 18-8. A spermatid during development of the acrosome. Shown is the nucleus (*N*) with the acrosomal granule (*aG*) and head cap (*hc*) at one pole of the nucleus. The enzymatic contents of the acrosome are released to disperse the outer cellular corona and assist the penetration of the sperm through the zona pellucida. The Golgi apparatus (*Gs*) from which the acrosome is formed is located nearby. (aer = endoplasmic reticulum; n = nucleolus; pG = peripheral region of Golgi.) (From F. R. Susi, C. P. Leblond and Y. Clermont, Changes in the Golgi apparatus during spermiogenesis in the rat. *Am. J. Anat.* 130:251, 1971.)

◁———————————————————

Fig. 18-9. Cross-section through the seminiferous tubule showing the elongate nucleus of a Sertoli cell (*S*) and its prominent nucleolus. Note the flattened dense nuclei of spermatids associated with the apical end of the Sertoli cell cytoplasm (*T*). The nearby younger spermatids have a small dense granule adjacent to the nucleus representing the developing acrosome (unlabeled arrows).

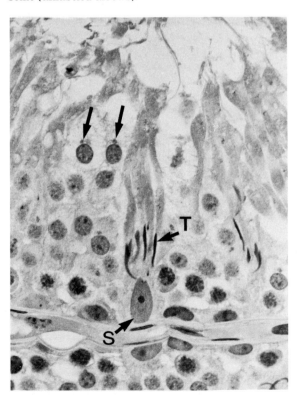

some releases a variety of enzymes including hyaluronidase which disperse the cells of the corona radiata from the outer surface of the zona pellucida and assist the sperm to penetrate the zona pellucida.

SERTOLI CELLS

The Sertoli cells (see Figs. 18-2, 18-4) are roughly columnar elements that extend from the basement membrane to the luminal surface of the seminiferous tubules (see Fig. 18-9). They are interposed between the developing germinal elements; indeed, the developing germ cells are embedded in cytoplasmic invaginations of the Sertoli cells. The large euchromatic nucleus of these cells, which is characterized by an elaborately infolded nuclear envelope and a complex nucleolus, is located in the basal cytoplasm. Other typical basal occupants are a well-developed smooth endoplasmic reticulum and Golgi apparatus, a modest rough endoplasmic reticulum, lipid droplets, glycogen granules, and actinlike filaments. In humans, peculiar inclusions (crystalloids) are also found. The apical cytoplasm of Sertoli cells contains numerous filaments and microtubules; mitochondria are located throughout. Between adjacent Sertoli cells are gap junctions and elaborate multiple tight junctions. The latter are located in the basal portions of the seminiferous epithelium and tend to isolate the spermatogonia from more luminal gametogenic cells.

Functionally, the Sertoli cells are probably the most diverse of the testicular elements. Their functions include (1) support, protection, nutrition, regulation, and release of the germinal elements; (2) phagocytosis of degenerated germinal cells and spermiogenic residual bodies; and (3) secretion of various products.

The protective role of the Sertoli cells is of particular importance. Because spermatogenesis is a process that begins at sexual maturity long after the establishment of immunorecognition, and because all germ cells subsequent to meiosis I are genetically different from somatic cells, spermatogenic proteins are "foreign" and could therefore initiate an immune response if they appeared in the general circulation. To prevent such a reaction, the germ cells are isolated by what has come to be known as the **blood-testis barrier.** Unlike the blood-brain barrier, which involves tight junctions between capillary endothelial cells, the principal components of this barrier are the Sertoli-Sertoli tight junctions. It is significant that the spermatogonia are outside this barrier. Not only are spermatogonia genetically identical with somatic cells and present since birth, but also they are responsive to various circulating factors; for example, they are among the elements that bind follicle-stimulating hormone (FSH) produced by the adenohypophysis. When spermatogonia divide to give rise to primary spermatocytes, the Sertoli-Sertoli junctions apparently "unzip" and rejoin subjacent to the newly formed spermatocytes. This barrier therefore divides the seminiferous tubules into two compartments: a **basal compartment** located between the basement membrane and the tight junctions, which contains spermatogonia, and an **adluminal compartment** located between the junctions and the lumen, which contains the other germinal cells.

The Sertoli-Sertoli junctions are of further significance in that Sertoli cells have been found to secrete all or most of the testicular fluid important for sperm transport into the excurrent duct system as well as a specific protein called **androgen-binding protein** (ABP) through stimulation by FSH and testosterone. The function of this protein is apparently to concentrate testosterone, a requirement for spermatogenesis, in the seminiferous tubules. The tight junctions therefore prevent leakage of testicular fluid, ABP-testosterone, and other substances from the tubules into the surrounding interstitium. A continuous production of fluid that cannot escape the confines of the tubules is responsible at least in part for the flow of released gametes out of the testis toward the excurrent ducts. The flow of ABP bathes the lining epithelium of the ductuli efferentes and epididymis and helps maintain their normal function.

Interstitial Tissue

The interstitial tissue of the testis (see Fig. 18-2) is a delicate, vascular, intertubular connective tissue in which the seminiferous tubules are embedded. It consists of one or more laminae closely adherent to the seminiferous tubules and looser intermediate regions containing the Leydig cells, fibroblasts, macrophages, mast cells, lymphocytes, collagen fibers, blood vessels, lymphatics, nerves, and a number of undifferentiated mesenchymal cells. The blood vessels here are continuous with the tunica vasculosa in the testicular capsule.

PERITUBULAR BOUNDARY TISSUE

All epithelia have a basement membrane and rest directly on a bed of connective tissue that is generally called the **lamina propria.** The seminiferous epithelium is no exception. The lamina propria of the seminiferous tubules has been given several names, including **tunica propria, limiting membrane,** and **peritubular boundary tissue.** It consists of collagen fibers embedded in an amorphous ground substance and elongated cells. These cells resemble fibroblasts; however, their cytoplasm contains many fine longitudinal filaments. Recent studies suggest that these filaments are composed of actin. Because these cells are known to be contractile, they have been termed **myoid cells.** Functionally, the myoid cells may be responsible for the rhythmic movements of the seminiferous tubules and aid in the transport of released spermatozoa and testicular fluid toward the rete.

LEYDIG CELLS

The interstitial tissue is an endocrine compartment of the testis in that it contains the hormone-producing **interstitial cells of Leydig.** There are millions of Leydig cells in the interstitial space between seminiferous tubules (Fig. 18-10). These polyhedral epithelioid cells have a large euchromatic nucleus with one or two prominent nucleoli, and an eosinophilic cytoplasm

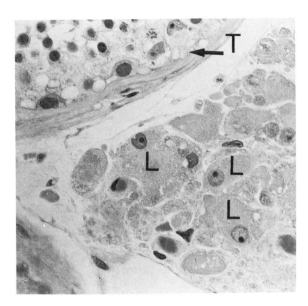

Fig. 18-10. Leydig cells (*L*) in the interstitial space between seminiferous tubules (*T*).

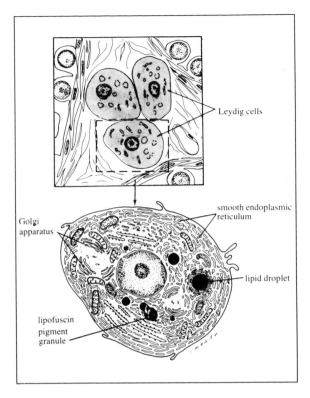

Fig. 18-11. The interstitial cells of Leydig. Above, a high magnification of an interstitial region of the testis as seen with the light microscope; it represents an enlargement of the region delimited by the square in Figure 18.2. Below, a typical Leydig cell as seen with the electron microscope.

that may contain lipid droplets or lipofuscin pigment. This pigment is especially prominent in the Leydig cells of older men. At the electron microscopic level, Leydig cells exhibit structural characteristics that are typical of steroid-secreting cells (Fig. 18-11), that is, an elaborate and abundant, tubular, smooth endoplasmic reticulum; many mitochondria that usually contain tubular cristae; lipid droplets; a prominent multiple Golgi apparatus; and numerous lysosomes or lipofuscin pigment granules. A characteristic feature of human Leydig cells is the presence of highly structured cytoplasmic crystals (**crystals of Reinke**). The significance of these crystals is not known.

Functionally, Leydig cells produce androgenic steroid hormones, mainly testosterone, which are responsible for male characteristics. The membranes of their extensive smooth endoplasmic reticulum and numerous mitochondria possess the enzymatic machinery neded for the synthesis of androgens from cholesterol or its precursors. Testosterone is required for (1) developmental testicular differentiation, (2) changes that occur at sexual maturity, and (3) the development and maintenance of spermatogenesis, the secondary sex organs, and the male secondary sex characteristics including facial and body hair patterns, depth of voice, muscular development, and male libido.

Leydig cells are under pituitary control through the gonadotropin, luteinizing hormone (LH). Without LH (e.g., following hypophysectomy) these cells lose their steroid machinery, cease to secrete testosterone, and atrophy. Testosterone produced by the interstitial cells completes a negative feedback loop with the hypothalamus, which regulates LH secretion (Fig. 18-12). Testosterone inhibits secretion of LH by inhibiting the release of GnRH, the common gonadotropin-releasing hormone, from the hypothalamus. In addition, a newly discovered peptide, **inhibin,** is believed to be secreted by the tubular epithelium and to exert a direct inhibitory effect on FSH secretion. It is not known whether inhibin affects the hypothalamus directly. Also, the pineal glands in many species of animals inhibit gonadotropin secretion by the direct action of pineal secretions on the hypothalamus or pituitary. However, the role of the pineal in control of human reproductive mechanisms have not been established.

Recent studies, mainly using the scanning electron microscope, demonstrate that peritubular lymphatics and Leydig cell clusters are intimately related. These associations may be important for a means of "bathing" the seminiferous tubules with high concentrations of testosterone for this steroid's "spermatotropic" effect.

STRUCTURE AND FUNCTION OF THE EXCURRENT DUCTS AND ACCESSORY GLANDS

As the tortuous seminiferous tubules approach the mediastinum testis, they lose their spermatogenic elements and are lined only by columnar Sertoli cells. In this location the Sertoli cells apparently differ somewhat from their counterparts in the germinal portions—that is, the pattern and distribution of certain organelles change, the number of tight junctions between cells is reduced, and cytoplasmic filaments are in abundance. In addition, the luminal diameters are greatly decreased in these regions. Functionally, it is thought that the cytoplasmic filaments maintain the narrow lumina, which may prevent a fluid reflux into the seminiferous tubules. The **seminiferous tubule termini** open into a series of straight tubules. These **tubuli recti** mark the beginning of the excurrent duct system that ex-

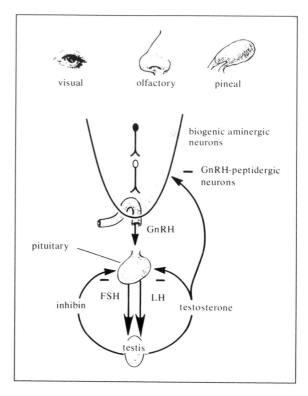

Fig. 18-12. Regulation of gonadotropin secretion in the male, showing the interactions of neural and hormonal feedback controls. Pituitary and testis are connected by a negative feedback link. Secretion of testosterone by the testis is stimulated by LH, whereas maturation and growth of the tubule cells are stimulated by FSH. The secretion of testosterone in turn inhibits the secretion of LH. It is likely that the major target of negative feedback is the hypothalamus, where GnRH, the common gonadotropin-releasing hormone, is inhibited. FSH = follicle-stimulating hormone; LH = luteinizing hormone; GnRH = gonadotropin-releasing hormone. (From J. B. Martin, S. Reichlin, and G. M. Brown, *Clinical Endocrinology*. Philadelphia: F. A. Davis, 1977. Reproduced with permission.)

tends to and includes the penile urethra. Situated at various loci along this system are the accessory glands; these ducts and glands are described in order of their occurrence from the testis outward.

Tubuli Recti

The tubular diameter markedly narrows in the straight tubules, and the epithelium becomes a simple cuboidal type. These tubules connect the seminiferous tubules with the rete testis (see Fig. 18-1).

Rete Testis

The rete testis is a labyrinthine network of channels located in the substance of the mediastinum (see Fig. 18-1). It is generally lined with a cuboidal epithelium, although the epithelium may vary from squamouslike to columnar. The cells possess a single flagellum. The underlying connective tissue is highly vascular.

Ductuli Efferentes

A series of approximately a dozen delicate, convoluted tubules in the shape of inverted cones extends from the rete testis to the head of the epididymis. These projections are called the **efferent ductules** (see Fig. 18-1). Each ductule is lined with an epithelium composed of two cell types: **principal cells** and **ciliated cells.** The former possess numerous microvilli on their luminal surfaces and many lysosomes in their cytoplasm; the cilia of the latter beat toward the epididymis. The luminal surface configuration of the epithelium has been described as "stellate" or "festooned" (Fig. 18-13). This appearance is caused by pocketlike invaginations formed by alternating regions of varying cell height. Surrounding each ductule subjacent to the basement membrane is a layer of circularly arranged smooth muscle and loose connective tissue containing elastic fibers.

Functionally, the efferent ductules are involved in sperm transport and fluid absorption. Move-

Fig. 18-13. The head of the epididymis in histologic section, showing cross sections of an efferent ductule (*upper left*) and the ductus epididymis (*lower right*).

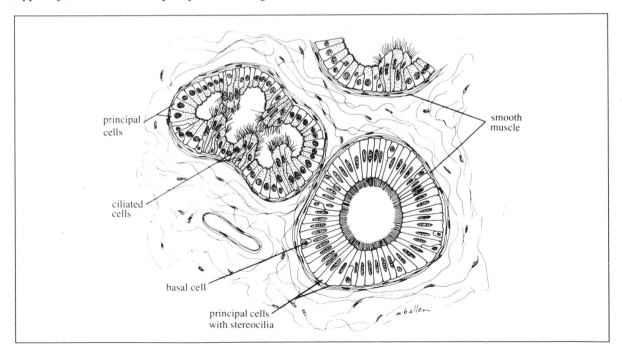

ment of spermatozoa is facilitated by ciliary action and muscular contraction. It is important to note that beginning with the ductuli efferentes, the remaining portions of the excurrent duct system are provided with varying thicknesses of muscular investment. Therefore, once the sperm are presented by testicular fluid flow to the excurrent duct system at the efferent ductule junctures, their subsequent transport is effected by muscular contraction. Absorption of a large proportion of the fluid produced in the testis occurs in the ductuli efferentes through the action of the principal cells. Their abundance of lysosomes probably functions in the degradation of absorbed materials. In addition, the microvilli and the scalloped epithelial border undoubtedly increase the surface area for enhancement of this process.

The efferent ductules are often considered to be part of the epididymis as an organ. However, where they fuse, the single tubular structure forming the next segment of the excurrent duct system is called the **ductus epididymidis.**

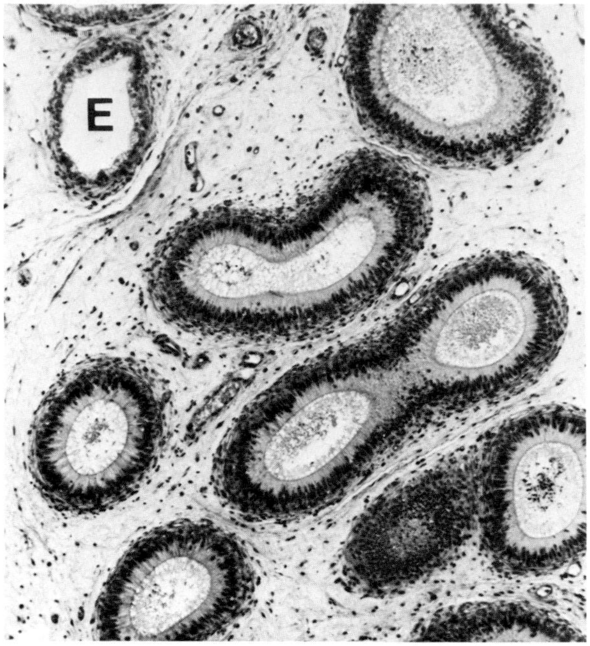

Fig. 18-14. Light micrograph of human epididymis. Various profiles of the duct are seen here, as well as a cross section of an efferent ductule (*E*).

Ductus Epididymidis

The ductus epididymidis is a single, highly coiled tube that lies longitudinally along the posterolateral surface of the testis (see Fig. 18-1). Together with the various tissue investments, these components form the structure called the **epididymis.** Although the coiled duct of the epididymis is not much longer than the testis, it has been estimated that its uncoiled length would be in excess of 6 m. The duct is lined with a pseudostratified columnar epithelium (see Figs. 18-13, 18-14) that consists of two cell types: **principal cells** and **basal cells.** The columnar principal cells contain a well-developed endoplasmic reticulum of both rough and smooth varieties and an elaborate Golgi apparatus. However, there appears to be little evidence for the elaboration of secretory granules. These cells also possess exceedingly long microvilli called **stereocilia** on their luminal surfaces that are visible in the

light microscope as well as the electron microscope (see Figs. 18-6, 18-13, 18-14). Numerous subluminal micropinocytotic vesicles and multivesicular bodies are also present. The basal cells rest on the basement membrane but do not reach the free surface. The epithelium is surrounded by layers of smooth muscle and vascular connective tissue.

Grossly, the epididymis is traditionally divided into **head** (caput), **body** (corpus), and **tail** (cauda). Although these regions do not correspond to areas of the duct that are histologically distinct, the epithelial height decreases from tall columnar principal cells with long microvilli in the head to cuboidal principal cells with somewhat shorter microvilli in the tail. In contrast, the smooth muscle investment increases from unilaminar in the head to trilaminar in the tail. The epididymal epithelium secretes glycerylphosphorylcholine, complex carbohydrates, and possibly steroids; at least, it has the capability for steroid biosynthesis.

Functionally, the duct of the epididymis is involved in several processes:

1. Fluid absorption and modification. It has been estimated that more than 90 percent of the testicular fluid is absorbed in the ductuli efferentes and ductus epididymidis; most of the epididymal absorption takes place in the upper segments where the microvilli are longest.
2. Sperm maturation. Testicular spermatozoa are not capable of full motility or fertilization of ova, whereas epididymal sperm are.
3. Sperm storage. The bulk of sperm storage occurs in the tail of the epididymis.
4. Sperm expulsion. The extensive smooth musculature in the tail region, the sperm reservoir, forcefully contracts during ejaculation.

Ductus Deferens (Vas Deferens)

The deferent duct (see Fig. 18-1) leaves the cauda epididymidis and passes superiorly along the posterolateral surface of the testis in a direction opposite to that of the epididymis to enter the **spermatic cord** and pass through the inguinal canal into the abdominal cavity.

The ductus deferens is a thick-walled tube consisting of a mucosa, muscularis, and adventitia (Fig. 18-15). The mucosa is composed of a pseudostratified columnar epithelium with stereocilia, similar to that found in the ductus epididymidis, and a prominent lamina propria rich in elastic fibers. The exceedingly robust muscularis consists of a trilaminar arrangement of smooth muscle; the inner and outer layers are longitudinal, whereas the intermediate layer is circular. This muscular investment as well as the elastic tissue causes the mucosa to be thrown into numerous longitudinal folds. The fibrous adventitia is continuous with the connective tissue of the spermatic cord. In addition to the ductus deferens, the spermatic cord contains testicular blood vessels and nerves surrounded by

Fig. 18-15. The ductus deferens in histologic cross section.

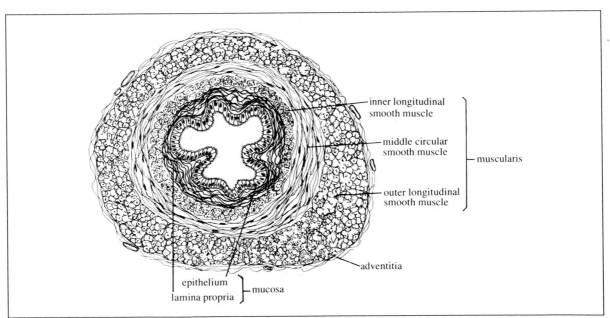

inner longitudinal smooth muscle

middle circular smooth muscle

muscularis

outer longitudinal smooth muscle

adventitia

epithelium
lamina propria — mucosa

longitudinal bundles of striated muscle called the **cremaster.** Contraction of these muscles raises the testes against the abdominal wall.

Functionally, the major role of the deferent duct is sperm propulsion during ejaculation brought about by the powerful contractions of its musculature. The portion proximal to the epididymal duct also plays a part in sperm storage.

After "hooking" over the ureter in the abdominal cavity, the ductus deferens dilates to form the **ampulla** of the ductus deferens (see Fig. 18-1).

Ampulla

In the ampulla, the longitudinal folds of the ductus deferens exhibit many evaginations into the subjacent tissues where the muscularis is much thinner. The epithelium is a pseudostratified columnar variety similar to that of the ductus deferens proper. However, the principal cells are secretory in nature. Therefore, the ampullae with their epithelial infoldings can be considered as accessory glands. Indeed, in some mammals these "ampullary glands" reach enormous size and complexity.

Opening into the ductus deferens immediately distal to the ampulla is the duct of the **seminal vesicle.**

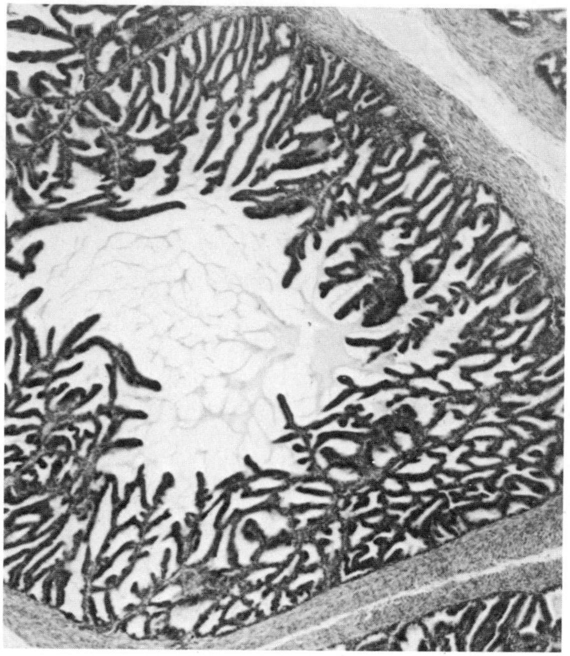

Fig. 18-16. Low-magnification light micrograph of human seminal vesicle. Note the highly infolded anastomosing mucosa.

Seminal Vesicle

The seminal vesicle, a glandular evagination of the ductus deferens (see Fig. 18-1), is actually a highly coiled tube embedded in connective tissue and smooth muscle whose mucosa is thrown into a complex series of primary, secondary, and tertiary folds and ridges (Fig. 18-16). The resulting outpocketings, therefore, all communicate with the main lumen. Like that of its parental ductus deferens, the wall of the seminal vesicle contains a mucosa, muscularis, and adventitia. The mucosa consists of a pseudostratified columnar epithelium and a lamina propria with numerous elastic fibers. The epithelium contains secretory principal cells and basal cells. The principal cells exhibit organelles typical of protein-secreting cells—that is, prominent rough endoplasmic reticulum, Golgi apparatus, and secretory granules. These cells secrete a yellowish, viscous liquid containing fructose, ascorbic acid, citric acid, phosphorylcholine, and prostaglandins. The muscularis contains inner circular and outer longitudinal fibers. The connective tissue adventitia also contains elastic fibers.

Although its name is suggestive of a sperm storage function, the seminal vesicle does not serve this purpose. Functionally, it contributes to the fluid medium of the semen. Its secretory products are important substrates for sperm metabolism. The prostaglandins may also exert influence on the female reproductive tract.

Ejaculatory Duct

The segment of the deferent duct that extends from its union with the seminal vesicle and traverses the prostate to open into the prostatic portion of the urethra is called the **ejaculatory duct.** Its folded mucosa with numerous glandular evaginations consists of pseudostratified columnar epithelium and underlying elastic connective tissue. A muscularis is lacking; undoubtedly the smooth muscle of the surrounding prostate serves this function.

Each ejaculatory duct opens into the prostatic urethra through its dorsal wall on a hill-shaped mound of tissue called the **colliculus seminalis** or **verumontanum.** The ejaculatory ducts open bilaterally to the prostatic utricle, which is also located in the "seminal hill."

Prostate

The prostate (see Fig. 18-1) is the sex accessory gland or glandular complex that is common to all male mammals. In humans it is the largest of the male accessory glands, with a weight of approximately 20 g. This organ is a compact mass of compound tubuloalveolar glands that opens into the prostatic urethra through numerous ducts. The epithelium is usually of the simple or pseudostratified columnar type but may vary depending on glandular activity or region (Fig. 18-17). Fine structurally, the cells exhibit typical secretory features; histochemically, they are strongly positive for acid phosphatase. The prostatic stroma and capsule are composed of dense fibroelastic connective tissue and smooth muscle. A usual feature of the human prostate, especially in older persons, is the presence of intraluminal bodies composed of concentric lamellae. These prostatic **concretions** are probably condensations of secretory material that may become calcified (Fig. 18-18).

Recent reexamination of human prostatic structure (Fig. 18-19), especially in relation to its pathologic changes, has revealed that this organ is actually a glandular complex composed of sev-

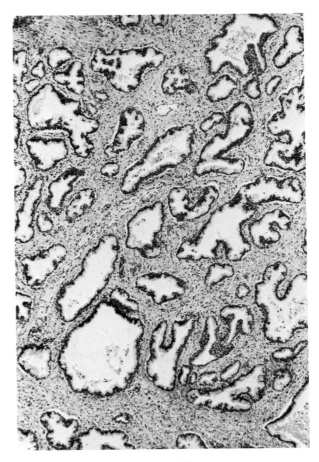

Fig. 18-17. Light micrograph of human prostate. The alveoli vary greatly in size and are usually quite sacculated. Note also the extensive fibromuscular stroma between alveoli.

eral discrete entities: the **prostate proper,** the **transition zone,** the **periurethral tissue,** and the **utriculus prostaticus.**

PROSTATE PROPER

The prostate proper, which makes up the bulk of the organ, is divided into two zones based on epithelial appearance and stromal arrangement. This portion has also been referred to as the "true" prostate. The zonation of this region is seen to particular advantage when the prostate is

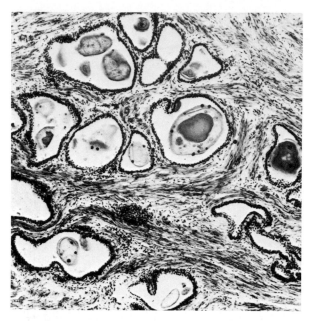

Fig. 18-18. Light micrograph of prostate from an elderly male. Note the numerous prostatic concretions in the lumens, the relatively thin epithelium, and the extensive fibromuscular stroma.

sectioned in a plane that is parallel to the long axis of the ejaculatory ducts (frontal plane; see Fig. 18-19C).

The **central zone,** which forms about 25 percent of the prostate proper, is roughly an inverted pyramid that is located posteriorly to the urethra (see Fig. 18-19A). This pyramidal region, whose base is located at the neck of the bladder, extends to about the center of the prostate where its apex surrounds the ejaculatory ducts as they open into the prostatic urethra through its dorsal wall. The epithelial component of this area is described as having a pseudostratified appearance, being composed of crowded cells with pale nuclei lying at different levels and a granular, eosinophilic cytoplasm that occasionally contains brown pigment granules. The glandular acini are very large with an irregular contour due to prominent intraluminal ridges. The smooth muscle component of the stroma is described as having a compact, streaming arrangement.

The **peripheral zone** makes up the remaining 75 percent of the prostate proper. This roughly heart-shaped region, with an anterior concavity (see Fig. 18-19A,B), is of pathologic importance because it is the major site of prostatic carcinoma. The epithelial component of this area is described as having a more regular, simple columnar pattern with rather small, basally located dark nuclei and a relatively clear cytoplasm. The glandular units of this zone are characterized by small, rounded, uniform acini of simple structure. The smooth muscle component of the stroma is described as having a loose, trabeculated pattern.

The ducts of the central zone open into the prostatic urethra through its posterolateral walls in the area of the verumontanum; the ducts of the peripheral zone open into the lower prostatic urethra (see Fig. 18-19A).

TRANSITION ZONE

The transition zone, recently described as a discrete entity of the prostatic complex, is located above the verumontanum immediately anterior to the peripheral zone and lying within the concavity of the latter's anterior face. The principal ducts of the transition zone enter the urethra laterally in the area of the verumontanum and just above the most superior ducts of the peripheral zone. From their points of entry into the urethra, the bilateral, glandular tissue masses of

Fig. 18-19. The human prostate. A. Composite of the prostatic complex as seen anteriorly. The bladder has been removed as well as surrounding periurethral sphincteric muscle and connective tissue so that the urethra could be opened anteriorly to reveal anatomic relationships. Located on the midline of the verumontanum is the opening of the utriculus prostaticus; just below and to each side of the utricle are the bilateral openings of the ejaculatory ducts. B. The prostatic complex as seen posteriorly. C. Frontal section of the prostate in anterior view showing the relationship of central and peripheral zones. (Redrawn through the courtesy and permission of Dr. J. E. McNeal.)

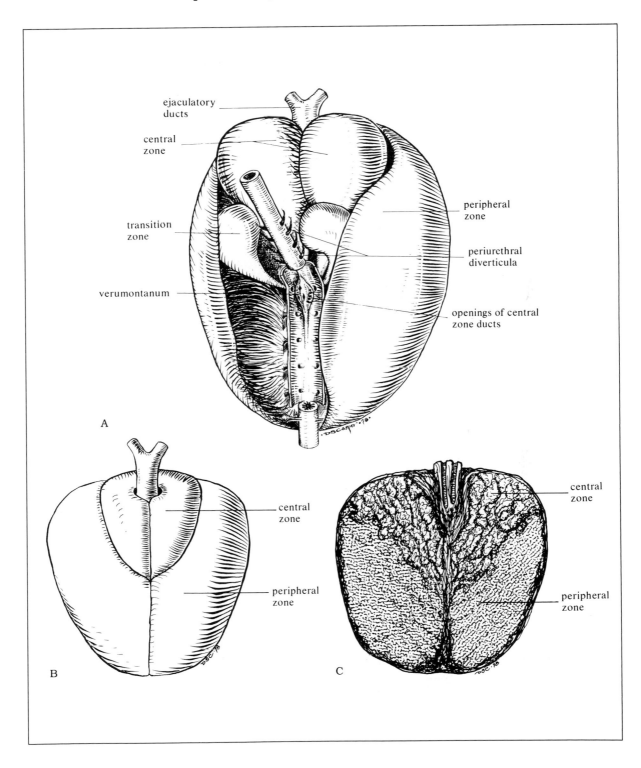

the transition zone angle forward and upward away from the prostate proper and parallel the axis of the upper prostatic urethra, which projects anteriorly and superiorly toward the bladder (see Fig. 18-19A). Indeed, these masses actually penetrate the smooth muscle tissue surrounding the urethra, the cylindrical sphincter that originates from the bladder neck muscle and extends toward the verumontanum. Histologically, the epithelial component of transition zone glands is similar to that of the posteriorly located peripheral zone tissue. The stroma of the transition zone, however, markedly differs from the stroma of the peripheral zone. Whereas the latter normally contains loosely woven and finely textured smooth muscle, the transition zone is characterized by extremely compact and coarse fibers. These fibers appear poorly oriented around transition zone acini and often form incomplete concentric rings parallel to the muscle fibers of the urethral sphincter. Furthermore, the glandular branches of the most medial portions of the transition zone frequently curve inward and penetrate the lateral aspects of the sphincter.

This region of the prostate is of extreme importance because it has recently been defined as the principal site involved in the evolution of benign prostatic hyperplasia (BPH). In BPH, large and discrete nodules of proliferative cells form that, in advanced development, can strangle the urethra and obstruct urinary flow. Prostates with numerous nodules may weigh in excess of 200 g. BPH may begin in men in their middle forties; by age 80 an estimated 80 percent of the male population is affected. Surgical treatment is common.

PERIURETHRAL TISSUE

The periurethral tissue is composed of small, poorly differentiated glandular diverticula of the upper prostatic urethra, that is, above the verumontanum (see Fig. 18-19A). This portion of the prostate is enclosed inside the cylindrical sphincter and separated by this mass of muscle from the transition zone. The lowest or most inferior of the periurethral ducts enters the urethra just above the main transition zone ducts. Previously, the periurethral tissue was thought to be involved in the production of nodular hyperplasia. Although nodules may also develop here and be of importance if they produce an obstructing midline nodule that bulges into the bladder neck, they are usually fewer in number and smaller in size than the nodules found in the transition zone. It is now recognized that periurethral nodules seldom form the main mass of BPH tissue; rather, most nodules in this condition arise from glands and stroma of the transition zone.

UTRICULUS PROSTATICUS

The prostatic utricle is the remnant of the fused müllerian ducts located in the verumontanum on the midline just above the entrance of the ejaculatory ducts (see Fig. 18-19A). Its glandular function has not been thoroughly examined.

Functionally, the prostate contributes to the fluid medium of the semen by producing a slightly acid, colorless fluid containing hydrolytic enzymes, including abundant acid phosphatase, citric acid, and large amounts of zinc. Determination of prostatic acid phosphatase activity has been a widely used means of assessing prostatic function; more recently, it has become a reliable and sensitive method for the identification of semen in vaginal fluid. The large quantity of zinc may be important in exerting (1) a stabilizing, energy-preserving effect on the spermatozoa while in the seminal fluid during ejaculation and (2) a protective effect against spermiophagic cells in the female reproductive tract, in that this metal inhibits sperm metabolism as well as phagocytosis and oxygen uptake in granular leukocytes and macrophages. However, the prostate apparently pays a price for its zinc-concentrating role in that it is often the site of chronic bacterial inflammation—a condition that may be allowed by inhibition of its own inflammatory cells.

Urethra

The urethra extends from the bladder through the penis (see Fig. 18-1). It is the final common pathway of the reproductive and urinary systems. Its wall is composed of elastic tissue and smooth muscle. The **prostatic portion** (pars prostatica) extends from the bladder to the base of the prostate. The **membranous portion** (pars membranacea) extends from the base of the prostate to the bulb of the corpus spongiosum of the penis. The **cavernous portion** (pars cavernosa) consists of bulbous, pendulous, and glandular segments corresponding to the bulb, body, and glans of the penis, respectively. The epithelial lining of the urethra varies from transitional (prostatic portion) to stratified or pseudostratified columnar (membranous and cavernous portions) to stratified squamous nonkeratinizing (glandular segment) varieties. This last type, which reflects its origin from surface ectoderm, is continuous with the stratified squamous keratinizing epithelium that covers the glans, prepuce, and surface of the penis.

Bulbourethral Glands

The bulbourethral glands (of Cowper) are two small glandular nodules located at the junction of the membranous and cavernous portions of the urethra, whose ducts generally open into the cavernous portion (see Fig. 18-1). These glands are of the compound tubuloalveolar variety and are lined with a cuboidal or columnar epithelium. The epithelium is surrounded by fibroelastic connective tissue and strands of smooth and striated muscle. The glandular cells are similar in appearance to mucus-producing cells, with basally flattened nuclei and clear cytoplasm. However, they produce a clear, viscous liquid containing numerous carbohydrate components. Functionally, they lubricate the urethra prior to ejaculation.

Urethral Glands

Throughout most of the urethra, especially in the cavernous portion, small cellular outpocketings occur in the lining epithelium. Mucous cell "nests" called **urethral glands** (of Littre) are found in these outpocketings. These glands may also have a lubricating function.

Preputial Glands

Covering the glans penis around its circumference is a fold of skin called the **prepuce,** which is often removed in humans (circumcision). On the inner aspects of this fold are numerous sebaceous glands called **preputial glands** (of Tyson), which are not associated with hair follicles.

STRUCTURE AND FUNCTION OF THE PENIS

The penis (Fig. 18-20; see also Fig. 18-1) is a highly vascular, cylindrical organ composed of three masses of erectile tissue: the paired, but intercommunicating, superior **corpora cavernosa penis** and the single, inferior **corpus cavernosum urethrae** or **corpus spongiosum.** The corpora cavernosa are located above the urethra and are surrounded by a thick, fibrous connective tissue capsule called the **tunica albuginea penis.** The corpus cavernosum urethrae, as its name implies, surrounds the penile urethra. Its fibrous investment is modest. Elastic tissue, smooth muscle, specialized sensory nerve endings, and a labyrinth of endothelial-lined channels in the erectile bodies continuous with arterial supply and venous drainage are the structural modifications that allow for the functioning of this organ.

In the normal resting state, the penis is flaccid due to a paucity of blood in the spaces of the erectile tissue. Upon arousal, the cavernous erectile bodies fill with blood and the penis becomes turgid. During the sex act or **copulation,** three successive phases in the male are defined: **erection, ejaculation,** and **detumescence.**

The mechanism of erection begins when erotic stimuli, through autonomic input, cause a loss of muscular tone in the walls of arterial connections to the endothelial-lined lacunae in the erectile tissue. As blood pours into these spaces, the lacunae expand and the venous drainage "backs up." Indeed, at some point the vascular pressure in the labyrinth, especially in the corpora cavernosa, compresses the draining veins against the resistant tunica albuginea (penis) so that blood

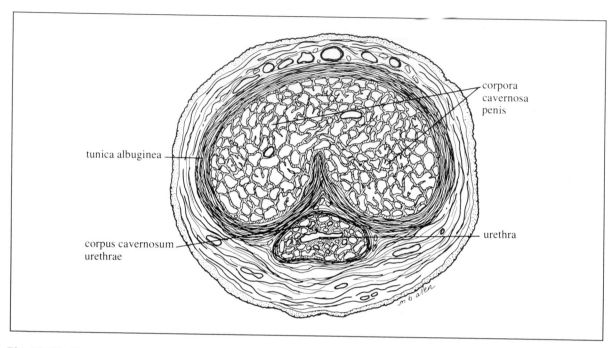

corpora
cavernosa
penis

tunica albuginea

urethra

corpus cavernosum
urethrae

Fig. 18-20. The human penis in histologic cross section.

is actually retained in the spongy tissue. Stimulation of nerve endings in the glans penis maintains this condition, thus producing an engorged structure whose primary function is to introduce the male gametes directly into the female reproductive tract.

Ejaculation is the process by which the semen is expelled. The sequence of events includes lubrication of the urethra by the secretions from the bulbourethral and urethral glands, discharge of the prostate, forceful contractions of the ductus epididymidis and ductus deferens to expel the spermatozoa, and finally discharge of the seminal vesicles. Also involved in this process are striated perineal muscles.

When ejaculation is complete or the stimuli are removed, the arterial smooth muscle regains its tone and blood flow into the erectile tissue is decreased. Gradually, venous drainage catches up and blood is withdrawn from the lacunae. However, since decompression of the small veins oc-

curs slowly and is accomplished only by removal of blood from the lacunae, detumescence is a gradual process.

NATIONAL BOARD TYPE QUESTIONS

For the following, select
  A. if only *1, 2, and 3* are correct.
  B. if only *1 and 3* are correct.
  C. if only *2 and 4* are correct.
  D. if only *4* is correct.
  E. if *all* are correct.

1. Sertoli cells
    1. originate from splanchnic mesoderm.
    2. secrete androgen-binding protein.
    3. rest on the basement membrane of seminiferous tubules.
    4. have tight junctions between them which constitute the blood-testis barrier.
2. Interstitial tissue of the testis contains
    1. Leydig cells.
    2. fibroblasts.

3. capillaries derived from the tunica vasculosa.
4. spermatogonia.

3. During spermiogenesis
   1. the second meiotic division occurs.
   2. the acrosome is formed.
   3. secondary spermatocytes are formed.
   4. the flagellum is formed.

4. The middle piece of the sperm contains
   1. mitochondria.
   2. microtubules.
   3. outer dense fibers.
   4. centrioles.

5. The ductus epididymis
   1. is the primary storage site for sperm.
   2. lacks basal epithelial cells.
   3. contains columnar epithelial cells with stereocilia.
   4. contains columnar epithelial cells with numerous secretory granules.

6. The prostate
   1. is a compound tubuloalveolar gland.
   2. contains a central zone especially vulnerable to carcinoma.
   3. contains a transition zone associated with benign hyperplasia.
   4. has a stroma lacking smooth muscle cells.

7. The male urethra is lined by
   1. simple cuboidal epithelium along the membranous portion.
   2. transitional epithelium along the prostatic portion.
   3. transitional epithelium along the cavernous portion.
   4. stratified squamous nonkeratinizing epithelium along the glandular segment of the cavernous portion.

8. Leydig cells
   1. synthesize testosterone
   2. contain abundant smooth endoplasmic reticulum.
   3. contain lipid droplets.
   4. contain mitochondria lacking tubular cristae.

9. During the second meiotic division
   1. DNA is replicated.

2. chromatids (monads) move to opposite poles of the cell.
3. crossing-over occurs.
4. haploid spermatids are produced.

10. During the first meiotic division
    1. chromatids (dyads) move to opposite poles of the cell.
    2. primary spermatocytes with tetraploid DNA are produced.
    3. secondary spermatocytes containing diploid DNA are produced.
    4. one secondary spermatocyte is formed from each primary spermatocyte.

11. Type B spermatogonia
    1. reside within the adluminal compartment of seminiferous tubules.
    2. produce primary spermatocytes by mitotic division.
    3. are stem cells which replenish type A spermatogonia by mitotic division.
    4. rest on the basement membrane of seminiferous tubules.

ANNOTATED ANSWERS

1. E.
2. A. Spermatogonia are located in the basal compartment of the seminiferous tubules where they rest on the basement membrane.
3. C. The meiotic divisions are complete. Spermiogenesis consists of a transformation of the spermatid into a spermatozoan without further cell divisions.
4. A. The centrioles occupy the neck region.
5. B.
6. B. The peripheral zone of the prostate is vulnerable to carcinoma. Stroma is fibromuscular throughout the prostate.
7. C. The membranous and cavernous portions are lined either by stratified or pseudostratified columnar epithelium.
8. A. As with other steroid-producing cells, their mitochondria have tubular cristae.
9. C. Replication of DNA and crossing-over occur during prophase of the first meiotic division.
10. A. Two secondary spermatocytes are pro-

duced for every primary spermatocyte completing the first meiotic division. See Table 18-2.

11. C. Type B spermatogonia rest on the basement membrane of the seminiferous tubule and divide mitotically to form preleptotene spermatocytes.

BIBLIOGRAPHY

Austin, C. R., and R. V. Short (eds.). *Reproduction in Mammals.* Cambridge: Cambridge University, 1972–1976. Books 1–6.

Beatty, R. A. The genetics of the mammalian gamete. *Biol. Rev.* 45:73, 1970.

Blandau, R. J., and D. Bergsma (eds.). *Morphogenesis and Malformation of the Genital System: Birth Defects.* Original Articles Series. New York: Liss, 1977. Vol. 13, no. 2.

Clermont, Y. The cycle of the seminiferous epithelium in man. *Am. J. Anat.* 113:35, 1963.

Clermont, Y. Kinetics of spermatogenesis in mammals: Seminiferous epithelium cycle and spermatogonial renewal. *Physiol. Rev.* 52:198, 1972.

Clermont, Y., and L. Hermo. Spermatogonial Stem Cells and Their Behavior in the Seminiferous Epithelium of Rats and Monkeys. In A. B. Cairnie, P. K. Lala, and D. G. Osmond (eds.), *Stem Cells of Renewing Cell Populations.* New York: Academic, 1976.

Clermont, Y., M. Lalli, and A. Rambourg. Ultrastructural localization of nicotinamide adenine dinucleotid phosphatase. (NADPase), thiamine pyrophosphatase (TPPase), and cytidine monophosphatase (CMPase) in the Golgi apparatus of early spermatids of the rat. *Anat. Rec.* 201:613, 1981.

Davajan, V., R. M. Nakamura, and M. Saga. Role of immunology in the infertile human. *Biol. Reprod.* 6:443, 1972.

Dym, M., and Y. Clermont. Role of spermatogonia in the repair of the seminiferous epithelium following x-irradiation of the rat testis. *Am. J. Anat.* 128:265, 1970.

Fawcett, D. W. The mammalian spermatozoon. *Dev. Biol.* 44:395, 1975.

Fawcett, D. W. Ultrastructure and Function of the Sertoli Cell. In D. W. Hamilton and R. O. Greep (eds.), *Handbook of Physiology.* Washington, D.C.: American Physiology Society, 1975. Vol. 5.

Fawcett, D. W., L. V. Leak, and P. M. Heidger, Jr. Electron microscopic observations on the structural components of the blood-testis barrier. *J. Reprod. Fertil.* 10(Suppl.):105, 1970.

Gilula, N. B., D. W. Fawcett, and A. Aoki. Ultrastructural and experimental observations on the Sertoli cell junctions of the mammalian testis. *Dev. Biol.* 50:142, 1976.

Gould, K. G. Application of in vitro fertilization. *Fed. Proc.* 32:2069, 1973.

Hamilton, D. W., and R. O. Greep (eds.). Male Reproductive System. In *Handbook of Physiology.* Washington, D.C.: American Physiological Society, 1975. Vol. 5.

Koehler, J. K. Human sperm head ultrastructure: A freeze-etching study. *J. Ultrastruct. Res.* 39:520, 1972.

Leblond, C. P., and Y. Clermont. Definition of the stages of the cycle of the seminiferous epithelium in the rat. *Ann. N.Y. Acad. Sci.* 55:548, 1952.

Moens, P. B. Mechanisms of chromosome synapsis at meiotic prophase. *Int. Rev. Cytol.* 35:117, 1973.

Moresi, V. Chromosome activities during meiosis and spermatogenesis. *J. Reprod. Fertil.* 13(Suppl.):1, 1971.

Ohno, S. Morphological Aspects of Meiosis and Their Genetical Significance. In E. Rosemberg and C. A. Paulsen (eds.), *Advances in Experimental Medicine and Biology: The Human Testis.* New York: Plenum, 1970.

Parvinen, M., K. K. Vihko, and J. Toppari. Cell interactions during the seminiferous epithelial cycle. *Int. Rev. Cytol.* 104:115, 1986.

Phillips, D. M. Substructure of the mammalian acrosome. *J. Ultrastruct. Res.* 38:591, 1972.

Rattner, J. B. Observations of centriole formation in male meiosis. *J. Cell Biol.* 54:20, 1972.

Rattner, J. B., and B. R. Brinkley. Ultrastructure of mammalian spermiogenesis: II. Elimination of the nuclear membrane. *J. Ultrastruc. Res.* 36:1, 1971.

Rimpau, J., and T. Lelley. Attachment of meiotic chromosomes to nuclear membrane. *Z. Pflanzenzuchtung* 67:197, 1972.

Rowley, M. J., J. D. Berlin, and C. G. Heller. The ultrastructure of four types of human spermatogonia. *Z. Zellforsch.* 112:139, 1971.

Setchell, B. P. Testicular Blood Supply, Lymphatic Drainage and Secretion of Fluid. In A. D. Johnson, W. R. Gomes, and N. L. Vandemark (eds.), *The Testis.* New York: Academic, 1970. Vol. 1.

Setchell, B. P., and G. M. H. Waites. The Blood-Testis Barrier. In D. W. Hamilton and R. O. Greep (eds.), *Handbook of Physiology.* Washington, D.C.: American Physiological Society, 1975. Vol. 5.

Solari, A. J., and L. L. Tres. Ultrastructure and Histochemistry of the Nucleus During Male Meiotic Prophase. In E. Rosemberg and C. A. Paulsen (eds.), *Advances in Experimental Medicine and Biology: The Human Testis.* New York: Plenum, 1970.

Steinberger, E. Hormonal control of mammalian spermatogenesis. *Physiol. Rev.* 51:1, 1971.

Susi, F. R., C. P. Leblond, and Y. Clermont. Changes in the Golgi apparatus during spermiogenesis in the rat. *Am. J. Anat.* 130:251, 1971.

19 Female Reproductive System

Objectives

You will learn the following in this chapter:

How to illustrate the stages of ovarian follicle development, from the primordial to the mature follicle

The formation of the corpus luteum from the postovulatory follicle and the factors that determine its maintenance or regression

How the mucosa of the oviduct is specialized for the sustenance and movement of the ovum

How to distinguish the histologic changes of the uterine endometrium during a normal menstrual cycle

The blood supply to the uterine endometrium and the mechanism by which the stratum functionalis hypertrophies, sheds, and regenerates

The endocrine regulation of ovarian and uterine events during the menstrual cycle

The primary endocrine and histologic events involved in the initiation of pregnancy and formation of the placenta

The special distinguishing features of the cervix and vagina

The distinguishing histologic features of the inactive and active mammary glands and what hormonal influences are responsible for breast development at puberty and during pregnancy, and lactation postpartum

---

The female reproductive system comprises a group of internal organs located within the pelvis consisting of the paired **ovaries** and **oviducts** (uterine or fallopian tubes), the **uterus,** and the **vagina** (Fig. 19-1). The mons pubis, the clitoris, and the labia minora and labia majora represent the **external genitalia.** The paired **mammary glands** or breasts, important adjuncts to the reproductive system, are also considered in this chapter.

The sexual organs usually rest in an immature state until the female is about 10 years of age. During the next few years pituitary hormones cause the reproductive organs to enlarge, the breasts to begin growth, fat to accumulate in the female phenotypic pattern, and axillary and pubic hair to appear. When these changes have occurred, the first **menses** begin at an average age of about 13. Hormones made in the mature ovaries interact with others released from the anterior pituitary under hypothalamic regulation in a cyclic nature that influences the lining of the uterus. Such a **menstrual cycle** averages 28 days or one lunar month (menses = month), although there is considerable individual variation. A mature **ovum** is released at the midpoint of the cy-

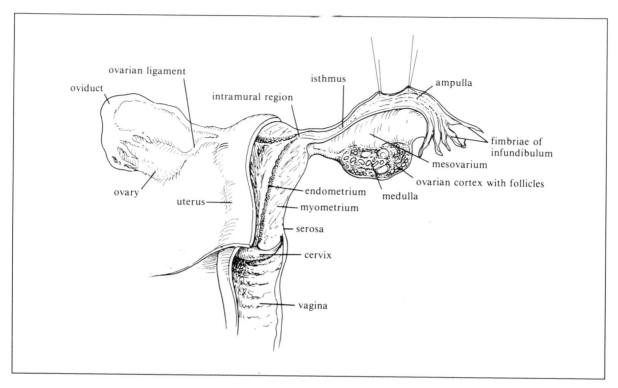

Fig. 19-1. Posterior view of the internal female reproductive organs. On the right, the organs have been hemisected to reveal internal structure.

cle; if fertilized it will implant in the uterine lining that has thickened as a result of hormones secreted by the ovary. If fertilization does not occur, the thickened uterine lining will break down and be shed, the phenomenon of **menstruation.**

THE INTERNAL REPRODUCTIVE ORGANS
The Ovaries

The two ovaries are solid, almond-shaped organs about 4 cm long, 2 to 3 cm wide, and 1 cm thick. The anterior wall of each ovary is attached to the back of the broad ligament by a short peritoneal fold, the **mesovarium,** which conducts vessels and nerves to the hilus. The ovarian ligament also attaches the ovary to the uterus. Arterial blood reaches each ovary predominantly through the **ovarian arteries,** which anastomose with the **uterine arteries** in the mesovarium of each ovary. Large vessels from the anastomosis enter the ovary through the hilus and branch extensively in the medulla in a coiled manner, where they are known as **helicine arteries.** These arteries then send forth smaller branches peripherally to feed the cortex, where they break up into capillaries between follicles. Veins accompany the arteries.

The ovaries develop from ridges within the intraembryonic coelom. The covering mesoderm differentiates into a cuboidal epithelium that persists in the adult, as distinguished from the typical squamous mesothelium lining the peritoneal cavity. Beneath the epithelium, cords of epithelial-type cells develop within the stroma. The primordial germ cells develop in the yolk sac

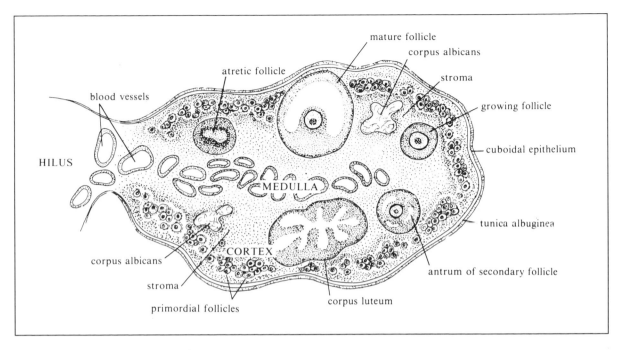

Fig. 19-2. Longitudinal section of a mature ovary.

and migrate to the developing ovary, where they are called **oogonia.** Following mitotic divisions that produce many **oocytes,** the germ cells enter prophase of their first meiotic division. The oocytes remain arrested in prophase until their time of ovulation after puberty.

The adult functional ovary (Fig. 19-2) is covered by a simple cuboidal epithelium that rests on a layer of dense connective tissue, the **tunica albuginea.** The organ is divisible into a central **medulla** and an outer **cortex.** The medulla is composed of loose connective tissue and an abundance of large blood vessels, the helicine arteries and accompanying veins. The cortex is composed of a compact, richly cellular **stroma,** whose spindle-shaped cells are arranged in a characteristic swirly pattern, and **ovarian follicles** in various stages of development and degeneration.

FOLLICLES

A follicle consists of an oocyte surrounded by a layer of epithelial cells. About 400,000 follicles are present in the ovaries at birth, and of these only about 400 are ovulated during the average reproductive life of a woman. On the average, one oocyte matures every 28 days; thus, very few ova are ultimately released. The other oocytes gradually degenerate (a process called **atresia** that begins even **before** birth) throughout the reproductive period. Therefore, a section of mature ovary will show follicles in many stages of growth and degeneration. Each month several follicles may begin to mature at once and then will degenerate so that usually only one finally produces a mature ovum. The four stages of follicular maturation (Fig. 19-3) are described in the following sections.

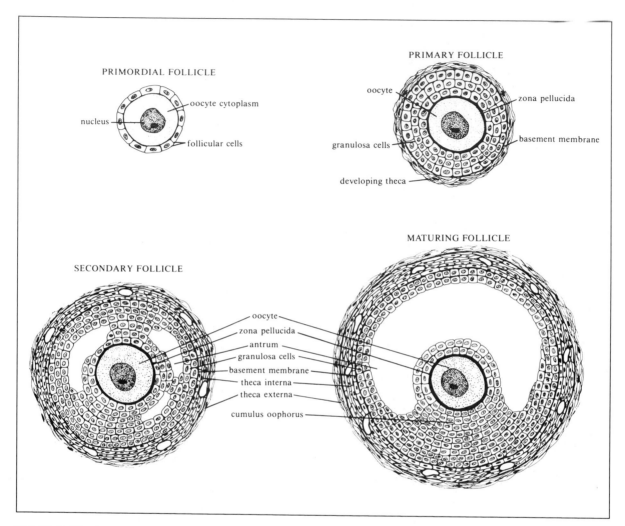

Fig. 19-3. The four stages of follicular development.

Primordial Follicle

As the name implies, primordial (unilaminar) follicles (Fig. 19-4) are the most primitive follicles, which have not yet begun to develop. They consist of a central oocyte about 20 μm in diameter, surrounded by a single flattened layer of epithelial (follicular) cells. These small follicles occur in large numbers just beneath the tunica albuginea. As follicles begin to mature, they migrate further inward toward the medulla.

Primary Follicle

As the follicle begins to grow, changes occur at three levels (Fig. 19-5):

1. The oocyte enlarges to 50 to 80 μm and develops multiple Golgi complexes and abundant free ribosomes. Microvilli on the oocyte surface penetrate the forming **zona pellucida,** a deeply staining, thick, neutral glycoprotein coat that appears to be the combined syn-

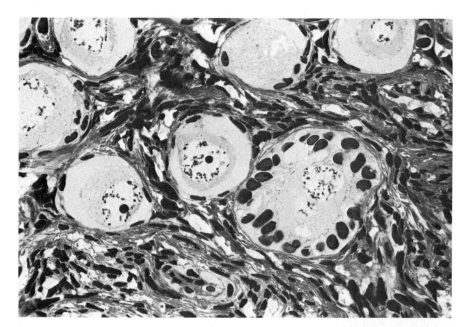

Fig. 19-4. A light micrograph of monkey ovary showing six primordial follicles and one follicle beginning the maturational process. Note the change in follicular cell morphology.

Fig. 19-5. A light micrograph of a primary follicle in a monkey ovary. Note the stratified nature of the follicular (granulosa) cells. A well-developed zona pellucida surrounds the oocyte. The connective tissue theca encapsulates the follicle. See Figure 19-3 for orientation.

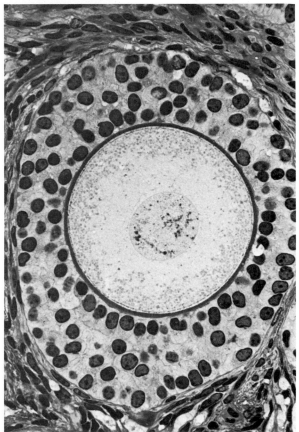

thetic effort of the oocyte and surrounding epithelial cells.

2. The single, flattened layer of follicular cells first becomes cuboidal and then divides to form a stratified layer of **granulosa cells** that rest on a basement membrane. Gap junctions between the adjacent granulosa cells and the granulosa cells and oocyte promote passage of nutrients and metabolites for the capillaries in the connective tissue to the developing oocyte.

3. The connective tissue surrounding the follicle begins to condense and form a **theca** (Greek, "box"), which encapsulates the follicle. At a later stage, this theca will differentiate into two functional layers.

Secondary (Antral) Follicle

When follicles reach about 0.2 mm in diameter, with six to twelve layers of granulosa cells, irregular fluid-filled spaces occur between the granulosa cells. These spaces become confluent and form a crescentic space, or **antrum,** filled with **liquor folliculi.** The follicle, largely as a result of increase in fluid, may reach a diameter of greater than 10 mm, although the oocyte has attained its final size. The oocyte comes to reside eccentrically in a mound of granulosa cells, the **cumulus oophorus,** which protrudes into the antrum, giving it a crescentic appearance. The theca, which is separated from the granulosa cells by the basement membrane, differentiates into two layers, an inner vascular **theca interna** and a fibrous **theca externa** (Figs. 19-6, 19-7).

Mature (Graafian) Follicles

In 10 to 14 days, the original primordial follicle has reached maturity (see Fig. 19-6) and occupies the entire thickness of the ovarian cortex, visibly bulging out on the free surface. Liquor folliculi begins to accumulate between cells of the cumulus oophorus, freeing the oocyte from all but one layer of loosely adherent cells, the **corona radiata.** Under endocrine control (to be described subsequently) a sudden increase in the amount of liquor folliculi immediately precedes ovulation. Androgens produced by the theca interna in all preovulatory follicles are converted to estrogens by granulosa cells which have an aromatizing enzyme induced by follicle-stimulating hormone (FSH).

OVULATION

Rupture of the follicle with release of the ovum occurs at approximately 28-day intervals. Ovulation usually occurs at the midpoint (days 10–14) of a typical 28-day cycle. Just prior to ovulation, the ovum and its adherent corona radiata are floating free in the liquor folliculi. The fluid within the antrum increases suddenly in volume, exerting pressure on the overlying thin rim of

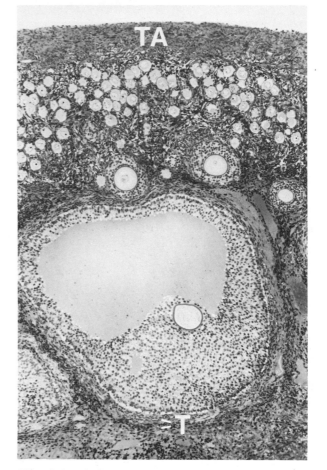

Fig. 19-6. A light micrograph of a monkey ovary. The dense connective tissue tunica albuginea (*TA*) encapsulates the organ. Beneath it are numerous primordial follicles. Deeper in the cortex is a nearly mature follicle with a well-developed antrum. The theca (*T*) surrounding the follicle has differentiated into two distinct layers. Three primary follicles are also visible between the mature follicle and the primordial follicles. See Figures 19-2 and 19-3 for orientation and further structural identification.

cortical tissue, which bulges up to form a small cone or **stigma.** The follicle ruptures through the stigma, and the ovum, surrounded by its corona radiata, escapes into the peritoneal cavity and is then quickly drawn into the oviduct (Fig. 19-8).

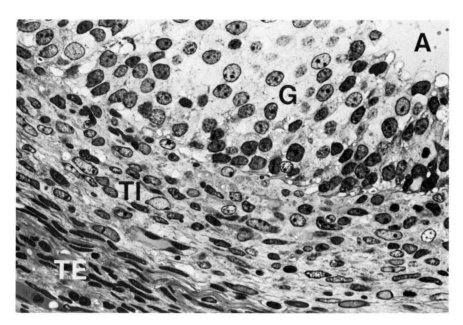

Fig. 19-7. A light micrograph of a monkey ovary showing some granulosa cells (*G*) and a portion of the antrum (*A*) of a mature follicle. The adjacent theca is composed of two layers, the theca interna (*TI*) and theca externa (*TE*).

Meanwhile, it completes the first meiotic division, casting off a small polar body, and enters the second meiotic division, which will be completed only after fertilization occurs. The ovum retains its capacity to be fertilized for approximately 24 hours. If fertilization does occur, the union of sperm and egg takes place in the oviduct. Following fertilization, the zygote takes 3 to 5 days to traverse the oviduct and arrive at the site of implantation in the uterine wall. The stages of ovulation can be observed in vivo in the rabbit when induced experimentally by **luteinizing hormone** (LH). The mechanism is described later.

CORPUS LUTEUM

Following ovulation, the follicle does not degenerate immediately but is transformed into a tempo-
rary endocrine organ, the **corpus luteum** (Fig. 19-9). The basement membrane separating granulosa cells and theca interna cells dissolves, allowing the fenestrated capillaries to grow in between the granulosa cells. By this time, estrogen produced by granulosa cells of preovulatory follicles has provoked the pituitary to release a surge of LH. The LH causes granulosa cells to hypertrophy and become laden with numerous small lipid droplets containing a yellow pigment. These cells are now called **granulosa lutein cells** and under the influence of LH begin producing progesterone in greater quantities relative to estrogen. The theca interna cells become luteinized to **theca lutein cells** which also produce progesterone (Figs. 19-9, 19-10).

If pregnancy does not occur, the corpus luteum functions for only 10 to 12 days and then degenerates. The cells get progressively smaller and connective tissue invades, transforming the endocrine organ into a small scar, the **corpus albicans** (Fig. 19-11).

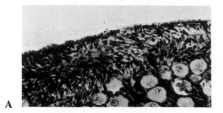

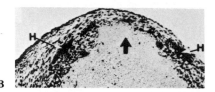

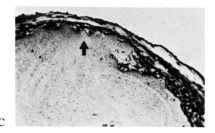

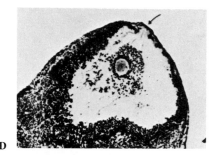

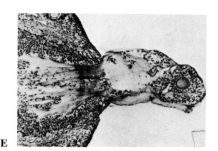

ATRETIC FOLLICLES

Most of the 400,000 oocytes that exist in the ovary at birth eventually degenerate. Several follicles begin to mature during each cycle, and of these usually only one is ovulated. Others degenerate, or undergo atresia, at various stages of maturation. Atretic follicles, therefore, may occur at any point in follicular development. Atretic primordial or primary follicles are characterized by eccentric oocytes with pyknotic (shrunken, dark) nuclei. Granulosa cells of atretic secondary follicles are shed into the antrum; they also have pyknotic nuclei. In advanced atresia, the only remnant of the follicle may be the tough zona pellucida.

EFFECT OF HORMONES ON THE OVARY

Two hormones from the anterior pituitary, FSH and LH, are involved in follicular growth, ovulation, and formation of the corpus luteum. FSH promotes growth of the follicles during the first half of the cycle, whereas LH controls the final burst of growth, increase in liquid folliculi, and rupture of the mature follicle. The formation of the corpus luteum is also under the direct control of LH.

The ovary itself produces two steroid hormones, **estrogen** and **progesterone.** At first, under FSH influence, granulosa cells convert the-

Fig. 19-8. Stages in the formation of the stigma in an ovulating follicle, rabbit ovary. A. Several hours before ovulation the stratum granulosum is still quite thick, as are the theca and tunica albuginea. B. One-half hour before ovulation hemostasis (*H*) appears in the region of the stigma. There is a significant thinning out of the follicular cells and stroma. C. A few minutes before rupture the follicular cells have almost disappeared, as has the stromal tissue in the region of the stigma (*arrow*). D. The stigmal cap lifts away (arrow) and the free cumulus oophorus streams toward the opening. E. Ovulation is completed but the viscous antral fluid still adheres to the site of rupture. (Courtesy of R. J. Blandau.)

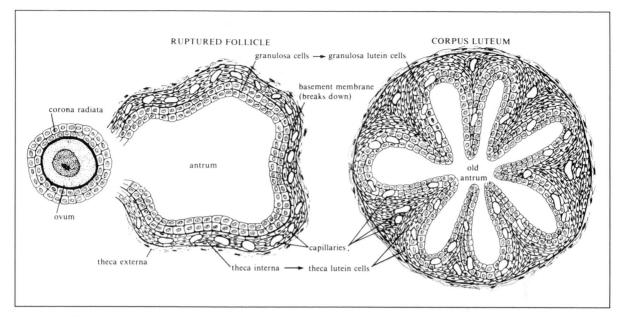

Fig. 19-9. Transformation of an ovulated follicle into a corpus luteum.

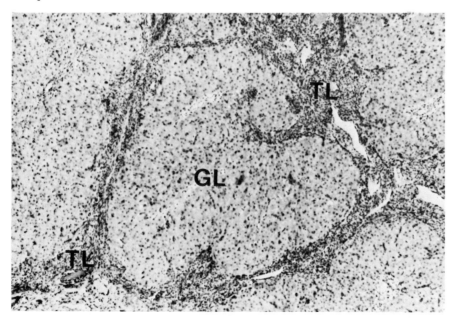

Fig. 19-10. A low-power light micrograph of a human corpus luteum. The predominant large granulosa lutein cells (*GL*) and the smaller, darker theca lutein cells (*TL*) occupy distinct regions within this large structure.

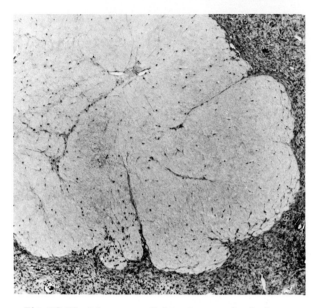

Fig. 19-11. A low-power light micrograph of a human corpus albicans. The degenerated corpus luteum has contracted and now consists of a fibrous mass composed primarily of collagen and fibroblasts.

Fig. 19-12. Regulation of gonadotropin secretion in the female, showing the interactions of neural and hormonal feedback controls. The development of the ovarian follicle is largely under control of FSH. Ovulation is brought about by LH. Estrogenic hormones have complex effects on the feedback control mechanisms of LH and FSH secretion. Depending upon dose, time course, and prior hormonal status, estrogens can either inhibit or stimulate the secretion of LH through effects at both hypothalamic and pituitary levels. Thus, there is evidence for both negative and positive feedback control. Progesterone also can either stimulate or inhibit GnRH secretion, but its effects at the pituitary level are relatively insignificant. Secretions of the GnRH-peptidergic neurons are in turn regulated by the biogenic-aminergic system, through which a variety of nonhormonal signals can influence reproductive function. Visual and olfactory stimuli and pineal factors can also influence gonadotropin secretion. FSH = follicle-stimulating hormone; LH = luteinizing hormone; GnRH = gonadotropin-releasing hormone. (From J. B. Martin, S. Reichlin, and G. M. Brown. *Clinical Endocrinology.* Philadelphia: F. A. Davis, 1977. Reproduced with permission.)

cal androgens to estrogen; later, under LH influence, granulosa cells produce progesterone. Estrogen secretion occurs throughout the 28-day cycle, peaking at ovulation. The high midcycle estrogen level stimulates hypothalamic secretion of GnRH, the common gonadotropin-releasing hormone. While GnRH seems capable of releasing both pituitary gonadotropins, it is more potent in releasing LH than FSH. Thus, after midcycle, FSH secretion declines and follicular growth ceases. The concomitant release of LH triggers ovulation of the mature follicle and its transformation into the corpus luteum. The regulation of gonadotropin secretion is illustrated and summarized in Figure 19-12.

Progesterone is secreted by the granulosa lutein cells of the corpus luteum. It is responsible

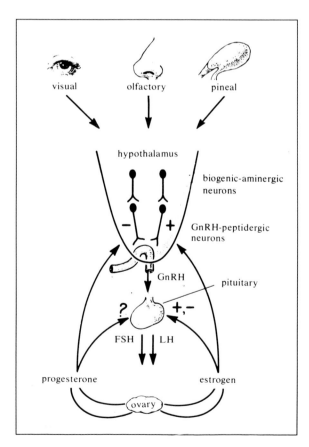

for changes in the glands and stroma of the uterine endometrium that occur in preparation for a possible pregnancy; these changes are discussed later in the chapter.

The Oviducts (Fallopian or Uterine Tubes)

The oviducts are paired muscular tubes that are 15 cm long and 6 to 8 mm in diameter. One end of the oviduct opens into the peritoneal cavity abutting the ovary, and the other end opens into the superior lateral part of the uterus. The oviduct is divisible into four major segments, starting at the ovary and working toward the uterus:

1. The **infundibulum** is the funnel-shaped opening close to the ovary. The mucosa is thrown up into long, fingerlike folds or **fimbriae** that closely embrace the ovarian surface.
2. The **ampulla** is the expanded intermediate section, also characterized by a highly folded mucosa, where fertilization usually occurs.
3. The **isthmus** is the narrow section adjacent to the uterine wall.
4. The **intramural region** or **pars interstitialis** is the part of the tube traversing the uterine wall.

The oviduct receives the ovum from the ovary, nourishes it and provides a chamber in which fertilization can occur, and then transports the ovum or zygote to the uterus. The tube has a three-layered organization along its length comprising:

1. **Mucosa.** The mucosa is a simple columnar epithelium consisting of two cell types, a **ciliated cell** and a narrow **peg cell.** All cilia beat toward the uterus and are partly reponsible, along with rhythmic contractions of the tube, for transport of the ovum. It has also been demonstrated that the corona radiata is required in order to form an attachment to the epithelium. Without it the ovum tends to spin in one place.

   Until recently, it was widely believed that both the numbers of ciliated cells as well as the rate of ciliary beat are greatly increased by steroid hormones, particularly progesterone, thus promoting transport of the ovum upon ovulation. However, more recent evidence shows that while this may be true for some animals, in humans the oviduct epithelium remains rather constant. The other cell type, the peg cell, is apparently secretory in nature and is thought to contribute nutritive material for the gametes. The epithelium is supported by a typical cellular lamina propria (Figs. 19-13, 19-14).
2. **Muscularis.** An inner circular layer and an outer longitudinal layer of smooth muscle give rise to muscular contractions, which help propel the ovum or zygote to the uterus.
3. **Serosa.** The oviduct is bounded by a sparse layer of connective tissue covered by a mesothelium.

The Uterus

The uterus is a pear-shaped, thick-walled organ that is flattened dorsoventrally. It is roughly 7 cm long, 5 cm wide at its broadest part, and 2.5 cm thick. The round part of the uterus is called the **body,** and the neck, which projects into the vagina, is termed the **cervix.** The uterus consists of three coats; from the outside in they are as follows:

1. The **serosa** is of typical organization and is continuous on either side of the uterus with the peritoneum of the broad ligament.
2. The **myometrium** is a muscular coat, 15 mm thick, consisting of smooth muscle and connective tissue. It has three poorly distinguishable layers. The middle layer, or **stratum vascularis,** contains numerous large blood vessels, the origin of which will be discussed later. The individual muscle cells of the nongravid uterus are about 60 μm long, but in pregnancy they increase to more than 500 μm.
3. The **endometrium** of the uterus undergoes cyclic changes in concert with ovarian hormones. It is lined by a simple columnar epithelium supported by lamina propria. Numer-

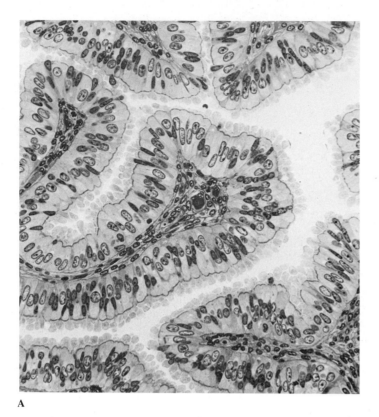

A

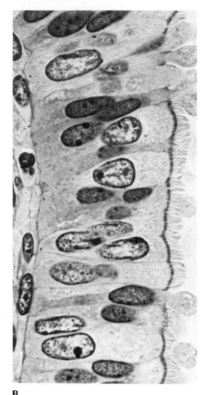

B

Fig. 19-13. Oviduct of a monkey. A. This light micrograph shows the highly folded mucosa of the ampulla. Note that there are two epithelial cell types, the
pale ciliated cells and the dark narrow peg cells. B.
A higher magnification of the epithelium. Note the
ciliated cells. Scattered among them are the peg cells,
which display apical blebs and are thought to secrete
a glandular product.

ous simple tubular glands composed of cells
similar to the surface lining penetrate the
lamina propria and reach almost to the myometrium. The endometrium can be divided
into two regions: the **stratum functionalis,** a
thick, superficial layer that undergoes periodic changes consisting of cyclic thickening
and shedding; and the **stratum basalis,** a
thin, deep layer unaffected by menstruation,
which remains to regenerate the functionalis
after it has been shed.

A knowledge of the uterine blood supply is essential in order to understand the mechanism by
which the functionalis hypertrophies, sheds,
and is regenerated (Fig. 19-15). The **uterine artery** branches into several **arcuate arteries,**
which run in the middle layer, or stratum vascularis, of the myometrium. These arcuates send
radial branches inward toward the endometrium; these branches are of two types:

1. **Straight** or **basal arteries** supply the stratum
   basalis of the endometrium, the deep portion
   that is unaffected by hormonal variation and
   remains after menstruation to regenerate the
   stratum functionalis.
2. **Coiled** or **spiral arteries** pass through the basalis to supply the functionalis. These vessels
   branch into arterioles that supply a capillary

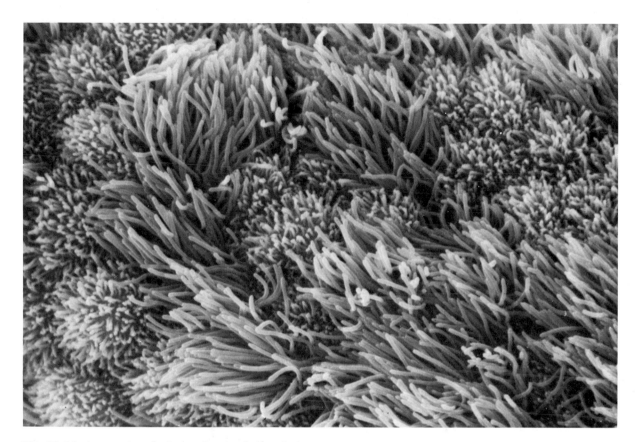

Fig. 19-14. A scanning electron micrograph showing a surface view of the monkey oviduct epithelium. Ciliated cells are interspersed with peg cells, which are covered with short microvilli. (Courtesy of R. J. Blandau.)

bed, which ramifies and anastomoses into thin-walled **lacunae.** The spiral arteries undergo repeated degeneration and regeneration and, as will be described, precipitate the actual shedding of the functionalis during the menstrual period.

During the child-bearing years, the endometrium passes through cyclic changes that are closely related to the maturation of an ovarian follicle, ovulation, and the establishment of a corpus luteum. These changes prepare the uterus for implantation. If implantation occurs, the en-

dometrium continues to develop. If a zygote does not implant, however, the endometrium breaks down and the tissue debris together with some blood is discharged as menstrual fluid. When the discharge ends, the uterine lining rapidly regenerates and a new cycle begins. The onset of menstruation is considered day 1 of the cycle, which can be divided into four segments (Fig. 19-16):

1. **Menstrual stage:** occupies the first 3 to 5 days
2. **Proliferative (estrogenic) stage:** termination of menstruation to 1 or 2 days postovulation
3. **Secretory (progestational or luteal) stage:** just after ovulation to the 26th or 27th day
4. **Premenstrual** or **ischemic stage:** 1 or 2 days in length, terminated by the onset of menstruation

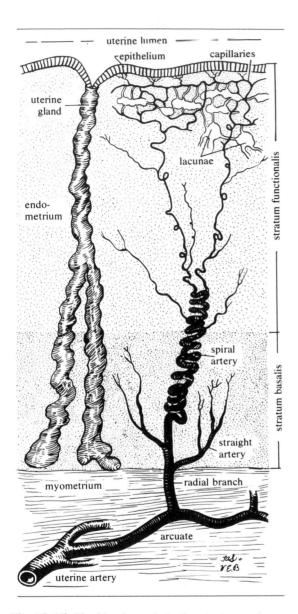

Fig. 19-15. The blood supply to the uterine endometrium. (From R. O. Greep and L. Weiss. *Histology* [4th ed.]. New York: McGraw-Hill, 1977. Reproduced with permission.)

After the stratum functionalis is shed during menstruation, it is reconstituted through these four stages, as described below.

1. Proliferative stage. The proliferative stage (Fig. 19-17A) represents regeneration of the endometrium from the narrow basal zone remaining after menstruation. Epithelial cells in the basal glands multiply and cover the raw surface of the mucosa. The glands increase in length, being generally straight and of uniform diameter, and coiled arteries grow into the regenerating tissue. The endometrium increases from a postmenstrual thickness of 0.5 mm to 2 or 3 mm, under the influence of estrogen produced by the growing ovarian follicles.

2. Secretory stage. A day or two after ovulation (Fig. 19-17B), the endometrium hypertrophies, reaching a thickness of 4 to 5 mm. The tissue becomes increasingly edematous and vascular, and the glands assume a corkscrew shape. The lumina of the glands dilate and become filled with a secretion rich in glycogen that will help to nourish the zygote during implantation.

3. Premenstrual stage. As a direct consequence of involution of the corpus luteum, the coiled arteries begin to constrict periodically, leading to stasis in the capillaries and periods of ischemia (Fig. 19-17C). The glands stop secreting, and the functionalis shrinks in size as a result of water loss. At this stage the functionalis appears more deeply stained because the cells of the stroma are more closely packed. This stage lasts only 1 to 2 days.

4. Menstrual stage. As the coiled arteries begin to constrict for longer periods of time, the walls of the capillaries they supply become ischemic

Fig. 19-17. Light micrographs of the human uterine endometrium. A. Proliferative stage. The developing glands are straight and relatively sparse. B. Secretory stage. The glands have become larger, assuming a corkscrew shape. C. Premenstrual stage. The stratum functionalis has shrunk due to water loss. It appears dark due to closer packing of stromal cells and hemostasis of blood.

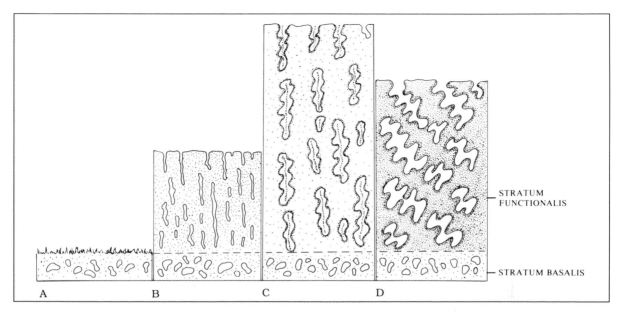

Fig. 19-16. Different stages of the uterine endometrium. A. End of menstrual stage. B. Proliferative stage. C. Secretory stage. D. Premenstrual stage.

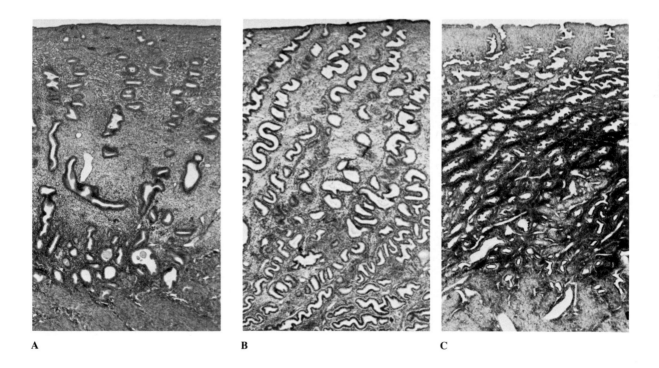

A   B   C

and rupture. The glands fragment, and blood, uterine fluid, and tissue debris are sloughed off from the endometrium and discharged through the vagina. Deep veins begin to bleed, and over a 4- to 5-day period the functionalis is lost. The cause of vascular constriction is hormone deficiency, in particular progesterone, precipitated by involution of the corpus luteum. It is important to remember that the straight arteries supplying the stratum basalis do not react to hormonal changes. This basal layer, therefore, remains viable, and when a new set of ovarian follicles begins to develop, mitosis of the epithelial cells in the glands of the stratum basalis regenerates the epithelial covering of the endometrium.

RELATIONSHIP OF MENSTRUATION TO OVULATION

1. The postmenstrual proliferative (estrogenic) stage correlates with follicular maturation.

Fig. 19-18. The relationship between ovarian and pituitary hormones, and their effect on the uterine endometrium. FSH = follicle-stimulating hormone; LH = luteinizing hormone.

The growing follicle secretes estrogen, which supports endometrial proliferation.
2. The secretory stage is mainly associated with growth of the corpus luteum, which secretes progesterone. Estrogen continues to be secreted during this stage.
3. Menstruation is precipitated by involution of the corpus luteum and withdrawal of progesterone (Fig. 19-18).

The Cervix

The cervix forms the lowest portion or neck of the uterus and encloses the cervical canal, 3 cm in length, which opens into the vagina. It is composed chiefly of dense connective tissue, with only about 15 percent smooth muscle. Its blood supply and mucosa show very little resemblance to the uterus proper. The mucosa of the canal, which is very complex, is arranged in a series of deep compound furrows formed from a single columnar mucus-secreting epithelium. Although the epithelial architecture does not change during the menstrual cycle, there are characteristic changes in both the quantity and consistency of

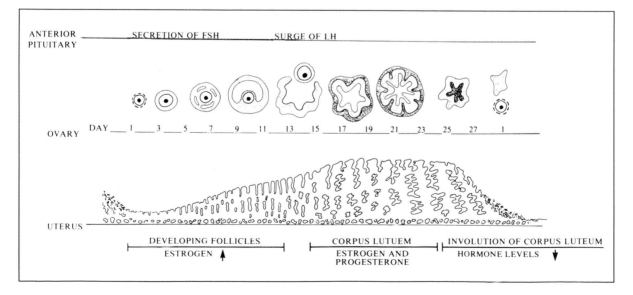

the cervical mucus that can be used as an indication of where an individual is in the cycle. The part of the cervix facing the vagina is lined by a stratified squamous nonkeratinizing epithelium.

PREGNANCY

Following ovulation, an ovum that is fertilized requires 3 to 5 days to reach the uterus, by which time it has developed into a **blastocyst.** During the next few days, during which the uterus is in the **luteal stage,** the blastocyst becomes embedded in the uterine mucosa and the chorion begins to secrete human chorionic gonadotropin (HCG), which prolongs the life of the corpus luteum beyond its normal, predetermined 10- to 12-day span. Since progesterone continues to be secreted, the endometrium is not shed and continues to develop into a more complex **gestational endometrium.** As the fetus develops, the **placenta** eventually takes over the production of progesterone, and when the corpus luteum of pregnancy finally involutes after several months, it leaves a large scar that may remain in the ovary for many years (**corpus albicans**).

The Placenta

Within the uterus the developing **zygote** develops through the **morula** stage to become a **blastocyst.** The blastocyst is characterized by a fluid-filled cavity and an inner cell mass both surrounded by a single layer of cells called the **trophoblast.** At this time the zona pellucida has disappeared and the blastocyst is prepared to attach to the uterine wall. Implantation begins when the blastocyst contacts the endometrium. During this first stage of implantation, the cells of the trophoblast proliferate and differentiate into an inner layer of **cytotrophoblast** cells, which are continuous with the inner cell mass, and an outer **syncytiotrophoblast** layer of fused cells.

The trophoblast enzymatically erodes the endometrial epithelial lining. By day 11 or 12 the blastocyst becomes completely embedded in the stroma of the compact layer of the endometrium.

The entry point of the blastocyst is initially indicated by a slight elevation in the endometrium where a small blood clot in the surface epithelium is visible. The entry is later reepithelialized by growth of surrounding epithelial cells. Although the blastocyst remains near the surface of the compact layer, the trophoblast continues to erode deeper into the endometrium. The stromal cells near the invading trophoblast hypertrophy and become filled with glycogen and lipids. They are now referred to as decidual cells. This stromal cell response to the trophoblast continues until the endometrial stroma of the entire uterus is involved. From that time it becomes known as the decidua. The zone between the blastocyst and the myometrium is the **decidua basalis;** the zone between the blastocyst and the endometrial epithelium is the **decidua capsularis.**

The syncytiotrophoblast begins secreting HCG which directs the corpus luteum to continue releasing estrogen and progesterone, two hormones that will ensure survival of the decidua. After 4 months the corpus luteum will deteriorate when the placenta is sufficiently developed to synthesize its own estrogen and progesterone. The syncytiotrophoblast also begins producing human chorionic somatomammotropin (HCS) which acts like prolactin (lactogenic hormone) to contribute to the growth of the mammary glands and subsequently to assist lactation.

Soon the inner cell mass becomes organized into a distinct embryonic disk with two germ layers: a layer of columnar cells known as the embryonic ectoderm and a layer of cuboidal cells known as the embryonic entoderm. The ectoderm expands to form the amniotic cavity. The entoderm expands to form the yolk sac. A third germ layer, the extraembryonic mesoderm, differentiates from the cytotrophoblast. Extracellular fluid-filled spaces produced by this mesoderm coalesce to form the extraembryonic coelom. The extraembryonic mesoderm proliferates and forms a lining along the interior surface of the trophoblast (surrounding the extraembryonic coelom) and along the external surfaces of the yolk sac and amniotic cavity. The trophoblast together with this internal lining of mesoderm is now called the **chorion.** The embryonic disk remains attached to the trophoblast at the site of the future placenta by a narrow cord of mesoderm called the **body stalk.**

During continued erosion by the trophoblast, maternal vessels (spiral arteries) in the decidua are ruptured and bleed into spaces around the syncytiotrophoblast. The chorion begins to grow and differentiate rapidly. Primary villi consisting of an inner core of cytotrophoblast and an outer lining of syncytiotrophoblast extend into these blood-filled intervillous spaces. Secondary villi are formed when the extraembryonic mesoderm grows into the cores of the primary villi. The villi in the body stalk region continue to proliferate dramatically until that region of the chorion, the **chorion frondosum,** is distinguished from the remainder of the chorion where villi have disappeared, the **chorion laeve.** Villi of the chorion frondosum continue to grow and branch. Most are suspended freely in the intervillous space but others called **anchoring villi** attach to the decidua to hold the developing placenta in position. The cytotrophoblasts and syncytiotrophoblasts continue to proliferate until they line the entire surface of the intervillous space including the decidua.

Capillaries differentiate from the mesoderm in the core of each villus and establish connections with capillaries in the wall of the chorion. Eventually umbilical veins in the body stalk, soon to become the umbilical cord, will carry oxygenated blood to the developing embryonic heart. Deoxygenated blood will return in the umbilical arteries. About the fourth month, the cytotrophoblast begins to disintegrate until by the fifth month only the syncytiotrophoblast layer remains. Thus, in the mature placenta the fetal blood is separated from the maternal blood in the intervillous spaces by the endothelial lining of the capillaries in the core of the villi, by a small amount of mucous connective tissue derived from the extraembryonic mesoderm, and by the syncytiotrophoblast which has become extremely thin. These three elements constitute the placental barrier (Fig. 19-19). This thin layer enhances the exchange of oxygen and nutrients between the maternal and fetal circulations and replaces diffusion across the extraembryonic coelom as the major metabolic link with the mother.

In addition, microvilli can be seen with the electron microscope on the surface of the syncytiotrophoblast to enhance its available surface area for various types of transport. Exchange of gases, ions, and small molecules across the placental barrier takes place by diffusion. However, the occurrence of vacuoles indicates that larger molecules are exchanged via pinocytosis or similar transport systems. Maternal antibodies are known to cross the placental barrier and confer immunity to the fetus in this manner. Consequently drugs used during pregnancy should be closely scrutinized for possible deleterious effects on the fetus. Any doubts about their effect should be sufficient reason to avoid their use. At birth separation of the placenta occurs along the spongy layer of the decidua basalis.

Umbilical Cord

Growth of the amniotic cavity within the extraembryonic coelom eventually brings the amnion and chorion into contact and they fuse except around the body stalk and yolk sac which the amnion surrounds and confines to within the eventual umbilical cord. The mesenchyme within the cord develops into mucous connective tissue filling the available space around the enclosed pair of umbilical arteries, a single umbilical vein, the vitelline duct, and remnants of the allantois. The umbilical arteries will carry the deoxygenated blood from the fetus to the chorion. Since blood pressure is not high in these arteries, their muscular walls will not be as thick as in typical adult arteries elsewhere. The umbilical vein (its partner deteriorated earlier) will carry oxygenated blood to the fetus.

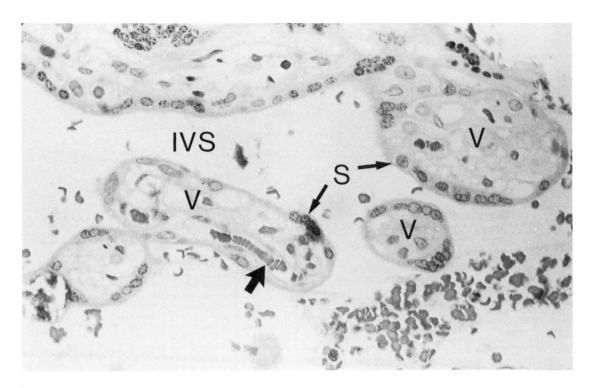

Fig. 19-19. Human placenta showing sections of villi (*V*). The villi are lined only by syncytiotrophoblast (*S*) as the cytotrophoblast has degenerated at this time. Within the connective tissue cores of the villi are fetal capillaries (*arrow*) containing blood cells. Maternal erythrocytes occupy the intervillous spaces (*IVS*).

The Vagina

The vagina (Fig. 19-20) is a musculofibrous sheath lined by a mucous membrane. Its wall consists of three coats: mucosa, muscularis, and fibrosa. Longitudinal ridges are present on both anterior and posterior walls, from which rugae extend laterally. The vagina is lined by a stratified squamous nonkeratinized epithelium, rich in glycogen, supported by a cellular lamina propria that may contain lymph nodules. The muscularis is not gathered into discernible layers but runs predominantly longitudinally and is continuous with the uterine myometrium. The fibrosa consists of dense connective tissue. There are no glands in the vagina; lubrication is a combined result of cervical mucus secretion and local secretion from the **glands of Bartholin** and the lesser mucous glands situated in the **vestibule,** the space at the vaginal orifice flanked by the labia minora.

THE MAMMARY GLANDS

At the sixth week of embryonic life, the ectoderm thickens along two lines running from axilla to groin. The epithelium along these "milk lines" can potentially grow down into the underlying mesenchyme to form mammary glands. In humans, only one pair of glands usually develops. The down-growing epithelial cells form a cluster from which up to 20 separate cords of epithelial

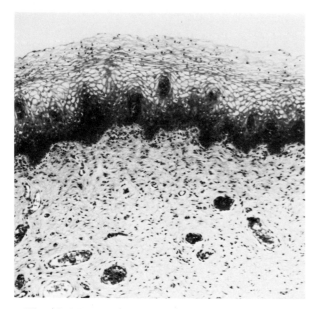

Fig. 19-20. The mucosa of the human vagina. The more superficial layers of the nonkeratinized stratified squamous epithelium appear pale due to leaching out of glycogen in histologic preparation. The connective tissue below is dense, collagenous, and highly vascular.

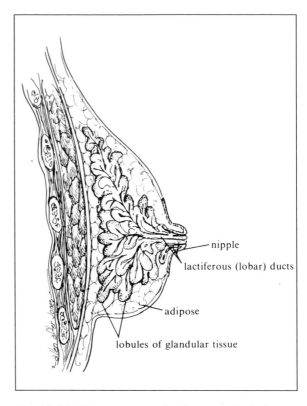

nipple

lactiferous (lobar) ducts

adipose

lobules of glandular tissue

Fig. 19-21. The mammary gland is composed of separate lobes, each of which is an independent compound alveolar gland whose ducts join into progressively larger ducts. Alveoli bud off the duct system in response to the hormonal changes of pregnancy and lactation.

cells invade the underlying tissue. Each cord develops into a lobe comprised of the rudiments of a compound tubular exocrine gland, which empties through its own lobar (lactiferous) duct into the nipple.

The lobes are separated by layers of connective tissue. Each lobe is provided with a **lactiferous duct** containing a local dilation beneath the areola and nipple, called the **lactiferous sinus.** After puberty, each sinus gives rise to several groups of smaller interlobular ducts. The development of the duct system and accumulation of fat account for enlargement of the mammary glands at puberty. No further mammary development occurs until pregnancy. During pregnancy, the smaller interlobular ducts give rise to the secretory portions of the glands called **alveoli.** Groups of alveoli drained by a small interlobular duct constitute a lobule (Fig. 19-21).

Areas of the Mammary Gland

STROMA

The interlobar and interlobular septa consist primarily of dense irregular collagen fibers and some elastic fibers. The septa contribute to the suspension of the mammary gland by being anchored in the sternum and epimysium of the pectoral muscles and inserting into the overlying dermis. The major duct system courses through these septa and is surrounded by circumferentially oriented collagen fibers. The smallest ductules and alveoli within each lobule are surrounded by loose connective tissue. Adipose tissue is interposed between the septa. Adipocytes are prominent in the inactive gland, but become depleted of fat during pregnancy and lactation, providing more space for developing alveoli.

A considerable amount of smooth muscle inserts into the nipple and areola. Free nerve endings are present in the dermis of the nipple as well. These are responsible for nipple erection during tactile and sexual stimulation and exposure to cold.

A significant lymphatic drainage is present around the lobules, but not within them. Larger lymphatics course through the connective tissue septa and drain the mammary glands into the axillary lymph nodes.

DUCTS

The lumina of the outer segments of the lactiferous ducts are continuous with the nipple surface and are lined by stratified squamous epithelium. The presence of melanocytes in the duct epithelium of this region confers a pigmentation not found in the deeper portions of the duct system. Melanocytes are also responsible for the

Fig. 19-22. The human mammary gland. A. Inactive state. The inactive mammary is composed primarily of dense irregular collagenous connective tissue and adipose cells. Only the ducts of the glandular tissue are present. B. Lactating state. The active mammary contains an extensive system of alveoli that replace most of the connective tissue.

A

B

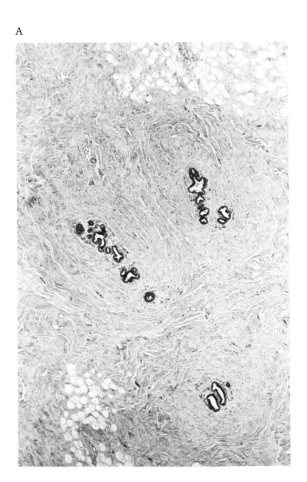

dark appearance of the nipple and areola. In the deeper regions of the ducts, the stratified squamous epithelium is progressively replaced by a double layer of cells consisting of a superficial columnar or cuboidal layer and a basal layer of myoepithelial cells. Myoepithelial cells propel milk through the ducts and into the sinuses.

PARENCHYMA

The nature of the parenchyma depends on whether the mammary gland is active (lactating) or inactive. In the inactive gland, the glandular tissue is sparse, consisting chiefly of little islands of ducts. Dense connective and adipose tissue compose the bulk of the tissue (Fig. 19-22A).

During pregnancy, the interlobular ducts bud and alveoli are formed. The connective and adipose tissue decrease strikingly in amount and are replaced by alveoli (Fig. 19-22B). The alveoli are lined by a simple cuboidal epithelium and contain the usual organelles found in a protein-synthesizing exocrine cell. In addition, their cytoplasm contains numerous lipid droplets that are extracted during tissue preparation, leaving a vacuolated cytoplasm. Myoepithelial cells beneath the basement membrane of the alveoli contract in the response to hormonal stimulation, ejecting milk into the ducts.

Milk consists of an aqueous suspension of proteins (primarily casein and lactalbumin), lipids (triglycerides), and carbohydrates. Most of these are synthesized by the alveolar epithelium. Other components, including vitamins, salts, and minerals, are selectively transferred from the blood. Milk immunoglobulins, especially secretory IgA, provide passive immunity for the suckling infant against various microorganisms. Secretory IgA concentrations are particularly high in colostrum.

Hormonal Influence on Breast Development

A rudimentary duct system develops in both males and females, as indicated previously. In the female, however, a rapid expansion of the duct system and an increase in connective and adipose tissue begins at puberty. The growth of the breasts at puberty and their differentiation during pregnancy are dependent not only on estrogen and progesterone, but also on a number of pituitary hormones including prolactin, somatotropin, ACTH, and thyrotropic hormone, as well as the pancreatic factor, insulin. The secretion of prolactin, which is absolutely essential for the maintenance of lactation, is maintained by a neurohumoral reflex. The afferent sensory stimulus set up by suckling relays to the hypothalamic nuclei, which manufacture prolactin-releasing factor. After birth, several days of nursing are required to stimulate full secretory development of alveoli. Cessation of suckling results in a decreased prolactin level and involution of the alveolar components of the mammary glands. After several months nearly all the alveoli will have been resorbed, and the duct system will remain as before lactation.

The act of suckling not only promotes prolactin release, ensuring maintenance of the functional lactating state, but also sends afferent stimuli to the hypothalamus, where the oxytocin-producing cells are located. This results in release of the hormone **oxytocin** from the neurohypophysis. Oxytocin stimulates contraction of the myoepithelial cells, ejecting milk from the alveoli into the duct system, where it becomes available for nursing.

NATIONAL BOARD TYPE QUESTIONS

For the following, select
    A. if only *1, 2, and 3* are correct.
    B. if only *1 and 3* are correct.
    C. if only *2 and 4* are correct.
    D. if only *4* is correct.
    E. if *all* are correct.

  1. Which of the following is (are) characteristic of a secondary follicle?
    1. It contains ovum which is in the prophase of its first meiotic division.

2. It is entirely vascularized.

3. It contains a fluid-filled antrum.

4. It secretes progesterone.

2. The corpus luteum can be maintained by which of the following?

1. Luteinizing hormone (LH)

2. Oxytocin

3. Chorionic gonadotropin

4. Follicle-stimulating hormone

3. Which of the statements regarding the human ovarian epithelium is (are) correct?

1. It is a simple columnar type.

2. The ratio of cell types is under endocrine control.

3. It contains both ciliated and secretory cells.

4. The rate of ciliary beat is under endocrine control.

4. The proliferative phase of the uterine endometrium is characterized by

1. increased secretion of uterine glands.

2. the endometrium reaching its full thickness.

3. temporal correspondence with formation of the corpus luteum.

4. rising levels of estrogen.

5. Which of the following statements regarding the mammary gland is (are) correct?

1. The inactive mammary contains only the duct portions of glands.

2. The lactating gland requires prolactin for ejection of milk.

3. Milk is rich in both lipid and protein.

4. Fat cells increase in size in the active mammary.

6. Regarding the blood supply of the uterine endometrium, which of the following is (are) correct?

1. The stratum basalis and stratum functionalis have a separate arterial supply.

2. The blood supply to the cervix is similar to that of the uterus proper.

3. The menstrual stage is initiated by prolonged constriction of the spiral arteries.

4. Spiral arteries remain intact through menstruation.

7. The syncytiotrophoblast

1. secretes chorionic gonadotropin.

2. is basal to the cytotrophoblast.

3. is formed from cells of the trophoblast.

4. is part of the inner cell mass.

8. The placental barrier in the mature placenta consists of

1. endothelium of fetal capillaries.

2. syncytiotrophoblast.

3. small amounts of mucous connective tissue in the villi.

4. cytotrophoblast.

9. What mechanism(s) is (are) responsible for the transport of the ovum or zygote down the oviduct?

1. Ciliary beating

2. Muscular contraction

3. Corona radiata

4. Chemotaxis

Select the one best response for the following.

10. Follicular atresia occurs

A. only after the first menstrual period.

B. only after menopause.

C. even before birth.

D. only in primordial follicles.

E. in all follicular stages except in mature (graafian) follicles.

Select the response most closely associated with each numbered item.

A. Hypothalamus

B. Pituitary

C. Both

D. Neither

11. Subject to positive and negative feedback in terms of estrogen influence on LH production

12. Cellular source of oxytocin production

ANNOTATED ANSWERS

1. B. The hallmark of a secondary follicle is the presence of an antrum. Oogonia enter the first meiotic division and remain arrested in prophase until ovulation. Complete vascu-

larization and production of progesterone are characteristic of the corpus luteum.

2. B. The corpus luteum is maintained by LH. In case of pregnancy, the corpus luteum continues to be supported by chorionic gonadotropins of the placenta.

3. B. The simple columnar epithelium of the oviduct contains ciliated cells, and peg cells, which are secretory. Both the ratio of cell types and rate of ciliary beating remain constant in humans.

4. D. Rising levels of estrogen induce the proliferation of the endometrium. The other statements refer to the secretory phase.

5. B. The resting mammary contains only the ducts of glandular tissue. During lactation the mammary contains fewer fat cells (making room for alveoli). Oxytocin causes the milk ejection reflex. The product is rich in lipid and protein as well as many other nutrients transferred from the mother's blood.

6. B. The stratum basalis and stratum functionalis have a separate blood supply. Only the functionalis layer is shed, initiated by constriction of spiral arteries. Eventually, this layer, including the arteries, is regenerated. The cervix is histologically different and undergoes only minor cyclic changes.

7. B. The cytotrophoblast is basal to the syncytiotrophoblast and continuous with the inner cell mass.

8. A. During the fourth month of gestation the cytotrophoblast begins to disintegrate until it has disappeared by the fifth month.

9. A. Transport of the ovum or zygote down the oviduct is promoted by ciliary beating and contractions of the muscularis. The corona radiata provides a means of attachment to the oviduct wall. There is no evidence that chemotaxis plays any role in this process.

10. C. Follicular atresia occurs as soon as follicles are present, even before birth, and occurs throughout the reproductive life of the woman (until menopause). Atresia can occur at any stage of follicle development, including the mature follicle.

11. C. Estrogen provides positive and negative feedback to both the hypothalamus and pituitary in its regulation of LH production.

12. A. Oxytocin is produced in the cells of the hypothalamus and is transported to the posterior pituitary where it is released.

BIBLIOGRAPHY

Adams, E. C., and A. T. Hertig. Studies on the human corpus luteum: I. Observations on the ultrastructure of development and regression of the luteal cells during the menstrual cycle. *J. Cell Biol.* 41:696, 1969.

Adams, E. C., and A. T. Hertig. Studies on the human corpus luteum: II. Observations on the ultrastructure of luteal cells during pregnancy. *J. Cell Biol.* 41:716, 1969.

Anderson, E., and D. Albertini. Gap junctions between the oocyte and companion cells in the mammalian ovary. *J. Cell Biol.* 71:680, 1976.

Baker, T. G. A quantitative and cytological study of oogenesis in the rhesus monkey. *J. Anat.* 100:761, 1966.

Balboni, G. C. Histology of the Ovary. In V. H. T. James, M. Serio, and G. Giusti (eds.), *The Endocrine Function of the Human Ovary*. London: Academic, 1976.

Banarjee, M. R. Responses of mammary cells to hormones. *Int. Rev. Cytol.* 47:1, 1976.

Beer, A. E., and R. E. Billingham. *The Immunobiology of Mammalian Reproduction*. Englewood Cliffs, N.J.: Prentice-Hall, 1976.

Blandau, R. J. (ed.). *The Biology of the Blastocyst*. Chicago: University of Chicago, 1971.

Blandau, R. J., and K. Moghissi. *The Biology of the Cervix*. Chicago: University of Chicago, 1973.

Brenner, R. M. The Biology of Oviduct Cilia. In E. S. E. Hafes and R. J. Blandau (eds.), *The Mammalian Oviduct*. Chicago: University of Chicago, 1969. P. 203.

Crisp, T. M., D. A. Dersouky, and F. R. Denys. The fine structure of the human corpus luteum of early pregnancy and during the progestational phase of the menstrual cycle. *Am. J. Anat.* 127:37, 1970.

Enders, A. C., and W. R. Lyon. Observations on the fine structure of lutein cells: II. The effect of hypophysectomy and mammotrophic hormones in the rat. *J. Cell Biol.* 22:127, 1964.

Enders, A. C., and S. Schlafke. Cytological aspects of trophoblast-uterine interaction in early implantation. *Am. J. Anat.* 125:1, 1969.

Finn, C. A., and D. G. Porter. *The Uterus. Handbooks of Reproductive Biology.* London: Paul Elek, 1974.

Gay, V. L., A. R. Midgley, and G. D. Niswender. Patterns of gonadotropin secretion associated with ovulation. *Fed. Proc.* 29:1880, 1970.

Greep, R. O. Histology, Histochemistry and Ultrastructure of the Adult Ovary. In D. E. Smith (ed.), *The Ovary.* Baltimore: Williams & Wilkins, 1962.

Gregoire, A. T., O. Kandil, and W. J. Ledger. The glycogen content of human vaginal epithelial tissue. *Fertil. Steril.* 22:64, 1971.

Guraya, S. S. Morphology, histochemistry and biochemistry of human oogenesis and ovulation. *Int. Rev. Cytol.* 37:121, 1974.

Guraya, S. S. Recent advances in the morphology, histochemistry and biochemistry of the developing mammalian ovary. *Int. Rev. Cytol.* 51:49, 1977.

Hafez, E. S. E. (ed.). *Scanning Electron Microscopic Atlas of Mammalian Reproduction.* New York: Springer-Verlag, 1975.

Hebb, C., and J. L. Linzell. Innervation of the mammary gland. A histochemical study in the rabbit. *Histochem. J.* 2:491, 1970.

Jones, R. E. (ed.). *The Vertebrate Ovary.* New York: Plenum, 1978.

Long, J. A. Corpus luteum of pregnancy in the rat—ultrastructural and cytochemical observations. *Biol. Reprod.* 8:87, 1973.

McCann, S. M. Luteinizing-hormone-releasing-hormone. *N. Engl. J. Med.* 296:797, 1977.

Martin, C. R. Hormones and Reproduction. In C. R. Martin (ed.), *Textbook of Endocrine Physiology.* Baltimore: Williams & Wilkins, 1976.

Mills, E. S., and Y. J. Topper. Some ultrastructural effects of insulin, hydrocortisone and prolactin on mammary gland explants. *J. Cell Biol.* 44:310, 1970.

Moghissi, K. S. The function of the cervix in fertility. *Fertil. Steril.* 23:295, 1972.

Odor, D. L. The ultrastructure of unilaminar follicles of the hamster ovary. *Am. J. Anat.* 116:493, 1965.

Patek, E., L. Nilsson, and E. Johannisson. Scanning electron microscopic study of the human fallopian tube: I. The proliferative and secretory stages. *Fertil. Steril.* 23:459, 1972.

Patek, E., L. Nilsson, and E. Johannisson. Scanning electron microscopic study of the human fallopian tube: II. Fetal life, reproductive life, and post menopause. *Fertil. Steril.* 23:719, 1972.

Schlafke, S., and A. C. Enders. Cellular basis of interaction between trophoblast and uterus at implantation. *Biol. Reprod.* 12:41, 1975.

Schmidt-Matthiesen, H. *The Normal Human Endometrium.* New York: McGraw-Hill, 1963.

Segal, S. J. The physiology of human reproduction. *Sci. Am.* 231:52, 1974.

Van Blerkom, J., and P. Motta. *Cellular Basis of Mammalian Reproduction.* Baltimore: Urban & Schwarzenberg, 1978.

Vickery, B. H., and J. P. Bennett. The cervix and its secretions in mammals. *Physiol. Rev.* 48:135, 1968.

Villee, D. B. Development of endocrine function in the human placenta and fetus. *N. Engl. J. Med.* 281:473, 1969.

Vorherr, H. *The Breast. Morphology, Physiology, and Lactation.* New York: Academic, 1974.

Winsatt, W. A. Some comparative aspects of implantation. *Biol. Reprod.* 12:1, 1975.

Wooding, F. B. P. The mechanism of secretion of the milk fat globule. *J. Cell Sci.* 9:805, 1971.

20 Organs of Special Sense

The special sense organs associated with other organ systems have already been discussed in detail. The olfactory mucosa is described with the nasal cavity in the chapter on the respiratory system, the taste buds with the tongue in the chapter on the accessory digestive organs, and the tactile receptors in the chapter on the integument. In this chapter we discuss the structure and function of the two remaining organs of special sense, the eye and the ear, both of which are anatomically independent of other organ systems and, due to their complexity, require special attention.

THE EYE

The human eye is a roughly spherical structure 2.5 cm in diameter that is suspended by a series of ligaments in a bony **orbit.** The bony orbit is lined with a periosteum. Six extrinsic ocular muscles give the eye a wide range of mobility to scan a field and to track moving objects. The orbit also contains the **lacrimal gland,** a serous gland which continually lubricates the anterior surface of the eye, the nerves and blood vessels supplying the eye, and a cushioned pad of fat and connective tissue. The lids shade the eyes and protect them from desiccation, and a duct system drains the continuous secretion from the lacrimal glands into the nasal cavity.

The eyeball itself is lightproof except for its anterior transparent surface, the **cornea.** Light passing through the cornea is refracted by a series of different media and focused by the convex lens as an inverted image on the photosensitive lining called the **retina** at the back of the eye.

It is common to compare the eye to a camera, since there is an analogy between the three basic layers of each. The camera body corresponds to the external **corneoscleral coat;** the black lining to the vascular **uvea;** and the image-recording film to the retina. In addition, the diaphragm of the camera has a counterpart in the **iris** of the eye, which controls both the amount of entering light and the resultant depth of field. The eye, however, is focused by changing the convexity of its lens, whereas a camera lens is moved back and forth. The geography of the eye (Fig. 20-1) is outlined below so that the interrelationship of the various parts can be appreciated before each area is treated in more detail.

Geography of the Eye

MAJOR LAYERS OF THE EYE

The three major layers of the eye are as follows:

1. **Corneoscleral layer** (tunica fibrosa). The fibrous outer supportive coat of the eye com-

prises the **sclera,** a dense connective tissue covering the posterior four-fifths of the eye, and the **cornea,** a transparent connective tissue covering the anterior fifth of the eye. The sclera and the cornea are histologically distinct structures that are continuous with each other at a transition zone termed the **limbus.**

2. **Uvea** (tunica vasculosa). The middle coat is composed of three continuous structures, the choroid, the ciliary body, and the iris. These structures function both to exclude light and to form a nutritive layer, housing blood vessels. The **choroid** is an extremely vascular, highly pigmented connective tissue lining the back of the eye as far as the scalloped edge of the retina (ora serrata). The **ciliary body** is the intermediate part of the uvea, extending from the ora serrata posteriorly to the edge of the iris anteriorly. Its epithelial covering and underlying connective tissue are highly folded in the area of the **pars plicata,** which is responsible for secretion of the **aqueous humor.** Beneath the connective tissue is the **ciliary muscle,** a smooth muscle that inserts onto the lens by *zonular fibers* and causes

Fig. 20-1. An eye cut in a meridional plane that passes through the equator of the eye horizontally, dividing the eye into an upper and a lower half.

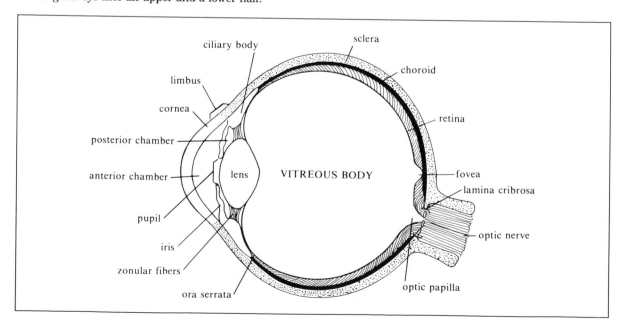

accommodation of the lens for the focusing of near objects. The **iris** is the most anterior part of the uvea, originating at the angle of the anterior chamber where the ciliary body terminates. It consists of a pigmented disk with a central aperture, the **pupil,** which rests on the lens and can vary in diameter in response to light.

3. **Retina** (tunica interna). The retina is a complex, photosensitive structure that is embryonically derived from the optic vesicle, an extension of the embryonic forebrain. It lines the back of the eye, terminating at the ora serrata, and is responsible for transducing light stimuli to nerve impulses, which are relayed through the optic nerve to the thalamus and then to the visual cortex.

INTERIOR CHAMBERS OF THE EYE

Anterior to the Lens

The interior portion of the eye lying in front of the lens is divided into two compartments. The **anterior chamber** of the eye is the space between cornea and iris, while the **posterior chamber** lies between iris and lens. Both chambers are filled with aqueous humor, a modified plasma filtrate that is extremely low in protein. The aqueous humor is secreted by the epithelium of the ciliary body (pars plicata), which lines the lateral aspect of the posterior chamber. The aqueous humor passes through the pupil to fill the anterior chamber and then percolates through a system of thin-walled vessels or **trabeculae** into one or more circular channels, called collectively **Schlemm's canal,** which drain into the ciliary vein. This drainage pathway is discussed later in the chapter in reference to the limbus. The flow rate of the aqueous humor is 2 μl per minute.

Posterior to the Lens

The large interior compartment of the eye bounded anteriorly by the lens and posteriorly by the retina is termed the **vitreous body.** The vitreous is a transparent, jellylike connective tissue comprising a small number of collagen fibrils embedded in a matrix of hyaluronic acid. This firm, transparent pad refracts light as well as cushioning and protecting the retina from shock and vibration that could cause it to detach from the choroid layer, leading to partial blindness. The vitreous becomes more fluid with advancing age. Occasionally, suspended debris causes motile opacities that float in front of the retina and appear as spots before the eyes.

The Corneoscleral Coat

SCLERA

The sclera is a tough, opaque fibrous coat about 0.5 mm thick that is continuous with the cornea and covers the posterior four-fifths of the eyeball. It consists of bundles of collagen fibrils that run parallel to the surface of the eye, branching and anastomosing to form a meshwork of great strength. The fibrils are embedded in a typical ground substance and maintained by fibroblasts. The dense sclera forms the point of attachment for the ligaments of the six voluntary extraocular muscles (Fig. 20-2), which are responsible for movements of the eyeball in its bony socket. In addition, the sclera maintains the eye, whose interior is composed largely of a gel (the vitreous body), in a rigid shape, which is of utmost importance optically.

The optic nerve fibers converge in a bundle at the posterior wall of the eyeball forming a slightly elevated **optic disk (optic papilla;** Fig. 20-3; see also Fig. 20-1). Immediately beyond the disk the nerve fibers exit from the eyeball by penetrating a perforated region of the sclera called the **lamina cribrosa** (L. *cribrum,* "sieve"). Also at this point, the outer layer of the sclera becomes continuous with the dural sheath of the optic nerve. Within the retina, optic nerve fibers are unmyelinated but beyond the lamina cribrosa they become myelinated, which accounts for the abrupt increase in bulk of the optic nerve compared with its nerve fibers emanating from the inner layer of the retina and converging at the optic disk. Although the sclera is poorly vascularized, it is penetrated by ciliary blood vessels traveling to the middle layer of the eye.

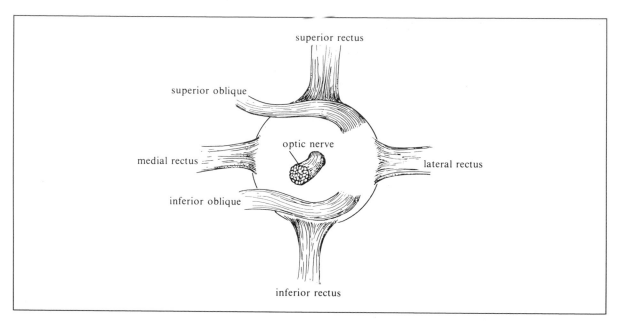

Fig. 20-2. The six voluntary extraocular muscles as seen from the posterior aspect of the eyeball.

CORNEA

The cornea (Fig. 20-4) is an avascular, transparent window forming the anterior fifth of the eye (see Fig. 20-1). It is composed of the following five layers, from outermost inward:

1. A **stratified squamous nonkeratinizing epithelium** forms the outer boundary. It is approximately five cells thick and has a unique, smooth surface. It is replete with an abundance of free nerve endings making it extremely sensitive.
2. **Bowman's membrane,** an acellular, densely packed layer of fine collagen fibrils, lies immediately beneath the epithelium.
3. The **stroma** represents 90 percent of the corneal thickness and is largely responsible for its shape, resistance, and transparency. It is composed of several layers of collagen fibrils in a precisely ordered configuration. Each layer of fibrils runs parallel to the surface of the cornea and for its entire length. The fibrils run at different angles to each other in successive layers, however, forming a transparent window of tremendous tensile strength. All of the fibrils are of uniform size and spacing and are embedded in a ground substance rich in chondroitin sulfate and keratin sulfate, which helps to make the cornea transparent and probably contributes to its ability to swell reversibly.
4. **Descemet's membrane** is an acellular, collagenous layer 10 μm thick with a small elastic component that allows it to accommodate in length to the cornea, when it temporarily swells, as will be described.
5. An **endothelium,** consisting of one layer of cuboidal cells, covers the posterior aspect of the cornea.

The transparency of the cornea is probably due to a combination of factors, including the smoothness of the epithelium, the absence of blood vessels, the uniform organization of collagen fibrils in the stroma, and the type of ground

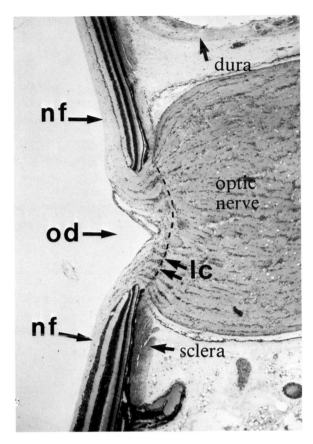

Fig. 20-3. Low-power micrograph of a section passing through the posterior wall of the eye where the optic nerve exits. At this point the inner sclera is perforated, forming the lamina cribrosa (*lc*) through which optic nerve fibers (*nf*) from the retina pass. The optic disk (*od*) is the point where the nerve fibers from the retina converge to form the optic nerve. The outer part of the sclera becomes continuous with the dural lining of the optic nerve.

substance. The bounding epithelium and endothelium help to maintain the state of hydration of the ground substance, which in turn maintains the spacing of the collagen fibrils. In the case of corneal abrasion, for instance, in which a small piece of epithelium is removed from the cornea, the ground substance under that region swells with concomitant disruption

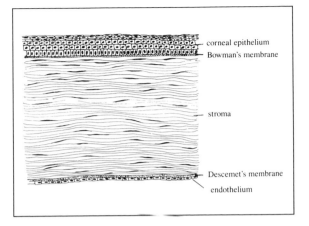

Fig. 20-4. A section through the human cornea revealing the characteristic five layers.

of spacing between collagen fibrils, which results in opacity. Fortunately, the corneal epithelium regenerates quickly, swelling diminishes, and transparency is restored. The cornea is both the first refractive surface contributing to the object image and also a rigid protective layer for the underlying tissues. The cornea is remarkable in its capacity to undergo transplantation into allogeneic recipients without immunologic rejection; the lack of blood vessels may prevent the host's immune cells from attacking the graft. The metabolic needs of the avascular cornea and the avascular lens are met by the aqueous humor, which carries nutrients and bathes the cornea and lens.

LIMBUS

The zone of transition between cornea and sclera is called the **limbus.** At this point the conjunctival epithelium, which is the mucous membrane covering both the anterior aspect of the sclera (**bulbar conjunctiva**) and the underside of the lids (**palpebral conjunctiva**), joins with the corneal epithelium, which is the covering for the anterior portion of the eye (Fig. 20-5). Both the palpebral and bulbar conjunctiva contain goblet cells which produce the lubricating mucus on the eyeball. The conjunctival epithelium is four

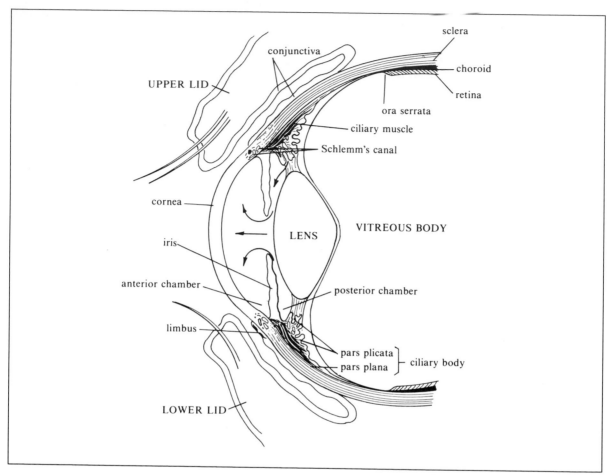

Fig. 20-5. An eye cut in longitudinal section showing the relationship of the eyeball in the conjunctiva. The conjunctiva lines the underside of the eyelids and continues as a reflection covering the anterior aspect of the sclera as far as the corneal epithelium. The arrows indicate the direction of flow of the aqueous humor. The aqueous humor is formed by the pars plicata of the ciliary body and fills the posterior chamber, percolating through the pupil to fill the anterior chamber. In the region of the limbus, at the angle of the anterior chamber, the aqueous humor drains into a trabecular meshwork and then into Schlemm's canal, which empties into the ciliary vein.

to five cells thick except at the limbus, where it suddenly doubles in thickness. Beneath the epithelium is a **trabecular meshwork** that is continuous with Descemet's membrane and the subjacent endothelium. Anterior and lateral to the network are one to several channels, lined by endothelium, that circumscribe the entire cornea and are known as **Schlemm's canal (si-nus venosus sclerae)**. As previously indicated, Schlemm's canal receives aqueous humor from the trabeculae and drains it into the anterior chamber into episcleral vessels. If drainage is blocked, intraocular pressure rises, resulting in a condition known as **glaucoma.** For more about the formation of aqueous humor, see Ciliary Body below.

The Uvea

CHOROID

The choroid is sandwiched between the sclera and the retina. It consists of a heavily pigmented layer of epithelial cells (pigment epithelium) that abut the retina and rest on a basement membrane (**Bruch's membrane**). Under this membrane is a heavily vascularized and pigmented connective tissue adjoining the sclera (Fig. 20-6).

Pigment Epithelium

The **pigment epithelium** is a single layer of cuboidal epithelial cells containing melanin pigment. The epithelium rests on a basement membrane that was formerly considered to demarcate

the outer limit of the choroid. The cytoplasmic processes of the pigment epithelial cells interdigitate with processes of the photoreceptor cells (rods and cones) of the retina and phagocytize worn-out membranous lamellae of the outer segments of the rods, which are being continuously renewed. Because the pigment epithelium is so closely associated with the retina, some texts treat it as a layer of the retina. On the other hand, Bruch's membrane of the choroid is actually the basement membrane of the pigment epithelium, making it illogical to assign an epithelium to one layer and its basement membrane to another. Furthermore, although the pigment epithelium interdigitates with rod and cone outer segments, there are no intercellular junctions between the two cell layers, which derive embryologically from different layers of the

Fig. 20-6. Low magnification of the wall of the eyeball excluding most of the sclera. The connective tissue stroma of the choroid is blackened by the presence of numerous interspersed pigment cells. The choroid is interrupted by several small blood vessels. Also visible where the choroid meets the retina is the pigment epithelium of the choroid. The layers of the retina are shown at higher magnification in Figure 20-8.

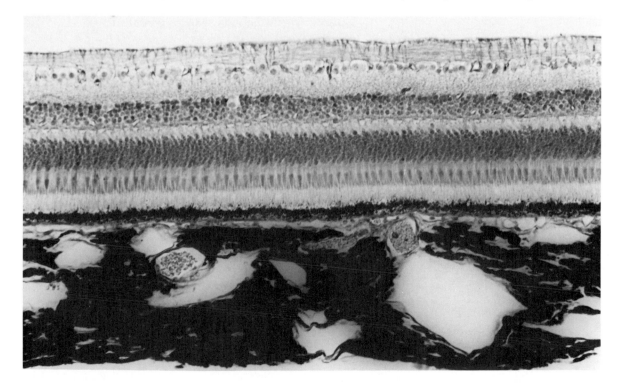

optic cup. In the case of a retina becoming detached, which leads to partial blindness, the pigment epithelium remains adherent to the underlying choroid and the retina peels off as a separate entity. For these reasons most texts now consider the pigment epithelium as part of the choroid, although it has been traditionally considered with the retina.

The epithelium is a simple cuboidal type and is characterized by prominent melanin granules (see Figs. 20-6, 20-10). The cells are joined to one another by typical terminal bars, including gap junctions and elaborate tight junctions, the latter constituting part of the blood-ocular barrier, to prevent any undesirable substances from diffusing out of the choroidal capillaries into the retina. The pigment functions to absorb light after it has passed through the photoreceptor cells so that it will not reflect back into the retina from the outer layers, interfering with the visual image. The apical ends of the pigment epithelial cells form cylindrical sheaths, which encompass the membranous tips of the rods and cones, and microvilli, which extend between photoreceptor cells.

Choroid Proper

The choroidal stroma is essentially a loose connective tissue containing a large number of blood vessels as well as pigment cells (melanophores), which vary in number according to an individual's genetic constitution (see Fig. 20-6). The innermost region of the choroidal stroma beneath the pigment epithelium contains an extensive **capillary network,** which provides nutrients for the outermost layers of the retina. The choroid functions as a nutritive layer, providing a pathway for blood vessels; it supports the retina and absorbs light that has passed through the retina.

CILIARY BODY

The ciliary body extends from the ora serrata, or edge of the retina, to the root of the iris (see Fig. 20-5). Seen as a whole mount, the ciliary body is a complete ring, to which the suspensory ligament of the lens is attached and which forms the point of origin for the iris. If a section is cut from the ring, it is seen to be triangular, with its apex pointing posteriorly to join the choroid. Its inner surface faces the vitreous body and the lens. The ciliary body has two distinct regions: the **pars plicata** and the **pars plana.** The pars plicata is the anterior portion, which is folded into numerous ridges referred to as **ciliary processes** from which the zonular fibers extend to the lens (Fig. 20-7). The tension of these fibers is regulated by the ciliary muscle which resides within the substance of the pars plicata. By comparison, the pars plana is the relatively flat posterior two-thirds of the ciliary body. The posterior extent of the pars plana abuts the anterior terminus of the retina forming an uneven junction called the **ora serrata** (see Fig. 20-5). The inner surface of the ciliary body is covered by a double-layered cuboidal epithelium sandwiched between two basement membranes. The innermost layer is an unpigmented epithelium; the outermost layer is highly pigmented (Fig. 20-8). Their apical membranes are joined together by zonula occludens–type junctions which constitute part of the blood-ocular barrier.

The connective tissue underlying the pars plicata is highly vascular and contributes to the formation of the aqueous humor, a plasma filtrate that is actively modified in composition by the overlying epithelial cells of the pars plicata. These epithelial cells are joined by tight junctions that form a barrier preventing the entrance of any large, extraneous molecules into the aqueous humor. Functionally, the aqueous humor helps to maintain intraocular pressure as well as acting as a clear refractive medium and as an avenue of exchange for metabolic nutrients and waste to and from the avascular cornea and lens.

Beneath the pars plicata and pars plana is a second and larger component of the ciliary body, the **ciliary muscle.** This smooth muscle is innervated by parasympathetic fibers of the oculomotor nerve, which relaxes tension on the suspensory ligament of the lens so that the lens increases in convexity to accommodate for near vision.

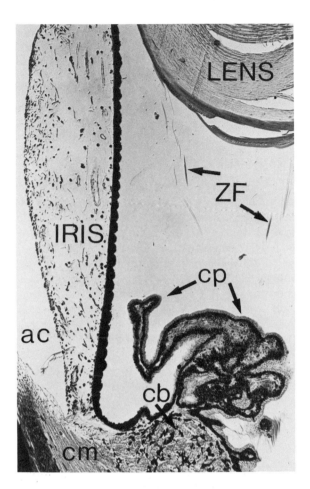

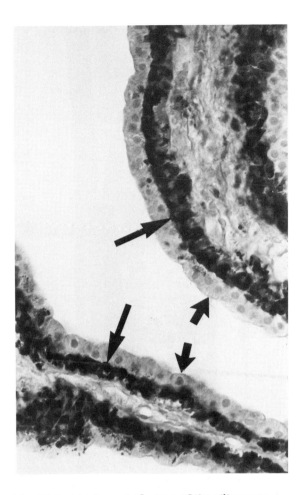

Fig. 20-7. An area of the eye showing a portion of the ciliary body (*cb*), iris and lens. A few short segments of zonula fibers (*ZF*) are visible where they span the distance between ciliary processes (*cp*) and lens. The pigmented epithelium, which appears black, forms the surface of the iris facing the posterior chamber of the eye. The anterior chamber (*ac*) is on the opposite side of the iris. The ciliary muscle (*cm*) is shown.

Fig. 20-8. A high magnification of the ciliary processes showing its double layer of cuboidal epithelium consisting of a surface unpigmented epithelium (*short arrows*) and an underlying pigmented cuboidal epithelium (*long arrows*).

IRIS

The iris is the most anterior portion of the uvea. It is shaped like a disk with a central aperture, the **pupil,** which rests on the anterior surface of the lens. The iris consists of a stroma of loose connective tissue covered by an anterior epi-

thelium continuous with the corneal endothelium, and a two-layered cuboidal posterior pigmented epithelium continuous with that of the ciliary body (see Fig. 20-9). A circularly arranged sphincter muscle, the **sphincter pupilla,** encircling the pupillary margin, causes constriction of the pupil under parasympathetic stimulation, while less distinct dilator muscle fibers run radially around the pupil and cause dilation in response to sympathetic stimulation. The nerves

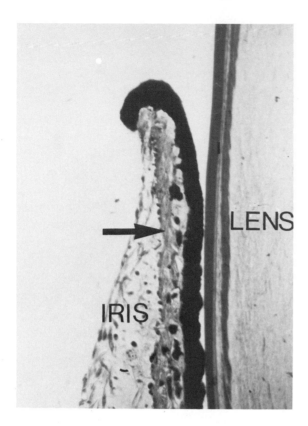

Fig. 20-9. Higher magnification of the iris near the pupil. Black pigmented epithelium constitutes the posterior surface of the iris. The pupillary sphincter muscle occupies the core of the iris (*arrow*).

that innervate the sphincter pupillae and ciliary muscles first pierce the sclera and travel between the sclera and choroid to their muscular destinations.

Eye color is a function of the number of pigment cells located in the stroma. Many pigment cells yield brown eyes, whereas fewer pigment cells give rise to green or blue eyes.

The pupil reacts to light as a variable diaphragm, which prevents overstimulation of the retina in bright light, while ensuring adequate illumination for night vision. The arterial supply of the iris is functionally adapted for change in dimensions as the pupil dilates and contracts. The arteries follow a spiral course that gives them slack; they also have an unusual histologic arrangement consisting of a thin intima and media but a very thick adventitia. This fibrous adventitia helps to ensure that the arteries will not suddenly yield to stretch or become compressed and occluded when the pupil accommodates to light.

The Retina

The retina is a complex membrane consisting of photoreceptor cells (**rods** and **cones**) that sense light intensity and color. The photoreceptor cells synapse with neurons, transducing these stimuli into nerve impulses that travel through the optic nerve to the lateral geniculate nucleus of the thalamus and finally to the visual cortex where the sensation of vision is created. Embryologically, the eye forms from an evagination of the diencephalon called the **optic vesicle.** The vesicle then invaginates like a balloon into which a fist is pressed. The resultant optic cup comprises two layers of neural ectoderm. The outer layer develops into the pigment epithelium of the choroid while the inner layer gives rise to the neural retina, which is actually a differentiation of the brain.

About 2.5 mm lateral to the **optic papilla,** where the optic nerve exits, is a shallow, round depression called the **fovea** (see Fig. 20-1). The fovea has a special structure, which can be better appreciated after study of the remainder of the retina, and is the site of most accurate vision. Conversely, the optic papilla, where the optic nerve exits, is characterized by a lack of photoreceptors and is commonly called the "blind spot." The remainder of the photosensitive retina is composed of the following nine layers, starting from the outside of the eye and working inward (Figs. 20-10, 20-11):

1. Rod and cone outer segments
2. External limiting membrane
3. Outer nuclear layer
4. Outer plexiform layer
5. Inner nuclear layer
6. Inner plexiform layer

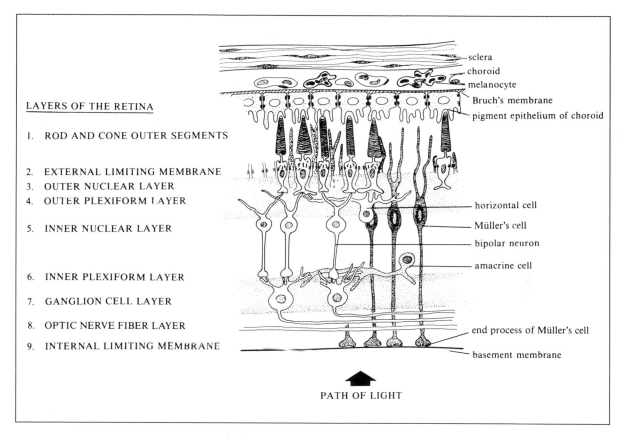

LAYERS OF THE RETINA

1. ROD AND CONE OUTER SEGMENTS

2. EXTERNAL LIMITING MEMBRANE
3. OUTER NUCLEAR LAYER
4. OUTER PLEXIFORM LAYER

5. INNER NUCLEAR LAYER

6. INNER PLEXIFORM LAYER

7. GANGLION CELL LAYER

8. OPTIC NERVE FIBER LAYER

9. INTERNAL LIMITING MEMBRANE

PATH OF LIGHT

Fig. 20-10. The retina showing its nine layers and connections using a few cells of each type as an example. Note that light must pass through the entire thickness of the retina before it finally triggers a photochemical reaction in the rod and cone outer segments. This "backward" retina is typical of all vertebrates.

7. Ganglion cell layer
8. Nerve fiber layer
9. Internal limiting membrane

It is interesting to note that the vertebrate retina is "backward," in that light must traverse eight layers before arriving at the rod and cone outer segments where the light energy is actually transduced into neural impulses.

RODS AND CONES

Layers 1 through 4 are formed predominantly from different regions of the photoreceptor cells, which are arranged in a layer with their long axes perpendicular to the retina.

Rods

The rods (Fig. 20-12) are cylinders 40 to 60 μm long that consist of three basic parts. The **outer segments,** which form the outermost layer of the retina, contain stacks of flattened cisternae of membrane that interdigitate with microvilli of the pigment epithelium of the choroid. **Connecting stalks** attach the outer segments to the cell bodies or **inner segments.** The average outer seg-

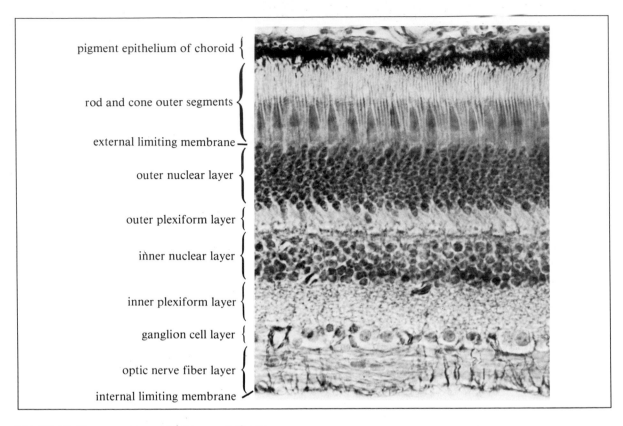

pigment epithelium of choroid {

rod and cone outer segments {

external limiting membrane —

outer nuclear layer {

outer plexiform layer {

inner nuclear layer {

inner plexiform layer {

ganglion cell layer {

optic nerve fiber layer {

internal limiting membrane

Fig. 20-11. Human retina at higher magnification.

ment contains more than a thousand uniform, membranous disks that are formed by repeated infoldings of the plasmalemma (see Fig. 20-12). These disks contain molecules of **rhodopsin** (visual purple), which give the retina a purple color in the dark; this color quickly bleaches out on exposure to light. Rhodopsin is composed of vitamin A aldehyde (**retinal**) complexed to a protein called **rod opsin.** Exposure to light changes the conformation of the rhodopsin molecule so that the component parts separate within the disk membrane. This photochemical reaction leads, in a manner that is incompletely understood, to a hyperpolarization of the rod cell membrane and triggers an action potential on a bipolar neuron, with which the rod axon synapses. The outer seg-

ment is thus the actual receptor end of the cell, which transduces the impulse created by light into a membrane hyperpolarization by virtue of the complex membrane protein, rhodopsin. Rods are responsible for sensing low levels of illumination and are indispensable for night vision.

A connecting stalk attaches the rod outer segment to the rod inner segment or cell body. The stalk is actually a modified cilium consisting of the nine usual doublet microtubules, but lacking a central pair. The part of the cell body closest to the connecting stalk is characterized by closely packed mitochondria and is called the **ellipsoid.** The cell body itself contains all the organelles required by a cell engaged in rapid protein synthesis. Rods must synthesize the protein required to make new membrane disks on a regular basis, since these disks are constantly added to the base of the outer segment, shed at the tip, and

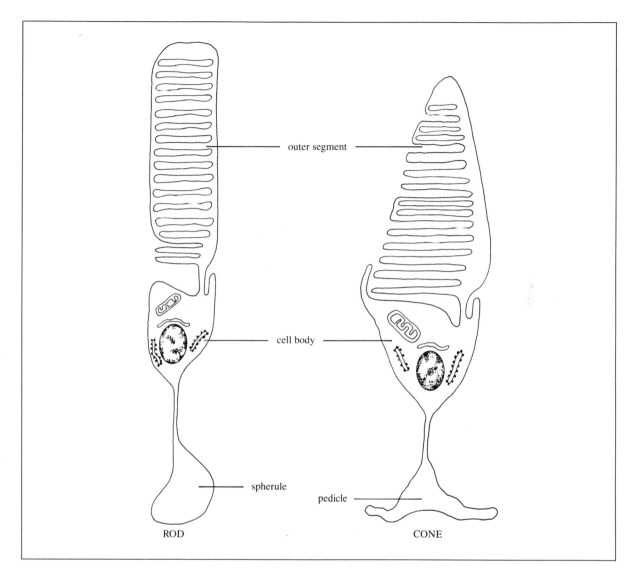

outer segment

cell body

spherule

pedicle

ROD

CONE

Fig. 20-12. Rods and cones are structurally similar in component parts, although the outer segments differ in shape and in the type of pigment present in the disk membranes. The axon terminal of the rod is a small spherule, whereas that of the cone is flared into a wide pedicle. The axons of rod and cone cells synapse with a variety of bipolar neurons.

phagocytized by the pigment epithelium. It takes about 10 days for a newly formed disk to work its way down the outer segment and to be shed.

Cones

Cones (see Figs. 20-11, 20-12) vary slightly in shape, depending on their location within the retina, but the majority are actually cone- or flask-shaped, consisting of a **conical outer segment** attached by a broad connecting region to a **bulbous inner segment.** The outer segment is composed of membranous infoldings which form a stack of disks, as in the rod. The cone disks differ from those of the rod, however, in several important features. Most obviously, the cone disks are broad near the inner segment and get progressively smaller in diameter as they approach the tip of the outer segment. In addition, they are not constantly renewed and shed as are those of the rod, but instead new protein is continually synthesized and shipped to all the disks. There are more pigments associated with the cone disks as well, but they are formed in a similar manner. Cone pigment is called **iodopsin** and is a complex of **retinal** and a **cone opsin.** The various pigments absorb light most efficiently at different wavelengths, giving rise to the perception of color. Whereas many rods can synapse onto one bipolar neuron (**summation**), cones may synapse individually or may summate very slightly. This lack of summation produces great visual acuity, since stimulating a given number of cones triggers a much greater number of nerve impulses than the equivalent number of rods. Cones, however, respond only to bright light and are not useful in night vision in which color perception is consequently lost.

The cone outer segment is connected to the inner segment by a modified cilium similar to that of the rod, but broader. The inner segment itself is similar to that of the rod.

OTHER LAYERS OF THE RETINA

The **external limiting membrane** of the retina (see Figs. 20-10, 20-11) is not a membrane at all, but a series of junctional complexes between **Müller's cells,** the major supporting glial cell, and the photoreceptor cells, with which they interdigitate.

The **outer nuclear layer** consists of rod and cone cell bodies. The cone nuclei form a single layer adjacent to the external limiting membrane, whereas the rod nuclei occupy several layers except at the fovea. The fovea centralis consists of a single layer of cones exclusively; no rods are present. Here, the cones synapse with individual bipolar neurons and occur with their highest packing density, creating the area of

greatest visual acuity. The fovea centralis is a small area within the **macula lutea** (yellow spot) where the cells and fibers of the inner retinal layers are diverted to expose the cones located there more readily to light. When viewed with an ophthalmoscope, the macula is both darker and more orange than the surrounding retina because the pigment epithelial cells located there contain more melanin plus a yellow pigment. In addition, no retinal blood vessels pass over this area to interfere with the passage of light. Visual acuity is enhanced by a greater packing density of cones in the fovea centralis.

The **outer plexiform layer** consists of rod and cone axons, dendrites of bipolar neurons, and processes of **horizontal cells.**

The **inner nuclear layer** contains nuclei of the bipolar neurons, nuclei from two types of association neurons (**horizontal cells** and **amacrine cells**), and nuclei of the insulating and supportive Müller's cells.

The **inner plexiform layer** consists of amacrine cell processes, bipolar axons, and ganglion cell dendrites.

The **ganglion cell layer** comprises multipolar ganglion cells and supporting glia. Branches of the central artery of the retina, which enters with the optic nerve, are present in this layer and nourish layers 5 through 9, while capillaries of the choroid nourish the first four layers.

The **nerve fiber layer** is composed of bundles of unmyelinated axons from the ganglion cells, which course in parallel to the retina and run to the optic disk and through the lamina cribrosa to form the optic nerve. Posterior to the lamina cribrosa the optic nerve is myelinated.

The **internal limiting membrane** is formed from the bulbous, expanded ends of the Müller's cells and their basement membrane. Thus the Müller's cells extend throughout the entire retina, since they form junctions with the rods and cones in the external limiting membrane, contribute to the nuclei in the inner nuclear layer, and terminate finally at the very outer border of the retina. Although other glia are also present in the retina, the Müller's cells are the predominant supporting cells.

The major difference between retinal and peripheral sensory pathways is in the location of the nerve cell bodies. In nonretinal sensory pathways, the cell body of the peripheral or first neuron resides in a dorsal root ganglion, and the cell body of the second neuron resides in the nucleus cuneatus or gracilis of the medulla (a conical expansion of the cervical spinal cord). Within the eye, the specialized receptors and nerve cell bodies of the first and second neurons are fully contained within the retina. The bipolar neurons are the first neurons connecting the photoreceptors (i.e., rods and cones) with the second neurons or ganglion cells whose axons exit the eye as the optic nerve and synapse in the lateral geniculate body of the thalamus.

The Lens

The lens (Fig. 20-13) is a transparent, biconvex body that has considerable flexibility. It lies between the iris and the vitreous body and is suspended at its most peripheral part, the **equator,** by zonular fibers originating from the ciliary body. The flexibility of the lens allows it to participate in the process of **accommodation,** during which it becomes more convex to bring near objects into focus. When the ciliary muscle is relaxed, the zonular fibers are stretched and the lens is under tension and relatively flattened so that distant objects are in focus. When the ciliary muscle contracts, the zonula fibers are pulled in an anteromedial direction, which causes relaxation of tension on the zonular fibers. With the zonular fibers relaxed, the elastic lens increases in convexity and thickens to bring close objects into focus on the retina. With increasing age, the lens loses its flexibility and cannot adjust its curvature to adequately focus light arriving from near objects.

The adult lens comprises three parts: the **capsule,** the **anterior epithelium,** and the **lens substance.** The capsule is actually a tough, elastic basement membrane that envelops the entire lens. Only the anterior surface of the lens, facing the pupil, is covered by a low cuboidal epithelium. Toward the equator of the lens, these

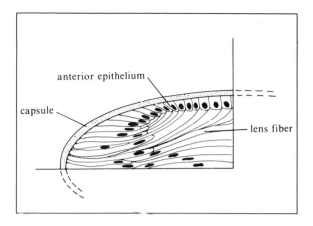

Fig. 20-13. One quadrant of the lens. New lens fibers form from cells of the anterior epithelium, which becomes columnar and then turn in a direction parallel to the lens surface as they transform into lens fibers.

cells become columnar, turn meridionally (from perpendicular to parallel to the lens surface; see Fig. 20-13), and are transformed into the **lens fibers** that form the bulk of the lens substance. During embryonic development, the first lens fibers are formed in an anteroposterior direction from a posterior epithelium. These first fibers, then, run from front to back of the lens, and in their formation the posterior epithelium becomes "used up." Succeeding fibers form as layers on top of the embryonic fibers by elongation of the **anterior epithelial cells** at the equator, which turn meridionally and transform into lens fibers. Lens fibers are laid down concentrically in this manner around the original central core of fibers that run in an axis perpendicular to the pupil. The old fibers become enucleate, but new fibers keep forming at the equator. Each fiber is a six-sided prism, 7 to 10 mm long, which extends across the entire diameter of the lens.

Although the lens is important for focusing light on the retina, the overall shape of the eyeball is critical also. If the eyeball is smaller than normal, the lens can focus more distant objects on the retina. This is "farsightedness" or **hyperopia.** If the eyeball is longer than normal, distant objects are more difficult to focus. This is called "nearsightedness" or **myopia.**

Blood Supply to the Eye

The blood supply to the eye arrives through the central artery and the ciliary arteries, both branches of the ophthalmic artery. The central artery travels within the optic nerve and emerges through the optic disk where it arborizes over the surface of the retina (except the macula lutea) to supply it with blood. With an ophthalmoscope the radial branching pattern of the central artery can be seen against the retina as its branches distribute away from the optic disk in all directions. Two long posterior ciliary arteries pierce the sclera just lateral to the entry of the optic nerve and travel forward between the choroid and sclera to supply the ciliary body and iris. The short posterior ciliary arteries only supply the choroid. The anterior ciliary arteries penetrate the sclera more anteriorly and anastomose with the long posterior ciliary arteries to form the greater arterial circle around the iris which is supplied with blood from small branches emanating from this circle.

Eyelids

The eyelids have two surfaces: (1) a moist mucosal surface (**palpebral conjunctiva**) to lubricate movement of the eyelids over the exposed anterior surface of the eyeball, and (2) an outer surface of thin skin containing only sparse adipose tissue. Within each eyelid are skeletal muscle fibers from the orbicularis oculi muscle, and within the upper lid are additional skeletal muscle fibers from the insertion of the levator palpebrae superioris muscle. The deep stroma of the eyelids contains dense collagen fibers forming tarsal plates which have large sebaceous glands (**meibomian** or **ciliary glands**) embedded in them. These sebaceous glands have ducts associated with each row of eyelashes. Another system of glands on the eyelid called **tarsal glands** have 15 to 20 accumulated ducts opening posterior to the eyelashes along the margin (free edge) of the eyelid. The oily secretion from the tarsal glands helps to seal the margins of opposing eyelids when they close over the surface of the eye, but

more importantly, the oily secretion forms a thin film over the lacrimal secretions covering the eyeball and thereby reduces evaporation of tears from the surface of the eye. In addition, near the medial canthus there is a single larger orifice in each lid. Each orifice leads into a canaliculus that drains tears (**lacrimal secretions**) away from the surface of the eyeball into the lacrimal sac. The **lacrimal sac** is drained by a **nasolacrimal duct** into the **nasal cavity.** The canaliculi are lined by stratified squamous epithelium.

THE EAR

The ear has two important sensory functions: (1) hearing and (2) detection of changes in acceleration or direction of movement of the head, and orientation of the head relative to gravity.

Parts of the Ear

The ear itself consists of three parts: the external, middle, and inner ears (Fig. 20-14).

1. The **external ear** consists of an elastic cartilaginous appendage (**auricle, pinna**) covered by skin for funneling sound waves down a canal, the **external auditory meatus,** to the eardrum or **tympanic membrane,** which vibrates upon impact of sound waves. This membrane separates the external ear from the middle ear. In the skin lining the outer portion of the meatus, sebaceous glands are found associated with hair follicles. Special apocrine sweat glands, **ceruminous glands,** produce a waxy substance (**cerumen**) that coats the meatus. Their ducts open directly into the meatus or into hair follicles. The external surface of the tympanic membrane is covered by stratified squamous epithelium. The surface facing the middle ear is a low simple cuboidal epithelium characteristic of the lining of the middle ear. A core of two layers of collagen is all that separates the two epithelial surfaces.

2. The **middle ear** contains three tiny bones (**ossicles**), which are arranged in series and span the distance between the tympanic membrane and the inner ear. The three ossicles are the **malleus** (hammer), the **incus** (anvil), and the **stapes**

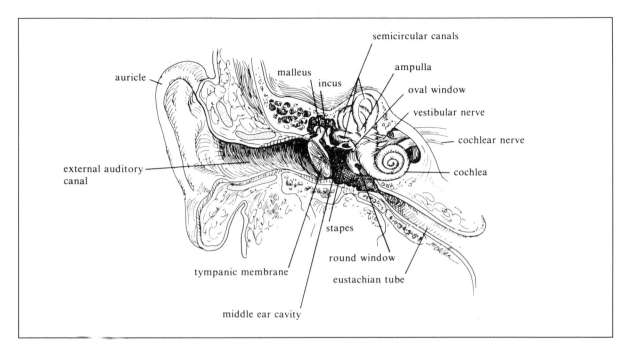

Fig. 20-14. Anatomic relationship of the outer, middle, and inner ears.

(stirrup). The malleus rests against the medial side of the tympanic membrane; the incus joins the malleus to the stapes. The stapes inserts like a piston onto the oval window in the temporal bone, which houses the inner ear. Sound waves cause vibrations of the tympanic membrane and are transferred along the ossicles to the inner ear, where the epithelial organ for hearing is located. Two muscles within the middle ear exert tension on the ossicles to influence relative vibrational sensitivities to low- vs. high-frequency sounds. The **tensor tympani** inserts onto the malleus and by contracting can pull the tympanic membrane inward, making it taut and therefore enhancing its sensitivity to high-pitched sounds. The **stapedius** inserts onto the stapes and by contracting reduces pressure on the inner ear, thereby enhancing sensitivity to low-frequency sounds. A canal, the **eustachian tube,** leads from the air-filled middle ear to open into the nasopharynx on its lateral wall.

3. The **inner ear** houses several groups of special neuroepithelial cells, some of which form the end organ for hearing and some of which are sensitive to linear and rotational movements of the head as well as its orientation with respect to gravity. The inner ear consists of a membranous portion housed within a cavity in the **petrous portion** of the temporal bone. The bone forms a close-fitting casing around it. A **perilymph fluid** fills the space between the membranous inner ear and its bony vault.

The Inner Ear

The bony cavity just medial to the middle ear is a part of the inner ear called the **vestibule.** An anterior extension of the vestibule called the **bony cochlea** contains the membranous **cochlear duct;** this duct in turn contains the epithelial **organ of Corti,** which is concerned with hearing. A posterior extension of the vestibule called the **bony labyrinth** contains the three membranous

semicircular canals, which are concerned with position and movement of the head in space and with respect to gravity (see Fig. 20-14).

THE COCHLEAR DUCT

The cochlear duct is contained within the bony cochlea, a spiral canal curling two and a half times around a central axis of spongy bone called the **modiolus.** The cochlear duct is suspended within the bony cochlea with perilymph-filled

spaces above (**scala vestibuli**) and below (**scala tympani**) (Fig. 20-15). Consequently, the cochlear duct is often referred to as the **scala media** because it occupies the central third of the bony cochlea. For all practical purposes the cochlear duct separates the perilymph within the two scalae from each other, except at a small opening near the apex of the cochlea called the **helicotrema.**

The floor of the cochlear duct is an elastic and collagenous **basilar membrane.** It extends from a periosteal thickening (**spiral ligament**) on the outer edge of the duct to a thin shelf of bone (**osseous spiral lamina**) on the inner edge of the

Fig. 20-15. A section through a single turn of the cochlea. (From W. Bloom and D. W. Fawcett, *A Textbook of Histology* [10th ed.]. Philadelphia: Saunders, 1975. Reproduced with permission.)

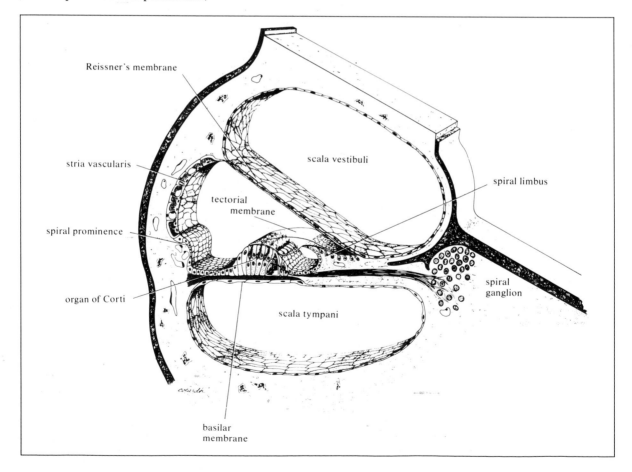

duct. The roof of the duct is formed by a double layer of squamous epithelial cells (vestibular membrane) extending obliquely across the duct from the osseous spiral lamina to the outer wall of the cochlea (see Figs. 20-15, 20-17).

The cochlear duct is filled with endolymph, a liquid that is similar in electrolyte composition to intracellular fluid, that is, higher in potassium relative to sodium. The perilymph filling the other scala is of a very different composition more nearly reflecting that of extracellular fluid that is, higher in sodium relative to potassium. The perilymph filling the scala vestibuli continues through the vestibule as far as the membrane-covered opening in the bony cochlea called the **oval window,** on the other side of which the footplate of the stapes presses from the middle ear. Consequently, sound waves impinging on the tympanic membrane are conveyed along the malleus and incus to the stapes, whose vibrational frequency and amplitude are transmitted to the perilymph within the scala vestibuli. These vibrations are transferred across the cochlear duct to the perilymph within the scala tympani and from there to the **round window,** the other side of which is the middle ear. The vibrational transfer across the cochlear duct stimulates the neuroepithelial cells within the organ of Corti, the end organ of hearing located within the duct.

NEUROEPITHELIAL CELLS

Hair cells are mechanoelectrical transducers found in the cochlea, in the three ampullae of the semicircular canals (sensors of angular acceleration), and in the **utricle** and **saccule** (both sensors of gravitational force and linear acceleration). Although hair cells have different anatomic surroundings in these six different locations, they are essentially the same cell type. The apical surface is characterized by a bundle of extremely long **microvilli** (sometimes referred to as **stereocilia**) of different lengths. The microvilli are arranged in a cone-shaped projection. The cone consists of rows of microvilli. Each row consists of microvilli of equal length, but each successive row has taller microvilli producing a bilateral

symmetric array. There exists a single true **cilium** or **kinocilium** with a terminal knob at one end of the plane of bilateral symmetry (Fig. 20-16).

When the orientation of the hair bundle is displaced in the direction along the axis of bilateral symmetry by the relative movement of endolymph, the hair cell is maximally depolarized and releases a neurotransmitter from the basal plasmalemma. Displacement of the hair bundle in a direction 90 degrees to the plane of bilateral symmetry produces no depolarization of the hair cell. Displacement at smaller angles than 90 degrees to the plane of bilateral symmetry produces progressively greater depolarization of the hair cell. (Since the transmitter released from the hair cell is released by secretory vesicles, the hair cell is often referred to as a **paraneuron.**) The released transmitter depolarizes an afferent neuron innervating the base of each hair cell. These nerves are components of the eighth cranial nerve, which carries sensory information back to the brain.

THE ORGAN OF CORTI

The organ of Corti (Figs. 20-17, 20-18) is a ribbon of innervated **neuroepithelial cells** (hair cells) that rests on the basilar membrane and runs the length of the cochlear duct. It is the site at which mechanical vibrations are translated into nervous impulses that are conveyed back to the brain along sensory nerves. The 15,000 hair cells resting on the basilar membrane are composed of functionally distinct groups. Each group is sensitive to a different limited range of frequencies. The sum of these increments spans the range between 20 Hz and 20 kHz.

Two types of neuroepithelial cells are recognized within the organ of Corti, in addition to supporting cells. There is a single row of inner, goblet-shaped hair cells and three to five rows of outer, columnar hair cells, both types resting on the basilar membrane. Their bases are innervated by afferent and efferent fibers from the cochlear division of the eighth cranial nerve (see Fig. 20-17).

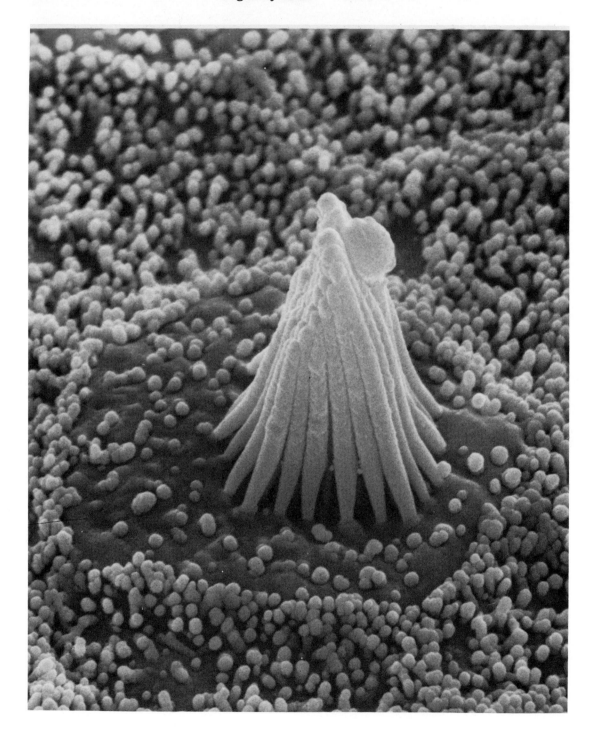

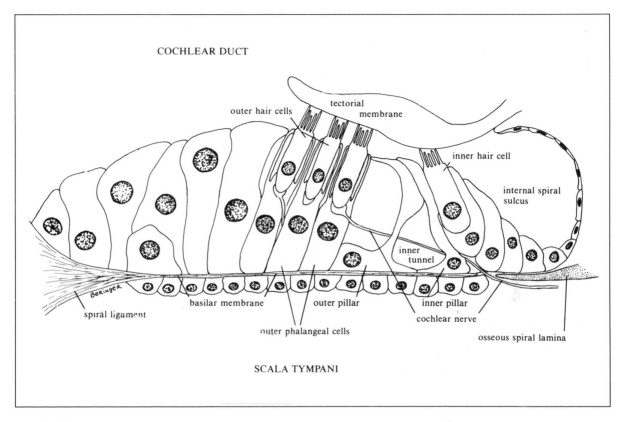

COCHLEAR DUCT

outer hair cells

tectorial
membrane

inner hair cell

internal spiral
sulcus

inner
tunnel

BERINGER

basilar membrane

outer pillar

inner pillar

cochlear nerve

spiral ligament

outer phalangeal cells

osseous spiral lamina

SCALA TYMPANI

Fig. 20-17. Organ of Corti (radial transection).

Fig. 20-16. Hair bundle from the inner ear of a bull-frog magnified 14,000 times. The bundle consists of about 50 stereocilia or long microvilli plus one true cilium, the kinocilium, with its bulbous swelling at its terminus. The hair bundle is shown in the resting position here. Pushing the hair bundle off this axis will cause the hair cell to relay an electrical signal to the brain. (Courtesy of Richard A. Jacobs and A. J. Hudspeth)

The long, hairlike microvilli are embedded in a proteinaceous, noncellular **tectorial membrane,** which is anchored at the inner angle of the cochlear duct and extends over the hair cells. When vibrations are transferred across the cochlea from the scala vestibuli to the scala tympani, the basilar membrane vibrates, causing the tectorial membrane to vibrate against microvilli of the hair cells (see Fig. 20-17). Different regions along the length of the organ of Corti vibrate according to specific sound frequencies. The hair cells whose microvilli are stimulated by the tectorial membrane induce nerve impulses in the cochlear nerves that innervate their bases. These afferent dendritic fibers of the cochlear nerve course through the basilar membrane between bony plates of the osseous spiral lamina to their nerve cell bodies in the **spiral ganglia,** located in the modiolus (see Fig. 20-15).

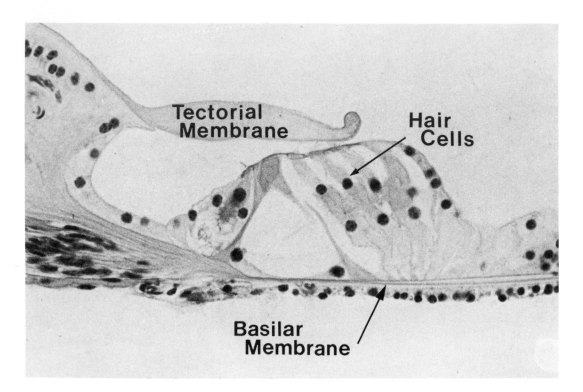

Fig. 20-18. A light micrograph of the organ of Corti.

MEMBRANOUS LABYRINTH

The posterior extension of the bony labyrinth houses the three membranous semicircular canals and two membranous sacs, an anterior **saccule** and a posterior **utricle.** These elements of the membranous labyrinth are filled with endolymph and are separated from the bony labyrinth by perilymph. The three semicircular canals open into the utricle so that endolymph is continuous throughout all these structures. Each semicircular canal has an expanded portion (**ampulla**), in which a group of neuroepithelial cells called a **crista** is located. Another mass of neuroepithelial cells, the **macula,** is located in the utricle and saccule.

The epithelium lining the membranous parts of the vestibule (utricle and saccule) and the semicircular canals is a simple squamous variety, except for the neuroepithelial cells and supporting cells of the maculae and cristae.

Ampullae

Each ampulla contains a transverse ridge of hair cells called a **crista.** The crista consists of two types of cells: flask-shaped and columnar hair cells, both with large, oval, deep-staining nuclei. The **cupula,** a gelatinous, flaplike structure, rests on the crista and extends across the lumen of the ampulla. Its specific gravity is similar to the endolymph that bathes it. The cupula responds to **angular acceleration** (i.e., changes in rotational velocity).

The semicircular canals occupy different planes at 90-degree angles to each other. During angular acceleration of the head in one of the planes occupied by either of the semicircular canals, the endolymph tends to remain stationary within the ampulla due to its own inertia, providing resistance to the cupula in the direction of rotation. Thus the cupula is pushed aside, exciting hair cells and initiating afferent nervous impulses that give information regarding angular movement to the brain.

Utricle and Saccule

Both the utricle and the saccule contain a 1-mm-wide mass of neuroepithelial cells called the **macula,** which monitors gravity and linear acceleration. These neuroepithelial cells or hair cells are of two general types, one being flask-shaped and the other columnar. Both have round nuclei. The basal surface is innervated by nerve fibers. The apical surface is characterized by long microvilli and a single kinocilium, as in the cells of the organ of Corti. The tips of these microvilli are embedded in a gelatinous mucopolysaccharide substance called the **otolithic membrane.** Numerous calcium carbonate–protein crystals called **otoconia** are embedded in the free surface of the otolithic membrane. The calcium carbonate crystals impart mass to the membrane, giving it a specific gravity greater than the endolymph in which it is bathed. When the head is tilted, the otolithic membrane tends to fall to its lowest center of gravity, moving the hairlike microvilli and kinocilium in the direction opposite to the direction of acceleration. Since the macula is vertical in the saccule and horizontal in the utricle, the saccule responds to vertical acceleration while the utricle responds to horizontal acceleration. Nerve fibers innervating these specific cells provide information to the brain regarding the direction and magnitude of tilt.

INNERVATION

The two divisions of the eighth cranial nerve provide both afferent and efferent fibers to the various structures of the inner ear. The **vestibular division** supplies innervation to the cristae within each ampulla of the semicircular canals and the maculae of the utricle and saccule, while the **cochlear division** innervates the hair cells of the organ of Corti.

Both vestibular and cochlear nerves are made up of bipolar neurons. The cell bodies of the vestibular nerve are in the **vestibular ganglion** in the internal auditory meatus; the cell bodies of the cochlear nerve are in the **spiral** or **cochlear** ganglion located in the modiolus.

NATIONAL BOARD TYPE QUESTIONS

Select the single best response for each of the following.

1. A beam of light illuminating the retina must first pass through the following structures in which sequence: (1) lens, (2) pigmented epithelium, (3) vitreous body, (4) rods and cones, (5) cornea.
   A. 2,4,5,1,3
   B. 5,3,2,4,1
   C. 5,1,3,4,2
   D. 5,2,1,4,3
2. The fovea centralis
   A. contains rods with high packing density.
   B. has an outer nuclear layer containing the nuclei of cones.
   C. is a small area within the optic disk.
   D. is the thickest portion of the retina.
3. Which of the following cells phagocytize rod outer segment discs?
   A. Bipolar neurons
   B. Amacrine cells
   C. Müller's cells
   D. Pigment epithelial cells of the choroid
4. Endolymph
   A. fills the cochlear duct.
   B. is higher in sodium than potassium.
   C. fills the scala vestibuli.
   D. fills the scala tympani.
5. Otoconia are located
   A. on the tectorial membrane.
   B. in ampullae of the semicircular canals.
   C. on the otolithic membrane.
   D. on the cupula.

For the following, select
- A. if only *1, 2, and 3* are correct.
- B. if only *1 and 3* are correct.
- C. if only *2 and 4* are correct.
- D. if only *4* is correct.
- E. if *all* are correct.

6. The utricle
   1. responds to changes in horizontal acceleration.
   2. responds to changes in vertical acceleration.
   3. contains a sheet of hair cells (macula) with a horizontal orientation.
   4. contains a sheet of hair cells (macula) with a vertical orientation.
7. Cristae within the ampullae of the semicircular canals
   1. consist of hair cells with hair bundles bathed in endolymph.
   2. are oriented at 90 degrees to each other.
   3. consist of hair cells with hair bundles in contact with the cupula.
   4. respond to changes in angular acceleration.
8. The blood-ocular barrier consists of zonula occludens—type intercellular junctions involving which of the following:
   1. Müller's cells
   2. Unpigmented epithelium of ciliary body
   3. Ganglion cells
   4. Pigmented epithelium of choroid
9. Neuroepithelial cells (hair cells)
   1. are maximally depolarized when the hair bundle is displaced in the direction along the axis of bilateral symmetry.
   2. have an apical hair bundle consisting entirely of microvilli.
   3. release a neurotransmitter during mechanoelectrical transduction.
   4. are exclusively columnar cells.
10. Which of the following structures contain pigment cells (melanocytes)?
    1. Iris
    2. Choroid
    3. Ciliary body
    4. Cornea
11. Which of the following structures is (are) devoid of blood vessels?
    1. Cornea
    2. Choroid
    3. Fovea centralis
    4. Ciliary body
12. The optic nerve
    1. consists of axons from bipolar neurons in the retina.
    2. consists of axons from ganglion cells in the retina.
    3. consists of unmyelinated axons.
    4. exits from the eyeball through a perforation in the sclera called the lamina cribrosa.

ANNOTATED ANSWERS

1. C. For further discussion, refer to Figures 20-1 and 20-10.
2. B. The fovea centralis is the thinnest portion of the retina containing densely packed cones with no rods.
3. D. The rod outer segments are intimately associated with the pigment epithelium. Refer to Figures 20-10 and 20-11.
4. A. Perilymph fills the scala vestibuli and scala tympani.
5. C. The otoconia are calcium carbonate crystals which respond to linear acceleration in the utricle and saccule.
6. B. Because the macula has a horizontal orientation in the utricle, it is sensitive to changes in horizontal acceleration.
7. E.
8. C. Since the vascular supply to the eye travels in the choroid and ciliary body, it is logical for occluding junctions to be located in those sites.
9. B. The inner row consists of goblet-shaped neuroepithelial cells. There is one kinocilium present in each hair bundle.
10. A. Pigment cells in the cornea would impede the transmission of light through it.
11. B. The absence of blood vessels in the cornea and fovea improves transmission of light

and gives greater access of light to the cones, respectively.

12. C. The optic nerve is composed of myelinated axons from the lamina cribrosa back to the brain.

BIBLIOGRAPHY

Cohen, A. I. Vertebrate retinal cells and their organization. *Biol. Rev.* 38:427, 1963.

Davson, H. *The Physiology of the Eye.* New York: Academic, 1972.

Dowling, J. E. Organization of vertebrate retinas. *Invest. Ophthalmol.* 9:655, 1970.

Fine, B. S., and M. Yanoff. *Ocular Histology.* New York: Harper & Row, 1972.

Hogan, M. J., J. A. Alvarado, and J. E. Weddell. *Histology of the Human Eye.* Philadelphia: Saunders, 1971.

Hudspeth, A. J. The cellular basis of hearing: the biophysics of hair cells. *Science* 230:745, 1985.

Kimura, R. S. The ultrastructure of the organ of Corti. *Rev. Cytol.* 42:173, 1975.

Polyak, S., G. McHugh, and D. K. Judd, Jr. *The Human Ear in Anatomical Transparencies.* New York: McKenna, 1946.

Rasmussen, G., and W. F. Windle (eds.). *Neural Mechanisms of the Auditory and Vestibular Systems.* Springfield, Ill.: Thomas, 1961.

Wersall, J. Studies on the structure and innervation of the sensory epithelium of the cristae ampullares in the guinea pig. *Acta Otolaryngol.* (Stockholm) 126 (Suppl.), 1956.

Index

Index